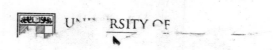
Case Studies in Communication Disorders

Designed for students of speech-language pathology, audiology and clinical linguistics, this valuable text introduces students to all aspects of the assessment, diagnosis and treatment of clients with developmental and acquired communication disorders through a series of structured case studies. Each case study includes questions which direct readers to important features of the case that will facilitate clinical learning. A selection of further readings encourages students to extend their knowledge of communication disorders. Key features of this book include:

- 48 detailed case studies based on actual clients with communication disorders
- 25 questions within each case study
- Fully-worked answers to every question
- 105 suggestions for further reading

The text also develops knowledge of the epidemiology, aetiology and linguistic and cognitive features of communication disorders, highlights salient aspects of client histories and examines assessments and interventions used in the management of clients.

Louise Cummings is Professor of Linguistics at Nottingham Trent University. She is a member of the Royal College of Speech and Language Therapists and is registered with the Health & Care Professions Council in the UK.

Case Studies in
Communication
Disorders

LOUISE CUMMINGS

Professor of Linguistics, School of Arts and Humanities,
Nottingham Trent University

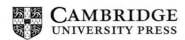

CAMBRIDGE
UNIVERSITY PRESS

CAMBRIDGE
UNIVERSITY PRESS

University Printing House, Cambridge CB2 8BS, United Kingdom

Cambridge University Press is part of the University of Cambridge.

It furthers the University's mission by disseminating knowledge in the pursuit of education, learning and research at the highest international levels of excellence.

www.cambridge.org
Information on this title: www.cambridge.org/9781107154872

© Louise Cummings 2016

First published 2016

Printed in the United Kingdom by Clays, St Ives plc

A catalogue record for this publication is available from the British Library

ISBN 978-1-107-15487-2 Hardback
ISBN 978-1-316-60838-8 Paperback

Contents

SECTION B LANGUAGE DISORDERS · 67

Transsexual voice

SECTION E   HEARING DISORDERS   **293**

Conductive hearing loss

Sensorineural hearing loss

Cochlear implantation

Central auditory processing disorder

SECTION F   PSYCHIATRIC DISORDERS   **321**

Childhood emotional and behavioural disorders

Schizophrenia

Bipolar disorder

Figures

Preface

Most authors use the preface of a book to emphasise the ways in which their volume is novel or makes an original contribution to an area of study or investigation. For the most part, I will observe this convention. *Case Studies in Communication Disorders* is certainly not the first volume to include case studies of clients with communication disorders. However, it is the first volume to treat case studies as a route into the study of communication disorders and as an instructional tool for prospective speech-language pathologists. While other volumes include case studies within text boxes where their purpose is to provide illustration, *Case Studies in Communication Disorders* immerses the reader in every aspect of a client's communication disorder. From medical history and client background through to assessment, diagnosis and treatment, this volume adopts a systematic case study approach which examines dimensions of communication disorders that are either neglected or treated superficially in other texts.

This book is also novel in three other respects. First, its coverage of the full range of developmental and acquired communication disorders is not replicated by other volumes. Many of these disorders – specific language impairment and aphasia are examples – are treated as standard by all texts. However, conditions such as Huntington's disease, AIDS dementia complex and foreign accent syndrome are rarely addressed by other texts, and yet pose significant communication problems for the clients who have them. Second, the current volume does not restrict the examination of communication disorders to speakers of English. Case studies of developmental phonological disorder in Portuguese, pragmatic language impairment in Swedish and cleft palate speech in Dutch are cases in point. Third, the book places emphasis on rigorous linguistic analysis and sound medical knowledge as the basis of understanding any communication disorder. The combination of these features confers uniqueness on the book and a breadth of coverage which will equip speech-language pathologists to deal with communication disorders of the future.

Each case study observes a similar structure. Information is presented in five units which examine the communication disorder at the centre of the case study, the client's history and communication status, speech and language assessments, and communication interventions. Of necessity, these sections are subject to variation between case studies. In some case studies medical history is examined in detail, while in other case studies developmental history is more significant to a client's communication difficulties and is discussed at length. Speech, language and hearing may all be addressed under communication status in some case studies, while in other case studies only one of these aspects of communication may be examined. Cognitive issues are often so integral to a client's communication disorder that they warrant a dedicated section in a case study. Linguistic data, which include phonetic transcriptions of single-word productions and extracts of conversation and narrative discourse, may be examined in depth in a 'focus on' section. This five-part structure reflects the complex array of factors that must be considered in the study of communication disorders, with some of these factors more prominent than others in certain case studies.

Each of the five units is followed by a series of questions. These questions are intended to challenge the reader in several respects. The reader is encouraged to consider the significance of certain linguistic features and clinical findings in the information that is presented. These questions also interrogate the basis of decision-making in speech-language pathology, from the choice of assessments to the adoption of a particular intervention approach or technique. Through engagement with these questions, the reader will develop analytical and problem-solving skills and identify possible gaps in his or her clinical knowledge. The questions can be attempted individually and are a valuable revision tool for exam preparation. Alternatively, they may be used as the basis of a group discussion in class. Responses and observations may be compared with those in an answer section at the back of the book.

Other features of this volume include over 100 suggestions for further reading. These items have been carefully selected not only to provide a comprehensive coverage of communication disorders but also to extend the reader's knowledge of these disorders. To this end, the suggestions contain articles which present state-of-the art discussions of developmental and acquired communication disorders. Several articles describe controversies in communication disorders or challenge the reader to reflect on the ways in which our knowledge of these disorders is still evolving. Among the three recommended readings for each communication disorder are books and articles that are suitable for introductory-level students and pieces that are appropriate for more advanced readers and researchers. Regardless of their experience and knowledge, all readers will find one or more articles that will stimulate their interest among the suggestions for further reading.

Acknowledgements

There are a number of people whose assistance I wish to acknowledge. I particularly want to thank Dr Andrew Winnard, Executive Publisher in Language and Linguistics at Cambridge University Press, for responding so positively to the proposal for this book.

I have received considerable assistance with data used in Case study 28 from Valeria Abusamra and Daniel Low (Universidad de Buenos Aires and Hospital Interzonal General de Agudos Eva Perón (San Martin), Buenos Aires, Argentina). I am indebted to them for their generosity. The following individuals and organisations have kindly given me permission to reproduce material: Cleft Palate Foundation; InHealth Technologies; MED-EL; and Elsevier. I also wish to acknowledge the assistance of Judith Heaney who collated the manuscript and prepared the index for the volume.

Finally, I have been supported by family members and friends who are too numerous to mention individually. I am grateful to them for their kind words of encouragement during my many months of work on this volume.

Section A

Speech disorders

Case study 1

Girl aged 6 years with cleft palate

Introduction

The following exercise is a case study of a girl ('Rachel') with cleft palate who was studied by Howard (1993). Rachel has grossly impaired speech and a severely reduced phonological system. Yet, she retains a high level of intelligibility. Her speech disorder has only been minimally responsive to prolonged therapy. The case study is presented in five sections: primer on cleft lip and palate; speech, language and hearing in cleft lip and palate; client history; focus on phonological analysis – part 1; and focus on phonological analysis – part 2.

Primer on cleft lip and palate

Cleft lip and palate is a congenital malformation of the upper lip and gum and hard and soft palates. A cleft of the lip can be complete, extending through the lip and into the nose, or incomplete, involving a variable degree of notching of the lip. A cleft lip may be unilateral or bilateral as is shown in Figure 1.1. A cleft of the palate may also be complete or incomplete. In a complete palatal cleft, the cleft extends the full length of the palate. In an incomplete palatal cleft, the cleft may involve just the uvula and soft palate. A palatal cleft may also be submucous (see Case study 2 for further discussion). Several methods of classifying cleft lip and palate have been proposed. A system that continues to be used in many cleft centres is the one proposed by Kernahan and Stark (1958). This system recognises the embryological division of the primary and secondary palates at the incisive foramen. If a palatal cleft occurs in front of the incisive foramen, it is called a primary palate or prepalate cleft. If a palatal cleft occurs behind the incisive foramen, it is called a secondary palate or simply palate cleft. Primary palate clefts may be unilateral (left or right), bilateral or median. Figure 1.2 shows different types of palatal clefts.

Some forms of cleft are more common than others. Cleft lip and palate is the most common diagnosis, accounting for 46% of cases. Isolated cleft palate and isolated cleft lip account for 33% and 21% of cases, respectively. Unilateral clefts are nine times as common as bilateral clefts. They also occur twice as frequently on the left side than on the right (Hopper et al., 2007). The epidemiology of cleft lip and palate has been extensively investigated. Matthews et al. (2015) examined the epidemiology of cleft lip and palate in Canada between 1998 and 2007. The mean birth prevalence was 0.82 per 1,000 live births for cleft lip with or without cleft palate, and 0.58 per 1,000 live births for cleft palate. Cleft lip with or without cleft palate was significantly higher in boys, with a boy to girl ratio of 1.75:1. Cleft palate was significantly greater in girls, with a boy to girl ratio in 2007 of 0.59:1. The incidence of oral clefts varies among different ethnicities. Saad et al. (2014) found that the incidence of any cleft disease was highest in the white (non-Hispanic) population in the state of California at 16.2. Lower incidence rates were

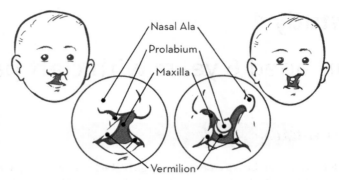

Figure 1.1 Unilateral and bilateral cleft lip and nose.
Reprinted with permission from the Cleft Palate Foundation (www.cleftline.org).

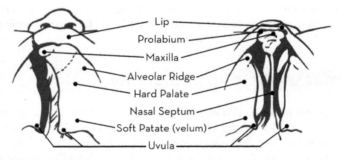

Figure 1.2 Unilateral and bilateral cleft palate.
Reprinted with permission from the Cleft Palate Foundation (www.cleftline.org).

reported in the Hispanic population (12.26), Asian/Pacific Islanders (11.57), the African American population (8.9) and the Native American population (8.15).

The exact causes of cleft lip and palate are still unknown. What is clear is that genetic factors and environmental teratogens increase the likelihood that a child will develop a cleft. Several genes have been implicated in the aetiology of orofacial clefts (Simioni et al., 2015). Cleft lip and palate is also a clinical feature of many genetic syndromes. The most common syndrome associated with cleft lip and palate is van der Woude syndrome. Isolated cleft palate is most commonly associated with microdeletions of chromosome 21, resulting in velocardiofacial, DiGeorge, or conotruncal anomaly syndromes (Hopper et al., 2007). Several teratogens and other environmental factors have been implicated in the aetiology of cleft lip and palate. Reduced folic acid levels, alcohol consumption, active and passive smoking, and antiepileptic drugs (e.g. topiramate) have all been associated with non-syndromic cleft lip and palate (Bezerra et al., 2015; Margulis et al., 2012; Sabbagh et al., 2015).

Unit 1.1 Primer on cleft lip and palate

(1) Respond with *true* or *false* to each of the following statements about cleft lip and palate:
   (a) Cleft lip and palate is an embryological malformation that arises in the first trimester of pregnancy.

    (b) Cleft lip and palate is a clinical feature of Pierre Robin syndrome.

    (c) An isolated cleft palate is more common in boys than in girls.

    (d) Cleft lip and palate is a clinical feature of Down's syndrome.

    (e) A bilateral cleft lip results in isolation of the prolabium.

(2) A cleft of the palate can be submucous in nature. Describe this type of cleft.

(3) Why do you think it is important for speech-language pathologists to know if a child has a syndromic cleft of the palate?

(4) There is considerable discussion about the optimal timing of surgical repair of a cleft of the palate. What *two* factors are central to the debate about the merits and disadvantages of early versus late palatal surgery?

(5) On account of its embryological significance, the incisive foramen is an important anatomical landmark in the classification of cleft lip and palate. Which of the following statements is *true* of the incisive foramen?

    (a) The incisive foramen is located in the maxilla bone.

    (b) The incisive foramen transmits blood vessels between the nasal cavities.

    (c) The incisive foramen is located in the mandible.

    (d) The incisive foramen transmits blood vessels and nerves between the nasal and oral cavities.

    (e) The incisive foramen is located in the midline of the palate posterior to the central incisors.

Speech, language and hearing in cleft lip and palate

Speech-language pathologists and audiologists must assess and treat the speech, language and hearing impairments that occur in cleft lip and palate. The primary speech defect is hypernasal speech related to velopharyngeal incompetence, although abnormal dentition and the presence of fistulae can also have phonetic consequences during speech production. Phonetic anomalies may have an adverse impact on a child's developing sound system (i.e. phonology). For example, the child who adopts a backed pattern of articulation in an effort to achieve closure and a build-up of air pressure in the vocal tract may eventually adopt backing as an organising principle within his system of sound contrasts. Such a child has a phonological disorder as well as a phonetic disorder. In a study of 80 children aged 6–15 years with cleft lip and palate, Albustanji et al. (2014) reported speech abnormalities including articulation and resonance deficits in 74% of subjects. Productive phonological processes in these children were consonant backing, final consonant deletion, gliding and stopping.

    Although speech can improve following palatal surgery, phonetic and phonological defects may persist for many years. Nyberg et al. (2014) examined the speech of 69 children who had a one-stage palatal repair at a mean age of 13 months. At 5 years of age, more than mild hypernasality, weak pressure consonants and perceived incompetent velopharyngeal function were present in 19 to 22% of children. This improved to less than 5% at 10 years of age. Audible nasal air leakage was present in 23% at 5 years and did not improve by 10 years. Frequent or persistent compensatory articulation was present in 30% at 5 years of age and in 6% at 10 years. At 5 years, 57% of children gave an impression of normal speech. This increased to 89% at 10 years. A high prevalence of distorted /s/ was present in these children at 5 and 10 years of age.

Children with cleft lip and palate often experience expressive language delay. Morris and Ozanne (2003) reported delayed expressive language in 9 of 20 cleft children aged 3 years. Eight of these children achieved a mean length of utterance (MLU) which was below average for their age. There is considerable evidence of delayed lexical development in children with cleft palate. Hardin-Jones and Chapman (2014) found that the size of the expressive lexicon of toddlers with cleft palate was significantly smaller than that of a noncleft group at 21 and 27 months of age. Discourse deficits have also been reported in children with cleft palate. Klintö et al. (2015) examined narrative retelling in 29 children with unilateral cleft lip and palate. An information score below 1 standard deviation from the norm value was obtained by 65.5% of these children. This compared with 30% in a comparison group of children. Several studies have found evidence of reading impairments in children with cleft palate. Conrad et al. (2014) found that subjects with non-syndromic cleft of the lip and/or palate performed significantly worse on a test of word reading than control subjects. Word reading deficits were not associated with measures of speech or hearing, but were correlated with auditory memory impairments.

Hearing loss is commonly found in children with cleft palate. In a retrospective audit of 123 newborns with cleft deformities, Tan et al. (2014) reported the incidence of hearing loss to be 24.4%. This was significantly higher than the hospital incidence of 0.3%. Hearing loss is most often conductive in nature and is associated with the development of otitis media with effusion. However, sensorineural hearing loss can also occur, particularly in children with syndromic cleft palate. Ventilation tube insertion is beneficial to the recovery of hearing in children with cleft palate and otitis media with effusion (Kuo et al., 2014). However, even after the placement of tubes, hearing loss may persist. Chen et al. (2008) reported that of 30 newborns who failed hearing screening and had tympanostomy tubes placed, 43% had persistent hearing loss. Factors, which predicted persistent hearing loss, were cleft palate alone, female infants and the presence of an associated syndrome.

Unit 1.2 Speech, language and hearing in cleft lip and palate

(1) Which of the following factors is associated with velopharyngeal incompetence in children with cleft palate?
   (a) short, immobile velum
   (b) glossoptosis
   (c) excessively capacious pharynx
   (d) micrognathia
   (e) adenoidectomy

(2) Explain why the oral plosives /p, b, t, d, k, g/ are often substituted by the glottal stop /ʔ/ in the speech of children with cleft palate.

(3) In their study of the expressive lexicon in children with cleft palate, Hardin-Jones and Chapman (2014) reported that toddlers with cleft palate produced significantly more words beginning with sonorants and fewer words beginning with obstruents in their spontaneous speech samples. Why do you think this is the case?

(4) Give *three* reasons why children with cleft palate are at risk of language delay.

(5) Respond with *true* or *false* to each of the following statements about otitis media with effusion (OME) in children with cleft palate:
    (a) OME is associated with inadequate ventilation of the inner ear.
    (b) OME is treated by a surgical procedure known as myringotomy.
    (c) OME is associated with malfunction of the Eustachian tube.
    (d) OME is normally only found in syndromic cleft palate.
    (e) OME is a cause of conductive hearing loss.

Client history

Rachel is 6 years old. She was born 11 weeks prematurely with a central cleft of the hard and soft palates. At 2;2 years, she underwent surgical repair of her palatal cleft. Rachel has a severe speech disorder, although her receptive language and expressive language have developed normally. Rachel has a history of fluctuating, mild to moderate, conductive hearing loss (average 45–55 dB). At 3;0 years, grommets were inserted. These were inserted again at 4;0 years. Auditory ability improved significantly following grommet insertion. At 5;11 years, T-tubes were inserted with reported improvements in hearing levels. Notwithstanding improvements in hearing, Rachel's performance in assessments of auditory discrimination for speech sounds remained inconsistent. There was no evidence of either oral apraxia or developmental apraxia of speech.

Rachel had received speech therapy for approximately three years by the time of the study. However, her speech problems had remained largely resistant to change and little progress had been made in therapy. There was also concern that Rachel had reached a plateau and that any further change in her speech would be difficult for her to achieve. Rachel had deficits across several aspects of speech production. She had difficulty initiating, maintaining and coordinating phonation. Her voice was breathy and she displayed high pitch. In relation to resonance, she exhibited hypernasality, nasal emission and nasal friction. A pharyngoplasty was performed at 5;5 years. However, it had had little effect in reducing her nasal emission. In terms of articulation, Rachel displayed glottalisation of consonants. There was also a lack of alveolar and post-alveolar segments in her speech. Rachel exhibited greater difficulty with the articulation of obstruents than nasals and approximants.

Unit 1.3 Client history

(1) Which feature of Rachel's history is frequently found in newborns with oral clefts?

(2) Is Rachel's cleft type consistent with the findings of studies of sex differences in clefting?

(3) Respond with *true* or *false* to each of the following statements about grommets and T-tubes:
    (a) Both devices are used to treat Eustachian-tubal insufficiency.
    (b) Grommets remain in situ for longer than T-tubes.
    (c) Both devices reside in the middle ear.
    (d) Both devices are naturally extruded by the tympanic membrane.
    (e) T-tubes are used when multiple grommet insertions have failed to provide adequate middle ear ventilation.

(4) Rachel had a breathy voice quality and other phonatory disturbances. Why are children with cleft palate at an increased risk of voice disorder?

(5) At 5;5 years, Rachel underwent a pharyngoplasty. Describe this procedure and state what it is intended to achieve.

Focus on phonological analysis – part 1

Audio- and video-recordings were made of Rachel's speech production during two clinical sessions over a period of five days. To obtain comprehensive coverage of the entire phonological system, the Sheffield Test of Phonetics and Phonology (Eastwood, 1981) was used. The nearly 100 words from this test were supplemented by words recorded during spontaneous speech and picture description tasks. A detailed phonetic transcription of all words was completed. Symbols from the IPA and extensions to the IPA were used in the transcription. Following transcription, the PACS framework (Grunwell, 1985) was used to carry out a phonological analysis of Rachel's speech. The data that was used in this analysis is examined in this unit and in the next unit.

Phonotactic structure

glasses	[ˈɴwæç̌ə̌ç̌]
string	[ˈfŋʔωɪɴ]
matches	[ˈmaʔjə̌ɦ̃]

Oral–nasal contrast

letter	[ˈɰeʔə]	nose	[ɴəʊç̌]
ladder	[ˈɰæʔə]	ring	[ʊɪɴ]
sugar	[ˈç̌ʊʔə]	fine	[f̩ːaɪɴ]
down	[ʔaʊɴ]	penny	[ˈp̚ʔeɴɪ]
dog	[ʔɒʔʰ]	singing	[ˈç̌ɪɴɪɴ]
cat	[ʔæʔʰ]	teaspoon	[ˈʔiç̌bʊɴ]

Bilabials

pig	[ʘɪʔʰ]	mud	[məʔʰ]
pen	[ʔeɴ]	mum	[məm]
tap	[ʔæʔʘ]	mouth	[maʊθ]
paper	[ˈp̚ʔeɪp̚ʔə]	thumb	[θəm]
big	[mɪʔʰ]	jam	[ʔjæm]
baby	[ˈɓeɪbɪ]	hammer	[ˈɦæmə]
bike	[maɪʔʰ]/[ɓaɪʔʰ]	shop	[ç̌jɒp̚p̚ʰ]

Unit 1.4 Focus on phonological analysis – part 1

(1) Describe the phonotactic structures of the words 'glasses', 'string' and 'matches'. Is Rachel able to replicate these structures in her spoken productions? What does your answer to this question reveal about Rachel's phonological knowledge?

(2) Is Rachel able to maintain a broad oral–nasal contrast in her use of alveolar segments? Use examples from the above data to support your response.

(3) Is Rachel able to maintain a broad oral–nasal contrast in her use of velar segments? Use examples from the above data to support your response.

(4) Is there any similarity in the way in which Rachel realises alveolar and velar segments and the way in which she realises bilabial segments? What additional clue does Rachel provide for listeners to assist them in the identification of target bilabial segments? Use examples from the above data to support your response.

(5) Not all of Rachel's bilabial segments are realised as glottal stops. In what other ways are bilabial segments realised within her speech? What do most of these realisations have in common? One realisation is particularly unusual. Which one is it, and why do you think it occurs?

Focus on phonological analysis – part 2

Several other aspects of the manner of articulation were examined in Rachel's speech. They included her ability to signal the stop–fricative–approximant continuum and the stop–affricate continuum. These continua tell us something about Rachel's ability to signal the difference between open and close sounds and, in the case of the stop–affricate continuum, the timing of release of closure. Contrasts of place of articulation and the voicing of segments were also examined.

Stop–fricative–approximant continuum and stop–affricate continuum

tap	[ʔæʔʰ]	zip	[ʨɪʔθ]
down	[ʔaʊɴ]	cup	[ʔʊʔʰ]
chair	[ʔjɛə]	go	[ʔəʊ]
jam	[ʔjæm]	yes	[jɛʔ]
sock	[ʨɒʔʰ]	why	[waɪ]
shop	[ʨjɒp̃ʰ]		

Place of articulation

baby	[beɪbɪ]	bucket	['bʊʔɪʔʰ]
toy	[ʔɔɪ]	Sue	[ʨu]
cat	[ʔæʔʰ]	daddy	['ʔæʔɪ]

tap	[ʔæʔƆ]	dog	[ʔɒʔʰ]
paper	[p͡ʔeɪp͡ʔə]	sugar	[ˈɕ͡ɬʊʔə]
kick	[ʔɪʔʰ]	shoe	[ɕ͡u]

Voicing

pig	[Ɵɪʔʰ]	bib	[bɪɓ̥ʰ]
baby	[ˈbeɪbɪ]	tea	[ʔi]
letter	[ˈɰe̝ʔə]	ladder	[ˈɰæʔə]
Sue	[ɕ͡u]	zoo	[ɕ͡u]
watch	[wɒʔɕ͡]	jam	[ʔjæm]
four	[fɔ]	a van	[ə ˈfæɴ]
feather	[ˈfeʊə]	laughing	[ˈæɟɪɴ]
dig	[ʔɪʔʰ]	chair	[ʔjɛə]
key	[ʔi]	fridge	[fʊɪʔħ]
go	[ʔəʊ]	cover	[ˈʔʊʊə]

Unit 1.5 Focus on phonological analysis – part 2

(1) Is Rachel able to signal a contrast between stop, fricative and approximant sounds? Use examples to illustrate how she signals this contrast.

(2) Does Rachel succeed in signalling a contrast between stops and affricates? Support your answer with examples from the above data.

(3) Prior to speech therapy, alveolar and postalveolar fricatives had pharyngeal realisations in Rachel's speech. Does Rachel effectively signal an alveolar–postalveolar contrast between these sounds following therapy? In what way does Rachel's post-therapy production of alveolar and postalveolar fricatives represent an improvement on her pre-therapy production?

(4) Is Rachel able to signal a voicing contrast for bilabial, alveolar and velar plosives? Does Rachel succeed in signalling a phonological contrast between /f/ and /v/?

(5) Which of the following statements best characterises Rachel's speech production?
   (a) Rachel is severely unintelligible on account of her use of segments that are phonetically distant from target phonemes.
   (b) Rachel is severely unintelligible because of a lack of consistency in her use of phonemes.
   (c) Rachel is severely unintelligible because she is unable to signal a number of phonological contrasts in her speech.
   (d) Rachel is more intelligible than expected because she makes consistent use of phonetically deviant phonemes.
   (e) Rachel is more intelligible than expected because she is able to signal a contrast between plosive and fricative sounds.

Case study 2

Girl aged 3;8 years with Kabuki make-up syndrome

Introduction

The following exercise is a case study of a girl ('Louise') aged 3;8 years with Kabuki make-up syndrome who was studied by Van Lierde et al. (2000). Kabuki make-up syndrome is a rare genetic syndrome which is characterised by a dysmorphic face, postnatal growth retardation, skeletal abnormalities, intellectual disability and unusual dermatoglyphic (fingerprint) patterns (Matsumoto and Niikawa, 2003). For those with the disorder, speech, language and hearing can be adversely affected. The case study is presented in five sections: history and clinical presentation; clinical assessment; communication and cognition profile; focus on speech production; and clinical intervention.

History and clinical presentation

Louise is the second child of healthy, non-consanguineous parents. Her sister, who is 2 years older, is healthy. After a complicated pregnancy, Louise was born at 37 weeks of gestation weighing 2.610kg. A fetal right chylothorax was detected at 20 weeks of pregnancy. (A chylothorax is the presence of lymphatic fluid in the pleural space secondary to leakage from the thoracic duct or one of its tributaries.) Karyotyping by amniocentesis was undertaken and was found to be normal. At birth, Louise was observed to have a high-arched palate with a submucous cleft. She also exhibited generalised hypotonia. The following postnatal investigations were normal: an electroencephalogram, a computed tomography scan of the brain, electromyography and metabolic screening. An internal strabismus with mild nystagmus was revealed during an ophthalmologic examination. Louise had transtympanic drains fitted at 11 months, 18 months and 2 years. At 2;4 years, a hearing examination revealed pure-tone thresholds within the normal range. This examination was repeated at 3;0 years and again revealed normal hearing. Oto-acoustic emissions were also detected. A team of geneticists and dysmorphologists diagnosed Louise at 3;1 years as having Kabuki make-up syndrome (KMS). The diagnosis was based on the presence of facial characteristics (e.g. arched eyebrows), a high-arched palate with submucous cleft, fingertip pads, a foot deformity, broad thumbs, a mild to moderate delay in motor development, and postnatal growth deficiency. At 3;4 years, an assessment of motor skills showed Louise to be at percentile 1 on the gross and fine motor scales of the Peabody Developmental Motor Scales (Folio and Fewell, 1983). A slight, general hypotonia was also observed.

Unit 2.1 History and clinical presentation

(1) There is evidence of an otological abnormality in Louise's clinical history. You should (a) state what that evidence is, (b) indicate what type of hearing loss (conductive or sensorineural) is associated with the otological defect in question and (c) explain how the placement of transtympanic drains can serve to correct the hearing loss.

(2) The history states that oto-acoustic emissions were detected during a hearing examination. What is the significance of these emissions?

(3) Is Louise's middle ear defect related to her palatal abnormality? If you answer 'yes', provide an explanation.

(4) Is there any evidence in the history to suggest that Louise may experience a speech disorder of neurogenic aetiology?

(5) KMS is a genetic disorder. The American Speech-Language-Hearing Association (ASHA) states that as genetic research continues 'it will become increasingly critical that audiologists and speech-language pathologists understand principles of genetics, genetic testing and genetic counselling' (ASHA, 2005a). Describe *one* way in which knowledge of the genetics of this syndrome might assist a speech-language pathologist in understanding the features of Louise's clinical history.

Clinical assessment

The Dutch version of the McCarthy Developmental Scales (Van der Meulen and Smrkovsky, 1986) was used to assess Louise's cognitive level. Language was assessed by means of the Dutch version of the Reynell Developmental Language Scales (Schaerlaekens et al., 1993). Louise's voice was assessed by an otorhinolaryngologist and two voice therapists. The otorhinolaryngologist conducted nasolaryngoscopy. The voice therapists used the GRBAS scale (Hirano, 1981) to assess Louise's voice. In order to determine the fundamental frequency of Louise's voice, she was asked to sustain the vowel /a/ for 4 seconds into a microphone. The instrumentation used in this analysis was the Multi-Dimensional Voice Program (model 4305) from Kay Elemetrics Corporation. A picture naming test which consisted of 135 black-and-white drawings of common objects and actions was used to assess Louise's articulation skills. The speech data obtained from this assessment were analysed independently of their relation to the adult targets as well as in relation to the adult standard forms. Three relational analyses were used: phonotactic analysis; phonetic analysis; and phonological process analysis.

Unit 2.2 Clinical assessment

(1) Which of the above tests is (a) a standardised assessment of receptive and expressive language, (b) a perceptually based assessment of voice and (c) an assessment of a child's IQ?

(2) One of the instrumental techniques used to assess Louise's voice was nasolaryngoscopy. Describe how this procedure is performed and what it may be used to assess.

(3) The fundamental frequency of Louise's voice was assessed. Which perceptual attribute of voice is fundamental frequency related to?

(4) Only *common* objects and actions were depicted by the drawings in the picture naming test. Why is this important?

(5) Which of the following statements best describes what is involved in a phonotactic analysis?

    (a) consonant and vowel productions are compared with target productions and analysed for error types at the segmental level

    (b) an analysis is undertaken of the child's productions to establish if they retain the correct syllable structure of words

    (c) the child's productions are analysed for error types beyond the segmental level

Communication and cognition profile

Louise was found to have normal cognitive functioning. Her mean cognitive score was 98. Louise scored at the 60th percentile for receptive language on the Dutch version of the Reynell Developmental Language Scales. She was able to understand a range of named objects, verbs and adjectives. She was also able to respond correctly to instructions that involved an action–object semantic relation. Certain 'wh' questions were understood and there was evidence of emerging comprehension of passive sentences. However, it was still difficult for Louise to understand sentences such as 'The dog is bitten by the rabbit'. Louise was able to understand utterances such as 'John pushes the baby. Who is naughty?', a number of spatial prepositions and some terms relating to the size of objects. She could also comprehend primary colours. Louise's expressive language skills exhibited strengths and weaknesses. She was at the 75th percentile in her ability to produce the names of items in the Reynell and to define concrete words (e.g. soap) and abstract words (e.g. being hungry). Louise performed at the 30–40th percentile on the expressive semantics subtest of the Reynell. She was able to express semantic relations of two elements (e.g. 'prepare dinner') during story telling based on pictures (e.g. setting the table). However, she was unable to capture the general theme of the depicted situations. Louise's worst area of expressive language (20th percentile) was her morphosyntactic abilities. Nouns, verbs and personal pronouns were the only word classes produced. She made use of singular and plural nouns, but did not use irregular plural forms. Louise also used some nouns with diminutive endings. Verbs only occurred in infinitive form. There were no examples of third-person singular verbs, past participles or future tense verbs. Compound sentences involving either coordination or subordination were completely absent. A negative sentence was occasionally produced. Louise's expressive output only contained sentences of two or three words, with an average of 2.4 words per sentence.

Nasolaryngoscopy failed to reveal any organic or functional voice disorder. Normal results were obtained on all perceptual and instrumental analyses of the voice. The results of the articulation assessment are examined below.

Unit 2.3 Communication and cognition profile

(1) Louise displayed relatively strong receptive language skills on the Reynell Developmental Language Scales. Based on the above description of these skills, how would you characterise her comprehension of each of the following items? *kiss the doll*; *beside*; *smallest*.

(2) Explain why Louise struggled to comprehend sentences like 'The dog is bitten by the rabbit' despite showing emerging comprehension of passive sentences.

(3) Louise was able to comprehend utterances such as 'John pushes the baby. Who is naughty?' Which of the following is suggested by her comprehension of these utterances?
    (a) Louise has intact comprehension of relative clauses.
    (b) Louise is able to understand semantic relations of two elements.
    (c) Louise is able to draw inferences based on language and world knowledge.
    (d) Louise has intact comprehension of subordinate clauses.
    (e) Louise has intact comprehension of locative prepositions.

(4) Louise's expressive language skills were most impaired in the area of morphosyntax. Based on the above description of these skills, which of the following forms was Louise able to produce and which forms did she not use? Explain your response in each case: *will come; cups; mice; dog; gone; she; run; walks; John likes oranges and Mary likes apples.*

(5) Louise was unable to capture the general theme of a depicted situation. Impairments of several cognitive and language skills might account for this difficulty. Which of the following deficits might explain Louise's specific difficulty in this area?
    (a) deficits in receptive syntax
    (b) deficits in theory of mind skills
    (c) deficits in expressive semantics
    (d) weak central coherence skills
    (e) deficits in high-level discourse comprehension skills

Focus on speech production

Phonetic inventory: Louise could correctly produce all Dutch vowels and 68% of Dutch consonants. She could not produce correctly the nasal /ɲ/ and the fricatives /f/, /v/, /ʃ/, /ʒ/ and /h/.

Phonotactic analysis: Target syllables were usually retained. A change in syllable structure occurred in only 10% of words.

Phonetic analysis: Compared to target productions at the segmental level, 55% of Louise's consonants were in error and 21% of her vowels. Consonant errors included omissions, substitutions, distortions and additions. Substitutions were the most common error type. The most common types of distortion errors were dentalisation, labiodentalisation, devoicing, weak articulation, mild to moderate hypernasality and moderate nasal emission. Vowel errors included lowering, backing, neutralisation (replacement by a schwa) and unrounding of a target rounded vowel.

Phonological process analysis: Syllable structure processes are present including cluster reduction (affecting /s/-, /t/- and /R/-blends), final and initial consonant deletion (the former chiefly affecting final /k/) and deletion of unstressed syllables. The following substitutions were in evidence, some of which are shown in the table below.

(a) /p/ → /f/; /b/ → /v/; /k/ → /X/; /k/ → /s/; /t/ → /f/
(b) /s/ → /t/; /z/ → /b/

(c) /k/ → /t/; /ɣ/ → /p/
(d) /f/ → /j/

Dutch word	English word	Phonemic norm	Client production
sigaret	cigarette	[siˠɑRɛt]	[sizɑRɛt]
boekentas	satchel	[bukəntɑs]	[pupətɑs]
fiets	bicycle	[fits]	[sis]
kapstok	clothes hanger	[kɑpstɔk]	[tɑtɔk]
zwart	black	[zwɑrt]	[vɑt]
gieter	watering-pot	[ˠitər]	[Ritə]
kraan	tap	[kra:n]	[ka:n]
kruis	cross	[krœYs]	[XœYs]
worsten	sausages	[wɔrstən]	[wəs]
borstal	brush	[bɔrstəl]	[bɔtəl]
wolken	clouds	[wɔlkən]	[wɔk]
jongen	boy	[jɔŋən]	[ɔŋə]
kop	head	[kɔp]	[tɑp]
klok	clock	[klɔk]	[slɔk]

Unit 2.4 Focus on speech production

(1) Louise's speech production displays mild to moderate hypernasality and moderate nasal emission. Which feature(s) of her clinical presentation might explain this articulatory deviance?

(2) Which phonological processes are exemplified by the substitutions in (a) to (d) above? Which of these processes occur in 'kruis' and 'kop' in the table?

(3) Give *one* example of each of the following phonological processes in the above data.
  Progressive assimilation
  Regressive assimilation
  Metathesis
  Syllable deletion
  Final consonant deletion

(4) What feature do the following productions have in common?
  Word initial /kr/ in 'tap' and 'cross'
  Word medial /rst/ in 'sausages' and 'brush'
  Final syllable /ən/ in 'clouds' and 'boy'
  Word initial /k/ in 'head' and 'clock'

(5) Two phonological processes are evident in each of the following productions. State what these processes are in each case.
  'worsten' /wəs/
  'wolken' /wɔk/
  'jongen' /ɔŋə/

Clinical intervention

Van Lierde et al. (2000) recommend the use of 'tailor-made' therapy with children who have KMS. They consider this approach to be warranted by the considerable variation that occurs in communication skills both between children with KMS and within individual children with this syndrome. The latter was particularly evident in Louise's case. She displayed a number of intact skills and areas of performance that were within normal limits. For example, Louise had normal cognitive functioning, good receptive language skills and her production of speech sounds was within normal limits for her age. There were also no vocal or laryngeal abnormalities. However, Louise also had considerable difficulties. For example, she had particularly poor expressive language skills in the area of morphosyntax. Although Louise's hearing was within normal limits, she had a history of otitis media that required the placement of transtympanic drains. She also had a submucous cleft palate, slight general hypotonia and poor gross and fine motor skills. Also, her speech sound production was highly variable, and she displayed persisting normal phonological processes, and processes that are uncharacteristic of normal development. Louise also exhibited hypernasality and moderate nasal emission. According to Van Lierde et al., this pattern of communication abilities and impairments cannot be explained by general developmental delay, structural deviations of the speech apparatus, hearing loss or specific language impairment. This pattern, these authors argue, is 'somewhat reminiscent' of a phonologic–syntactic disorder.

Unit 2.5 Clinical intervention

(1) Which of the following interventions might play a part in Louise's 'tailor-made' therapy?
    (a) an intervention that targets social communication
    (b) an intervention that targets expressive morphosyntax
    (c) an intervention that targets velopharyngeal insufficiency
    (d) an intervention that targets theory of mind skills
    (e) an intervention that targets semantic memory

(2) Is there any basis for the inclusion of a treatment that is based on principles of motor learning of the type used to treat apraxia of speech? Justify your response.

(3) The presence of persisting normal phonological processes, and processes which are uncharacteristic of normal development, suggests the need for some type of phonological treatment as part of Louise's wider communication intervention. Name *one* such treatment. Also, what evidence is there to support the efficacy of the phonological treatment that you have chosen?

(4) The presence of hypernasality and nasal emission suggests that Louise has velopharyngeal dysfunction (VPD). Blowing and sucking exercises are often used in the treatment of VPD. Are these techniques considered to be effective in the treatment of VPD?

(5) One of the reasons it is so difficult to decide on an appropriate course of intervention in Louise's case is that the diagnosis of her communication disorder is not without

complication. In this way, Van Lierde et al. state that her communication problems do not occur (a) as part of a general developmental delay or (b) are a form of specific language impairment. Explain why the diagnoses in (a) and (b) are not appropriate in Louise's case.

Case study 3

Girl aged 13 years with developmental dysarthria

Introduction

The following exercise is a case study of a 13-year-old girl ('CB') with spastic dysarthria who was studied by Marchant et al. (2008). CB has a medical diagnosis of spastic hemiplegic cerebral palsy. She received speech and language therapy for her communication disorder between 6 and 11 years of age. The case study is presented in five sections: primer on developmental dysarthria; client history and communication status; focus on spastic dysarthria; intervention; and speech outcome.

Primer on developmental dysarthria

Hodge (2014) defines developmental dysarthria as 'a group of speech disorders caused by dysfunction of the immature nervous system that delays speech onset and impairs the strength, speed, accuracy, coordination and endurance of the muscle groups used to speak. Depending on the extent of impairment, one or more of the speech processes of respiration, phonation, resonance, articulation and prosody may be affected' (26). A child with developmental dysarthria may have reduced breath support for speech (*respiration*), with the result that only short utterances are possible. The vocal folds may fail to adduct normally during *phonation*, causing the child to speak with a breathy voice. Closure of the velopharyngeal port may not be adequate during speech production, with the result that the child produces hypernasal speech (*resonation*). Impairments of the strength, speed and accuracy of articulatory movements may lead to the production of weak and distorted consonants and vowels (*articulation*). The child with dysarthria may be unable to vary the pitch and loudness of the voice, both of which can compromise intonation (*prosody*). The resulting speech impairment may be mild in nature, and have few implications for a child's intelligibility. Alternatively, the speech disorder may be so severe that no intelligible speech production is possible. In cases of anarthria, an alternative means of communication may need to be found for the client.

A large range of medical conditions, illnesses and events can give rise to developmental dysarthria. Cerebral palsy is the single largest cause of developmental dysarthria. However, other causes of this motor speech disorder include traumatic brain injury (TBI), infections (e.g. encephalitis), cerebral neoplasms, birth anoxia, brain damage related to metabolic disorders (e.g. phenylketonuria), cranial nerve damage in syndromes (e.g. Möbius syndrome) and neurodegenerative disorders (e.g. Duchenne's muscular dystrophy and Friedreich's ataxia). On account of these diverse aetiologies, it is difficult to obtain figures for the prevalence and incidence of developmental dysarthria. Typically, such figures are reported in relation to particular clinical groups within the dysarthria population. In this way, Morgan et al. (2010) reported a low incidence of dysarthria (1.25) in a cohort of 1,895 children following TBI. In children with severe TBI, this incidence figure rose to 205. Mei and Morgan (2011) reported the incidence of post-surgical dysarthria in 27 children with posterior fossa tumour to be 30%. Sigurdardottir and Vik (2011) found severe dysarthria in 16% of 152 Icelandic children with congenital cerebral palsy. Developmental dysarthria should be distinguished from acquired dysarthria in childhood. It is only in the former type of dysarthria that the neurological injury has its onset prior to the acquisition of speech skills.

Unit 3.1 Primer on developmental dysarthria

(1) Each of the following diseases, injuries or disorders is a cause of developmental dysarthria. For each one, indicate if it is a traumatic, infectious or genetic cause of dysarthria:
  (a) meningitis
  (b) closed head injury
  (c) Friedreich's ataxia
  (d) Prader–Willi syndrome
  (e) congenital rubella

(2) Each of the following statements describes a speech feature of developmental dysarthria in children. Relate each statement to an impairment of one or more of these five speech production subsystems: *respiration; phonation; resonation; articulation; prosody.*
  (a) A child with dysarthria uses fricative strictures in place of stops.
  (b) A child with dysarthria places stress on the wrong syllables in words.
  (c) A child with dysarthria has a strained–strangled voice.
  (d) A child with dysarthria produces heavily nasalised vowels.
  (e) A child with dysarthria speaks in short, truncated utterances.

(3) Cerebral palsy is the single largest cause of developmental dysarthria. Name *three* disorders in children with cerebral palsy other than dysarthria which are assessed and treated by speech-language pathologists.

(4) Respond with *true* or *false* to each of the following statements:
  (a) Developmental dysarthria is a neurogenic speech disorder.
  (b) Children with Down's syndrome have spastic dysarthria.
  (c) Dysarthria is a post-surgical feature of cerebellar tumour in children.
  (d) Dysarthria is related to vagus nerve damage (CN X) in Möbius syndrome.
  (e) Children with Prader–Willi syndrome have a flaccid dysarthria.

(5) Some dysarthrias in children improve over time. Other dysarthrias in children deteriorate over time. Still other dysarthrias remain static over time. For each of the following conditions, indicate whether the associated dysarthria improves, deteriorates or remains static over time:
  (a) traumatic brain injury
  (b) Duchenne's muscular dystrophy
  (c) Möbius syndrome
  (d) cerebral palsy
  (e) Bell's palsy

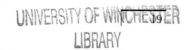

Client history and communication status

CB is a 13-year-old girl with spastic hemiplegic cerebral palsy. She has spastic dysarthria. CB attends a mainstream school, and is a native speaker of New Zealand English. Speech is her primary means of communication. Her vision and hearing are within normal limits, and her cognitive skills are sufficient for study participation. Although CB had not received speech and language therapy (SLT) for her dysarthria for one year prior to the study, she received continuous SLT between the ages of 6 and 11 years. However, her parents reported limited success from this intervention. There was little information available on the nature of this intervention other than that it took place for only 30 minutes once a week. Parental report suggested that it involved sound production drills. CB is currently receiving instruction in the use of an augmentative communication device. However, she is resistant to using it, and wishes to continue using speech as her primary means of communication.

An oromotor analysis of CB was undertaken. CB displayed severely restricted lingual and labial movement. This included inadequate tongue elevation, tongue lateralisation, tongue retraction, lip pursing and lip seal. The Goldman–Fristoe Test of Articulation (Goldman and Fristoe, 1986) was conducted. This revealed significantly impaired consonant accuracy, particularly in fricative and affricate production. Perceptual analysis by a listener experienced in dysarthria research confirmed a severe spastic dysarthria, characterised by excessively slow rate, strained–strangled phonation, and imprecise consonant and vowel articulation. CB's expressive language was assessed by means of the Language Assessment Remediation and Screening Procedure (LARSP; Crystal, 1997), the conversation analysis profile (Fey, 1986) and the profile in semantics (Crystal, 1997). These assessments revealed a severe language delay. The results of the LARSP indicated a severe syntactic delay. CB's attempts at more complex sentences were highly unintelligible and could not be analysed. During conversational exchanges, CB's reduced speech intelligibility led to frequent communicative breakdowns. This resulted in the use of simplified sentences, and the repetition and rephrasing of utterances. Communication partners frequently sought clarification of CB's utterances. This increased the occurrence of her responsive utterances, and reduced the frequency of her attempts to communicate.

Unit 3.2 Client history and communication status

(1) CB was receiving instruction in the use of an augmentative communication device. Give *two* examples of such a device, one low-tech and the other high-tech. In assessing the suitability of a device for CB, a number of non-communicative factors need to be considered. Name *four* such factors.

(2) CB was resistant to using an augmentative communication device and wished to use speech as her primary means of communication. How typical is this attitude of AAC users with cerebral palsy?

(3) CB has spastic dysarthria. At what level of the motor pathway for speech is there neurological damage to cause this type of dysarthria?

(4) CB displayed strained–strangled phonation. What is the phonatory basis of this type of voice production?

(5) Explain the sequence of events which leads from CB's reduced speech intelligibility to her assumption of a passive role in communication.

Focus on spastic dysarthria

Spastic dysarthria is more common than other forms of dysarthria in cerebral palsy (Nordberg et al., 2012). Hodge (2014) describes the pathophysiological signs and speech features of spastic dysarthria in children. Pathophysiological signs include slow movements that are limited in range, muscle weakness, excessive muscle tone, muscle rigidity, persisting primitive oral–pharyngeal reflexes and hyperactivity of reflexes that normally persist into adulthood (e.g. jaw stretch, gag). The speech features of this form of dysarthria include vowel and consonant articulation errors, hypernasality, slow speaking rate and short breath groups. During the production of utterances, there are uncontrolled changes in voice quality. The pitch of the voice is lower than expected for the child's age. Speakers with spastic dysarthria exhibit extended word durations. Abnormal resting postures of the lips, tongue and jaw are common.

These speech features of spastic dysarthria have been confirmed in a number of studies. Platt et al. (1980) examined the speech intelligibility and articulatory impairment of 50 adult males with cerebral palsy. Spastic cerebral palsy and dysarthria were present in 32 of these subjects. The performance of these subjects on two intelligibility measures – accurate recognition of single words and a prose intelligibility rating – was impaired. Indices of articulatory impairment – DDK syllable rates and percentage of correctly articulated phonemes – were also reduced in these subjects. Specific phonemic features in the dysarthric speech of these subjects included anterior lingual place inaccuracy, reduced precision of fricative and affricate manners, and an inability to achieve the extreme positions in the vowel articulatory space. In a later study, Wit et al. (1994) compared the performance of two children with TBI-related spastic dysarthria to that of two children with perinatal-onset spastic dysarthria on a number of maximum performance tasks. The three tasks examined maximum sound prolongation, fundamental frequency range and maximum repetition rate. The performance of the children with perinatal-onset spastic dysarthria on all three tasks was poorer than that of their peers with normal speech. The subjects with TBI-related spastic dysarthria performed within normal limits on maximum sound prolongation and fundamental frequency range. However, their maximum repetition rate was extremely slow.

Unit 3.3 Focus on spastic dysarthria

(1) Which of the following are pathophysiological signs of spastic dysarthria?
    (a) hypertonia
    (b) fasciculations
    (c) sucking reflex
    (d) atrophy
    (e) hyperreflexia
(2) The speaker with spastic dysarthria exhibits hypernasality. In what *two* ways is palatal elevation disrupted in spastic dysarthria to result in this speech defect?

(3) Some of Platt et al.'s subjects had perinatal-onset spastic dysarthria. What is the likely cause of these subjects' dysarthria?

(4) Which of Wit et al.'s findings accounts for the reduced pitch of children with spastic dysarthria?

(5) Respond with *true* or *false* to each of the following statements:
   (a) Vowel centralisation is a feature of spastic dysarthria.
   (b) Reduced DDK rates are related to slow articulatory movements.
   (c) Inaccuracy of anterior lingual placement in spastic dysarthria is evident in the articulation of /k, g/.
   (d) Cul-de-sac resonance is a feature of spastic dysarthria.
   (e) The articulatory control needed for frication is difficult to achieve in spastic dysarthria.

Intervention

CB received a six-week intervention that consisted of phonetic placement therapy (PPT) and surface electromyography (sEMG)-facilitated biofeedback relaxation therapy. PPT focused on articulation, with five consonant sounds selected for treatment: /t/, /s/, /f/, /ð/ and /ʃ/. The selection of these sounds was based on several factors, including CB's developmental stage, the effect of the sound upon intelligibility, and the results of the Goldman–Fristoe Test of Articulation. All sounds were targeted during each PPT session. However, one sound was the focus of the session and received 30 minutes of treatment. CB was informed of the target sound at the start of the session, and was given an auditory and visual representation of it. A mirror was used to help CB place her articulators. Speech drills and specific feedback were employed. CB was also required to provide feedback about her sound productions. Traditional articulation hierarchies were used, with CB progressing to the next level when an accuracy rate of 80% was achieved for a specific target. For all targeted speech sounds, CB did not progress beyond the sounds-in-words level.

sEMG-facilitated biofeedback relaxation therapy was used with the aim of reducing CB's orofacial spasticity. A portable biofeedback device was used during therapy. In a quiet room at home or at school, CB was seated upright and surface electrodes were applied to the skin. Electrodes were placed in three locations: under the chin, on the left top lip and on the right top lip. These locations corresponded, respectively, to the submental (floor of mouth) muscles, the left superior orbicularis oris muscle, and the right superior orbicularis oris muscle. The submental and orbicularis oris muscles were selected for treatment in order to establish if a reduction in muscle tone could improve the articulation of consonants and vowels. The first 20 minutes of treatment focused on the reduction of submental amplitude measures during rest and non-speech postures. The equipment's software provided visual feedback in the form of an animated character. To control this character, CB received the following instructions: 'I want you to make the man sit on his chair for 10 seconds. Remember, to do this you need to try and stay relaxed.' The aim was to achieve a consistent response at different thresholds. This process was repeated multiple times for all lingual and labial postures.

Unit 3.4 Intervention

(1) Five consonant sounds were selected for therapy. Aside from the factors described above, explain why these sounds were chosen for treatment. Your answer should address *two* phonetic features of these sounds.

(2) Traditional articulation hierarchies were employed during PPT. Explain what is involved in these hierarchies.

(3) The aim of sEMG-facilitated biofeedback relaxation therapy was to improve the articulation of consonants and vowels through a reduction in muscle tone during non-speech postures. What assumption underlies this aim? Is this assumption valid?

(4) The orbicularis oris muscles were targeted in sEMG-facilitated biofeedback relaxation therapy. Which of the following are *true* statements about these muscles?
  (a) The function of the orbicularis oris muscles is to retract the lips at the corners.
  (b) The orbicularis oris muscles receive innervation from the facial nerve (CN VII).
  (c) The orbicularis oris are paired upper (orbicularis oris superior) and lower (orbicularis oris inferior) muscles.
  (d) The orbicularis oris muscles receive innervation from the vagus nerve (CN X).
  (e) The orbicularis oris is primarily involved in mastication.

(5) CB's intervention was designed in order to adhere to the principles of motor learning. Describe *two* such principles. Give *one* example of how each of these principles was implemented in CB's treatment.

Speech outcome

The effects of PPT and sEMG were variable, with positive and negative findings resulting from both therapies. At rest, there were no significant differences in sEMG amplitudes across the treatment phases. However, there was a trend towards reduced submental amplitude post-sEMG treatment. There were also considerably smaller standard deviations for all submental values post-sEMG, indicating greater stability. During non-speech postures, amplitude measures decreased significantly for both tongue protrusion and lip pursing tasks post-sEMG.

These therapies also produced variable perceptual effects. There was a significant increase in single-word intelligibility post-PPT that was maintained following sEMG-facilitated biofeedback. However, on Duffy's perceptual rating scale (1995), there was no change to any articulatory parameters or to overall intelligibility. Imprecise consonants and overall intelligibility were rated as severely deviant. Vowel distortions were also considered to be markedly deviant. Phonemes were still rated as prolonged following both therapies. The subject's self-perception of her speech impairment remained unchanged following intervention. CB still had moderate concern about her speech disorder.

Acoustic measures of vowel and consonant articulation were also made following intervention. There were significant changes in the second formant (F_2) for /æ/ and /u/ following PPT and sEMG, respectively. However, there were no changes in any other formant values. In terms of consonant articulation, there were no significant differences in

CV durational measures across any of the targeted syllables. There was only one significant decrease in alternate motion rates, and that was for /kə/ post-sEMG. There was also a significant decrease in inter-syllable gap durations for /pə/ and /tə/ following both PPT and sEMG.

Unit 3.5 Speech outcome

(1) Both treatments in this study failed to bring about improvement in sentence- or paragraph-level intelligibility. Is this finding consistent with the evidence based on the efficacy of interventions available to individuals with developmental dysarthria?

(2) Within an ICF framework for measuring health and disability (World Health Organization, 2001), clinicians must consider the impact of a communication disorder on an individual's quality of life and participation in daily activities. Is there any evidence that CB's functioning or psychological well-being was enhanced by the treatments she received in this study?

(3) Amplitude measures decreased significantly for both tongue protrusion and lip pursing tasks post-sEMG. However, this did not lead to any corresponding improvement in CB's overall intelligibility. How might these findings be explained?

(4) Alternate motion rates did not decrease significantly following PPT. How might these rates be assessed? Why is this finding not entirely unexpected?

(5) The intervention that CB received lasted for six weeks. In terms of the improvement in intelligibility that was achieved by CB at the end of the study, is there any evidence that an intervention of longer duration might have been more effective?

Case study 4

Boy with developmental apraxia of speech

Introduction

The following exercise is a case study of a boy ('Zachary') who was studied by Powell (1996). Zachary's speech delay was first noted at 30 months of age. Subsequent assessment revealed a pattern of speech behaviours which was consistent with a diagnosis of developmental apraxia of speech and oral apraxia. The case study is presented in five sections: primer on developmental apraxia of speech; client history; neurological, adaptive and cognitive evaluation; speech, language, hearing and oral mechanism evaluation; and intervention and outcome.

Primer on developmental apraxia of speech

Developmental apraxia of speech (DAS), which is also known as childhood apraxia of speech (CAS) and developmental verbal dyspraxia (DVD), is a complex motor speech disorder which has its onset in early childhood. A position statement published by the American Speech-Language-Hearing Association (2007) defines CAS as:

a neurological childhood (pediatric) speech sound disorder in which the precision and consistency of movements underlying speech are impaired in the absence of neuromuscular deficits (e.g., abnormal reflexes, abnormal tone). CAS may occur as a result of known neurological impairment, in association with complex neurobehavioral disorders of known or unknown origin, or as an idiopathic neurogenic speech sound disorder. The core impairment in planning and/or programming spatiotemporal parameters of movement sequences results in errors in speech sound production and prosody.

Although DAS has been extensively investigated, little is still known about the epidemiology of the disorder. Shriberg et al. (1997) stated that DAS occurs in 1–2 children per 1,000. The prevalence of DAS is considerably higher in certain metabolic and genetic disorders. Shriberg et al. (2011) reported the prevalence of CAS in the metabolic disorder galactosaemia to be 18 per 100. This is 180 times the estimated risk for idiopathic CAS. DAS is more commonly found in boys than in girls. Hall et al. (1993) found an average male:female ratio of approximately 3:1 in a review of 24 group studies and 11 single-subject studies. DAS has been reported in several chromosomal and genetic syndromes including cri du chat syndrome, Down's syndrome and 7q11.23 duplication syndrome (Kumin, 2006; Marignier et al., 2012; Velleman and Mervis, 2011). The presence of DAS in these syndromes and many others confirms the neurogenetic origins of the disorder.

The speech features of DAS are well characterised. Children with DAS produce a range of consonant errors. These errors include the deletion of initial and final consonants, cluster reductions, voicing errors and substitutions (Lewis et al., 2004; Jacks et al., 2006). The vowel system in DAS is often severely disordered. Lewis et al. (2004) found that 100 per cent of the children with CAS in their study produced vowel errors. Davis et al. (2005) charted the vowel inventory and accuracy patterns of three children with suspected DAS over a three-year period. Vowel accuracy was impaired in all children, although accuracy did show a moderate increase from the first data recording to the final data recording. Errors consisted mainly of vowel substitutions and de-rhoticisation. No consistent pattern of errors was found in the substitutions. Prosodic disturbances, including anomalies of rate, intonation and stress, have been reported in children with DAS (Odell and Shriberg, 2001). Children with DAS also display reduced diadochokinetic rates and poor sequencing of sounds and syllables (Moriarty and Gillon, 2006). There is often an accompanying oral apraxia (Alcock et al., 2000). Language problems are also present, with receptive language skills superior to expressive skills (Aziz et al., 2010; Grigos and Kolenda, 2010).

Unit 4.1 Primer on developmental apraxia of speech

(1) Which feature of ASHA's position statement on CAS sets the disorder apart from developmental dysarthria?

(2) Why do you think the epidemiology of DAS has received little investigation?

(3) Which of the following is *not* a feature of DAS?
   (a) inconsistency of speech errors
   (b) articulatory groping
   (c) circumlocution
   (d) receptive–expressive language gap
   (e) errors increase with word and utterance length

(4) Why might consonant voicing errors occur in DAS?

(5) Why might speakers with DAS reduce their rate of speech?

Client history

A developmental and medical history was taken, using Zachary's mother as an informant. Zachary was a full-term baby who had a normal delivery. He developed influenza when he was 8 months old. This caused diarrhoea and a high fever. Zachary became dehydrated during his illness as he would not consume liquids. He developed middle ear infections and chickenpox when he was 3 years old. At 30 months of age, a speech delay was noted. As a result, a communication evaluation was conducted. The speech-language pathologist reported that Zachary's behaviours were consistent with DAS and oral dyspraxia. Zachary was enrolled in a course of speech and language therapy. However, his progress was reportedly slow. At 38 months of age, Zachary underwent a comprehensive multidisciplinary evaluation.

Unit 4.2 Client history

(1) Zachary developed influenza at 8 months and chickenpox at 3 years of age. What implications might these infections have had for Zachary's development?

(2) Is there any evidence that Zachary might be at risk of conductive hearing loss?

(3) A speech delay was noted when Zachary was 30 months old. Which of the following speech and language skills are acquired by normally developing children by 30 months of age?

    (a) production of the consonant sounds /ʧ, ʃ/

    (b) use of plural nouns (e.g. 'dogs')

    (c) production of the consonant sounds /j, v/

    (d) use of negative forms (e.g. 'I can't')

    (e) comprehension of certain questions (e.g. 'What do you do when you are sleepy?')

(4) The speech-language pathologist reported that Zachary's behaviours were consistent with DAS and oral dyspraxia. Describe *three* behaviours which are indicative of oral dyspraxia.

(5) At 38 months of age, Zachary underwent a comprehensive multidisciplinary evaluation. Aside from speech and language, describe *three* areas which should be examined by such an evaluation.

Neurological, adaptive and cognitive evaluation

As part of his neurological evaluation, Zachary had a CT scan and an EEG. The scan results were normal, while the EEG was 'mildly diffusely slow for age'. The paediatric neurologist concluded that Zachary exhibited 'developmental delay, language greater than motor, of unknown etiology'. At 47 months of age, Zachary underwent a second neurological examination. His sensory examination was normal. Zachary's motor skills were characterised as 'generally normal, although he [was] minimally hypotonic and [had] a generalized decrease in coordination with running'. The neurologist concluded that Zachary was 'afflicted with an organic static, probably prenatal encephalopathy resulting in a developmental expressive aphasia, tongue apraxia, and possibly a mild developmental delay'.

On the Vineland Adaptive Behavior Scales (Sparrow et al., 1984), Zachary performed in the low range relative to same-age peers on 'daily activities required for personal and social sufficiency'. His intellectual functioning was in the low average to borderline range on standardised testing. At 63 months of age, Zachary's non-verbal intellectual functioning was evaluated. Zachary was required to place blocks into a wooden frame to complete visual problems. These problems increased in complexity from simple concretistic matching to conceptual items that required reasoning and problem-solving skills. Zachary displayed some incoordination on this task, especially when smaller or irregularly shaped blocks were used. When Zachary had to combine two or more smaller blocks into a larger one that could be fitted into the frame, his responses were frequently mirror images of the stimuli.

Unit 4.3 Neurological, adaptive and cognitive evaluation

(1) Is there any evidence that Zachary may have a generalised dyspraxia in addition to his apraxia of speech?

(2) Zachary's motor skills were reported to be minimally hypotonic. What is hypotonia? In what motor speech disorder in children can hypotonia be a feature?

(3) Zachary's adaptive functioning was assessed by means of the *Vineland Adaptive Behavior Scales*. Name *two* neurodevelopmental disorders which this assessment may be used to diagnose. Is there any evidence that Zachary has these disorders?

(4) What *two* sets of skills are required in order to place blocks into a wooden frame so that they match a visual pattern?

(5) Zachary struggled to bring two or more smaller blocks together in order to fit them into the frame. This task requires skills beyond those that you identified in your response to question (4). What are these skills?

Speech, language, hearing and oral mechanism evaluation

Zachary's language skills were assessed using standardised tests on four occasions between 4;0 years and 6;1 years. On all occasions, his comprehension was in the extremely low to low average range. At 5;1 years, Zachary's score on the Peabody Picture Vocabulary Test (PPVT; Dunn and Dunn, 1981) placed him in the 8th percentile. One year later at 6;1 years, Zachary's score on the PPVT placed him in the 14th percentile. Zachary appeared to follow most verbal commands that did not require a verbal response. His comprehension was facilitated by the use of gestures alongside verbal commands. In relation to expressive language, Zachary had fewer than 10 single words at 4 years of age. He imitated single words inconsistently, and produced car-like noises as he played with a toy car. Zachary had such limited expressive speech skills that an articulation test could not be performed. At 4 years of age, he was only able to produce six consonants ([m], [p], [b], [d], [k], [h]) and four vowels ([i], [o], [ɑ], [u]). Syllable structure was adversely affected, with Zachary producing words with a CV structure or reduplicated CVCV structure. His speech displayed frequent homonymous forms.

An examination of the oral mechanism revealed that Zachary's speech structures were symmetric and functioning. There were no apparent organic abnormalities of the oral structures that might interfere with speech production. However, oral motor functioning was difficult for Zachary. He was able to perform most simple voluntary movements. Exceptions were puffing his cheeks, lateralising and elevating his tongue inside his mouth, and pushing the examiner's finger when it was placed against his cheek. It was unclear to what extent Zachary's comprehension problems compromised his performance on these tasks. The production of alternating nonsense syllables was also difficult for him. Zachary had one episode of otitis media at 3 years of age. He passed pure-tone hearing screening.

Unit 4.4 Speech, language, hearing and oral mechanism evaluation

(1) Zachary's scores on the PPVT placed him in the 8th percentile at 5;1 years and the 14th percentile at 6;1 years. Explain what these percentiles mean.

(2) By 4 years of age, Zachary had fewer than 10 single words. How much of a developmental delay does this represent?

(3) Zachary's speech displayed frequent homonymous forms. What does this mean?

(4) Name *three* behaviours which suggest the presence of an oral dyspraxia.

(5) What type of communication intervention would be appropriate in Zachary's case?

Intervention and outcome

For over a year, Zachary received individual speech and language therapy at two different institutions. The content of this therapy was consistent with some of the published literature on DAS. However, it resulted in only modest gains in Zachary's communicative competence at which point Powell (1996) undertook an alternative intervention. This new intervention emphasised the early stimulation of unknown aspects of phonology with a view to encouraging broadening of the phonetic inventory and distribution of sounds. It was delivered in four, one-hour treatment sessions per week (Zachary's previous treatment involved two, 30-minute sessions per week). Therapy sessions were modular in nature. One such module, which is taken from Powell (1996: 325), is shown below.

Warm-up activity

Stimulate imitation of sounds and/or syllables using pictured stimuli. Note that activity should initially be play-like and relatively indirect. Successful imitations may be acknowledged. To maintain a high level of motivation, the use of phonetic placement cues is avoided.

Sample targets:	Stimulus photo:
[pʌpʌpʌ]	Popcorn being popped
[gʌgʌgʌ]	Drinking water
[f:::]	Balloon leaking air
[ʒ:::]	Sewing machine
[ʃʃʃ]	Train
[ɝ:::]	Growling dog or bear
[m:::]	Bowl of ice cream

Goal 1

Elicitation of a new sound in CV or VC syllables (imitation) using visual, tactile or auditory cues as needed. Example: Imitation of [iz], [ɑz], [uz], [æz] using a drill-play paradigm.

Goal 2

Stabilisation of inconsistently used sounds in words. Vary the position and phonetic context. Stimulus items may also be used to reinforce vocabulary development. Example: Elicited production of [k] in words: 'key', 'keep', 'eek', 'peek', etc. Fade cues and increase speed to encourage automaticity.

Goal 3

Generalisation of 'known' sounds in 'known' positions at a more conversational level. Tasks may be relatively flexible provided frequent opportunities are provided for the production of targeted sounds. Example: 'Shopping' activity where items on sale are chosen on the basis of their sound shapes: 'pie', 'map', 'tea', 'baby', etc. Design of the activity may also address language goals.

Goal 4

Maintenance of previously taught sounds embedded in language stimulation activity. The activity may be less structured than the preceding in terms of phonological stimuli. The focus of this goal may be on language skill with planned opportunities to monitor production of previously generalised targets.

Cool-down activity

Repeat the warm-up activity or some similar variant

At the outset of this intervention, Zachary had only 11 consonants in his phonetic inventory. After three months of this new treatment, his phonetic inventory had increased to 17 consonants. Not only had the size of his phonetic inventory increased, but its complexity had also increased. Zachary's consonant inventory had initially included stops, nasals and glides. By 5;1 years, his inventory had increased in complexity to include fricatives and affricates. By 5;4 years, its complexity had increased further by the addition of the liquid /l/. The complexity and range of syllabic structure also increased following this new intervention. Before intervention, Zachary only produced CV syllables and reduplicated CVCV strings. However, by 5;4 years he was also using VC, CVC, CCVCV and CVCC syllables.

Unit 4.5 Intervention and outcome

(1) In what respect does the new intervention that Zachary received differ from other therapies for sound production disorders in children?

(2) To what extent do you think the intensity of Zachary's earlier treatment contributed to its limited success?

(3) The type and frequency of feedback are acknowledged by clinicians to play an important role in interventions for DAS. What kind of feedback is used in this new intervention? What other forms of feedback can facilitate speech production in children with DAS?

(4) Zachary's language skills, particularly his expressive language skills, are severely impaired. How does this new intervention embed language stimulation alongside its speech goals?

(5) Respond with *true* or *false* to each of the following statements:
   (a) This new intervention uses multi-sensory cues to facilitate production of speech targets.
   (b) This new intervention does not address speech prosody.

(c) This new intervention provides Zachary with multiple opportunities for the production of target sounds.

(d) This new intervention aims to enhance the range and strength of articulatory movements.

(e) This new intervention prioritises speech goals over language goals.

Case study 5

Total glossectomy in a man aged 69 years

Introduction

The following exercise is a case study of a man ('GS') who was studied by Morrish (1988). GS underwent a total glossectomy for the treatment of a carcinoma at the base of his tongue. His post-operative speech production was examined in detail. The case study is presented in five sections: primer on oral cancer and glossectomy; speech and swallowing following glossectomy; client history; focus on articulation and intelligibility; and focus on instrumental and acoustic analyses.

Primer on oral cancer and glossectomy

Glossectomy is the surgical removal of whole or part of the tongue (total and partial glossectomy, respectively). The procedure is typically performed to treat tongue cancer, although in a smaller number of cases it may also be used to correct congenital macroglossia (Choi et al., 2013). The tongue is the most common intraoral site for oral cancer worldwide (Moore et al., 2000). In 2013, there were 13,590 estimated new cases of oral tongue cancer in the United States and 2,070 estimated deaths. The most common type of tongue cancer is a squamous cell carcinoma. Less commonly found carcinomas of the tongue include adenoid cystic carcinoma and mucoepidermoid carcinoma (Leong et al., 2007; Luna-Ortiz et al., 2009). As well as tobacco smoking and alcohol consumption, other risk factors for tongue cancer include certain viruses (e.g. Epstein–Barr virus and human papilloma virus (HPV) 16 and 18), cultural practices – prevalent in parts of India – such as reverse smoking (the burning end of cigars is within the mouth) and dipping (placing a mixture of Khaini tobacco and slaked lime in the lower gingival groove), and sexual behaviours including oral sex (although this is likely to be related to HPV infection) (Heck et al., 2010; Stich et al., 1992; Zheng et al., 2010).

On account of the serious implications of glossectomy for speech and swallowing, this operation is performed as a last resort when other treatment options (e.g. radiotherapy) have failed to treat a tumour. The defect that is created by glossectomy is reconstructed with a local closure, a local flap or a free flap. A local closure is used when the defect is small. If the defect is relatively large, then it is closed with the use of a flap. To form local flaps, tissue can be raised from the neck (platysma muscle), chest (pectoralis muscle) and forehead (frontalis muscle). Free flaps can be formed using tissue from the radial forearm, inside of the thigh (gracilis flap) and the abdomen (rectus abdominis muscle). The oral surgeon must consider a range of factors in the choice of flap, including the size of defect to be reconstructed, the aesthetic appearance of the tongue and the functional outcome for the patient in terms of speech and swallowing. The radial forearm free flap has emerged as the standard for partial glossectomy as it provides the desired bulk and contour for reconstruction. For total glossectomy, the more bulky anterolateral thigh flap and rectus abdominis can achieve greater propulsion of food into the pharynx during swallowing, the greater volume of these flaps compensating for the lack of motor function (Allan et al., 2015).

Advanced carcinoma of the tongue can necessitate additional surgical procedures including laryngectomy, mandibulectomy and pharyngectomy. These procedures also have serious implications for swallowing and the production of speech and voice. Van Lierop et al. (2008) studied eight patients who underwent total glossectomy. Three patients also required a total laryngectomy for a tumour involving the pre-epiglottic space or larynx. Five patients had a marginal mandibulectomy, one underwent segmental mandibulectomy and one required partial pharyngectomy. For patients with advanced squamous cell carcinoma of the tongue, Sinclair et al. (2011) reported reduced disease recurrence at 12 months postoperatively for patients who underwent total laryngoglossectomy (40%) compared to total glossectomy (61%). Disease-free survival at 12 months was also higher in patients with total laryngoglossectomy (50%) than in patients with total glossectomy (40%). However, intelligible speech was less often achieved by patients with total laryngoglossectomy (10%) than by patients with total glossectomy (30%).

Unit 5.1 Primer on oral cancer and glossectomy

(1) Respond with *true* or *false* to each of the following statements about glossectomy:
  (a) Glossectomy is used before radiotherapy and chemotherapy to treat tongue cancer.
  (b) Glossectomy may be used to treat macroglossia in children with Down's syndrome.
  (c) Glossectomy and laryngectomy are often used in combination to treat early-stage tongue cancer.
  (d) Total glossectomy is often accompanied by oesophagectomy.
  (e) Glossectomy may be used to treat macroglossia in children with Beckwith–Wiedemann syndrome.

(2) Quality of life is an important concept in the management of clients who undergo glossectomy. Which *two* factors are consistently reported by these clients to be most significant to their quality of life?

(3) Which of the following is *not* associated with the aetiology of tongue cancer?
  (a) tobacco use
  (b) cytomegalovirus infection
  (c) exposure to sunlight
  (d) HPV infection
  (e) alcohol consumption

(4) A range of different flaps may be used to correct the defect that is caused by glossectomy. Give *one* advantage and *one* disadvantage of the use of a bulky flap following total glossectomy.

(5) Studies have shown that incidence rates of oral cavity cancer vary considerably by country. Why do you think this is the case?

Speech and swallowing following glossectomy

Clients who undergo glossectomy are under the care of a multidisciplinary team. Included in this team are oral surgeons, radiation and medical oncologists, otolaryngologists, prosthodontists and speech-language pathologists. It is the role of the speech-language pathologist to assess and treat swallowing and speech problems in clients with glossectomy. SLP management of the client should begin at the point of diagnosis and continue until the best possible speech and swallowing outcomes have been achieved. However, the duration and intensity of intervention can vary markedly between healthcare systems and treatment centres.

Even the very best surgical results following glossectomy will involve some degree of compromise of swallowing and speech function. Dziegielewski et al. (2013) examined functional outcome data in 12 patients who underwent total glossectomy with laryngeal perseveration. These investigators also conducted a systematic review of the literature. Fifty per cent of the patients in this study, and 24% with systematic review, were still using gastrostomy tubes at one year post-surgery. In patients who could swallow, swallowing transit times more than doubled, but aspiration did not occur. On average, spoken sentence intelligibility was 66%. The best swallowing and speech functional outcomes occurred in patients who attended over 80% of swallowing and speech rehabilitation sessions. Vega et al. (2011) examined 39 patients who underwent glossectomy (24 total glossectomy, 15 subtotal glossectomy). Oral feeding was resumed in 33 (85%) of these patients. Speech was judged to be good or acceptable in 27 (87%) patients. Improved speech and swallowing outcomes following glossectomy are associated with flap reconstructions which have sufficient bulk and vertical height to allow for contact with the palate (Rigby and Hayden, 2014).

Speakers who undergo glossectomy can achieve relatively good intelligibility through the use of unusual labial, mandibular and pharyngeal speech compensations (Kazi et al., 2007). A number of these compensations occurred in the speech of seven German patients who were studied by Barry and Timmermann (1985). These patients were aged 32 to 62 years and each underwent a partial glossectomy. Plosive sounds involving the tongue were substituted by fricatives, glottal stops or bilabial stops. Kaipa et al. (2012) examined speech produced by a 31-year-old female in the three-month period following glossectomy. Acoustic analysis revealed improvements in the vowel space area during this time. However, there was deterioration in the perception of this speaker's consonants, with anterior sounds being perceived more correctly than medial and posterior sounds. Bressmann et al. (2009) assessed speech acceptability in 22 patients with partial glossectomies. These investigators found that the amount of tongue tissue resected predicted 41 per cent of the variance in post-surgical speech acceptability. Moreover, a defect size of more than 20.4 per cent of tongue tissue was found to be the critical cut-off point for poorer speech acceptability.

Unit 5.2 Speech and swallowing following glossectomy

(1) Which of the medical and health professionals described above manages the following aspects of care of clients with tongue cancer?
   (a) This professional oversees the surgical removal of the larynx.
   (b) This professional oversees the assessment and treatment of dysphagia.
   (c) This professional oversees the type of radiotherapy to be administered.

(d) This professional oversees the use of prosthetic devices by clients.

(e) This professional oversees the surgical removal of the tongue and defect reconstruction.

(2) Many patients who have a glossectomy need to use a gastrostomy tube for a period of time after surgery. Describe what this tube is, and explain why it is necessary in patients who have a glossectomy.

(3) The German speakers with partial glossectomy who were studied by Barry and Timmermann (1985) produced the following sound substitutions for the voiceless alveolar plosive: /t/ → [ʔ] and /t/ → [p]. Explain the basis of these substitutions.

(4) Barry and Timmermann's subjects make a number of other substitutions for plosive sounds that involve the tongue. These substitutions include /d/ → [s], /k/ → [x] and /g/ → [ɣ]. Explain the basis of these substitutions.

(5) Bressmann et al. (2009) found that the *amount* of tongue tissue resected was significant in post-surgical speech acceptability. Which other factor plays an important role in speech acceptability following glossectomy?

Client history

Subject 'GS' is a 69-year-old white man who underwent total glossectomy eight years earlier. This procedure was necessitated by a diagnosis of invasive squamous cell carcinoma at the base of the tongue. The epiglottis was preserved and there was no mandibular involvement. Dentition also remained unaffected, although GS's lower teeth had been replaced by dentures. The defect created by glossectomy was reconstructed using a forehead flap. Frontalis muscle was introduced through the cheek. There was no free edge to this flap – it was entirely set in. Following glossectomy, GS received speech therapy for two years. Notwithstanding the radical nature of GS's surgery, a speech and language therapist judged his speech to be good.

Unit 5.3 Client history

(1) Are the age, ethnicity and sex of GS typical of clients who are diagnosed with oral squamous cell carcinoma?

(2) Respond with *true* or *false* to each of the following statements about GS's tumour:
  (a) GS has the least common type of tongue cancer.
  (b) GS has been diagnosed at an early stage in tumour development.
  (c) GS has the most common type of tongue cancer.
  (d) GS has a type of tongue cancer which is mostly found in young adults.
  (e) GS has a tumour at the base of the tongue when most tumours affect the oral tongue.

(3) Is there a high or a low probability that GS resumed oral feeding after total glossectomy? What factors are influential in your decision?

(4) A forehead flap was used to reconstruct the defect caused by glossectomy. This is a type of local flap. What does this mean?

(5) A speech therapist judged GS to have a good speech outcome. Aside from features of his flap reconstruction, what other factor do you think contributed to this outcome?

Focus on articulation and intelligibility

To determine GS's intelligibility, 16 phonetically naive subjects listened through head-phones to an audio-recording of 10 randomly devised sentences. All sentences were played once in full and then singly, with no repetition permitted. Subjects also listened to an extract of conversation with GS. Repetition of the recording was permitted, although subjects were advised not to spend more than five or six minutes on this task. Subjects then orthographically transcribed what they heard. The transcription had to be 100% correct in order for a subject to be said to have understood what GS said. Intelligibility scores across the sentences and conversational passage were high at 65% and 58%, respectively. There was considerable variability between listeners, however, with intelligibility scores on the conversational passage ranging from 15% to 71%. A second intelligibility test was conducted. Because it had been observed that GS used a bilabial place of articulation for all plosive sounds, the focus of this test was on his production of initial plosive consonants. Subjects listened to audio-recordings of GS as he produced the following CVC monosyl-lables – kit, beat, tick, deep, dip, bill, peat, keep, pit, gill and teak. Although the bilabial plosives /p, b/ were identified at a rate better than chance, the alveolar plosives /t, d/ and the velar plosives /k, g/ did not even reach chance, and were overwhelmingly identified as bilabial plosives.

In the absence of a tongue, GS used a complete bilabial closure to articulate all plosive sounds. To establish if he varied this closure to signal different plosives, a close-up video analysis of GS during speech production was performed. The degree of bilabial protrusion, jaw retraction/protrusion and jaw elevation/lowering was measured in millimetres as deviations from a rest position. The same CVC monosyllables as above were used during this examination. Although there was little difference between alveolar and velar plosives, there was a consistent and statistically significant difference between bilabial and alveolar plosives in terms of jaw lowering. A lower posture was adopted for bilabial plosives. These same plosives also showed a statistically significant difference in terms of jaw protrusion, with bilabial plosives more protruded than alveolar plosives. There was a slight statistically significant difference between bilabial and alveolar plosives in terms of bilabial protrusion. GS used a more protruded posture for /t, d/ than for /p, b/.

Unit 5.4 Focus on articulation and intelligibility

(1) Intelligibility scores were based solely on audio-recordings of GS's speech. Ratings of intelligibility normally increase when speakers can be seen as well as heard. Is that likely to happen in this case?

(2) Video analysis revealed that GS used bilabial protrusion, jaw protrusion and jaw lowering to signal differences between bilabial and alveolar plosives. How would you characterise these articulatory adjustments on GS's part?

(3) The substitutions used by Barry and Timmermann's German speakers as they attempted to produce alveolar and velar plosives were examined at page 34. Is GS's

production of these same plosive sounds similar to, or different from, the productions of these speakers?

(4) How might the substitutions produced by GS and Barry and Timmermann's subjects be explained in terms of the surgical procedures that these subjects underwent?

(5) To the extent that GS naturally developed compensatory articulations following glossectomy, what role might speech-language pathology have for such a client?

Focus on instrumental and acoustic analyses

Instrumental analyses using electromyography (EMG) and a strain gauge apparatus were used to confirm the results of the video analysis of GS's speech. During EMG, surface electrodes were placed on either side of the philtrum from where they measured the activity of the orbicularis oris muscle. GS read CV monosyllables in which the vowels were neural for lip position. There was a high statistical difference in the activity of the orbicularis oris muscle during the articulation of /t, d/ and /p, b/, with greater activity observed during alveolar plosives. Through use of the strain gauge apparatus it was confirmed that jaw lowering was greater for /p, b/ than for /t, d/. These instrumental techniques confirmed that GS was using certain postures consistently during the production of bilabial and alveolar plosives, and that these postures were detectable during video and instrumental analyses, even if they were not always perceived by listeners.

Videofluoroscopy was used to assess GS's articulation of high and low vowels. For high vowels, the pharynx widens and the grafted flap rises slightly. There is slight protrusion of the jaw which retains a close position. The soft palate closes firmly and is raised to a position well above Passavant's ridge. For low vowels, pharyngeal narrowing is achieved by a strong retraction of the anterior wall and the epiglottis. The flap rises and bunches and is carried back with the anterior wall of the pharynx to approximate the posterior wall. The jaw moves downwards and backwards, with downward movement exaggerated in comparison with normal speakers. GS's production of vowels and consonants also underwent acoustic analysis. GS repeated randomly ordered CVC words which were analysed on a sound spectrograph. Formant frequencies were measured and compared with those from a normal speaker. GS was unable to differentiate between high and low vowels acoustically. Spectrograms were also made of all the CVC words used in the intelligibility tests. Several acoustic characteristics were examined. However, none were judged to correspond to GS's articulatory differences between bilabial and alveolar plosives.

Unit 5.5 Focus on instrumental and acoustic analyses

(1) During electromyography, GS read CV monosyllables in which the vowels were neutral for lip position. Why is a neutral lip position important in the context of this examination?

(2) GS's production of high and low vowels was assessed through the use of videofluoroscopy. Which of the following statements is *true* of this technique?
   (a) Videofluoroscopy can be used to assess velopharyngeal function.
   (b) Videofluoroscopy makes use of a palatal plate that contains electrodes.
   (c) A radio-opaque bolus must be swallowed during videofluoroscopy.

(d) Videofluoroscopy measures nasal airflow during speech production.

(e) Videofluoroscopy may be used in the assessment of dysphagia.

(3) A structure which is not normally active during articulation was used by GS during the production of vowels. What is that structure? What function does it serve during vowel production?

(4) GS was unable to use any acoustic feature to distinguish alveolar from bilabial plosives. Given that this is the case, what earlier finding is unsurprising?

(5) Although GS's post-surgical anatomy and physiology could not achieve an acoustic differentiation of alveolar from bilabial plosives, it is not the case that GS's vocal tract has been acoustically neutralised as a result of surgery. In what respect is this latter statement correct?

Case study 6

Man aged 39 years with stroke-induced dysarthria

Introduction

The following exercise is a case study of a 39-year-old man ('AB') who was studied by Grunwell and Huskins (1979). AB suffered a cerebrovascular accident in December 1972 which resulted in dysarthria and other neurological sequelae. The case study is presented in five sections: primer on acquired dysarthria; client history and clinical presentation; speech evaluation; focus on mixed dysarthria; and assessment issues.

Primer on acquired dysarthria

'Acquired dysarthria' is a collective term for a group of motor speech disorders which are caused by damage to the central and/or peripheral nervous systems. Typically, these disorders have their onset in adulthood, although acquired dysarthria may also arise in childhood. The perceptual anomalies that occur in acquired dysarthria reflect impairments in one or more speech production subsystems, namely, articulation, resonation, phonation, respiration and prosody. Acquired dysarthria may minimally disrupt speech intelligibility. Alternatively, the disorder may compromise speech production to such an extent that the client is severely unintelligible and must use an alternative means of communication.

The incidence and prevalence of acquired dysarthria in the general population is largely unknown. To understand the epidemiology of this motor speech disorder, it is necessary to examine its incidence and prevalence in relation to specific clinical populations. Adults who sustain a cerebrovascular accident or stroke are most at risk of acquired dysarthria. Using the Registry of the Canadian Stroke Network's database, Flowers et al. (2013) estimated the incidence of dysarthria in a sample of 221 patients with acute ischaemic stroke to be 42%. Another significant cause of acquired dysarthria in children and adults is traumatic brain injury (TBI). Safaz et al. (2008) reported the presence of dysarthria in 30.2% of 116 persons with TBI who were followed at a single centre in the five-year period between 2000 and 2006. Aside from stroke and TBI, other neurological disorders associated with acquired dysarthria include multiple sclerosis, Parkinson's disease, and motor neurone disease (also known as amyotrophic lateral sclerosis). The incidence and prevalence of acquired dysarthria in several of these disorders has also been investigated. Danesh-Sani et al. (2013) reported the presence of dysarthria in 42.1% of 500 patients aged 11 to 69 years with multiple sclerosis. Perez-Lloret et al. (2012) estimated the prevalence of dysarthria in 419 patients with Parkinson's disease to be 51%.

All aspects of speech production may be compromised in dysarthria. In terms of *articulation*, a speaker with dysarthria may produce weak and distorted consonant and vowel sounds. Problems with *resonation* may arise on account of mistiming of the closure of the velopharyngeal port. A breathy voice may reflect inadequate glottal valving of the pulmonary airstream during *phonation*. A speaker with dysarthria may produce short, truncated utterances on account of impaired *respiration*. In terms of *prosody*, a speaker with dysarthria may place stress on the wrong syllables within words, and the wrong words within sentences. Each of these speech production difficulties are related to neuromuscular deficits which affect the range, speed, force and timing of movements of the articulators and other organs of speech.

Dysarthria may occur in isolation in clients. However, it is often the case that it is found alongside dysphagia and other neurogenic communication disorders, principally aphasia and apraxia of speech. In their study of 221 clients with acute ischaemic stroke, Flowers et al. (2013) found that the highest co-occurrence of any two impairments was 28% for the presence of dysphagia and dysarthria. Dysarthria in combination with dysphagia and aphasia was present in 10% of these clients. A combination of dysarthria, sialorrhoea (drooling) and dysphagia was present in 136 (33%) of 419 patients with Parkinson's disease examined by Perez-Lloret et al. (2012). These additional disorders are significant in that they can make a differential diagnosis of dysarthria difficult (particularly if apraxia of speech is present), and they provide additional obstacles to the successful rehabilitation of clients.

Unit 6.1 Primer on acquired dysarthria

(1) Which of the following conditions is a cause of acquired dysarthria?
  (a) Duchenne's muscular dystrophy
  (b) cerebral haemorrhage
  (c) cerebral palsy
  (d) Wilson's disease
  (e) Möbius syndrome

(2) The following statements describe cases of acquired dysarthria in children and adults. For each statement, indicate if the dysarthria has a traumatic, infectious, neoplastic and/or iatrogenic aetiology.
  (a) A 10-year-old child develops speech problems following excision of a posterior fossa tumour.
  (b) A woman experiences speech problems following a prolonged illness with herpes simplex encephalitis.
  (c) A 15-year-old boy has reduced intelligibility following a head injury.
  (d) A man who sustains recurrent laryngeal nerve damage during thyroidectomy has speech production difficulties following surgery.
  (e) A 12-year-old boy has unintelligible speech following cranial irradiation for a medulloblastoma.

(3) Dysarthria is a feature of neurodegenerative disorders such as multiple sclerosis, Parkinson's disease and motor neurone disease. Which of the following types of dysarthria are associated with these disorders?
  (a) ataxic dysarthria
  (b) hypokinetic dysarthria

    (c) mixed flaccid-spastic dysarthria

    (d) flaccid dysarthria

    (e) mixed ataxic-spastic dysarthria

(4) The following statements describe impairments in dysarthria. Relate each statement to *one* of the following speech production subsystems: *articulation; resonation; prosody; respiration; phonation.*

    (a) The velum is unable to elevate to achieve closure with the pharyngeal wall.

    (b) The tongue achieves fricative strictures in place of stops.

    (c) Limited breath support for speech disrupts fluency.

    (d) Devoicing of voiced consonants is related to delays in the onset of voicing.

    (e) Stress is placed on the wrong syllables in words.

(5) For the severely unintelligible client with dysarthria an alternative communication system needs to be established. Describe *three* factors which speech-language pathologists need to consider in their assessment of a suitable system for a client.

Client history and clinical presentation

AB is 39 years old. In December 1972, he had a cerebrovascular accident (an intracerebral haematoma). He has a history of hypertension. Following his CVA, he presented with right-sided weakness. He displayed right upper and lower facial weakness, some dysphasia, dysphonia and dysarthria of brainstem origin. AB's wife reported that his speech had been somewhat nasal and difficult to understand prior to his CVA. In January 1974, AB's speech musculature was examined. It was found to be bilaterally affected, with greater impairment on the right. There was spastic weakness of the lips and tongue. The palate was atrophied and foreshortened. The palatal impairment was attributed to flaccid weakness. All articulatory movements, but especially those involving the palate, were impaired. AB was given a speech diagnosis of mixed dysarthria owing to the presence of both bulbar and suprabulbar signs.

Unit 6.2 Client history and clinical presentation

(1) AB suffered a cerebrovascular accident. Describe the type of CVA he experienced.

(2) AB displayed both spastic and flaccid weakness. What are the lesion sites which give rise to this type of weakness?

(3) Which of the following are clinical signs of lower motor neurone damage?

    (a) hypotonia

    (b) pathological reflexes

    (c) fasciculations

    (d) atrophy

    (e) hypertonia

(4) What evidence is there that AB displayed velopharyngeal incompetence (VPI) following his CVA? Is there any evidence that VPI was a feature of AB's premorbid communication?

(5) AB has sustained bilateral cortico-bulbar damage. Explain why bilateral cortico-bulbar lesions are required to produce a significant dysarthria.

Speech evaluation

AB's speech production underwent a comprehensive assessment. The slow movement of the articulators contributed to a general slow speaking rate. There was articulatory imprecision in the production of consonants and vowels which was related to slowness of movement and weakness of articulation. AB frequently failed to reach target positions. This resulted in errors of vowel quality and the use of a fricative stricture in place of a stop. In terms of phonation, AB displayed a breathy voice. The loudness of the voice did not vary. There was also a lack of pitch variation, and the pitch of the voice was abnormally high. AB exhibited audible nasal emission, which was evident on a spectrogram as a high frequency noise trace. Excessive nasal resonance was evident during voiced segments.

The interaction of these deviant features reduced the intelligibility of AB's speech. AB's uneconomical use of air meant that he was only able to speak in short phrases. His slow rate of articulatory movements also contributed to the restricted length of his utterances. The lack of variation in pitch and loudness and poor breath control compromised the use of stress, rhythm and intonation. Breathy voice and excessive nasal resonance limited AB's ability to produce qualitative distinctions between vowels. A reduction in intra-oral air pressure compromised consonant production, particularly plosives and fricatives.

Unit 6.3 Speech evaluation

(1) Which of the following is a feature of AB's speech production?
  (a) monoloudness
  (b) scanning speech
  (c) monopitch
  (d) reduced loudness
  (e) hypernasality

(2) AB was reported to make 'uneconomical use of air'. Describe *two* ways in which this description applies to AB's speech production.

(3) A spectrogram was used in the assessment of AB's speech production. It is one of several techniques which can be used to analyse dysarthric speech. Several others are listed below. For each technique, indicate if it is a type of perceptual, acoustic or physiological assessment:
  (a) intelligibility rating
  (b) videofluoroscopy
  (c) spectrogram
  (d) electroglottography
  (e) phonetic transcription study

(4) Describe *two* ways in which the articulation of plosive sounds is compromised in AB.

(5) Explain how disturbances at the phonatory level produce prosodic anomalies in AB's speech.

Focus on mixed dysarthria

AB's speech disorder was diagnosed as a mixed flaccid-spastic dysarthria. Individual deviant speech parameters could be attributed to spasticity and/or flaccidity. AB's slow rate of speech and articulatory imprecision could be attributed to spasticity which limits the range, force and speed of articulatory movements. Poor adduction and abduction of the vocal folds, manifested in a breathy voice and audible inspiration, was suggestive of a flaccid condition of the vocal folds. However, an indirect laryngoscopy was not performed and so this impression could not be confirmed. AB's breathiness might also be explained by spasticity. A spastic condition of the vocal folds, manifested in extreme tension of the folds and their reduced elasticity, could also explain AB's problems with high monopitch and monoloudness.

AB's palatal abnormality, which is responsible for his nasal emission and hypernasality, can be attributed to the combined effects of spasticity and flaccidity. The effect of spasticity on the palate is to produce a tendency towards downward movement. Flaccidity makes the palate too weak to counteract this movement. Because a flaccid weakness of the palate tended to predominate in AB, he had an incompetent velopharyngeal sphincter. AB's spasticity was exacerbated by the increased muscular effort needed to counteract the effects of his weak and fatiguing speech musculature. His general body tension rose as he made more effort to speak. As he made more effort to speak, the imbalance created by the asymmetrical nature of his spasticity was also exaggerated. The effect of these factors was heard as increasing inefficiency and weakening of articulations, the loss of control over coordination of breathing and phonation leading to increasing air wastage, and continuous nasal escape related to a breakdown of control over velopharyngeal valving.

Unit 6.4 Focus on mixed dysarthria

(1) AB appeared to have both flaccid and spastic involvement of the laryngeal musculature. Impairment of which of the following cranial nerves accounts for a flaccid weakness of the laryngeal musculature?
   (a) vagus nerves (CN X)
   (b) facial nerves (CN VII)
   (c) trigeminal nerves (CN V)
   (d) hypoglossal nerves (CN XII)
   (e) auditory nerves (CN VIII)

(2) Describe *three* effects of spasticity on AB's articulatory movements.

(3) Name *one* articulator in which there is combined flaccid and spastic involvement. Describe the effects of flaccidity and spasticity on this articulator. What type of prosthetic intervention might be appropriate in the case of this articulator?

(4) That a flaccid condition of the vocal folds is responsible for AB's phonatory abnormalities was suggested by the noticeable lower motor neurone involvement of the palate bilaterally. Explain the basis of this suggestion.

(5) The clinical impression of flaccidity of the vocal folds could not be confirmed by means of an indirect laryngoscopy. Explain what is involved in this procedure.

Assessment issues

The assessment of AB's speech focused on the functioning of speech production subsystems and the impact of deviant speech parameters on AB's intelligibility. The functioning of physiological mechanisms such as phonation and respiration and the impact of impairment of these mechanisms on speaker intelligibility correspond to the 'body' and 'activity' levels of the International Classification of Functioning, Disability and Health (ICF; World Health Organization, 2001). Lowit (2014: 400) states that '[a]t the body level, the functioning of the various speech subsystems, i.e. respiratory, laryngeal, and velopharyngeal function and oral musculature are investigated. In terms of the activity level, a variety of data elicitation methods are available to assess intelligibility, ranging from evaluations of single words and phrases to reading passages and spontaneous speech.' The evaluation of these levels typically proceeds by means of published assessment protocols such as the Frenchay Dysarthria Assessment-2 (FDA-2; Enderby and Palmer, 2008), which examines speech production under the following 11 sections: reflex; respiration; lips; jaws; palate; larynx; tongue; intelligibility; rate; sensation; and associated factors.

Today, dysarthria assessment is as likely to consider the impact of this speech disorder on an individual's participation in daily activities (the third level of the ICF framework) as it is on a speaker's intelligibility. During an assessment of dysarthria, it is at least as important for clinicians to consider the impact of dysarthria on an individual's self-esteem, quality of life and social participation as it is to assess the effect of respiratory, phonatory and articulatory impairments on a client's intelligibility. The need for assessment of the impact of dysarthria on a client's psychological wellbeing and participation could not be clearer. Piacentini et al. (2014) reported that dysarthria-related quality of life is significantly compromised in patients with multiple sclerosis and dysarthria, while Skolarus et al. (2014) found that dysarthria is a predictor of participation restrictions in stroke survivors. A number of clinical tools have been validated for the purpose of assessing impact and participation, not all of which are designed specifically for clients with dysarthria. (The reader is referred to Lowit (2014) for a list of scales for the assessment of the psychosocial effects of communication disorders.)

Unit 6.5 Assessment issues

(1) Which of the following statements are *true* of dysarthria assessment according to the ICF framework?
   (a) The ICF framework addresses an individual's functioning and disability related to dysarthria within the context of activities and social roles.
   (b) The ICF framework considers poor respiratory support in dysarthria under body structure and function.
   (c) The ICF framework only addresses the relationship between physiological impairments and speech intelligibility in dysarthria.
   (d) The ICF framework considers environmental factors that can help or hinder participation in activities by the person with dysarthria.
   (e) The ICF framework does not address the speed, range and force of articulatory movements for speech production in dysarthria.

(2) Explain why an assessment of the intelligibility of the speaker with dysarthria should use different listeners, and scripted and unscripted speech tasks.

(3) What anomalies might you expect to record under the reflex and jaw sections of the FDA-2 in speakers with dysarthria?

(4) Describe how AB's dysarthria might adversely affect his participation in daily activities.

(5) AB's speech exhibited monopitch and monoloudness. Which of the following components of the ICF framework would these speech features come under? *body structure and function; activity and participation; personal and environmental factors.*

Case study 7

Man aged 35 years with Wilson's disease

Introduction

The following exercise is a case study of a 35-year-old man ('R') who was studied by Day and Parnell (1987). R was diagnosed at 23 years of age with Wilson's disease. He has had a 10-year contact with speech-language pathology since his diagnosis. The case study is presented in five sections: primer on Wilson's disease; client history and presentation; speech intervention: part 1; speech intervention: part 2; and speech outcome.

Primer on Wilson's disease

Wilson's disease is an autosomal recessive disorder that affects copper metabolism, leading to toxic accumulation of copper in the liver, central nervous system and kidneys (Beinhardt et al., 2014). The disorder is also known as 'hepatolenticular degeneration', a term which reflects damage to the liver ('hepato') and the lenticular nucleus of the basal ganglia ('lenticular') as a result of copper deposits. Wilson's disease is caused by mutations in the ATP7B gene (Lorincz, 2010). The prevalence of the disorder is estimated to be 1:49,500 (Møller et al., 2011). Lai and Tseng (2010) estimated the annual incidence rate to be 0.27 per 100,000. There is evidence of gender differences in Wilson's disease, with more men than women developing the neuropsychiatric form of the disorder, and more women than men developing the hepatic form (Litwin et al., 2012). There is a good, long-term prognosis for those individuals with Wilson's disease who receive adequate care (Beinhardt et al., 2014).

Neurological and psychiatric symptoms are a common feature of Wilson's disease. In a sample of 126 patients with the disease, Mihaylova et al. (2012) reported neurological signs in 82 subjects. The most frequently observed signs were tremor and dysarthria. Rigidity, bradykinesia and pyramidal signs were found in over 25% of patients. Dystonia, chorea, athetosis, ballismus and epilepsy were rarely observed in these patients. Moores et al. (2012) examined 48 adult patients with Wilson's disease, 21 of whom presented with neurological symptoms. Diagnostic magnetic resonance imaging revealed basal ganglia and brainstem abnormalities and atrophy in 64%, 64% and 36%, respectively. At follow-up, 50% exhibited basal ganglia lesions and 55% displayed atrophy. Individuals with Wilson's disease have an increased lifetime prevalence of psychiatric disorders, including major depressive disorders and bipolar disorders (Carta et al., 2012).

There has been little systematic investigation of dysarthria in Wilson's disease. This is despite the fact that dysarthria is a common neurological symptom of the disorder. Machado et al. (2006) reported dysarthria in 91% of a sample of 119 patients with Wilson's disease. An early study of 20 patients with Wilson's disease reported the presence of a mixed dysarthria, with prominent ataxic, spastic and hypokinetic features (Berry et al., 1974). The 10 most common speech production errors in these individuals were reduced stress, monopitch, monoloudness, imprecise consonants, slow rate, excess and equal stress, low pitch, irregular articulatory breakdown, hypernasality and inappropriate silences. Speakers with Wilson's disease exhibit an impaired speech rate and impaired control of speech rate (Pernon et al., 2013). Dysarthria in Wilson's disease has been found to correlate with lesions of the putamen and caudate (Starosta-Rubinstein et al., 1987).

Unit 7.1 Primer on Wilson's disease

(1) Wilson's disease is an autosomal recessive disorder. Using your knowledge of genetics, explain what is meant by the term 'autosomal recessive disorder'.

(2) Individuals with Wilson's disease can exhibit bradykinesia. Which of the following statements best captures this neurological sign?
   (a) Bradykinesia describes rapid, erratic movement in Wilson's disease.
   (b) Bradykinesia describes slowness of movement in Wilson's disease.
   (c) Bradykinesia describes involuntary, writhing movement in Wilson's disease.
   (d) Bradykinesia describes an intention tremor in Wilson's disease.
   (e) Bradykinesia describes a postural tremor in Wilson's disease.

(3) Depending on the underlying neuropathology, some forms of acquired dysarthria are *static* in nature (they may change in their features but not in severity over time). Other forms of acquired dysarthria are *progressive* in nature (they worsen over time as the underlying disorder which causes them deteriorates). Still other forms of acquired dysarthria *ameliorate* over time (they display improvement as the underlying disorder which causes them improves). Is dysarthria in the well-managed client with Wilson's disease likely to remain static, deteriorate or improve over time?

(4) Damage to which of the following neuroanatomical areas and structures appears to be related to the presence of dysarthria in Wilson's disease?
   (a) insula
   (b) basal ganglia
   (c) inferior frontal gyrus
   (d) occipital lobe
   (e) planum temporale

(5) There are a number of perceptual anomalies in the speech of individuals with Wilson's disease. Several of these anomalies are listed below. For each one, indicate if it is related to *articulation, resonation* or *prosody*.
   (a) excess and equal stress
   (b) hypernasality
   (c) monoloudness
   (d) imprecise consonants
   (e) monopitch

Client history and presentation

In 1974, when R was aged 23 years, he began to experience dysarthria, drooling, dysphagia, decreased mental function and some dystonia. Subsequently, he went on to develop right foot drop, postural changes, clumsiness of the upper extremities and marked personality changes. These changes manifested as intermittent periods of depression. R was diagnosed as having Wilson's disease. His older sister had been diagnosed two years earlier with the disorder and had died shortly thereafter.

Following diagnosis, R was prescribed Penicillamine (an agent used for the mobilisation and elimination of copper) and was placed on a low-copper diet. However, R did not comply with either his drug or dietary regimen. Between 1974 and 1976, he contacted a number of specialists in psychiatry, internal medicine and speech-language pathology for assistance with his problems. These contacts were of limited duration with the exception of a period of psychiatric treatment for depression which lasted 18 months. R's speech deteriorated significantly during his psychiatric treatment. In April 1976, a psychiatrist remarked that 'speech (had) deteriorated almost to the point of being completely nonunderstandable . . . a direct result of the neurological damage associated with the (Wilson's) disease'. The psychiatrist also expressed the view that 'while (R's) speech might improve slightly, the chances of significant improvement (were) poor'. In the same year, R attempted suicide by means of a drug overdose. He was hospitalised in a mental health facility after a short period in an intensive care unit. His marriage failed during this time.

When R first attended the Columbia Speech and Hearing Clinic at the University of Missouri in 1976, he was already profoundly dysarthric. His speech was described as 'unintelligible for the most part'. His speech was non-functional, and he relied on written messages and sign language for communication. However, these other modes of communication were also of limited effectiveness. R also presented with drooling and dysphagia, had a fixed, grimace-like expression, and had oral and facial rigidity. On account of his severe speech disorder, R had been unable to work for two years. Accordingly, he received full disability compensation under social security.

Unit 7.2 Client history and presentation

(1) State *three* features of R's history prior to diagnosis, which are consistent with the clinical profile of Wilson's disease.

(2) R displayed poor compliance with his drug and dietary regimen. Which feature of R's clinical presentation directly contributed to his poor compliance? Does this same feature have any implications for the management of this client in speech-language pathology?

(3) Do you think R is at risk of aspiration pneumonia? Provide support for your answer.

(4) Why do you think written messages and sign language, like speech, were of limited effectiveness for R?

(5) R's severe speech disorder had effectively eliminated his occupational functioning. Name *one* other aspect of R's functioning which a speech disorder of this severity is likely to have compromised.

Speech intervention: part 1

At the Columbia Speech and Hearing Clinic, R received intervention for his dysarthria during 22 of 28 consecutive semester sessions over a 10-year period. A range of therapeutic techniques were used to improve intelligibility. Progress was monitored through the use of intelligibility ratings performed by familiar and unfamiliar listeners. During the 10-year period of R's intervention, specific areas of emphasis and therapy procedures, and the length and complexity of target utterances were varied to meet R's changing needs and abilities. Medical supervision of R was maintained throughout this entire time. Even though certain drug and dietary controls were prescribed, R displayed poor compliance with them.

Between admission in 1976 and the winter semester in 1977, R's speech intelligibility in clinic increased significantly. Oral-motor exercises which were aimed at improving the flexibility and precision of the oral structures were attempted initially. However, these produced little gain and were consequently abandoned. There was also an early emphasis on increased vocal volume and differentiation of vowel productions. However, this also made little contribution to the improvement of intelligibility. The focus of therapy then turned for several years to the production of single consonants and consonant blends and clusters. The production of multisyllabic words and word-final consonants was particularly difficult for R and made a large contribution to his reduced intelligibility. R was encouraged to engage in self-monitoring of his productions and, with the assistance of the therapist, to achieve consistency in his standards of judgement. His reliance on gestural communication, which was largely confusing and unsuccessful, was discouraged. Throughout this time, R refused to consider the use of an augmentative or alternative communication system.

Unit 7.3 Speech intervention: part 1

(1) R's progress in therapy was monitored through the use of intelligibility ratings by familiar and unfamiliar listeners. Under which of the following conditions is R's speech likely to be rated as most intelligible?
    (a) A familiar listener rates R's production of an unseen list of words.
    (b) An unfamiliar listener rates R's speech production during conversation.
    (c) A familiar listener rates R's production of an unseen list of sentences.
    (d) An unfamiliar listener rates R's production of an unseen list of phrases.
    (e) A familiar listener rates R's speech production during a conversation where the topic is known.

(2) Therapy was continually adjusted to meet R's changing needs and abilities. Why is this type of ongoing adjustment important in the context of R's dysarthria?

(3) Oral-motor exercises were attempted early in R's therapy. Which of the following are *true* statements about these exercises?
    (a) Oral-motor exercises aim to improve the strength and range of articulatory movements.
    (b) Oral-motor exercises focus on the accurate production of speech targets.
    (c) Oral-motor exercises are contra-indicated in progressive dysarthria.
    (d) Oral-motor exercises include tasks such as tongue protrusion and elevation.
    (e) Oral-motor exercises focus on the accurate production of non-speech targets.

(4) Describe *two* aspects of this intervention which may have been adversely affected by R's psychiatric problems.

(5) R displayed maladaptive compensatory behaviour in response to his severe speech disorder. What is this behaviour? Why is it described as 'maladaptive'?

Speech intervention: part 2

After intervention on the production of individual speech sounds proved to have limited benefit for speech intelligibility, the focus of intervention shifted to the use of suprasegmental guidelines on a continuous basis in contextual speech. The first two of these four guidelines emphasised the use of slowed rate and syllable-by-syllable production. This had a marked, positive effect on speech intelligibility for R. In fact, so considerable was the increase in R's intelligibility that he was able to secure part-time employment in 1980 for the first time since his diagnosis. In addition to these techniques, R was encouraged to make use of adequate respiratory support and appropriate pausing. He also received instruction in the use of stress and intonation patterns. However, these latter techniques were not as effective at improving intelligibility as slowed rate and syllable-by-syllable production. The third guideline encouraged the use of overarticulation within R's compensatory techniques. This required R to exaggerate articulatory movements. The fourth and final guideline, which complemented the third guideline, encouraged R to make use of increased mouth opening. This also increased R's intelligibility considerably. Notwithstanding these gains, R's motor speech skills were still highly vulnerable to the effects of physical fatigue. He was advised to rearrange his schedule in order to obtain sufficient rest, especially prior to therapy sessions. Because this advice was not always acted upon, R's compliance with this recommendation became a precondition for his enrolment in further therapy.

R's intelligibility was also compromised by hypernasality. R's hypernasal speech did not respond to traditional therapy techniques. Accordingly, a palatal lift appliance was recommended, which R used for approximately two years. By 1983, R's hypernasality had improved so much that even on days when he did not wear his palatal lift to therapy, his hypernasal speech had diminished considerably. Eventually, R was able to maintain improvements in his velopharyngeal control in the absence of the device, only resorting to its use during periods of fatigue.

Although R made considerable speech gains in clinic, he failed to generalise the use of his compensatory guidelines to communicative situations outside of clinic. Consistent with the therapeutic goal of helping R achieve optimal intelligibility and functional speech that was appropriate to his communicative needs in a range of settings, R was encouraged to assume ever greater responsibility for self-evaluation of his intelligibility and his use of the guidelines. Daily logs, which included ratings of intelligibility and consistency in use of the guidelines, were used for this purpose. Both R and his communicative partners completed these logs on a consistent basis. There was some deterioration in R's speech performance in the summer semester in 1985 when these logs were not completed. R married for the second time in 1983. R's wife occasionally attended therapy sessions in order to become acquainted with objectives and techniques which she could implement at home. It is expected that with greater involvement of R's wife in providing support, behaviour maintenance and feedback to R, he might be able to be discharged permanently from therapy.

Unit 7.4 Speech intervention: part 2

(1) Practice on speech sound production was minimally effective in terms of improving R's intelligibility. Accordingly, the focus of therapy changed to the implementation of

suprasegmental guidelines. Which of the following speech production subsystems is targeted by these guidelines?

(a) resonation
(b) articulation
(c) phonation
(d) respiration
(e) prosody

(2) Explain how slowed rate serves to increase the intelligibility of R's speech.

(3) Traditional therapy techniques did not improve R's hypernasality. Name *one* such technique. What is known about the efficacy of this particular technique?

(4) R achieved a satisfactory result in terms of resonation through the use of a palatal lift appliance. Explain how this appliance works to reduce hypernasal speech.

(5) Generalisation of improved speech skills beyond the clinic was an area of difficulty for R. What *two* main approaches were adopted to ensure that generalisation was achieved?

Speech outcome

R received intervention for his dysarthria over a 10-year period. At the outset of therapy, R was judged to have only 5% intelligibility (rated sentence by sentence) in connected speech. By the end of therapy, this had increased to an average of 95% intelligibility. During his 10-year period of intervention, R experienced several episodes when there were significant decreases in his intelligibility. These episodes could be accounted for by factors in R's lifestyle which he did not adequately manage and by R's underlying neurological disorder. When audiotaped samples of R's conversational speech from 1977 and 1985 were analysed and ranked according to the relative prominence of deviant speech features, it was found that whereas reduced intelligibility was first-ranked in 1977, it had dropped to fifth-ranked in 1985. This reflected R's success in using his compensatory techniques to achieve the major goal of treatment, optimal intelligibility and functional speech. The most prominent deviant speech features recorded in 1985 were imprecise consonants and prolonged phonemes. R's improved communicative status has enabled him to engage in full-time employment for the last three years. He has been remarried for two years and is the father of an infant son.

Unit 7.5 Speech outcome

(1) What contribution did R's articulation of individual speech sounds make to his overall intelligibility by the end of therapy?

(2) Throughout the 10-year period of R's intervention, his intelligibility decreased on certain occasions. Describe *two* factors which contributed to these episodes of reduced intelligibility in R.

(3) Increasingly, speech-language pathologists are asked to defend the cost-effectiveness of their interventions to clients. How would you defend the cost-effectiveness of the intervention that R has received?

(4) Charting R's speech progress over an extended period of time posed a number of challenges. Describe *two* such challenges.

(5) The decision to continue therapy in order to maximise the intelligibility of R's speech was motivated in part by his refusal to accept a form of augmentative or alternative communication. What does this decision reveal about how therapy can best be conducted?

Case study 8

Man aged 71 years with apraxia of speech

Introduction

The following exercise is a case study of a man aged 71 years who was studied by Peach and Tonkovich (2004). This client developed apraxia of speech (AOS) following a cerebrovascular accident. His case is somewhat unusual in that his AOS was caused by a subcortical haemorrhage of the basal ganglia. Most cases of AOS reported in the literature arise on account of cortical damage. The client also had stroke-induced aphasia. The case study is presented in five sections: primer on apraxia of speech; medical history; early post-stroke period; language assessment; and focus on speech.

Primer on apraxia of speech

McNeil et al. (2009: 264) state that 'apraxia of speech is a phonetic-motoric disorder of speech production'. This definition is extended to include the locus of breakdown in speech production – AOS is caused when well-formed phonological frames are not efficiently translated into the kinematic patterns that are used for carrying out intended movements. This inefficiency is manifested as temporal and spatial segmental and prosodic distortions both within and between articulators. The durations of consonants and vowels and the time between sounds, syllables and words may be extended as a result. The perceptual consequences may be heard as sound substitutions, the mis-assignment of stress, and other phrase- and sentence-level prosodic abnormalities. The location of speech errors within utterances is relatively consistent and the type of errors is invariable. (It should be noted that some researchers (e.g. Staiger et al., 2012) state that the invariability or consistency of speech errors is contentious at best, and should not be included as a criterion in the diagnosis of AOS.) AOS is not related to deficits of muscle tone or reflexes. It is also not related to deficits of sensory and language processing. AOS rarely occurs in pure or isolated form. When it does, it is not accompanied by deficits of basic motor physiology, perception or language.

Little is known about the epidemiology – prevalence and incidence – of AOS. Duffy (2005) reported that AOS accounted for 7.6% of all motor speech disorders diagnosed in the Mayo Clinic Speech Pathology practice between 1987 to 1990 and 1993 to 2001. This figure was based on 6,101 evaluations of people with a primary speech pathology diagnosis of a neurologic motor speech disorder. AOS is most frequently caused by cerebrovascular accidents. However, there is also a neurodegenerative form of AOS called primary progressive AOS (Duffy et al., 2015). There is still no consensus on the neuroanatomical location of the lesion(s) that are associated with AOS. However, potential regions include

Broca's area, the lateral premotor cortex, subcortical structures and the anterior insula, all in the left hemisphere (Robin and Flagmeier, 2014). As described above, pure AOS is a rare occurrence. AOS is much more likely to be found alongside dysarthria, aphasia and/or oral apraxia. Botha et al. (2014) reported that non-verbal oral apraxia is very common among patients with progressive AOS, and that the severity of AOS is predictive of oral apraxia. The presence of these other conditions makes a differential diagnosis of AOS difficult. However, there is evidence that specialist speech and language therapists display high intra-rater and inter-rater reliability in diagnosing the presence and severity of AOS in clients with communication difficulties following stroke (Mumby et al., 2007).

Unit 8.1 Primer on apraxia of speech

(1) Which of the following are *true* statements about apraxia of speech?
   (a) AOS is a disorder of language encoding.
   (b) The production of vowels and consonants is compromised in AOS.
   (c) AOS arises on account of muscle atrophy and reduced tone (hypotonia).
   (d) Automatic speech production is superior to volitional speech production in AOS.
   (e) Prosodic abnormalities in AOS are caused by respiratory difficulties.

(2) It was described above that AOS can be caused by cerebrovascular accidents and neurodegenerative disorders. Name *three* other causes of AOS.

(3) A Cochrane systematic review of AOS stated that 'there are no good epidemiological data on the prevalence of apraxia of speech' (West et al., 2005: 3). Which of the following statements best explains the lack of epidemiological data on AOS, according to the Cochrane reviewers?
   (a) AOS is a rare disorder and epidemiological studies are not a priority for funding in consequence.
   (b) Epidemiological studies of AOS are not a priority for funding because the disorder has few implications for an individual's quality of life.
   (c) Epidemiological studies are hampered by a lack of a universally agreed definition of AOS.
   (d) Epidemiological studies of AOS are not a priority for funding because the disorder has few implications for an individual's ability to communicate.
   (e) Epidemiological studies are hampered by difficulty in making a differential diagnosis of AOS, dysarthria and aphasia.

(4) Botha et al. (2014) found that non-verbal oral apraxia is very common among patients with progressive AOS. Why do you think this is the case?

(5) Depending on the condition that causes AOS, the speech disorder may be *static* or *progressive* in nature. Name *one* condition which causes static AOS, and *one* condition which causes progressive AOS.

Medical history

The client is a 71-year-old, right-handed man. He presented with an acute loss of speech and right hemiplegia following a cerebrovascular accident. Prior to his CVA, his medical history was unremarkable. Three days post-onset a CT scan was performed. It revealed a large, left frontal haemorrhage that probably originated in the region of the basal ganglia and extended into the frontal white matter. The lower half of the primary motor cortex, the posterior portion of the inferior frontal gyrus, the insula and the postcentral opercular structures were not involved.

Unit 8.2 Medical history

(1) Which of the following statements best captures the type of CVA that this client sustained?
   (a) The client sustained a cerebral embolism of the left cerebral hemisphere.
   (b) The client sustained a brainstem stroke.
   (c) The client sustained a cerebral embolism of the right cerebral hemisphere.
   (d) The client sustained a cerebral haemorrhage of the dominant hemisphere.
   (e) The client sustained a cerebral haemorrhage of the non-dominant hemisphere.

(2) The client developed a right hemiplegia as a result of his stroke. Describe *three* implications of a right hemiplegia for SLT assessment and intervention.

(3) This client's stroke probably originated in the region of the basal ganglia. Which of the following are *true* statements about the basal ganglia?
   (a) Damage to the basal ganglia only has implications for motor control.
   (b) The basal ganglia include the caudate, putamen and globus pallidus.
   (c) The basal ganglia are a number of cortical nuclei.
   (d) Damage to the basal ganglia can result in dyskinesias.
   (e) The basal ganglia are involved in language processing and motor planning and control.

(4) The CT scan revealed that the lower half of the primary motor cortex was not compromised by this client's haemorrhage. Has this neuroanatomical area any implications for motor speech production?

(5) Which of the following types of aphasia is this client most likely to experience?
   (a) Wernicke's aphasia
   (b) conduction aphasia
   (c) subcortical aphasia
   (d) Broca's aphasia
   (e) primary progressive aphasia

Early post-stroke period

Ten days after his stroke, the client was admitted to rehabilitation. He was alert but inconsistently responsive when an initial speech-language evaluation was performed. The client exhibited muteness and occasionally used simple gestures to refer to his inability to speak and understand questions. He used undifferentiated pointing responses to tasks that required auditory word discrimination and the matching of visual words to pictures. The client displayed no appropriate responses to questions in either formal or informal conversational contexts. Occasionally, when functional commands were presented in an appropriate context, he was able to follow them. Writing was impaired, with the non-preferred hand used to produce an unintelligible scribble.

A programme of speech-language intervention was initiated. During the next two weeks, the client exhibited minimal vocalisation, and spontaneously used a few grammatically well-formed sentences. Bucco-facial apraxia compromised his imitation of oral movements. He began to respond successfully to tasks that elicited automatic verbal responses by the end of the fourth week post-stroke. However, his speech remained aphonic. His inability to imitate speech consistently frequently frustrated him. There was moderate impairment of word recognition and auditory comprehension of yes–no questions. By pointing to an alphabet board, he was able to spell one simple word out of three.

His speech output at five weeks post-stroke was much improved from his initial appearance. However, he continued to be dysfluent – there was reduced phrase length and poor grammatical complexity – and he had substantial difficulty initiating speech. He was echolalic and perseverative. In conversation, there were occasional, but more frequent grammatically well-formed sentences of normal lengths. Although he was able to read sentences aloud, he did so with substantial difficulty. Through the use of self-cuing he was able to increase the consistency of vocalisation during speech production. There was mild impairment of auditory comprehension for word recognition. Limb apraxia made it difficult for him to follow commands using parts of his body. The client's naming was poor and was influenced by linguistic variables such as frequency of occurrence, open versus closed class and concrete versus abstract. Verbal paraphasias were also observed.

Unit 8.3 Early post-stroke period

(1) Is there any evidence that this client has phonatory apraxia? Provide support for your answer.

(2) Respond with *true* or *false* to each of the following statements:
   (a) The client uses gesture to compensate for his lack of spoken language.
   (b) The client has impaired auditory comprehension of language.
   (c) The client does not have non-verbal oral apraxia.
   (d) The client is unaware of his communication difficulties.
   (e) The client exhibits deficits of written language.

(3) Three linguistic variables were found to influence the client's naming. Give *one* example of each of these variables, and indicate how each variable may be manifested in the client's naming.

(4) By the end of the fourth week post-stroke the client began to produce verbal responses to tasks. Is there anything significant about the responses that the client produced?

(5) Is there any evidence that the client exhibits semantic deficits during naming? Provide evidence to support your answer.

Language assessment

The first formal assessment of the client's speech and language skills was undertaken at 6 weeks post-onset, when the Boston Diagnostic Aphasia Examination (BDAE;

Goodglass and Kaplan, 1983a) was conducted. The client's speech production was aphonic and effortful. He displayed trial and error behaviour, groping articulatory movements and attempts at self-correction. His speech displayed dysprosody which was unrelieved by extended periods of normal rhythm, stress and intonation. He had difficulty initiating utterances and his speech was perceived to contain phoneme substitutions. His description of the cookie theft picture from the BDAE is shown below:

(Examiner: What's happening with her?) With her? She's overflowing the sink . . . and . . . he's /s/ . . . (Examiner: How 'bout over there?) Over there? He /kæraher/ it in /e/ /ki/ it's a . . . (expletive) . . . /fo folling/ it's cookie jar . . . he's about to fall off . . . and hurt hisself.

The client's performance on the various subtests of the BDAE revealed a mild to moderate aphasia. The Rating Scale Profile of Speech Characteristics revealed that articulatory agility and paraphasia in running speech were the two most impaired areas, while repetition and auditory comprehension were areas of relative strength. The client's melodic line, phrase length, grammatical form and word-finding were disrupted, but were not as severely impaired as articulatory ability and paraphasia. This pattern of deficits did not correspond to any of the classical aphasia syndromes. The client's performance on each subtest of the BDAE is shown below:

Auditory Comprehension:
    Word discrimination (69/72)
    Body part identification (17/20)
    Commands (12/15)
    Complex ideational material (8/12)

Oral Expression:
    Oral agility (10/12)
    Verbal agility (14/14)
    Automatised sequences (5/8)
    Repetition of words (8/10)
    Repeating phrases (high probability) (8/8)
    Repeating phrases (low probability) (7/8)
    Word reading (30/30)
    Responsive naming (29/30)
    Visual confrontation naming (102/105)
    Body part naming (29/30)
    Oral sentence reading (8/10)

Reading Comprehension:
    Symbol and word discrimination (10/10)
    Word recognition (8/8)
    Comprehension of oral spelling (7/8)
    Word–picture matching (9/10)
    Reading sentences and paragraphs (9/10)

Writing:
    Mechanics of writing (1/3)
    Primer-level dictation (14/15)
    Written confrontation naming (3/10)

Unit 8.4 Language assessment

(1) Give *one* example from the cookie theft picture description of each of the following features:
   (a) The client produces phoneme substitutions.
   (b) The client omits the indefinite article in noun phrases.
   (c) The client displays efforts to self-correct.
   (d) The client associates the wrong semantic roles with verbs.
   (e) The client repeats part of the examiner's questions with correct prosody.

(2) How might the client's prosodic difficulties be related to other features of his verbal output?

(3) The client's pattern of deficits did not correspond to any of the classical aphasia syndromes. Five such syndromes are listed below. For each syndrome, indicate *one* feature which sets it apart from the client's particular language problems.
   (a) Wernicke's aphasia
   (b) conduction aphasia
   (c) Broca's aphasia
   (d) anomic aphasia
   (e) global aphasia

(4) The following items are taken from the BDAE. Each item is used to assess either limb/hand praxis or bucco-facial/respiratory praxis. Assign each of these items to one of these two categories.
   (a) The client is asked: 'How would you show there is too much noise?'.
   (b) The client is asked: 'Let me hear you cough'.
   (c) The client is asked: 'How would you pretend to stop traffic?'.
   (d) The client is told: 'Pretend to sip through a straw'.
   (e) The client is asked: 'How would you show that you are too cold?'.

(5) Why do you think the client's written confrontation naming is considerably worse than his visual confrontation naming?

Focus on speech

A detailed assessment of the client's speech was undertaken. The client orally read a series of word lists that sampled 45 voiced and unvoiced stop, fricative, affricate, nasal, semi-vowel and consonant cluster phonemes. Each phoneme or blend was sampled in initial, medial and final positions of words. Single phonemes were examined in words which were one to two syllables in length, while blends were examined in words of one to three syllables. Two experienced judges undertook broad phonemic transcriptions of a total of 1,057 audiotaped responses. Two types of phoneme errors were excluded from the analysis. First, phonemes which were produced in place of a target phoneme in a word were not included in the analysis. Second, substitutions of voiceless for voiced cognate phonemes were also omitted. These exclusions resulted in 77 (25%) of the total errors undergoing analysis. It was found that significantly more substitution errors were produced than other error types, followed by additions, repetitions, the use of intrusive schwa and finally omissions. Significantly more phoneme errors occurred in word initial position than in word medial and final positions. There were similar percentages of errors across different phoneme groupings (consonant cluster, fricative, nasal, etc.).

Unit 8.5 Focus on speech

(1) Monosyllabic and multisyllabic words were used to elicit the production of phonemes by the client. From your knowledge of AOS, would you expect speech errors to be more common or less common in monosyllabic versus multisyllabic words?

(2) The client has difficulty initiating speech. In view of this, where would you expect most speech errors to occur? Select one of the following as your answer: word initial position; word-medial position; word-final position.

(3) Why do you think all substitutions of voiceless phonemes for voiced cognate phonemes were omitted from the analysis?

(4) One of the speech errors produced by the client is the use of intrusive schwa. This is a relatively common speech feature of AOS. Why do you think this feature occurs?

(5) The authors of this study argue that the client's profile of speech errors is similar to, but not identical with, the profile observed in patients with AOS due to cortical lesions. Describe how the speech errors of speakers with cortical AOS differ from the speech errors of this client.

Case study 9

Woman aged 32 years with foreign accent syndrome

Introduction

The following exercise is a case study of a 32-year-old, Dutch-speaking woman ('TDF') who was studied by Van Borsel et al. (2005). TDF presented at the neurological department of a university hospital with speech problems of sudden onset. Although her history revealed noteworthy neurological events, her speech problems were considered to be of psychogenic origin. The case study is presented in five sections: primer on foreign accent syndrome; client history and medical investigations; language and oral motor evaluation; focus on articulation and prosody; and focus on accent.

Primer on foreign accent syndrome

Kuschmann and Lowit (2012) define foreign accent syndrome (FAS) as a 'motor speech disorder in which a variety of segmental and suprasegmental errors lead to the perception of a new accent in speech' (738). To date, there have been no epidemiological investigations of this speech disorder, although there is general consensus that the condition is rare. Typically, the disorder has a neurogenic aetiology. FAS has been reported in adults following cerebral infarction (Sakurai et al., 2015; Trax and Mills, 2013), traumatic brain injury (Lippert-Gruener et al., 2005) and the development of brain tumours (Tomasino et al., 2013). The speech disorder has also been documented in adults with neurodegenerative disorders such as multiple sclerosis (Chanson et al., 2009). Less commonly, a psychogenic aetiology is presumed to underlie the disorder. Verhoeven et al. (2005) described FAS in the case of a Dutch-speaking adult with conversion disorder. A developmental form of FAS has been described in two child patients by Mariën et al. (2009).

Linguistic investigations of FAS have focused primarily on the production of segments and use of intonation in speakers with the disorder. Verhoeven and Mariën (2010) described pronunciation problems at the segmental level in a female speaker of Belgian Dutch who developed a French/German foreign accent after a left hemisphere stroke. Many of this speaker's vowels had clear creaky voice. There was a substantially smaller vowel space and less acoustic differentiation between [i], [ɪ] and [e]. There was a tendency to devoice fricatives and stops. Velar fricatives were pronounced as velar stops, and the glottal fricative was almost consistently realised as a glottal stop in word-initial position. The alveolar trill was systematically pronounced as a uvular trill, which is a typical feature of French learners of Dutch.

Intonation and other aspects of speech prosody have been extensively examined in FAS. Katz et al. (2008) reported inaccurate and highly variable lexical stress assignment in a

46-year-old, monolingual female who presented with FAS of unknown aetiology. This client's sentence-level intonation also showed occasional deviations from typical American English patterns. Kuschmann and Lowit (2012) studied the pragmatic use of intonation in four speakers with FAS. Specifically, the use of phonetic parameters (fundamental frequency, intensity and duration) and phonological categories (pitch accents and de-accentuation) to signal information status was examined. Although speakers with FAS were able to use phonetic parameters to differentiate between given and new information, they frequently placed pitch accents on given information instead of de-accenting these elements. The foreign qualities of the Dutch-speaking adult described by Verhoeven et al. (2005) extended beyond pronunciation to include features of the lexicon, syntax and pragmatics.

Unit 9.1 Primer on foreign accent syndrome

(1) Respond with *true* or *false* to each of the following statements about the aetiology of FAS:
    (a) A client may present with FAS in the absence of a known aetiology.
    (b) FAS is most often associated with psychogenic factors.
    (c) Cerebral neoplasms are part of the neurogenic aetiology of FAS.
    (d) FAS may be related to the onset of neurodegenerative disease in adults.
    (e) FAS in a client may be associated with neurogenic and psychogenic factors.

(2) The speaker with FAS who was studied by Tomasino et al. (2013) displayed no signs of dysarthria, apraxia of speech, or aphasia. How typical is this case of FAS in general?

(3) The speaker with FAS who was studied by Verhoeven and Mariën (2010) was described as producing pronunciation errors that resulted from articulatory 'overshoot' of the active articulator (i.e. the active articulator overshoots its target). What *two* features of this client's speech are examples of articulatory overshoot?

(4) The speaker described in question (3) also produces the following speech errors: [k > x] and [t > s]. How would you characterise these errors?

(5) The speakers with FAS who were studied by Kuschmann and Lowit (2012) frequently placed pitch accents on given information. Explain why this is problematic in terms of signalling information status during communication.

Client history and medical investigations

TDF first visited the neurological department of the authors' university hospital because of speech problems of sudden onset. Her medical history contained several, noteworthy features. Since the age of 6, TDF had a right-sided neurosensory hearing loss with sloping configuration. A head trauma and whiplash injury were sustained nine years earlier. This caused chronic headache with variable lateralisation which was predominant in the occipito-nuchal and parietal region. An otorhinolaryngologist had been consulted one month earlier for a hoarse voice following a minor head trauma. However, a clinical ENT examination was normal: no structural abnormalities were revealed by flexible laryngoscopy and the voice sounded normal to the otorhinolaryngologist. It was shortly after this ENT consultation that TDF's speech problems appeared suddenly during an evening out with friends. TDF was described as being mute for some time after the onset of her speech difficulties. A clinical neurological examination was also normal. There were no motor or sensory impairments. Pathological reflexes were absent, and tendon reflexes were symmetrical. The results of coordination, posture and gait tests were normal. A whole brain CT scan was also normal.

TDF experienced significant psychiatric problems. She was being treated for depression and suicidal ideation at the time of the study. This was related to family problems. Specifically, TDF's husband had rapidly progressing Huntington's disease. Yet, she had been kept unaware of the family history in relation to this condition. TDF had concerns about the implications of this disease for her 10-year-old son who had a learning disorder. TDF took two antidepressants, sertraline and trazodone. However, neither drug is known to have any effect on speech either singly or in combination. A further drug, prazepam, was also administered to TDF. (Prazepam is a benzodiazepine which is used in the treatment of anxiety disorders.) This drug can cause slurred speech when given in high doses. However, TDF did not receive high doses of this drug.

Unit 9.2 Client history and medical investigations

(1) TDF had neurosensory hearing loss with sloping configuration. What does 'sloping configuration' mean?

(2) TDF's history reveals two episodes of head injury. Is either episode a likely cause of TDF's speech problems? Provide support for your answer.

(3) A clinical ENT examination of TDF, which included the use of flexible laryngoscopy, revealed no structural laryngeal abnormality. In this case, is a diagnosis of psychogenic dysphonia warranted?

(4) TDF's drug regimen included prazepam. What motor speech disorder is caused by this drug when it is taken in high doses?

(5) The following conditions are associated with FAS. However, one of them is not consistent with FAS of sudden onset, such as TDF experienced. Which condition is it?
(a) cerebral infarction
(b) traumatic brain injury
(c) conversion disorder
(d) neurodegenerative disorder
(e) cerebral haemorrhage

Language and oral motor evaluation

The results of a number of language assessments indicated that TDF did not have aphasia. The maximum score was obtained on the Dutch version of the Token Test (Van Dongen et al., 1976) and on a Dutch aphasia battery, the Stichting Afasie Nederland test (Deelman et al., 1981). TDF had intact comprehension of written language on the Dutch version of the Aachener Aphasie test (Graetz et al., 1992). TDF could recite without error the days of the week, months of the year, and could count numbers from 1 to 20. Word and sentence repetition was also intact. There were no word-finding difficulties during confrontation naming or a word retrieval test. TDF could also read aloud without difficulty. Video-recorded speech samples revealed some grammatical difficulties. Some auxiliaries, articles and prepositions were omitted, giving TDF's speech a telegraphic quality at times. Grammatical errors, including the use of singular for plural nouns, incorrect verb conjugation and incorrect word order, were present but not pervasive. There was no paralysis, paresis or oral apraxia during oral motor testing.

Unit 9.3 Language and oral motor evaluation

(1) TDF displayed intact performance on the Dutch version of the Token Test. Which of the following linguistic abilities are assessed by means of this test?
  (a) sentence repetition
  (b) auditory verbal comprehension
  (c) semantic categorisation
  (d) irregular word reading
  (e) lexical retrieval

(2) Which aspect of TDF's language performance suggests that (a) phonological long-term memory and (b) phonological short-term memory are intact?

(3) TDF's expressive language displays similarities to a certain symptom of aphasia. What is that symptom?

(4) Does the absence of oral apraxia in TDF's case necessarily exclude apraxia of speech?

(5) Which *two* neurogenic communication disorders are effectively excluded on the basis of the assessments conducted in this unit?

Focus on articulation and prosody

Video-recorded speech samples of TDF were phonetically transcribed and analysed. The samples included recitation of automatic series, word and sentence repetition, reading aloud, confrontation naming, word retrieval, monologue and conversation. TDF displayed no struggle behaviour during speech. The use of auditory masking and delayed auditory feedback during reading aloud did not diminish TDF's accent. A number of articulatory errors were noted, some of which are shown below:

/maːntɑx/ for /maːndɑx/ ('Monday')
/ɑltɛi/ for /ɑltɛit/ ('always')
/di/ for /dri/ ('three')
/awaji/ for /hawaji/ ('Hawaii')
/spreːkə/ for /spreːkən/ ('talk')

Other, less common error patterns were the production of the trill sound /r/ with insufficient trill, and the substitution of /ɣ/ or /x/ for /h/. Several errors occurred on a single occasion: /ʃ/ for /s/, /j/ for /r/, /ŋ/ for /n/, /r/ for /n/, the addition of /ɣ/ in word-initial position, and vowel changes such as /ə/ for /ɔ/ and /ɛ/ for /u/.

TDF displayed a number of prosodic anomalies. Word and sentence stress were aberrant and TDF displayed a tendency towards scanning speech. Stress was placed on the wrong syllables in words. Incorrect word stress occurred on 18.1% of two-syllable words, 35.1% of three-syllable words, 62.5% of four-syllable words, and 30% of words of five or more syllables. The speech tasks with the highest level of incorrect word stress were confrontation naming (61.1%) and word retrieval (51.7%). Incorrect sentence stress occurred in 6.8% of the sentences produced. Stress was placed on the wrong word in these sentences.

Unit 9.4 Focus on articulation and prosody

(1) The use of auditory masking and delayed auditory feedback did not diminish TDF's accent. In what speech disorder do auditory masking and delayed auditory feedback have a facilitative effect?

(2) TDF did not display struggle behaviour during speech production. In what motor speech disorder is there considerable struggle behaviour?

(3) Characterise the type of articulatory errors that occur during the production of the following words: *Monday; always; three; Hawaii; talk.*

(4) TDF is described as displaying a tendency towards scanning speech. What is scanning speech?

(5) TDF sometimes placed stress on the wrong words in sentences. Describe *one* pragmatic or discourse function which may be disrupted as a result of the incorrect use of stress in sentences.

Focus on accent

The perception of a foreign accent in TDF was confirmed by a listener experiment. A total of 33 third-year students in speech-language pathology, none of whom were familiar with foreign accent syndrome, listened to a speech sample of 6 minutes 25 seconds' duration. The speech sample contained fragments of automatic speech, word repetition, reading aloud, monologue, conversation and confrontation naming. The subjects were asked to decide if the speech sample was from a native speaker of Dutch and, if not, which language was the speaker's mother tongue. All subjects expressed the view that TDF's speech was unusual, with 69.7% stating that Dutch was not the speaker's native language. Linguistic features which were judged to be significant in this assessment were prosodic abnormalities (improper word stress, scanning, strange intonation), grammatical errors (deletion of articles, improper word order, errors of pluralisation), use of short sentences and the occurrence of 'strange sounding' sounds.

Although nine different accents were perceived in total, most subjects indicated that TDF was likely to be a native of an Eastern European country. TDF's personal history revealed no source for this accent. TDF was born in the Dutch-speaking part of Belgium to parents who were native speakers of Dutch. TDF was raised in a Dutch-speaking environment and attended Dutch schools. She had never lived abroad, and had only ever undertaken short journeys, mainly to Spain. She studied French at introductory level at school. TDF's husband was also a native Dutch speaker.

TDF was seen one year later when she accompanied her husband to a neurological consultation. Her speech was nearly normal at this stage. Her foreign accent had gradually resolved within five months of onset. A second listener experiment was conducted with 13 students in speech-language pathology, none of whom had participated in the first listener experiment. Although all 13 subjects judged TDF's speech to be unusual, only one stated that TDF was not a native speaker of Dutch. However, this subject was unable to identify TDF's mother tongue.

Unit 9.5 Focus on accent

(1) The perception of a foreign accent in TDF's case was based on linguistic features as well as on prosodic and articulatory features. Which language level was particularly influential in this regard?

(2) Van Borsel et al. (2005) describe FAS as a listener-bound epiphenomenon, that is, as a product of the listener and not a syndrome in its own right. What feature of the listener experiments provides support for this view?

(3) The dominance of prosodic disturbances in FAS is somewhat problematic for the view that FAS is a speech disorder associated with left hemisphere damage. Explain why this is the case.

(4) Kuschmann and Lowit (2015) have argued that a combination of scripted and unscripted data is required in order to obtain a comprehensive picture of the intonation abilities of a speaker with FAS. How is this realised in the listener experiments in this study?

(5) TDF's foreign accent resolved spontaneously within five months of onset. What does this suggest about the origin of TDF's speech disorder?

Section B

Language disorders

Language in dementia

Language in other neurodegenerative disorders

Case study 10

Boy aged 7 years with developmental phonological disorder

Introduction

The following exercise is a case study of a 7-year-old boy ('Jarrod') with developmental phonological disorder who was studied by Holm and Crosbie (2006). Jarrod is a monolingual, Australian English-speaking child. His phonological impairment is severe in nature. The case study is presented in five sections: primer on developmental phonological disorder; client background; medical, developmental and educational history; speech, language and cognitive evaluation; and focus on articulation and phonology.

Primer on developmental phonological disorder

Developmental phonological disorder (DPD) is a type of speech sound disorder. The American Speech-Language-Hearing Association (2015) states that:

speech sound disorders which impact the way speech sounds (phonemes) function within a language are traditionally referred to as phonological disorders. They result from impairments in the phonological representation of speech sounds and speech segments – the system that generates and uses phonemes and phoneme rules and patterns within the context of spoken language. The process of perceiving and manipulating speech sounds is essential for developing these phonological representations.

The phonological impairment in DPD can compromise speaker intelligibility to varying degrees, with some children so severely affected that they are completely unintelligible to all but the most familiar listeners. DPD exists in the absence of a known aetiology. So while children with hearing loss, craniofacial anomalies (e.g. cleft lip and palate), neurological damage and intellectual disability in the presence of syndromes (e.g. Down's syndrome) can also have problems with the production of speech sounds, their speech sound disorder has an identifiable organic aetiology which differs from the functional or unknown aetiology of DPD.

The prevalence of DPD and speech sound disorders varies according to different investigations. In a study of 1,494 4-year-old Australian children, Eadie et al. (2015) reported that the prevalence of idiopathic speech sound disorder was 3.4%. McKinnon et al. (2007) obtained a lower prevalence of speech sound disorder, 1.06%, in a study of 10,425 primary school students in Australia. In the United States, Shriberg et al. (1999) estimated the prevalence of speech delay (a type of speech sound disorder) to be 3.8% in 1,328 monolingual English-speaking 6-year-old children. A consistent finding across all studies is that many more boys than girls develop speech sound disorders. Shriberg et al.

reported that speech delay was approximately 1.5 times more prevalent in the boys (4.5%) than in the girls (3.1%) in their study. Children with speech sound disorders often have comorbid conditions such as reading disability and language impairment. In their sample of 1,494 Australian children, Eadie et al. (2015) reported that comorbidity with speech sound disorder was 40.8% for language disorder and 20.8% for poor pre-literacy skills. Sices et al. (2007) reported that 53% of 125 children aged 3 to 6 years with moderate to severe speech sound disorder had comorbid language impairment.

Speech errors in children with speech sound disorders have been extensively investigated. McLeod et al. (2013) analysed the speech features of 143 children aged 4 to 5 years who were assessed following parent/teacher concern regarding their speech skills. A standard score below the normal range for the percentage of consonants correct on the Diagnostic Evaluation of Articulation and Phonology (Dodd et al., 2002) was obtained by 86.7% of children. Consonants produced incorrectly were consistent with the late eight phonemes. Common phonological patterns in these children were fricative simplification (82.5%), cluster simplification (49.0%) and cluster reduction (19.6%), gliding (41.3%) and palatal fronting (15.4%). Interdental lisps on /s/ and /z/ were produced by 39.9% of children, while dentalisation of other sibilants and lateral lisps were identified in 17.5% and 13.3% of children, respectively.

Unit 10.1 Primer on developmental phonological disorder

(1) Which of the following children has a speech sound disorder of idiopathic origin? Which speech sound disorder is related to a structural anomaly, and which is related to a neurological impairment?
   (a) A 6-year-old girl with a cleft palate says [jɛʔ] for 'yes'.
   (b) A 9-year-old child with Down's syndrome says [bæ] for 'black'.
   (c) A 5-year-old boy produces speech errors following the onset of seizures.
   (d) A 7-year-old girl with a history of otits media reduces consonant clusters.
   (e) A 7-year-old boy with normal development consistently replaces fricatives with stops.

(2) Why do you think the prevalence of speech sound disorders varies between studies?

(3) What does the comorbidity of speech sound disorder, language impairment and reading disability tell us about these disorders?

(4) In the children studied by McLeod et al. (2013), incorrect consonant production was largely consistent with the 'late eight phonemes'. What are these phonemes?

(5) McLeod et al. also identified several phonological patterns in the speech of the young children in their study. Three such patterns were cluster reduction, palatal fronting and gliding. Which of the following single-word productions corresponds to these patterns?
   (a) /pleɪn/ → [peɪn] 'plane'
   (b) /bɛd/ → [bɛ] 'bed'
   (c) /lɛg/ → [jɛg] 'leg'
   (d) /bənana/ → [nana] 'banana'
   (e) /ʃɪp/ → [sɪp] 'ship'

Client background

Jarrod was born in New Zealand but moved to Australia at 2 years of age. He lives with his mother and 10-year-old sister. He sees his father regularly. His mother has a partner, with whom Jarrod does not have a close relationship. Jarrod has regular contact with extended family members. English is the only language spoken at home. Jarrod's mother works part-time as a bookkeeper, and his father is a full-time builder. Jarrod's father had a speech disorder as a child, and attended speech therapy. He still produces some speech errors. His maternal grandfather has a history of dyslexia. Jarrod's sister has bilateral integration problems, in that she struggles to integrate information from the left and right side of the brain.

Jarrod is described by his mother as being a happy, healthy boy who has a good sense of humour. His mother reports him as enjoying a number of activities – playing with his friends and on the computer, watching television and movies. She believes his speech problems have held him back but that he has still been able to forge friendships. For example, he plays with other children in the neighbourhood, and attends other children's parties. Jarrod's teacher also acknowledges that he has friends and that he participates happily in classroom activities. However, she says that he does not have particularly good social interactions. This is reflected in a report written by his teacher about an Intensive Language Class that Jarrod attends. Jarrod was described as having 'poor social skills as a result of poor communication skills'. The report also noted that Jarrod was aware of his communication problems and was sensitive about them. Jarrod has been teased by other children about his speech difficulties.

Within a known conversational context, Jarrod's mother and teacher could usually understand him. However, without context he was difficult to understand, and unfamiliar listeners, his mother reported, did not understand him. Jarrod did not get frustrated when he was not understood. He readily repeated himself or reformulated his message and would use gesture and drawings to help understanding. Despite his problems, he was not inhibited about communicating. For example, he was willing to address the school at assembly, even though he was not understood, and he answered questions in class and participated in group discussions.

Unit 10.2 Client background

(1) Jarrod's family background is particularly significant. What is the significance of his background?

(2) On the basis of maternal report, what *two* behaviours set Jarrod apart from the behavioural phenotype of autism spectrum disorder?

(3) Unlike Jarrod's mother, the teacher reports that Jarrod has some problems with social skills and social interaction. How do Jarrod's problems in this area differ from the social difficulties in autism spectrum disorder?

(4) What feature suggests that Jarrod's phonological disorder is particularly severe?

(5) Which *two* non-verbal strategies has Jarrod developed in order to compensate for his poor speech skills? What metalinguistic device does Jarrod use to aid listener understanding?

Medical, developmental and educational history

Jarrod's mother had an uneventful pregnancy and labour. Jarrod was born full-term and had an average birth weight. With the exception of 'clicky' hips, no other medical condition was identified at birth. Jarrod was breastfed for 6 months, and had no feeding difficulties. His gross motor development milestones were normally achieved. However, an occupational therapy assessment revealed some fine motor difficulties, although his writing abilities were good for his age. At 15 months, Jarrod was diagnosed with asthma, for which he has been using a Ventolin and Flexotide nebuliser. He has been hospitalised twice for the treatment of asthma. Jarrod has also been diagnosed with attention deficit hyperactivity disorder (ADHD) and has been taking Ritalin for approximately two months. Jarrod's mother and teacher report an improvement in his attention with this medication. At 2 and 4 years of age, Jarrod had grommets inserted for the treatment of otitis media. At 4;1 years, his hearing was tested and was judged to be adequate for the development of speech and language. Jarrod's mother and teacher have not reported any ongoing hearing difficulties.

Jarrod attended preschool. During the year in which he turned five, he was enrolled in a Special Education Development Unit. He attended a mainstream class the following year. When he was assessed for this study, he was enrolled in an Intensive Language Class of children with identified communication problems. The teacher of this class prepared a report on Jarrod at the end of the school year. Her comments identified several areas in which Jarrod had improved: organisational skills; self-esteem; attention; and fine motor skills. Jarrod had also developed a good understanding of the role of phonics and could recognise phonic sounds in isolation. He displayed a fair understanding of mathematical processes and was reported to enjoy mathematical activities. However, he had significant difficulties with reading and displayed reversal problems in both letters and numbers. The teacher remarked that Jarrod had a good sense of humour, enjoyed coming to school and liked narrative activities (listening to stories and engaging in retell).

Unit 10.3 Medical, developmental and educational history

(1) What evidence is there in the developmental period that Jarrod has normal oromotor control?

(2) Jarrod was diagnosed with attention deficit hyperactivity disorder (ADHD). The comorbidity between ADHD and speech sound disorder has been examined in a number of studies including McGrath et al. (2008) and Lewis et al. (2012). What have these studies revealed about the comorbidity of these disorders?

(3) Jarrod had grommets inserted on two occasions to treat otitis media. Describe what grommets are and explain how they are used to treat this middle ear pathology.

(4) Parental and educational reports in units 10.2 and 10.3 give us an insight into the impact of Jarrod's phonological disorder. The following statements capture different aspects of this impact. Use information in these units to provide support for these statements.

  (i) Jarrod's phonological disorder has not resulted in restrictions of his activities or participation.

  (ii) Jarrod's phonological disorder has placed him at risk of social devaluation.

(iii) Jarrod's phonological disorder has had adverse consequences for his psychological well-being.

(5) Jarrod's teacher reported that he had significant reading difficulties. Is this typical of children with speech sound disorder?

Speech, language and cognitive evaluation

Jarrod was extensively evaluated. A wide range of assessments was used: seven speech assessments; an oromotor assessment; three psycholinguistic assessment tasks; three phonemic awareness assessments; an assessment of activity and participation; and an assessment of non-verbal cognitive abilities. Several of these assessments and their results are described below.

Speech assessments

Diagnostic Evaluation of Articulation and Phonology (DEAP: Dodd et al., 2002): The DEAP is a standardised assessment which contains Australian normative data. Several subtests of the DEAP were administered including an articulation assessment, a phonology assessment, connected speech picture description, and an inconsistency assessment. An additional word list was also used to supplement the items in the DEAP. The purpose of this list was to provide extra word shapes, stress patterns and consonant clusters, among other features. On the DEAP articulation assessment, Jarrod produced most consonants word initially. Three others /v, ∫, ʧ/ appeared either medially or finally. /ʤ/ was produced as an error, while /z, ʒ/ were not produced at all. All vowels were present except for /ɪə/. There were a number of non-Australian-English sounds, and some distortion of consonants and vowels. On the DEAP phonology test, Jarrod had 44% phonemes correct. On the DEAP inconsistency assessment, Jarrod named 25 pictures on three occasions, producing 22 of the words (88%) differently on at least two of these occasions.

Hodson Assessment of Phonological Patterns – 3rd edn (HAPP-3; Hodson, 2004): The HAPP-3 is an American standardised test that is norm-referenced and criterion-referenced. It is used to elicit spontaneous productions of 50 target words for the Comprehensive Phonological Evaluation. Jarrod's expressive phonology performance on the HAPP-3 was below the 1st percentile. A 40% cut-off on the HAPP-3 is used to determine the phonological patterns which need to be considered first. This cut-off was achieved for five phonological deviations: omissions of consonants in sequences (92%); omissions of postvocalic singletons (69%); liquid deficiencies (89%); strident deficiencies (98%); and velar deficiencies (91%). The most prevalent substitution strategies were gliding and glottal stop replacement/insertion. Stopping and prevocalic voicing were the next most frequently occurring strategies. Fronting was also present as were some unusual substitutions of nasals for each other.

Systemic Phonological Protocol (SPP; Williams, 2003): The SPP assesses all English consonants using single-word naming of black-and-white drawings on cards. The assessment recommends the use of a detailed elicitation cueing hierarchy which could not be implemented in the present case. Instead, a reduced number of words was elicited through forced choice (i.e. 'Is it X or Y?').

Language assessment

Clinical Evaluation of Language Fundamentals-4 (CELF-4; Semel et al., 2003): Jarrod achieved a Core Language Score of 111 (average 85–115). His Receptive and Expressive Language Scores were 103 and 112, respectively. Jarrod obtained a Language Content Score of 94 and a Language Structure Score of 111. These scores are all within the average range.

Oromotor assessments

Verbal Motor Production Assessment for Children (VMPAC; Hayden and Square, 1999): The VMPAC is used to assess the motor speech system at rest, and during vegetative, volitional non-speech and speech tasks. The three main areas of the test are global motor control, focal oromotor control and sequencing. This assessment revealed that Jarrod's global motor control was age appropriate. However, he performed below the 5th percentile for neuromuscular integrity. Difficulties included jaw control, jaw–lip movement and tongue control.

Psycholinguistic assessments

Children's Test of Nonword Repetition (CNRep; Gathercole and Baddeley, 1996): Jarrod was required to repeat single non-words which were played to him on an audio cassette. He performed very poorly on this assessment.

Auditory Lexical Discrimination Tests (ALDT; Locke, 1980): Jarrod viewed 12 pictures in turn and was asked to decide if two or three spoken stimuli had been said correctly.

Same-Different Test (SDT; Bridgemann and Snowling, 1988): Jarrod's auditory discrimination was tested by presenting him with a pair of spoken words or non-words. He had to indicate if they were the same or different. When pairs of words or non-words differed by a single feature (e.g. [jeɪs]/[jeɪt]), Jarrod made few errors. However, he had difficulty with this task when pairs differed by a sequence of sounds (e.g. [vʌts]/[vʌst]).

Phonemic awareness assessments

Preschool Inventory of Phonological Awareness (PIPA; Dodd et al., 2000): PIPA is a standardised assessment of early phonological awareness development. Jarrod completed three subtests of PIPA: rhyme awareness; phoneme isolation; and letter knowledge. Jarrod obtained a standard score of 3 on rhyme awareness and phoneme isolation, which is a poor performance on tasks that are usually mastered in the preschool years.

Queensland University Inventory of Literacy (QUIL; Dodd et al., 1996): QUIL is an Australian standardised assessment of phonological awareness. Jarrod completed the following subtests: non-word spelling; non-word reading; syllable segmentation; spoken rhyme recognition; and phoneme manipulation. Jarrod was able to segment syllables. However, he performed at the bottom of the normal range on rhyme recognition, and did not score on non-word reading and spelling and on phoneme manipulation.

Sutherland Phonological Awareness Test-Revised (SPAT-R; Neilson, 2003): The SPAT-R is a standardised test that provides a diagnostic overview of phonological awareness skills for early literacy development. Jarrod scored 18 on the SPAT-R, when the average score range for his age is 33 to 45.

Non-verbal cognitive abilities

Wechsler Intelligence Scale for Children-IV (WISC-IV; Wechsler, 2003): Jarrod was assessed on the WISC-IV at 7;0 years of age. He achieved a Verbal Comprehension Index of 81 (10th percentile) and a Perceptual Reasoning Index of 111 (76th percentile).

Unit 10.4 Speech, language and cognitive evaluation

(1) The HAPP-3 was used to establish the consonant substitution strategies in Jarrod's speech. For each of the following productions, indicate which substitutions have occurred:
  (a) 'leaf' [jeɪ]
  (b) 'fork' [ɔ]
  (c) 'snake' [meɪʔ]
  (d) 'black' [bwæʔ]
  (e) 'thumb' [θʌŋ]

(2) The data generated by SPP was used to perform a relational analysis in which Jarrod's error productions for adult target sounds were mapped in terms of phoneme collapses. Two phoneme collapses were found to characterise Jarrod's organisation of his word-final sound system: Jarrod deleted all consonants word-finally or glottalised voiceless stops. The following sets contain some of Jarrod's single-word productions. Which set exemplifies these particular phoneme collapses?
  (a) [ɟɪŋ] 'thing'; [daɪdʌ] 'tiger'; [wɒʔ] 'watch'; [jɛç] 'yes'
  (b) [dɛdoʊ] 'yellow'; [dɜʔ] 'skirt'; [baɪdʌ] 'spider'; [wɪm] 'swim'
  (c) [ɟeɪ] 'teeth'; [jæm] 'lamb'; [bɒh] 'box'; [bɔɪ] 'boy'
  (d) [buʔ] 'book'; [jeɪ] 'cheese'; [boʊʔ] 'boat'; [jæʊ] 'clown'
  (e) [fɔ] 'four'; [hoʊm] 'home'; [ɟɪʔden] 'kitchen'; [ʔʌɪç] 'ice'

(3) Jarrod performed very poorly on non-word repetition tasks in the CNRep. What phonological processing ability does this finding suggest is impaired in Jarrod?

(4) In unit 10.3, Jarrod was reported to have significant difficulties with reading. Which assessment finding explains these difficulties?

(5) Respond with *true* or *false* to each of the following statements:
  (a) Jarrod's speech difficulties are related to intellectual disability.
  (b) An oromotor element to Jarrod's speech disorder cannot be excluded.
  (c) Jarrod's speech disorder displays inconsistency.
  (d) Jarrod has a language disorder as well as a speech disorder.
  (e) Jarrod's language scores are consistent with his non-verbal cognitive abilities.

Focus on articulation and phonology

Jarrod's single-word productions on the articulation subtest of the Diagnostic Evaluation of Articulation and Phonology (Dodd et al., 2002) underwent phonetic transcription. The phonemic targets are for the pronunciation of Australian English. Where symbols have superscript, it represents an impression that a sound or sound sequence is either epenthetic or a transition between sounds. Short extracts of Jarrod's connected speech are transcribed below the table.

Word	Phonemic target	Client production
pig	/pɪg/	[beɪ]
bird	/bɜd/	[bɜː]
teeth	/tiθ/	[dᵊi]
door	/dɔ/	[dɔ]
car	/ka/	[pʰa]
girl	/gɜl/	[gɜʊ]
moon	/mun/	[nəüʔɪ]
knife	/naɪf/	[naɪh]
fish	/fɪʃ/	goldfish [doʊbe̞ə̞]
van	/væn/	[beɪ̃n]
thumb	/θʌm/	[θʌɲᵈ]
teddy	/tedi/	[dedi]
sock	/sɒk/	[jːɒk]
zebra	/zebrə/	[jebwʌː] [jegbʌː]
sheep	/ʃip/	[ʃˑʲip]
chair	/ʧeə/	[jeə]
jam	/ʤæm/	[ʤæm]
legs	/legz/	[jeɡ̞]
ring	/rɪŋ/	[ɹɪ̃ŋ]
watch	/wɒʧ/	[mbwɒʔ]
yellow	/jeloʊ/	[jædoʊ̞]
house	/haʊs/	[hæʊ]
five	/faɪv/	[baɪ]
foot	/fʊt/	[b̞ɒʔ]
crab	/kræb/	[b̞b̞wa̰]
boy	/bɔɪ/	[bɔɪ̞]
orange	/ɒrɪnʤ/	[ɒwẽŋ]
snake	/sneɪk/	[fneɪʔ]
television	/teləvɪʒən/	[tstʌʔædbedẽ̞ɲ̞]
ear	/ɪə/	[ʔe̞əh]

Connected speech during articulation test

'No I didn't say "bear". I said "pig"' [nɒ aɪ dɪʔi jeɪ. be̞ ʌɪ̞jed. dɛ̞ː]
'that one' [ðæʔ wʌn]
'I don't know' [ʔaɪ dɔ̃ʔ noʊ]
'do (an/um?) clean around' [dy. ʌ̃n. ɹɪ̃ŋ gʌwæ̃ð]

Unit 10.5 Focus on articulation and phonology

(1) Give *one* example of each of the following phonological processes in Jarrod's single-word productions. Which of these processes affects syllable structure? Which of these processes are normally suppressed by 7 years of age?
  (a) prevocalic voicing
  (b) stopping of /v/
  (c) gliding
  (d) fronting
  (e) final consonant deletion

(2) Give *one* example of each of the following features in Jarrod's single-word productions:
  (a) Jarrod produces nasalised vowels.
  (b) Jarrod produces vowels with creaky voice.
  (c) Jarrod extends phonemes beyond their normal duration.
  (d) Jarrod substitutes oral plosives with glottal stops.
  (e) Jarrod uses gliding in word-medial position.

(3) On some occasions Jarrod reduces consonant clusters, while on other occasions he deletes them altogether. Give *one* example of each pattern in the above data.

(4) Respond with *true* or *false* to each of the following statements:
  (a) Weak syllable deletion is a feature of Jarrod's phonology.
  (b) Jarrod substitutes alveolar fricatives with [j] in word-initial position.
  (c) Final consonant deletion affects both plosives and fricatives.
  (d) Velar assimilation is a feature of Jarrod's phonology.
  (e) Jarrod does not produce voiced and voiceless affricates.

(5) State *two* phonological processes in connected speech which are also found in Jarrod's single-word productions. Give *one* example of each process in connected speech. What is noteworthy about Jarrod's production of the word 'pig' in both these contexts?

Case study 11

Portuguese-speaking girl aged 7 years with phonological disorder

Introduction

The following exercise is a case study of a 7-year-old girl ('D') with phonological disorder who was studied by Yavaş and Hernandorena (1991). D is a monolingual, Portuguese-speaking child who comes from the city of Pelotas in the southern state of Rio Grande do Sul in Brazil. The case study is presented in five sections: primer on phonological disorder in languages other than English; client history; speech evaluation; focus on systematic sound preference; and assessment issues.

Primer on phonological disorder in languages other than English

The majority of research which has been conducted into phonological disorder has been based on English-speaking children. It is important, however, to consider if features of phonological disorder in English are also found in children who speak other languages. This has implications not only for theories of language acquisition, but also for the assessment and treatment of children with phonological disorders. Recently, investigators have begun to examine phonological disorder in a range of European and non-European languages including Spanish (Goldstein et al., 2004), French (Brosseau-Lapré and Rvachew, 2014), German (Fox and Dodd, 2001), Putonghua (Modern Standard Chinese) (Hua and Dodd, 2000), Arabic (Bader, 2009), Hebrew (Ben-David et al., 2010) and Turkish (Topbaş, 2006). Some of these investigations have revealed that features of phonological disorder in English are also found in other languages. For example, Hua and Dodd (2000) examined the phonological systems of 33 Putonghua-speaking children with speech disorder. These children displayed the characteristics of phonologically disordered children who speak other languages, such as persisting delayed processes, unusual error patterns, variability, restricted phonetic or phonemic inventory, and systematic sound or syllable preference.

Other investigations have highlighted language-specific features of phonological disorder. Brosseau-Lapré and Rvachew (2014) calculated feature-match ratios for the production of target consonants in English- and French-speaking children with phonological disorder. They found that French-speaking children had significantly lower match ratios for the sound class features [+ consonantal], [+ sonorant] and [+ voice]. French-speaking children produced more syllable structure errors, followed by segment errors and a few distortion errors, while English-speaking children made more segment than syllable structure and distortion errors. Brosseau-Lapré and Rvachew concluded that the results 'highlight the need to use test instruments with French-speaking children that reflect the phonological characteristics of French at multiple levels of the phonological hierarchy' (98). Topbaş (2006) examined the phonological systems of 70 phonologically disordered, Turkish-speaking children aged 4;0 to 8;0 years. They found that while the stopping of affricates is a common developmental pattern in English, the stopping of fricatives, especially /s/ and /z/, was the more common developmental pattern in Turkish. This reflects the fact that affricates are acquired earlier than fricatives in Turkish. Topbaş stated that 'it can be inferred that the most frequent error patterns are dependent on the phonological structure of the language. Although universal tendencies exist, the ambient language effect is apparent in all languages' (520).

Unit 11.1 Primer on phonological disorder in languages other than English

(1) As well as examining Turkish-speaking children with phonological disorder, Topbaş (2006) undertook a normative study of phonology in 665 Turkish-speaking children aged 1;3 to 8;0 years. This study revealed the following order of phonological acquisition in these children: stops > nasals > affricates > glides/liquids > fricatives > flap. Describe *one* respect in which this order conforms to the universal pattern of acquisition and *one* respect in which it differs from this pattern.

(2) The following single-word productions were recorded by Hua and Dodd (2000) in a study of 33 Putonghua-speaking children with speech disorder. What type of phonological process does each production exemplify?
   (a) /ɕiɛ/ [tiɛ] 'shoe'
   (b) /tsʰae/ [tae] 'vegetable'
   (c) /pʰiŋ kuo/ [pʰiŋ puo] 'apple'
   (d) /tʂʰuaŋ/ [tsʰuɑ] 'bed'
   (e) /ɕiɛ/ [tɕiɛ] 'shoe'

(3) Brosseau-Lapré and Rvachew (2014) found that French-speaking children with phonological disorder produced more syllable structure errors than segment errors, while the opposite pattern obtained in English-speaking children with phonological disorder. Which of the following phonological processes affects syllable structure?
   (a) fronting
   (b) cluster reduction
   (c) weak syllable deletion
   (d) gliding
   (e) final consonant deletion

(4) In a study of the phonological systems of Turkish-speaking children, Topbaş (2006) found that most phonological processes were suppressed between 3;6 and 4;0 years. Reduplication, prevocalic voicing and fronting were the earliest processes to be suppressed, while liquid deviation and cluster reduction were still in evidence after four years. How does this compare to English?

(5) Which of the studies examined in this unit uses distinctive features to analyse the speech of children with phonological disorder?

Client history

D is a 7-year-old, Portuguese-speaking, Brazilian girl. She is monolingual. Her physical development was normal. She has a normally functioning oral mechanism and normal hearing. There is no evidence of neurological problems relevant to speech production. D is a very extroverted and cooperative child.

Unit 11.2 Client history

(1) Why is it important for a speech-language pathologist to know if D is monolingual or bilingual?

(2) D's physical development was normal. Name *three* motor milestones that fall within an assessment of physical development.

(3) D had a normally functioning oral mechanism. Name *one* structural anomaly that this description may be taken to exclude.

(4) D did not exhibit neurological problems relevant to speech production. Also, her oral mechanism functioned normally. What *two* motor speech disorders are effectively excluded in D's case?

(5) D was described as being very extroverted and cooperative. Which of the following conditions is excluded by this description?
    (a) autism spectrum disorder
    (b) intellectual disability
    (c) attention deficit hyperactivity disorder
    (d) developmental dyslexia
    (e) specific language impairment

Speech evaluation

D's speech was extensively evaluated. She produced spontaneous descriptions of thematic pictures. From these descriptions, a sample of 210 words was obtained for analysis. This sample did not contain imitated responses. Some of D's single-word productions are shown below along with their phonemic norms.

Portuguese	English	Phonemic norm	Client production
1			
caixa	box	[káyʃa]	[tátʃa]
2			
igreja	church	[igréʒa]	[idédʒa]
3			
queixo	chin	[kéʃu]	[tétʃu]
4			
acho	I think	[áʃu]	[átʃu]

(cont.)

Portuguese	English	Phonemic norm	Client production
5			
relógio	clock	[ʀelóʒyu]	[ʀelóʤu]
6			
azulejo	tile	[azúleʒu]	[atúleʤu]
7			
bicho	animal	[bíʃu]	[bíʧu]
8			
chave	key	[ʃávi]	[táʧĩ]
9			
chapeu	hat	[ʃapɛ́w]	[tapɛ́w]
10			
janela	window	[ʒanɛ́la]	[tanɛ́la]
11			
ajuda	help	[aʒúda]	[atúda]
12			
marchar	to march	[marʃár]	[matá]
13			
achei	I found	[aʃéy]	[atéy]
14			
cachorro	dog	[kaʃóʀu]	[tatóʀu]
15			
guarda-chuva	umbrella	[guardaʃúva]	[dadatúta]
16			
gusto	I like	[gɔ́stu]	[dɔ́tu]
17			
fogão	oven	[fugãw]	[tudãw]
18			
banco	bank	[bãnku]	[bãntu]
19			
querido	dear	[kirídu]	[tirídu]
20			
aqui	here	[akí]	[atí]
21			
guizado	ground beef	[gizádu]	[didádu]

Unit 11.3 Speech evaluation

(1) Several of D's single-word productions are shown below. For each production, characterise the simplification in terms of one or more phonological processes:

(a) [bãnku] → [bãntu] 'bank'

(b) [ʃávi] → [táʧĩ] 'key'

(c) [ʃapɛ́w] → [tapɛ́w] 'hat'

    (d) [gizádu] → [didádu] 'ground beef'
    (e) [bíʃu] → [bíʧu] 'animal'

(2) Give *one* example of each of the following combinations of phonological processes in D's single-word productions:
    (a) stopping and fronting
    (b) fronting, cluster reduction and affrication
    (c) stopping and devoicing
    (d) stopping, devoicing and affrication
    (e) fronting, stopping and devoicing

(3) Give *one* example of a syllable simplification process in the above data.

(4) Give *one* example of a vowel simplification in the above data.

(5) Respond with *true* or *false* to each of the following statements:
    (a) D realises all nasalised vowels in her productions.
    (b) D engages in initial consonant deletion.
    (c) D engages in fronting in word-initial and word-medial positions.
    (d) D engages in cluster reduction in word-initial position.
    (e) D engages in stopping in word-initial, word-medial and word-final positions.

Focus on systematic sound preference

A different interpretation of the substitutions examined in the above data is that D is making use of a systematic sound preference. Clinical phonologists have long considered systematic sound preference to be evidence of disordered phonology (e.g. Grunwell, 1985). Yavaş and Hernandorena (1991) stated that '[a] case of systematic sound preference is in evidence when a group of sounds with the same manner of articulation is represented by one or two sounds in the production of the child' (79). Fricatives are the focus of D's systematic sound preference. In percentage terms, D replaced 89.3% of fricatives with [t] and [d]. She replaced the remaining 10.7% of fricatives, all /ʃ/ and /ʒ/ targets, with the affricates [ʧ, ʤ], respectively. This level of fricative substitution, Yavaş and Hernandorena argue, well exceeds the minimum proposed by Weiner (1981) of 70% occurrence of all the possibilities where one or two sounds could replace a class of sounds. D's substitutions thus qualify as a systematic sound preference.

Unit 11.4 Focus on systematic sound preference

(1) How are /ʃ/ and /ʒ/ realised by D in the single-word productions in (1) to (7) in unit 11.3? What is noteworthy about the context in which these realisations occur?

(2) Are the realisations of /ʃ/ and /ʒ/, which were identified in response to question (1), maintained in the single-word productions in (8) to (10)? If not, how are these sounds realised in these productions? What is noteworthy about the context of the realisations in (8) to (10)?

(3) In response to question (1), you may have decided that D is realising /ʃ/ and /ʒ/ as [ʧ] and [ʤ], respectively, in syllable initial within word position. Is this pattern of

realisation maintained in the productions in (11) to (15)? If not, explain how /ʃ/ and /ʒ/ are differently realised in these productions.

(4) Why do you think /ʃ/ and /ʒ/ are differently realised in (11) to (15)? As a clue to help you, you should examine the context in which these realisations occur. Now try to generate a general rule that captures the realisations of /ʃ/ and /ʒ/ across all the productions in (1) to (15).

(5) A different type of sound substitution process is present in the single-word productions in (16) to (21). What is the name of this process? This process appears to be entirely separate from the process at work in (1) to (15). One piece of evidence which suggests that this is the case is that where the realisations of /ʃ/ and /ʒ/ did not observe the voicing contrast (i.e. /ʒ/ was realised as [t] on occasion), a voicing contrast is consistently observed in (16) to (21). What other feature of (19) to (21) in particular suggests that the process at work in these single-word productions is quite separate from D's systematic sound preference?

Assessment issues

D's systematic sound preference was apparent because Yavaş and Hernandorena undertook a detailed phonological analysis of her speech. In English, such an analysis is generally performed through the use of standardised phonological assessments such as the Diagnostic Evaluation of Articulation and Phonology (DEAP; Dodd et al., 2006) and the Hodson Assessment of Phonological Patterns – 3rd edn (HAPP-3; Hodson, 2004). These assessments permit speech-language pathologists to examine target sounds in all word positions and to compare the performance of a child to his or her peers. Their reliability and validity make them the mainstay of phonological assessment. Their ease of clinical administration has also guaranteed these assessments a place in the SLP's toolkit – the DEAP, for example, is individually administered and involves a 5-minute Diagnostic Screen and up to four specific assessments. The results of these assessments can be used to plan phonological intervention in child clients. For example, the HAPP-3 manual includes a chapter about phonological intervention principles and procedures. These standardised phonological assessments may be supplemented by informal techniques, such as the recording and transcription of spontaneous speech during conversation or narrative production tasks.

The ready availability of phonological assessments in English is very far removed from the situation found in other languages. In languages other than English there is a dearth of such assessments. One reason for this lack of assessment development is the limited availability of phonological norms in other languages. Da Silva et al. (2012) state that '[f]or many languages there is still a lack of norms and adequate assessments to assess phonological development in children suspected of having a disorder' (249). This situation has adverse implications not only for the phonological assessment of monolingual speakers of other languages with phonological disorder, but also for the assessment of bilingual and multilingual speakers with speech sound disorder. In a survey of 333 speech-language pathologists who worked with children with speech sound disorder, Skahan et al. (2007) reported that most respondents used English-only standardised tests when evaluating non-native English speakers. In a survey of 231 Australian speech-language pathologists, McLeod and Baker (2014) found that when assessing multilingual children with speech sound disorder, informal assessment procedures and English-only tests were commonly used, with SLPs relying on family members or interpreters to assist. Normative data on the phonologies of languages other than English, including Swahili (Gangji et al., 2015) and Brazilian Portuguese (da Silva et al., 2012), are beginning to emerge. The result has been the recent standardisation of tests for the assessment of phonology in a number of languages (e.g. Lousada et al. (2012) for European Portuguese).

Unit 11.5 Assessment issues

(1) Was a formal or informal assessment procedure used to assess D's phonology? What factor do you think motivated this choice of assessment procedure?

(2) The DEAP and HAPP-3 are reliable, valid, norm-referenced assessments of phonology. What do the terms 'reliable', 'valid' and 'norm-referenced' mean in this context?

(3) McLeod and Baker (2014) found that speech-language pathologists made extensive use of informal assessment procedures when assessing multilingual children with speech sound disorder. Describe *two* disadvantages in using these procedures.

(4) Describe *one* difficulty which speech-language pathologists might encounter when using a phonological assessment developed for English with children who are native speakers of other languages.

(5) Goldstein (2007) examined the phonological skills of Puerto Rican and Mexican Spanish-speaking children with phonological disorders. Why are studies of this type important in terms of assessment development?

Case study 12

Boy aged 4;8 years with specific language impairment

Introduction

The following exercise is a case study of a boy ('DF') with specific language impairment who was studied by Tompkins and Farrar (2011). DF was recruited from a speech and hearing centre preschool programme in Florida which admitted children who qualified for language services. The case study is presented in five sections: primer on specific language impairment; client history and cognitive-linguistic profile; focus on narrative production; focus on maternal language in SLI; and impact and outcomes in SLI.

Primer on specific language impairment

Specific language impairment (SLI) is a specific developmental disorder. As its name suggests, the disorder is *specific* to language, with other domains of development (motor, cognitive, etc.) proceeding along normal lines. (SLI is to be distinguished from a *pervasive* developmental disorder such as autism spectrum disorder in which several domains of development are compromised.) Children with SLI have an impairment of language in the absence of conditions that are normally associated with language disorders. These conditions include hearing loss, intellectual disability, sensory impairments, neurological impairment and emotional disturbance. Notwithstanding the absence of these conditions, children with SLI present with a severe disorder of language which can persist into adulthood, and which has serious consequences for the academic achievement, and social and occupational functioning of affected individuals (Whitehouse et al., 2009a, 2009b).

The prevalence of SLI has been investigated in several studies. There has been considerable variation in the figures reported by investigators. Tomblin et al. (1997) estimated the prevalence of SLI in a population of monolingual English-speaking kindergarten children in the United States to be 7.4%. A much lower prevalence figure of less than 1% was reported by Hannus et al. (2009) in a study of SLI in Finnish children aged 0 to 6 years. Reilly et al. (2010) reported that 251 (17.2%) of 1,462 4-year-old Australian children met criteria for SLI. The prevalence of SLI is higher in boys than in girls and in certain special populations. Tomblin et al. reported the prevalence of SLI in the boys and girls in their study to be 8% and 6%, respectively. In a study of 147 pupils attending language resource units, Archibald and Gathercole (2006) reported the prevalence of SLI to be 13%, with receptive–expressive SLI and expressive-only SLI accounting for 13% and 10% of the sample, respectively.

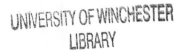

Language in SLI can be disrupted at several levels including phonology, morphology, syntax and semantics. Aguilar-Mediavilla et al. (2002) examined the phonology of 3-year-old children with SLI. They found that these children used more syllabic and non-syllabic cluster reduction and initial and final consonant deletions than age controls. Children with SLI also deleted medial consonants significantly more often than age controls and deleted unstressed syllables in initial position significantly more than control subjects. Grammatical morphology is an area of difficulty for children with SLI, with regular past tense *–ed*, regular third-person singular *–s* and copula/auxiliary 'be' forms used less frequently by these children than by control subjects. Complex syntax such as the comprehension and production of relative clauses and complement clauses is also impaired. (The reader is referred to Ellis Weismer (2014) for further discussion of grammatical morphology and complex syntax in SLI.) Lexical semantic deficits are also evident in SLI. Children with SLI produce more naming errors than normally developing children (McGregor et al., 2002), and have weak receptive vocabulary as measured by word–picture matching (Laws et al., 2015). Pragmatic deficits have also been reported in SLI (see Cummings (2009, 2014a, 2014b) for discussion). When these deficits are severe or the predominant language deficit, children are diagnosed with a subtype of SLI called pragmatic language impairment.

Unit 12.1 Primer on specific language impairment

(1) SLI has been described as a 'diagnosis by exclusion'. Explain what this expression means.

(2) State *one* factor which may account for the variation in prevalence of SLI across different studies.

(3) The following utterances were produced by two children with SLI who were studied by Moore (2001). Each child is aged 4;2 years. Describe *two* respects in which Child B's utterance is grammatically more sophisticated than Child A's utterance, notwithstanding the similarity in these children's chronological ages:
Child A: 'And her painting now'.
Child B: 'He's marrying my dad'.

(4) The following utterances were produced by children with expressive SLI who were studied by Moore (2001). For each utterance, indicate the syntactic error that the child has made. One grammatical morpheme is used consistently by these children. What morpheme is it?
(a) 'Her's painting a flower'.
(b) 'He eating'.
(c) 'She building block'.
(d) 'Why he fall in the car?'.
(e) 'Yeah, he sleeping right here'.

(5) Respond with *true* or *false* to each of the following statements:
(a) Pragmatic deficits in SLI are always secondary to structural language deficits.
(b) Phonology is often the only deviant aspect of language in SLI.
(c) Children with SLI have reduced receptive and expressive vocabularies.
(d) Children with SLI may have primary pragmatic impairments.
(e) Lexical acquisition is relatively unimpaired in children with SLI.

Client history and cognitive-linguistic profile

Before DF was recruited to the study, his file was reviewed. DF came from an English-speaking, middle-class family. His mother had 16 years of education. DF had passed hearing screenings and had no previous medical conditions that might account for his language problems.

DF's language skills were assessed using the Structured Photographic Expressive Language Test 3 (SPELT-3; Dawson et al., 2003). DF achieved a score of 72 on this assessment, which placed him below the age of four according to the SPELT age equivalency scores. DF's receptive vocabulary was assessed using the Peabody Picture Vocabulary Test – 3rd edn (PPVT-3; Dunn and Dunn, 1997). His score on the PPVT-3 was in the normal range. The Leiter International Performance Scale-Revised (Roid et al., 2003) was used to assess DF's non-verbal cognitive ability. This assessment measures visualisation, reasoning, memory and attention. DF scored within normal limits on the Leiter-R.

Unit 12.2 Client history and cognitive-linguistic profile

(1) Name *two* conditions which can be excluded as a cause of DF's language problems.

(2) DF's history revealed that he came from a middle-class family and that his mother had 16 years of education. What is the significance of socioeconomic status and maternal education in this case?

(3) The SPELT-3 is designed to elicit specific morphological and syntactic structures. Some of these structures are listed below. For each structure, indicate whether it relates to morphology or syntax. Why is the SPELT-3 particularly suited to an assessment of children with SLI?
  (a) present progressive
  (b) conjoined sentence
  (c) wh-question
  (d) regular and irregular past
  (e) relative clause

(4) DF's score on the PPVT-3 was in the normal range. How might this finding be explained?

(5) Although DF's non-verbal cognitive ability is within normal limits, there is increasing evidence that children with SLI have cognitive limitations that may not be tapped by IQ tests. Name *one* such limitation.

Focus on narrative production

DF and his mother were recorded undertaking two narrative production tasks. During an autobiographical memory narrative task (narrative 1), DF's mother encouraged him to narrate events that had occurred during a family camping holiday. During a storybook narrative task (narrative 2), DF was encouraged to tell a story based on a wordless storybook *Frog Goes to Dinner* (Mayer, 1974). In this story, a boy and his family go to a fancy restaurant for dinner. The boy's mischievous pet frog goes along with them.

Narrative 1

MO: Remember we went camping in the big tent?
MO: Or the little, the pop up.
MO: Remember our camper we went in?
DF: No.
MO: Remember we made fires?
DF: No.
MO: You don't remember the fires?
MO: And you got to carry a walkie-talkie.
DF: Yeah.
MO: Yeah?
DF: I get to hold the black walkie talkie.
MO: And you got to hold the black walkie talkie.

Narrative 2

MO: Uh oh, look at that.
DF: Frog!
DF: He going to jump into that.
MO: Yeah, that's not going to be good, is it?
DF: No.
MO: Not uh.
DF: I know that the frog would do it.
MO: Yeah, what's he looking for?
DF: A frog.
MO: He's looking for a frog?
MO: Do you think the frog is going to jump on his face?
MO: Oh!
DF: I know the frog going to jump on his face too.

Unit 12.3 Focus on narrative production

(1) DF's narratives reveal some of his difficulties with morphosyntax. Give *three* examples of morphosyntactic deficits in these narratives.

(2) DF's storybook narrative is more informative than his autobiographical memory narrative. Why do you think this is the case?

(3) During the storybook narrative, there is evidence that DF understands his mother's use of deixis and that he can use deictic expressions in his own utterances. Give *one* example where this occurs.

(4) These short narratives contain several instances of mental state language. Give *three* examples of this language. In order to produce and comprehend mental state language, DF must possess a certain cognitive capacity. What is this capacity?

(5) DF appears to be able to respond to a range of questions from his mother. Describe *four* types of questions that are employed by DF's mother in the above narratives.

Focus on maternal language in SLI

Aside from providing information about DF's language skills, the narratives in unit 12.3 can also tell us about the ways in which maternal language may be modified to facilitate language development in children with SLI. Increasingly, investigators are examining maternal language use with a view to understanding the influence of maternal linguistic behaviours on the conversational participation of children with SLI. Majorano and Lavelli (2015) examined 15 Italian-speaking children with SLI during shared book reading with their mothers. The informativeness of maternal utterances – coded on the basis of sophisticated word use – and use of scaffolding were analysed. Mothers of children with SLI produced a higher percentage of directly informative utterances with gestural scaffolding than did mothers of chronological age-matched children. Children's lexical development three months after the study was related to direct maternal informativeness in both groups of children, and to gestural scaffolding only in children with SLI. Barachetti and Lavelli (2011) examined repairs produced by mothers of children with SLI during shared book-reading conversation. Repairs were defined as any utterance that aimed to correct a child's problematic answer. Mothers of children with SLI produced significantly more high-supportive repairs than mothers of age-matched children. In children with SLI, supportive repairs significantly affected the occurrence of minimally acceptable answers, while non-supportive repairs affected significantly the occurrence of inadequate answers.

Some studies have failed to establish an effect of maternal language use on the responsiveness and participation of children with SLI. Rezzonico et al. (2014) examined the number and type of recasts used by mothers of French-speaking children with SLI during four different activities – joint reading, symbolic play, question-guessing game and clue-guessing game. Mothers of children with SLI provided more recasts than mothers of typically developing children. Moreover, these took the form of phonological recasts as opposed to lexical recasts which were more likely to be used by mothers of typically developing children. Recasts were used more frequently during joint reading. Notwithstanding these differences in recast use, no significant difference was observed in the children's responses. McGinty et al. (2012) examined the relationship between mothers' question use and the participation of preschool children with SLI during shared reading. Mothers' question use did not facilitate higher levels of verbal participation by these children. Moreover, children's level of verbal participation did not influence the topic directiveness or cognitive challenge of mothers' question use.

Unit 12.4 Focus on maternal language in SLI

(1) At the end of the autobiographical memory narrative (narrative 1), DF produces his first extended utterance. Describe his mother's response to this utterance. What function is this response intended to serve?

(2) In the storybook narrative (narrative 2), DF's mother uses two strategies to respond to his utterances. Identify what those strategies are.

(3) What functions are served by the strategies that you identified in your answer to question (2)?

(4) Respond with *true* or *false* to each of the following statements about maternal language use in SLI:

     (a) Maternal recasts and repairs are only found in specific languages and cultures.

     (b) Maternal utterances can influence children's lexical development but not their syntactic development.

     (c) Recasts and repairs are used more frequently in storytelling contexts than in other linguistic and non-linguistic contexts.

     (d) Maternal scaffolding can include non-verbal behaviours as well as linguistic utterances.

     (e) Maternal question use is not always influenced by the verbal participation of children with SLI.

(5) Rezzonico et al. (2014) examined the use of phonological and lexical recasts by the mothers of French-speaking children with SLI. Are there examples of these recasts in the narratives between DF and his mother? Provide evidence to support your answer.

Impact and outcomes in SLI

At 4;8 years, DF will soon enter the school system. At this stage, his severe expressive language problems may have a number of serious consequences including poor academic attainment and problems in establishing peer relationships. DF may also be at an increased risk of victimisation and bullying. These possible consequences of DF's language disorder are suggested by the findings of studies that have reported significant, adverse academic and psychosocial impacts of SLI in children. Moreover, these impacts continue to be experienced by individuals with SLI long after the completion of compulsory education at the age of 16 years. Typically, this takes the form of reduced vocational opportunities and problems with social relationships. Some of these studies' findings are examined in this unit.

For school-age children, SLI can have significant psychosocial and academic impacts. Redmond (2011) examined peer victimisation levels in 7- to 8-year-old children with SLI, children with attention deficit hyperactivity disorder (ADHD) and typically developing children. Clinical status was found to be associated with elevated levels of victimisation, particularly for children with SLI. For typically developing children and children with ADHD, there was a potential buffering effect for number of close friendships. However, this did not exist for children with SLI. Conti-Ramsden et al. (2009) examined the educational outcomes of 120 adolescents with a history of SLI at the end of compulsory education. The results of national educational examinations were analysed. At least one of the expected qualifications was obtained by 44% of young people with SLI (88% of adolescents with typical development obtained the same level of qualifications). Among the adolescents with SLI, 24% was not entered for any examinations at the end of compulsory education (only 1% of adolescents with typical development was not entered for any examinations). After controlling for IQ and maternal education, literacy and language skills were predictive of educational attainment.

For young people with SLI, the completion of compulsory education and entry into the workplace bring new, additional challenges. Conti-Ramsden and Durkin (2012) interviewed 50 19-year-olds with SLI about their education and employment experiences since finishing compulsory secondary education. Young people with SLI were on average less successful than peers without SLI, obtaining approximately two, mostly vocational qualifications in the first few years post school. For those who continued in education at 19 years, they were most commonly in lower educational placements than their typically developing peers. A larger proportion of young people with SLI were not in education, employment or training at 19 years of age. Whitehouse et al. (2009a) examined the adult psychosocial outcomes of children with SLI, pragmatic language impairment (PLI) and autism spectrum disorder (ASD). Individuals with SLI were more likely than individuals with PLI and ASD to pursue vocational training and to work in jobs that do not require a high level of language/literacy ability. All groups had problems establishing social relationships, and some individuals in each group experienced affective disturbances.

Unit 12.5 Impact and outcomes in SLI

(1) Explain how DF's poor expressive language skills may have an adverse impact on his ability to forge social relationships with his peers.

(2) Explain how DF's poor expressive language skills may have an adverse impact on his classroom participation.

(3) The various impacts of specific language impairment are complex, and are unlikely to be a direct, causal relationship in each case. What intervening variable is likely to mediate the relationship between SLI and poor vocational outcomes?

(4) Whitehouse et al. (2009a) identified affective disturbances in some individuals with SLI. Which of the following is an affective disturbance in SLI?
   (a) schizophrenia
   (b) depression
   (c) personality disorder
   (d) anxiety disorder
   (e) bipolar disorder

(5) What clinical value do the findings of impact and outcome studies have beyond improving our understanding of SLI?

Case study 13

Boy with pragmatic language impairment

Introduction

The following exercise is a case study of a boy ('Tony') who was studied longitudinally by Conti-Ramsden and Gunn (1986) between 3;4 and 7;0 years. Tony had a profile of language strengths and weaknesses which was consistent with a diagnosis of semantic-pragmatic disorder. In present-day terminology, his problems would be characterised as pragmatic language impairment or social communication disorder (American Psychiatric Association, 2013). In what follows, Tony's abilities in pragmatics, verbal comprehension, syntax and phonology and non-verbal tasks are examined at three points in time during the period in which he was intensively studied. The case study is presented in five sections: history and initial assessment; language profile at 3;10 to 4;4 years; language profile at 5;2 to 5;7 years; language profile at 6;5 to 7;0 years; and focus on pragmatics.

History and initial assessment

Tony is the second of three children of Ghanaian parents. He was born in England, UK. His mother is a staff nurse and his father is an insurance clerk. Although Tony's parents speak Twi as their native language, they are both fluent speakers of English, and have always spoken English to him. Tony attended an English speaking playgroup. His older and younger sisters have no communication problems. When Tony was first referred for assessment by professionals to a Regional Child Development Centre at 3;4 years, his family had been living in England for over 10 years. Tony's parents reported that he was a good baby who did not demand much attention. His general development was normal. Although his early communicative development appeared normal to his parents, they noticed that he stopped communicating some time during his second year and also did not appear to respond to language. His parents became increasingly concerned about his lack of spontaneous language. At the same time, Tony was reciting some pop songs and nursery rhymes in their entirety. Many of his parents' developmental observations were confirmed at Tony's initial assessment. His hearing was within normal limits and he had excellent self-help skills (e.g. he dresses himself and can undertake independent toileting). Tony had poor eye contact, did not relate to children or adults, and did not initiate conversation or respond in conversation. He produced echolalic speech and did not respond to simple instructions (e.g. selecting objects by name). His non-verbal intelligence was above average. Tony displayed limited symbolic play, and would link two items (e.g. put the doll to bed) but then lose interest. When given paper and a pencil, he did not draw. He was extremely good with puzzles.

Unit 13.1 History and initial assessment

(1) Are there any risk factors for language disorder in Tony's personal history?

(2) Tony appeared to experience a regression in his communication skills during his second year. In which of the following conditions might a similar regression occur?
   (a) attention deficit hyperactivity disorder
   (b) Landau–Kleffner syndrome
   (c) Down's syndrome
   (d) autism spectrum disorder
   (e) specific language impairment

(3) One of the communicative changes that Tony's parents observed was that he did not respond to language. At initial assessment, Tony did not respond to simple instructions and his hearing was observed to be within normal limits. Which of the following conditions are suggested by these behaviours and findings?
   (a) developmental apraxia of speech
   (b) auditory agnosia
   (c) developmental dysarthria
   (d) verbal perseveration
   (e) developmental dyslexia

(4) A number of Tony's behaviours are consistent with a diagnosis of autism spectrum disorder. Name *five* such behaviours.

(5) Tony has clear deficits in the areas of socialisation, communication and imagination. However, his development in at least one other domain appears to be intact. What is that domain?

Language profile at 3;10 to 4;4 years

During this period, Tony's eye contact improved, although he still did not initiate interaction or conversation. He does not point to indicate or request something, and does not bring anything to show it to another person. Tony cannot use language to communicate his needs and screams when he is communicatively frustrated. At a chronological age of 4 years, Tony has a verbal comprehension score on the Reynell Developmental Language Scales (Reynell, 1977) that is three standard deviations below the mean (age equivalent below the 1 year level). He can now yield objects on verbal request (e.g. Ball?) and is beginning to respond to his name. His receptive vocabulary in the last two to three months has grown to over 80 everyday objects. However, this is only in a structured setting with tangible reinforcement. Tony's echolalia continues. His phonology is intact in spontaneous speech. He can sing 'Happy Birthday' and the 'Grand Old Duke of York', and he can count up to 20. His first spontaneous utterances include single words like 'hot' of dinner, which is uttered to himself rather than directed at someone. Tony's symbolic play has improved in that he can now enact simple domestic situations with miniature toys. He can copy a peg board perfectly, can recall four out of five objects (visual memory), can recognise and match numbers and symbols up to 10, and can sort, match and sequence for size. Tony has good motor skills and likes music. He will let one child take him by the hand and tow him around. There are no positive results from an EEG.

Unit 13.2 Language profile at 3;10 to 4;4 years

(1) Tony does not point to indicate or request something, and does not bring anything to show it to another person. What cognitive capacity do these behaviours suggest might be impaired?

(2) Is there evidence of a discrepancy between Tony's receptive language skills as measured by the Reynell and by the number of words in his receptive vocabulary?

(3) Which condition, which was considered as an explanation of Tony's regression in communication skills in unit 13.1, now appears increasingly unlikely to be a suitable diagnosis? Justify your response.

(4) Tony was able to copy a peg board perfectly. Which of the following skills must be intact in order for this to be achieved?
   (a) visual perception skills
   (b) theory of mind skills
   (c) fine motor skills
   (d) inhibitory skills
   (e) visual motor coordination skills

(5) Tony's non-verbal skills (apart from his non-verbal communication skills) are clearly superior to his verbal skills. Which of the following disorders is consistent with this pattern?
   (a) developmental dysarthria
   (b) specific language impairment
   (c) developmental phonological disorder
   (d) developmental apraxia of speech
   (e) attention deficit hyperactivity disorder

Language profile at 5;2 to 5;7 years

At this stage in the study, Tony displayed further improvements in pragmatics, verbal comprehension and syntax and phonology. Tony is beginning to use spontaneous initiations in conversation both at school and at home (e.g. 'open it'; 'go outside, mummy'; 'take it off'). There is also some use of ellipsis in conversation, but Tony still never asks questions. Three tests of verbal comprehension were conducted at this stage. These tests were the auditory comprehension component of the Preschool Language Scale (Zimmerman et al., 1979), the verbal comprehension component of the Reynell, and the Test of Reception of Grammar (Bishop, 1983). The age equivalent on these tests was 4;6, 3;4 and 4;6, respectively. Tony still refers to himself as 'Tony' and displays pronoun reversals (e.g. I/you and my/yours). Tony has excellent auditory memory and could remember 11 food purchases in the correct sequence the following day. He can now imitate other children in puppet play and can make Lego models following detailed visual instructions. Tony's writing is improving and he appears to prefer to write than to speak. His mechanical reading ability is well above his age.

Unit 13.3 Language profile at 5;2 to 5;7 years

(1) To which of the following types of speech acts do Tony's spontaneous initiations in conversation belong?
  (a) assertive (e.g. predictions)
  (b) directive (e.g. orders)
  (c) commissive (e.g. promises)
  (d) declaration (e.g. excommunications)
  (e) expressive (e.g. greetings)

(2) We are told that Tony's mechanical reading ability is well above his age. What does 'mechanical reading ability' mean? Which of Tony's cognitive skills supports this ability?

(3) Tony is starting to use ellipsis. What does this suggest about Tony's understanding of his hearer's knowledge state?

(4) In unit 13.1, a number of behaviours were considered which are consistent with a diagnosis of autism spectrum disorder. Which behaviour are we told about for the first time in this unit which is also consistent with a diagnosis of ASD?

(5) The investigators account for the discrepancy in age equivalents on the Preschool Language Scale (PLS) and the Reynell Developmental Language Scales (RDLS) in terms of the complexity of the stimulus items. Specifically, in the RDLS, stimulus items deal with a number of concepts simultaneously, while in the PLS, concepts such as colour, number and prepositions are tested separately. To what extent are the multiple conceptual demands of the RDLS likely to exceed Tony's memory capacities?

Language profile at 6;5 to 7;0 years

Towards the end of this longitudinal study, Tony presented as a normal child in simple, predictable situations and routines. He is now able to initiate, respond and maintain conversations. If complex verbal reasoning is involved, Tony still has difficulty in maintaining a topic. When excessive pragmatic or semantic demands are placed on him, Tony becomes agitated and screams or shouts. He still has impaired verbal comprehension. For example, at a chronological age of 6;11 years, Tony has an age equivalent on the RDLS and PLS of 4;11 and 6;6 years, respectively. He still has difficulty understanding words that involve feelings (e.g. 'happy', 'sad'). Tony can now use complex sentence structures (e.g. sentences with direct and indirect objects), although he still has difficulty marking and maintaining tense appropriately in conversation. He is functioning above his age in terms of reading, writing and spelling. Tony tends to be obsessional and has difficulty coping with situation change. He has difficulty understanding humour but can treat simple activities as 'jokes' (e.g. he thought it was funny to copy a child who was whispering in the classroom). When told exactly what to do, Tony can be a very good actor. However, he is unable to spontaneously change or add anything to the instructions.

Unit 13.4 Language profile at 6;5 to 7;0 years

(1) Tony has difficulty understanding words that involve feelings. Impairments of which of the following cognitive skills might account for this difficulty?
   (a) cognitive theory of mind
   (b) inhibition of prepotent responses
   (c) working memory
   (d) affective theory of mind
   (e) planning

(2) Some of Tony's behaviours are still strongly suggestive of the symptomatology of autism spectrum disorder. Name *one* such behaviour.

(3) Tony is displaying problems interpreting humour. Which peer behaviour might he be at risk of misunderstanding in consequence?

(4) Which verbal behaviour on Tony's part suggests a lack of cognitive flexibility?

(5) We are told that Tony presents as a normal child in simple, predictable situations and routines. What construct do pragmatists and theorists draw upon to explain an individual's ability to operate under these conditions?

Focus on pragmatics

This unit examines several short conversational extracts that were recorded throughout the longitudinal study. These extracts illustrate at the level of conversation some of Tony's difficulties that were described in earlier units. The extracts all unfold between Tony (TO) and his teacher (TE):

Extract 1 Tony at 3;9 years

TE: Hello everyone.
    Hi Ken (*greeting taxi driver who had brought Tony*)
TO: Hi Ken (*in perfect imitation*)

Extract 2 Tony at 4;5 years

TE: Who cut your hair? (*Tony has a new haircut*)
TO: Daddy cut your hair.
TE: What are they? (*points to pictures of eggs*)
TO: Eggs.
TE: How many eggs?
TO: Two eggs.
TE: What does the cow say? (*points to next picture*)
TO: Cow says moo and all farm animals.

Extract 3 Tony at 4;5 years

TE: Whose turn is it?
TO: Tony's (*referring to self*)

Extract 4 Tony at 5;1 years

(Teacher has brought a fresh bunch of flowers and has put them in a vase)

TO: (*points to vase*) Flowers.
　　(*Tony is playing with water and a toy frog*)
TO: (*talking to himself*) Wind it up (*winds it up*)
　　Jump inside (*throws it in*).

Extract 5 Tony at 5;4 years

TO: Alex has new socks.
TE: What is Alex doing?
TO: Playing with a bus.
TE: Whose is it?
TO: Mine.

Extract 6 Tony at 6;2 years

(Tony feels sick and wants the teacher to ring home)

TO: Judy talk mummy.
TE: How?
TO: Orange (*referring to orange drink that may have made him feel sick*)
　　Tony is sick.
　　Can I talk to mummy?
TE: What do I do to talk to mummy?
　　What shall I do to talk to mummy?
TO: Because I am sick.

Extract 7 Tony at 6;2 years

(Teacher and child are playing with a doll called Carl. The doll has fallen)

TE: Is Carl frightened?
TO: Yes.
TE: Why is he frightened?
TO: He is falling down, he cried, he is sore mouth.
TE: What happened?
TO: Carl is crying.
TE: Why?
TO: Because he is frightened.
TE: Why has he got a sore mouth?
TO: Because you are falling (*to doll*). Why are you getting on the floor?

Extract 8 Tony at 6;6 to 6;9 years

(Specific questions taken from material developed by the Liverpool Language Unit therapists, chosen to illustrate difficulties working things out)

TE: Why do you have to be quiet when there's a baby in the room?
TO: 'Cos she's crying.
TE: What would happen to a flower if it didn't get any water?
TO: 'Cos it spilt.
TE: What would happen to your teeth if you were always eating lots of sweets?
TO: 'Cos I go to the dentist.

Unit 13.5 Focus on pragmatics

(1) Several pragmatic anomalies occur in the extracts above. Give *one* example of each of the following behaviours in these extracts:
(a) immediate echolalia
(b) pronoun reversal
(c) inappropriate use of proper noun for reference to self
(d) lack of ellipsis
(e) inappropriate use of proper noun for reference to others

(2) Even these pragmatic anomalies do not occur with complete consistency. Can you find instances in the data where ellipsis and a pronoun for self-reference are used appropriately?

(3) Notwithstanding his pragmatic difficulties, Tony can use language to perform a range of functions or speech acts. Several of these are listed below. Give *one* example of each of these functions in the above data:
(a) Tony can use language to convey information.
(b) Tony can use language to name things.
(c) Tony can use language as a commentary on his actions.
(d) Tony can use language to make requests.
(e) Tony can use language to ask questions.

(4) There is evidence in these extracts that Tony has reasonably intact theory of mind (ToM) skills. State where this occurs in the data. What type of ToM skills – cognitive or affective ToM – appear intact in the data that you have chosen.

(5) Tony's comprehension of wh-interrogatives is impaired. His poor comprehension reveals a difficulty in understanding certain concepts. Describe *two* concepts which appear to be problematic for Tony.

Case study 14

Swedish-speaking girl with pragmatic language impairment

Introduction

The following exercise is a case study of a young Swedish girl ('Lena') who was studied by Sahlén and Nettelbladt (1993) between the ages of 5;6 and 8;0 years. Lena was diagnosed as having semantic-pragmatic disorder, a subgroup within the group of specific and severe developmental language disorders. Nowadays, this group of children is labelled as having pragmatic language impairment or social communication disorder, the latter a diagnostic term used in DSM-5 (American Psychiatric Association, 2013). The case study is presented in five sections: history, hearing and cognitive evaluation; language profile at 5;6 years; language profile at 6;6 years; language profile at 8;0 years; and focus on pragmatics.

History, hearing and cognitive evaluation

Lena attends a language preschool unit for children with severe and specific developmental language disorders in Lund, Sweden. Staff at the unit reported that Lena at times behaves oddly. During pregnancy, Lena's mother had several infections of the upper respiratory tract and urinary tract. Apart from these infections, gestation was otherwise normal. Lena achieved motor milestones normally. At 2 to 3 years of age, there was a suspicion of autism. However, Lena's behavioural problems were later interpreted to be related to her language disorder. Lena experienced recurrent episodes of otitis media with effusion. However, screening audiometry, pure-tone audiometry and brainstem response audiometry all produced normal results. Some of Lena's family members have communication problems. Her two brothers – one older and one younger – are both receiving language training because of severe developmental language disorders. Lena's mother has a hearing impairment of unknown aetiology and wears a hearing aid at work. At 5;10 years, Lena underwent a speech discrimination test. She scored 78 to 86% (a score of > 90% is normal). The Raven's Coloured Progressive Matrices (Raven, 1962) and the Swedish version of the Wechsler Intelligence Scale for Children (WISC; Wechsler, 1976) were used to test Lena at 7;6 and 8;0 years, respectively. On the WISC, there was a discrepancy between verbal and performance scores, with the latter score higher (Verbal: Stanine 2 (low); Performance: Stanine 4 (low average)). On the Raven's Coloured Progressive Matrices, Lena's results were clearly above the mean.

Unit 14.1 History, hearing and cognitive evaluation

(1) Lena's history and clinical presentation are consistent with a diagnosis of specific language impairment (SLI). Which of the following features of her profile suggest a diagnosis of SLI?

    (a) normal audiological assessment

    (b) odd behaviour at school

    (c) non-verbal cognitive ability in the normal range

    (d) reduced verbal IQ

    (e) maternal infections during gestation

(2) The history states that Lena experienced recurrent episodes of otitis media with effusion. What type of hearing loss might this have predisposed her to?

(3) Which feature of Lena's history indicates that her developmental problems are *specific* to language?

(4) There is evidence of aggregation of communication disorders in Lena's family. What communication disorder is particularly significant with respect to a possible aetiology for Lena's problems with language?

(5) Lena's speech discrimination test result was below normal. Which of the following aspects of language is this test result most likely to have adverse implications for?

    (a) phonology

    (b) syntax

    (c) semantics

    (d) pragmatics

    (e) discourse

Language profile at 5;6 years

Lena underwent a wide-ranging assessment of her language skills at 5;6 years. Her repetition of sentences was poor. She seemed not to understand the sentences she was asked to repeat or to remember them. For example, when asked to repeat 'I cycle around the big house every night', she uttered 'Cycle every house' and 'I cycle every house'. Her ability to repeat word lists was also compromised. When asked to repeat the list 'mitten-bird-lamp', she said 'mitten-bird-chair', and the repetition of 'running-reading-swimming' took the form 'running-water-swim'. Lena relied heavily on visual feedback to help her discriminate phonemes. The following distinctions were problematic for her: /ɯ-y/, /ʃ-s/, /d-g/ and /b-p/. There were phonological problems in the use of liquids and consonant clusters. In terms of prosody, Lena exhibited 'childish' intonation due to too many sentence accents and exaggerated pitch variation. The retrieval of words from a given semantic category was difficult for her. For example, Lena was only able to produce two words in the food category (*apple* and *banana*), and when she was asked what kind of clothes she was wearing, she replied 'shirt, braids, black and black [*points to her trousers and shoes*] and pink [*points to a pink ribbon in her hair*]. Lena could classify pictures of objects correctly, but was unable to provide a superordinate lexical item for semantic categories (e.g. clothes). Language comprehension was assessed to be at the 3- to 4-year level. Where no visual support was given, Lena's participation on tasks that required comprehension of logical–grammatical constructions was poor. There was poor comprehension of prepositions, and attributive, possessive and comparative constructions. In spontaneous speech, there were errors in the use of prepositions. The use of finiteness and correct word order was also problematic. No sentence connectors were used. Lena's narrative retelling was fragmentary. When new topics were introduced, she made inconsistent use of indefinite and definite articles to refer to them and overused deictic expressions.

Unit 14.2 Language profile at 5;6 years

(1) The repetition of word lists is problematic for Lena. Which of the following occurs during Lena's repetitions?
   (a) phonemic paraphasia
   (b) perseveration
   (c) echolalia
   (d) semantic paraphasia
   (e) circumlocution

(2) Lena has difficulty with the production of consonant clusters. However, there is also evidence in her expressive output of the intact use of certain consonant clusters. Identify *four* such clusters.

(3) Lena has impaired lexical semantics. Are Lena's difficulties in this area of language largely expressive or receptive in nature? Provide evidence to support your answer.

(4) Lena is heavily dependent on visual cues to compensate for her poor language skills. Which *two* language levels are effectively compensated by the use of these cues?

(5) Lena produces 'fragmentary' narratives. Explain how this may be related to her lack of sentence connectors.

Language profile at 6;6 years

A second, comprehensive analysis of Lena's language was undertaken when she was 6;6 years. It was observed at this time that Lena had better understanding of instructions and that her echolalia was less evident. However, she still exhibited pragmatic problems and had difficulty concentrating on demanding tasks. Some of these problems were apparent in her responses to questions from the examiner (E).

Exchange 1

E: What would happen if you went out now without shoes?
L: You may go out in your shoes.
E: Yes, why?
L: You may not run and put on your shoes – may go out in the garden – then you get colours to play on – riding on horses.

Exchange 2

E: Why was her head aching? [*Examiner shows a picture of a girl falling from a sledge*]
L: Because she go in and ask with mother.

All tactile/kinaesthetic, visual/visuospatial, motor and non-verbal auditory tasks were performed adequately. Repetition of nonsense syllables, sequences with semantic content and tongue-twister words was poor. Sentence repetition was improved but still not age adequate. The repetition of word lists was also improved, with Lena retaining a maximum of three words. During narrative retelling, Lena related only three out of 10 events in the story, and even then not in a logical order. Since assessment at 5;6 years, Lena's phoneme discrimination had deteriorated, with eight distinctions now problematic for her. This necessitated a referral for an audiological examination where otitis media with effusion was confirmed. Three weeks later, when hearing was judged to be normal, the phoneme discrimination tasks were repeated. On this occasion, Lena failed on six distinctions. Unlike her assessment at 5;6 years, Lena was able to name all the clothes she was wearing. However, she was unable to give the names of clothes that were not present in the situation. Her comprehension of language was still not age adequate (4- to 5-year level), and she refused to undertake certain comprehension tasks. Her attempts to rhyme resulted in semantic errors (e.g. 'eel' was produced as a rhyme to 'whale'), as did her attempts to name pictures (e.g. for 'wheelchair' she produced 'old wagon bike'). Slight phonological problems still persisted. In terms of grammar, Lena occasionally omitted function words and she produced errors in the use of finiteness and prepositions during sentence repetition tasks and in spontaneous production. Sentence connectors were beginning to emerge.

Unit 14.3 Language profile at 6;6 years

(1) In exchanges 1 and 2, Lena is asked wh-questions which she clearly does not under-stand. Which of the following concepts must Lena possess in order to address these questions satisfactorily?
   (a) causation
   (b) space
   (c) time
   (d) consequence
   (e) personhood

(2) In exchange 1, Lena's responses are clearly tangential to the questions she is asked. However, a certain type of script appears to dominate her responses. What is this script?

(3) Aside from its irrelevance, Lena's response in exchange 2 is problematic in *three* further respects. What are these respects?

(4) In unit 14.2, an explanation of Lena's 'fragmentary' narratives in terms of her lack of use of sentence connectors was considered. At 6;6 years, Lena is still experiencing difficulty with the production of narratives. Does the same explanation appear to account for her narrative difficulties at this age?

(5) In unit 14.2, visual cues were seen to compensate for certain of Lena's poor language skills. Is there any evidence of visual (or other) cues functioning in a compensatory role in the information provided above?

Language profile at 8;0 years

A third and final assessment of Lena's language skills was undertaken at 8;0 years. As the intelligibility of her speech improved, and her willingness to participate in dialogue increased, her conversational difficulties have become even more evident. She is eager to respond to the examiner and almost never refuses to answer. She is poorly oriented to her own person, place and time, and cannot say how many brothers and sisters she has or tell the time of day. Lena still does not engage with demanding tasks. Although the repetition of nonsense syllables is still problematic (Lena does not appear to understand what she should do), the repetition of sequences with semantic content is age appropriate. Lena can retain three words during the repetition of word lists but there can be interference from other lists or when new words are introduced. There are more omissions during the repetition of sentences than in spontaneous speech. During narrative retelling, Lena's own experience tends to dominate, with familiar people taking the role of actors in the story. This is evident in the following extract from a narrative retelling task:

E: What happened one morning in the summer?
L: My Misse and Murre [*Lena's two cats*] they could climb up the tree in their sharp claws.

Lena was able to remember the 10 events in the story when given questions. At this stage, there are no errors of phoneme discrimination. Lena still struggles to produce words within a given semantic category. However, she is now able to produce superordinate lexical items. There continues to be considerable difficulty with the comprehension of logical–grammatical constructions and there is still no ability to rhyme. There is good performance on the Token Test (De Renzi and Vignolo, 1962), a test of language comprehension. Lena's naming is very poor for her age. Most naming errors are semantic in nature:

Target word	Lena's production
pyramid	the kings
fern	heather
funnel	strainer
hasp	locked
sphinx	pyramid lion man

There are still some grammatical problems such as the omission of function words and semantically inappropriate use of sentence adverbials and subjunctives. Lena's phonology has normalised. Her articulation sounds childish on account of a tendency to palatalise consonants, and her prosodic problems (e.g. exaggerated pitch variation) still persist.

Unit 14.4 Language profile at 8;0 years

(1) Lena's naming errors are interesting, with a range of associations linking her productions to the target word. What type of verbal behaviour is Lena exhibiting when she produces *pyramid lion man* for 'sphinx'? Are there any other examples of this behaviour in the data in unit 14.3?

(2) During the production of narratives, Lena's own experience tends to dominate over the actors and events in the story. Why might this occur?

(3) Give *one* example of each of the following patterns in Lena's naming errors:
    (a) Lena's production is related to the target word by *function*.
    (b) Lena's production is related to the target word by *physical similarity*.

(c) Lena's production is related to the target word by *semantic field*.

(d) Lena's production is related to the target word by *world knowledge*.

(4) Can Lena make appropriate use of cohesive devices during the production of narratives? Support your answer with evidence.

(5) Based on the above data, how would you characterise Lena's comprehension of language? Provide evidence to support your answer.

Focus on pragmatics

At 8;0 years, Lena participated in the following exchange with the examiner. The examiner is asking Lena a series of questions based on general knowledge:

E: What do you usually see on the ground when it is autumn?

L: Mosquitoes and birds and crows.

E: What season comes after autumn?

L: Winter and then spring then autumn and then spring . . . usually many days are passing.

E: What is it like in the winter?

L: (*pause*) You just build a snow man.

E: Mm . . . and in the spring?

L: At day nursery when was winter then everybody went out and played and she throw snowballs on the wall and it was red.

E: But look, if I tell you that right now there are already some flowers outside and small, small buds on the trees and so on . . .

L: Flowers . . . on the apple trees I think are beautiful to see.

E: So what season is it when it is like this outside?

L: (*pause*) Mm . . .

E: Is it winter then?

L: No . . . spring! This is probably not spring (*picks up a pen on the table*). What sort of pen is this?

Unit 14.5 Focus on pragmatics

(1) Respond with *true* or *false* to each of the following statements:
   (a) Lena observes the dyadic structure of conversation.
   (b) Lena has limited appreciation of adjacency pairs.
   (c) Lena never produces the first part in an adjacency pair.
   (d) Lena produces tangential responses to questions.
   (e) Lena produces a number of directives in this exchange.

(2) Lena makes use of topicalisation in the above exchange. Where does this occur? In view of Lena's language problems, what function might topicalisation serve for her?

(3) Does Lena display problems with world knowledge during this exchange with the examiner? Provide evidence to support your answer.

(4) Are there any referential anomalies in Lena's utterances in this exchange? Provide evidence in support of your answer.

(5) Give *one* example of each of the following in the above exchange:

(a) Lena produces an over-informative response to the examiner's question.
(b) Lena continues to talk on a topic which has been terminated.
(c) Lena engages in an abrupt change of topic.
(d) Lena needs time to process wh-interrogatives.
(e) Lena shows limited awareness of the examiner's knowledge state.

Case study 15

Man aged 47 years with developmental dyslexia

Introduction

The following exercise is a case study of a man ('JR') aged 47 years who was studied by Temple (1988). JR is an adult with developmental dyslexia. His case is somewhat unusual in that children with developmental dyslexia are seldom studied as adults. JR recalled having difficulty with reading from the start of school. He presented himself as an adult for assessment because he had heard about dyslexia and wanted to have a better understanding of his problems with reading and spelling. The case study is presented in five sections: primer on developmental dyslexia; client history; cognitive and language assessment; focus on reading; and focus on spelling.

Primer on developmental dyslexia

The International Dyslexia Association (2002) states:

Dyslexia is characterized by difficulties with accurate and/or fluent word recognition and by poor spelling and decoding abilities. These difficulties typically result from a deficit in the phonological component of language that is often unexpected in relation to other cognitive abilities and the provision of effective classroom instruction. Secondary consequences may include problems in reading comprehension and reduced reading experience that can impede growth of vocabulary and background knowledge.

This definition of dyslexia, which has been adopted by the National Institute of Child Health and Human Development and many US state education codes, places due emphasis on two features of developmental dyslexia: difficulties with reading and spelling cannot be accounted for by any environmental deprivation, and are not on account of a wider cognitive or intellectual disability. Notwithstanding 'provision of effective classroom instruction' and normal intellectual abilities, individuals with developmental dyslexia have significant problems with reading and writing which place them at risk of academic failure, vocational underachievement and other language disorders.

Developmental dyslexia is one of the few communication disorders with a well-developed epidemiological base. According to Shaywitz and Shaywitz (2003), the prevalence of dyslexia is estimated to be 5% to 17% of school-age children in the United States. Contrary to the findings of a number of studies, these investigators claim that dyslexia affects boys and girls comparably. The condition is both familial and heritable. Shaywitz and Shaywitz state that up to 50% of children of dyslexic parents, 50% of siblings of dyslexic children, and 50% of parents of dyslexic children may have the disorder. There is a high rate of comorbidity in children with dyslexia. Margari et al. (2013) examined

448 children between the ages of 7 to 16 years with a diagnosis of learning disorders. For children with a diagnosis of specific learning disorders, which included reading, writing and mathematics disorders, attention deficit hyperactivity disorder (ADHD) was present in 33%, anxiety disorder in 28.8%, developmental coordination disorder in 17.8%, language disorder in 11% and mood disorder in 9.4%. Studies have consistently reported phonological processing deficits in children with dyslexia in English and in languages with other orthographies (see Christo (2014) for discussion). Along with genetic and neurobiological factors, phonological processing deficits are part of a complex, multifactorial aetiology of dyslexia.

Unit 15.1 Primer on developmental dyslexia

(1) Which of the following are *true* statements about the epidemiology of developmental dyslexia?
   (a) The prevalence of dyslexia is higher in the prison population than in the general population.
   (b) Many epidemiological studies of dyslexia report a boy-to-girl gender ratio of 3:1.
   (c) The incidence of dyslexia decreases every year between the ages of 5 and 10.
   (d) There is a lower prevalence of dyslexia in children with ADHD than in the general population.
   (e) Dyslexia is found in all ethnic groups and socioeconomic classes.

(2) The children with reading and spelling problems in each of the following scenarios would *not* receive a diagnosis of developmental dyslexia. For each scenario, explain why a diagnosis of developmental dyslexia would not be appropriate.
   (a) A 10-year-old child with Down's syndrome can only read a few single words.
   (b) A teenager develops reading and spelling problems after sustaining a traumatic brain injury.
   (c) A child who has congenital sensorineural hearing loss does not have age-appropriate reading and spelling skills.
   (d) A boy with Landau–Kleffner syndrome loses the ability to read some of his favourite books.
   (e) A 10-year-old girl with fetal alcohol syndrome has the reading level of a preschool child.

(3) Developmental dyslexia has adverse implications for the functioning of individuals. Many of these implications are experienced throughout adulthood. Describe *three* areas of functioning that may be compromised in adulthood by developmental dyslexia.

(4) Which of the following are *true* statements about the aetiology of developmental dyslexia?
   (a) More than one genetic factor interacts to cause susceptibility to dyslexia.
   (b) There is no evidence of familial clustering in dyslexia.
   (c) Phonological processing deficits are a proximal cause of dyslexia.
   (d) There is no evidence of neurobiological differences between children with and without developmental dyslexia.
   (e) Genetic factors are a distal cause of developmental dyslexia.

(5) What light can comorbid conditions shed on our understanding of developmental dyslexia?

Client history

JR is 47 years old, and is right-handed. He is self-employed and has his own building firm. He remembers experiencing difficulty with reading from his early years at school. However, there were no reported problems with either mathematics or woodwork. When JR left school, he undertook a carpentry and joinery course at a technical college. He achieved the intermediate level, and then joined the army. JR's difficulties with reading and spelling persisted into adulthood, and a friend assists him with paperwork related to his business. JR referred himself for assessment, as he had heard about dyslexia and wanted to better understand the nature of his problems. An examination of JR's medical history revealed no serious illness, head injury or neurological disorder. He suffers from hay fever and migraine. JR has four children. One child has autism. Two other children had reading and spelling problems at school. In one of these children, a left-handed daughter, these problems were particularly marked.

Unit 15.2 Client history

(1) Explain how JR's case is consistent with what is known about the vocational outcomes of adults with developmental dyslexia.

(2) JR did not report difficulties with mathematics at school. On the basis of this report, what can we conclude about JR's intellectual functioning?

(3) How would you characterise JR's academic achievement?

(4) Which *two* features of JR's medical history are important in terms of a diagnosis of developmental dyslexia?

(5) Is there any aspect of JR's family situation which is significant in terms of the aetiology of dyslexia?

Cognitive and language assessment

JR was assessed on the Raven's Progressive Matrices. He scored at the 50th percentile for his age. When JR described his problems, he said that he sometimes has difficulty expressing his thoughts clearly in speech and occasionally has difficulty finding the words he needs to explain situations. JR thinks clearly, but his thoughts can appear muddled when he attempts to express himself. JR spoke slowly, carefully and clearly in conversation. On an object naming test (Oldfield and Wingfield, 1965), JR correctly identified 33 of 36 objects. His description of the cookie theft picture (Goodglass and Kaplan, 1983b) is presented below:

Presumably the housewife is washing-up and doesn't appear to realize that the sink is overflowing . . . at least her eyes are not in that direction. The children are having a mishap attempting to take some cake from the top shelf of the cupboard . . . assume it's a sunny day because she has a sleeveless dress on and the window is open. There doesn't appear to be a cooker in the kitchen.

JR displayed good oral fluency. In a 1-minute category fluency test, JR was able to produce the names of 22 animals and 38 things. However, his initial letter fluency was poorer.

He was only able to generate 12 words beginning with 'f' in one minute, and 8 words beginning with 's'. His recitation of the alphabet was poor with several hesitations and two omissions. JR recalled that it took him until the age of 9 years before he could recite this sequence. His short-term memory, as assessed by digit span, was 5 forward and 2 backward.

Unit 15.3 Cognitive and language assessment

(1) How would you characterise JR's performance on the Raven's Progressive Matrices?

(2) JR reports that he occasionally has difficulty finding the words he needs to explain situations. Do JR's test results suggest that he has anomia?

(3) Considerable information can be gleaned about JR's skills and problems from his description of the cookie theft picture. Several of these are listed below. Give *one* example of each skill and problem.
 (a) JR is able to use specific features of the scene to draw inferences.
 (b) JR uses a word that does not accurately capture the children's behaviour.
 (c) JR is unable to read a printed word that is displayed in the scene.
 (d) JR displays intact theory of mind skills.
 (e) JR is able to use his script knowledge to make inferences about the objects he would expect to see in the scene.

(4) Are JR's semantic memory and phonological memory impaired? Provide evidence to support your answer.

(5) JR has a forward digit span of 5. What does this indicate about his verbal working memory?

Focus on reading

JR's ability to read words, non-words and words written in different ways was examined. JR achieved a score equivalent to a reading age of 12 years and 6 months on the Schonell single-word reading test. The upper limit on this test is 15 years, and JR's performance became noticeably slower from the 8-year-old level onwards. The reading of several words revealed certain types of errors. These errors included morphological paralexias (the base lexical item is read correctly, but a bound morpheme is dropped, added, or substituted), visual paralexias (errors in which the response shares at least 50% of letters in common with the target word), and neologistic responses. Some of JR's responses are shown below:

pivot → 'pirate'
grotesque → 'grotique' /grɔtikə/
fascinate → 'fascinated'
systematic → 'sympathetic'
metamorphosis → 'metaporous' /mɛtapoˈrʌs/

JR was also assessed on Nelson and O'Connell's (1978) irregular word reading test. The words in this test cannot be read using grapheme-to-sound rules. JR was able to read the following seven words correctly: *ache, psalm, nausea, aisle, courteous, quadruped* and *catacomb.*

On Nelson and O'Connell's long regular word test, in which words can be read by the systematic application of grapheme-to-sound rules, JR was able to read nine of 10 high-frequency words, but only four unfamiliar, low-frequency words. There was one error on this test (*adventurously* → 'adventurous'). JR's reading of regular and irregular words using Coltheart et al.'s (1979) list was also examined. Four irregular words were incorrectly read, but none of these errors were regularisations, in which systematic grapheme-to-sound rules had been applied. The errors were three visual paralexias and one omission. Overall, JR read 312 of 379 words (82%) correctly. Forty-two errors (63%) were neologisms, with 31 of these errors occurring on words of nine or more letters. Visual and morphological paralexias accounted for 24% and 12% of errors, respectively.

To examine reading of non-words, three balanced lists of words and non-words were presented to JR. He consistently read non-words more poorly than words. With increasing length, the difference between word and non-word reading became more marked. Also with increasing length, the number of lexicalisations (the reading of non-words as words) decreased. Finally, JR's ability to read different typed and handwritten stimuli was also examined. This included typewritten letters in lower-case, poorly handwritten letters, and typewritten letters in lower case and in the reverse order. Only one error, a morphological paralexia, occurred when typewritten letters in lower-case were presented. When normal subjects are presented with poorly handwritten letters, they score about 90% correct. However, JR only scored 48% correct, with most errors taking the form of visual paralexias. This dropped even further to 24% correct under the condition in which typewritten, lower-case letters were presented in reverse order.

Unit 15.4 Focus on reading

(1) What types of errors occur on the reading of the following words?
pivot; grotesque; fascinate; systematic; metamorphosis

(2) There are a number of different models of how words may be read aloud. On a phonological model, letter strings are parsed into graphemes which are then translated via a system of rules into a series of phonological segments. These segments are then blended together. What evidence is there that this phonological route of reading is problematic for JR?

(3) Words can also be read aloud by accessing the semantic system. Specifically, a visual word representation reaches threshold and activates an entry in the semantic system. This, in turn, accesses an oral phonological representation of the target word. Certain words *must* be read via the semantic system. What are these words, and is JR able to read them?

(4) Why do you think JR reads high-frequency regular words well and low-frequency regular words poorly, when both can be read by applying impaired grapheme-to-sound rules?

(5) JR's reading performance can be summarised as follows: relatively good word reading; visual paralexias; morphological paralexias; and non-word reading poorer than word reading. This performance is consistent with phonological dyslexia. Which of the following statements best explains the high number of visual paralexias that are used by clients with phonological dyslexia?

(a) Visual paralexias are an inevitable consequence of impaired application of grapheme-to-sound rules.

(b) Visual paralexias arise because of inappropriate threshold activation of visually similar words in the semantic system.

(c) Visual paralexias arise because visual word representations in the semantic system cannot be accessed.

(d) Visual paralexias arise because of suppression of the phonological reading route.

(e) Visual paralexias arise because clients with phonological dyslexia attend only to the sound representation of words.

Focus on spelling

JR's spelling of regular and irregular words and non-words was also assessed. JR attained a spelling age of 10 years 2 months on the Schonell single-word spelling test. He was dictated words for written spelling. JR spelled 47% of the irregular words correctly and 80% of the regular words. This difference was significant. Some of JR's spelling errors on regular and irregular words are shown below.

Regular words
    'library' → *libary*
    'victim' → *victum*
    'effort' → *efort*
    'fabric' → *faberic*
Irregular words
    'cuisine' → *quizine*
    'menace' → *maness*
    'leopard' → *lepard*
    'ritual' → *richual*
    'health' → *heath*

A lexical decision task was orally dictated to JR for written spelling. He was able to spell 84% of the words correctly, and 52% of non-words. Once again, this difference was significant. This result was unexpected given JR's performance on the spelling of regular words.

Unit 15.5 Focus on spelling

(1) Is JR's spelling performance better than or worse than his reading performance? Provide support for your answer.

(2) Some of JR's spelling errors on irregular words were phonologically valid even as they were incorrect. Others involved a vowel error or the omission of a letter. Identify the type of spelling errors that occurs on each of the following words: *cuisine; menace; leopard; ritual; health.*

(3) What does JR's relatively strong performance on the spelling of regular words suggest? Is this consistent with what we know about JR's reading skills?

(4) The results on the lexical decision task were described as 'unexpected' given JR's performance on the spelling of regular words. Explain why this is the case. What wider conclusion can we draw about the phonological spelling route from JR's spelling of regular words and non-words?

(5) Is the graphemic (whole-word) spelling route intact in JR? Provide evidence to support your answer.

Case study 16

Boy aged 5;6 years with FG syndrome

Introduction

The following exercise is a case study of a boy ('JB') who was studied by McCardle and Wilson (1993). JB was diagnosed as having FG syndrome. FG syndrome is an X-linked disorder which is characterised by intellectual disability, hypotonia, dysmorphic facial features, broad thumbs and halluces, anal anomalies, constipation and abnormalities of the corpus callosum (Lyons et al., 2009). Young boys with the syndrome have a behaviour phenotype which includes hyperactivity, affability and excessive talkativeness, along with socially oriented, attention-seeking behaviour (Graham et al., 2010). The case study is presented in five sections: history and medical assessment; cognitive and developmental assessment; language assessment at 25 to 34 months; language assessment at 44 to 54 months; and language assessment at 67 months.

History and medical assessment

JB is a white boy who was first seen at 2 years of age for investigation of developmental delay and dysmorphic facies. He is the first child of a 20-year-old woman. JB was full-term and there was nothing remarkable about his prenatal and neonatal courses. Delayed milestones were first observed when JB underwent a well-baby check at one year. Following this assessment, JB went on to sit at 15 months, to walk at 26 months and to use phrases at 3 years. When JB was 11 months old, he had an episode of aspiration pneumonia. Between 2 and 3 years of age, JB experienced hearing loss secondary to recurrent acute otitis media.

JB's family history was significant in several respects. He had a younger brother with similar facial features, a cardiac anomaly (ventriculoseptal defect), imperforate anus and agenesis of the corpus callosum. This child underwent repair of his ventriculoseptal defect but died in the immediate postoperative period. Callosal agenesis was confirmed by an autopsy. There were no other CNS abnormalities. JB's maternal uncle died of congenital heart disease at 10 months of age. He also had characteristic facies. Two other family members, JB's mother and maternal grandmother, had low set, poorly developed ears and prominent foreheads. JB's mother did not have a history of developmental problems.

JB underwent a wide-ranging medical examination. His dysmorphic facies included telecanthus (widened area of skin between the eyes), frontal bossing, a triangular shaped skull, small upturned nose, 'carp mouth', and small, underdeveloped, low-set ears. There was no cleft palate. A cardiac examination revealed a systolic murmur, but JB had a normal ECG. There were no rectal or genital anomalies. JB had long slender fingers, hypermobile thumbs and a shortened fourth metacarpal on the left. A paediatric neurologist reported generalised gross and fine motor dysfunction but no other abnormalities. A CAT scan revealed complete agenesis of the corpus callosum. JB had normal bone age and orbital hypertelorism (excessive distance between the orbits). Blood and body chemistries were normal. JB tested negative for fragile X. His karyotype was 46, XY with normal banding. JB is ambidextrous. He displayed a friendly, inquisitive personality during his interaction with the authors of the study.

Unit 16.1 History and medical assessment

(1) JB's developmental milestones are significantly delayed. Use your knowledge of normal child development to characterise this delay.

(2) JB developed aspiration pneumonia at 11 months of age. This should raise a concern for the speech-language pathologist who assesses JB. What is this concern?

(3) Between 2 and 3 years of age, JB experienced hearing loss secondary to recurrent acute otitis media. What type of hearing loss is this? What other aspect of JB's clinical presentation suggests that otological development may not be normal?

(4) JB has a complete agenesis of the corpus callosum. Which of the following statements best describes the corpus callosum?
   (a) The corpus callosum is a bundle of nerve fibres that connects Broca's area to Wernicke's area.
   (b) The corpus callosum is a part of the brainstem that contains the nuclei of a number of cranial nerves.
   (c) The corpus callosum is a large band of myelinated fibres that connects the two cerebral hemispheres.
   (d) The corpus callosum is part of the primary motor cortex.
   (e) The corpus callosum contains cells which produce the neurotransmitter dopamine.

(5) Speech-language pathologists must have knowledge of karyotypes in order to understand the genetic and chromosomal disorders of their clients. JB has a normal karyotype: 46, XY. Imagine a male client has the following karyotype: 47, XY, + 21. Which of the syndromes below does this client have?
   (a) Williams syndrome
   (b) Cri-du-chat syndrome
   (c) Prader–Willi syndrome
   (d) Down's syndrome
   (e) Fragile X syndrome

Cognitive and developmental assessment

At 3;6 years, JB was assessed using the Bayley Scales of Infant Development (Bayley, 1969). This assessment revealed JB to be in the mild range of mental retardation (intellectual disability). During block manipulation, a mild tremor was noted. When undertaking visual–motor/visual–perceptual tasks, JB was observed to be awkward. Because he was unable to anticipate his own adjustments, JB often knocked down his own construction. His gross motor skills were also awkward, and he frequently tripped. At 3;10 years, JB was assessed using the Denver Developmental Screening (Frankenburg et al., 1968). The results of this assessment were highly varied. JB had personal-social skills at the 4;6 year level. His fine motor skills were at the 3;0 year level. His gross motor skills were solid to the 2;0 year level, with some successes at the 3;0 year level.

A more extensive set of assessments was undertaken at 4;5 years. JB's functioning was described as being in the 'educably mentally retarded range' with some strengths in verbal areas. Visual motor integration and non-verbal conceptual and reasoning skills were noted as problematic areas for JB. On the McCarthy Scales of Children's Abilities (McCarthy, 1972), JB was more than two standard deviations below the mean for his age in all areas except verbal functioning. His performance was lowest on the general cognitive scale, falling more than three standard deviations below the mean. At 5;4 years, JB achieved a mental age of 2;9 years on the Merrill-Palmer Scale of Mental Tests (Stutsman, 1948). This assessment revealed similar strengths and weakness in JB and confirmed his deficit in visual–motor deficits. His scores on the Beery Developmental Test of Visual Motor Integration (Beery, 1989) were commensurate with a 2;10 year level of functioning. Language testing at 5;6 years showed that JB had language skills at the 4;3 year level. JB had difficulties in what the authors of the study described as pragmatic–integrative semantic aspects of language. Overall, these combined tests revealed that verbal skills and self-help areas were strengths for JB, while gross motor skills, fine motor skills and visual motor integration were consistently weak.

Unit 16.2 Cognitive and developmental assessment

(1) Poor visual motor integration was a consistent finding in these various assessments. Explain JB's deficit in this area in terms of his callosal defect.

(2) Gross and fine motor skills were also consistently weak for JB. Give *two* examples of each of these skills.

(3) At 4;5 years, JB was found to have poor non-verbal conceptual and reasoning skills. A possible explanation of JB's difficulties in this area is that he may have bilateral representation of language, thus reducing the non-verbal capacities of the non-dominant (right) hemisphere. What evidence is there to suggest that JB may indeed have bilateral representation of language?

(4) JB's verbal skills were stronger than other aspects of development. However, deficits were noted in what the authors of the study described as pragmatic–integrative semantic aspects of language. Given what you know about the pragmatic interpretation of utterances, why might this aspect of language be compromised in a client with agenesis of the corpus callosum?

(5) Which aspect of JB's performance suggests that a diagnosis of autism spectrum disorder would not be appropriate in his case?

Language assessment at 25 to 34 months

At 25 months, JB's language skills were assessed. JB was found to have a seven-month delay in his receptive language skills and an 11-month delay in his expressive language skills. At 34 months, JB's language skills were assessed again. The gap between his chronological age and his language level had widened. On the Preschool Language Scale (Zimmerman et al., 1979), JB was found to have a 14-month delay in both his receptive and expressive language skills. At 34 months, JB was observed to have mild-to-moderate hearing loss in at least one ear. Immittance audiometry was indicative of a middle ear effusion. JB also experienced periodic wax build-up in both ears. JB's mother reported a significant increase in his vocabulary every time his ears were irrigated.

Unit 16.3 Language assessment at 25 to 34 months

(1) Given what is known about JB's receptive language skills at 34 months, is it likely that he will be able to comprehend sentences that have an *agent–action–object* structure (e.g. 'The mummy feeds the baby')?

(2) Given what is known about JB's expressive language skills at 34 months, is it likely that he will be able to use relational terms such as *more* and *no* (e.g. more juice)?

(3) At 34 months, JB underwent immittance audiometry. Which of the following are *true* statements about this audiological assessment?
    (a) Immittance audiometry is used to test cochlear function.
    (b) Tympanometry is a form of immittance audiometry.
    (c) The contraction of the stapedial muscle to acoustic stimuli cannot be measured by immittance audiometry.
    (d) In the presence of middle ear effusion, there is a greater degree of energy reflected by the eardrum during immittance audiometry.
    (e) Immittance audiometry is used to evaluate middle ear function.

(4) JB has middle ear effusion. Which of the following are *true* statements about this middle ear pathology?
    (a) Middle ear effusion is a common finding in children with a cleft palate.
    (b) Middle ear effusion arises through a lack of adequate ventilation of the inner ear.
    (c) Middle ear effusion leads to sensorineural hearing loss.
    (d) Middle ear effusion can be treated through the use of pressure equalising tubes inserted into the tympanic membrane.
    (e) Middle ear effusion does not have implications for speech and language development.

(5) It is clear that at this early stage of JB's development, his significant receptive and expressive language problems will have implications for his functioning in a number of domains. Describe the impact of his language problems on *two* such domains.

Language assessment at 44 to 54 months

JB's language skills were assessed again at 44 months. His expressive and receptive language skills at this stage were still delayed by 14 months. Additionally, JB displayed mildly disordered articulation which included phoneme substitutions, particularly /t/ for /k/, and some distortions. JB also exhibited a rapid rate of speech and nasal resonance. JB used pantomimic gestures to augment his words and phrases. He tapped or tugged listeners to get their attention, and then delivered his message or request. In one episode where JB wanted one more turn at pushing an equipment card around the room, JB held up one finger of his left hand, then motioned with his right hand in a sweeping circle. At the same time, he uttered 'I wanna push. More push please.' JB was affectionate, talkative and quite active during the assessment.

At 54 months of age, JB had a delay of 21 months in his receptive language skills. His expressive language delay had increased to 24 months. Although his articulation had improved, it was still abnormal, and he had mild but noticeable hypernasality. A cognitive assessment placed him in the mild range of mental retardation (intellectual disability). JB still did not have mastery of colours, shapes and number concepts. JB's sentences were telegraphic, although their content was usually clear. For example, when asked what one should do when tired, JB responded 'I go sleep uncle room, I sleep uncle bed'.

Unit 16.4 Language assessment at 44 to 54 months

(1) What evidence is there that JB may have a mild dysarthria alongside his language problems?

(2) JB has developed strategies for compensating his poor language skills. Describe *two* such strategies.

(3) Notwithstanding his poor structural language skills, there is evidence that JB has a relatively well-developed sense of the pragmatic aspects of language. What is this evidence?

(4) Describe *three* linguistic immaturities in the spoken utterance that JB produced at 54 months.

(5) What class of words is JB omitting in his expressive language to produce the appearance of telegraphic speech?

Language assessment at 67 months

At 67 months, JB achieved a receptive language score on the Preschool Language Scale that placed him 14.5 months below his chronological age. He scored at the 5-year level on some items (e.g. right-left discrimination of his body parts). JB was beginning to show evidence of the understanding of opposites and prepositions as well as agent–action relationships. His expressive language score on the Preschool Language Scale placed him at the 51-month level. On a task of verbal fluency, JB was able to name six animals. He responded correctly to 4 of 5 opposite analogies and to questions about remote events. Although his syntax and ability to express himself were not typical of a 4-year-old child, JB was able to convey clear message content. He was able, for example, to explain through words and pantomimic gesture that it is important to be sure there are 'no cars' when crossing the street. JB does not use conjunctions to link phrases. When asked to produce the names of objects, he produced the following errors: *watch* ('Daddy have a pretty'); *match* ('fire, burns'); *chicken* ('duck'); *shovel* ('rake'). Pauses and fillers are common. Some of JB's language problems are evident in the following exchange with the examiner (EX):

EX: Tell me about your dog.
JB: It go woof woof. I have a doggie, yep.

EX: What's your doggie's name?

JB: Spot. Spot doggie puppy dog. They go pee-pee. Go pee-pee (*pointing to the floor*)
Smell (*holding nose, laughing*)
I go fight doggie (*kicking the air*)
Puppy dog go bite.

Unit 16.5 Language assessment at 67 months

(1) JB undertook a verbal fluency task in which he was asked to produce the names of animals. Is this task assessing JB's semantic memory or phonological memory?

(2) What evidence is there that JB has a word-finding difficulty?

(3) In the short conversational exchange with the examiner, JB produces a number of linguistic forms which are immature for a child of his chronological age. Describe *three* such forms.

(4) JB's first turn in the conversational exchange with the examiner contains a pragmatic anomaly. What is this anomaly?

(5) What evidence is there that JB has relatively intact knowledge of the semantic categories of words?

Case study 17

Boy with Floating-Harbor syndrome

Introduction

The following exercise is a case study of an Italian boy who was studied by Angelillo et al. (2010). This boy has Floating-Harbor syndrome (FHS). FHS is diagnosed on the basis of a triad of clinical signs: specific dysmorphic facial features; short stature with delayed bone age; and speech and language disorders (Pouliquen et al., 2012). The gene(s) that is (are) responsible for the syndrome is (are) currently unknown. Although the majority of FHS cases appear to be sporadic, some appear to follow autosomal dominant inheritance (Lopez et al., 2012). The case study is presented in five sections: medical history and evaluation; cognitive and language profile; speech evaluation; speech and language intervention; and outcome of intervention.

Medical history and evaluation

The boy was born to non-consanguineous parents by caesarean section at 38 weeks' gestation. The pregnancy was uncomplicated and the family history was unremarkable. His birth weight was 2.7 kg and his length was 46 cm. The neonatal course was normal. Apgar scores were 8 and 9 at 1 and 5 minutes, respectively. He began to walk at approximately 14 months. Growth retardation was noted during the first years of life. At 3 years of age, an endocrine assessment for short stature was undertaken. At this stage, his height was 86 cm (<3rd centile) and his weight was 12 kg (<3rd centile). His bone age was 1 year and 9 months. The boy's thyroid function was normal. There was a significant growth hormone (GH) deficit and therapy with recombinant GH was commenced.

The boy was noted to have the typical facial features of Floating-Harbor syndrome. He had a triangular face, a bulging, narrow forehead, a broad, bulbous nose with a prominent nasal bridge, a wide columella and smooth, short philtrum, a thin upper lip, a wide mouth, long eyelashes, posterior rotated ears, a short neck, a low posterior hairline and small hands. A chromosomal examination was conducted and was found to be normal. Hearing and vision were also normal. A microdeletion of 22q11 was excluded. Echocardiography, computerised tomography of the head and magnetic resonance imaging were all normal. Several tests of blood chemistry (e.g. ToRCH assay) produced negative results.

Unit 17.1 Medical history and evaluation

(1) The boy had normal Apgar scores. Speech-language pathologists need to know how these scores are calculated and their significance for the health of a neonate. Briefly describe what these scores mean.

(2) The boy's height and weight at 3 years of age placed him below the 3rd centile. What does this mean?

(3) As part of his facial dysmorphology, the boy was observed to have a wide columella and smooth, short philtrum. What are these facial structures?

(4) A chromosomal examination revealed no abnormalities. Which of the following tests is used to perform such an examination?
   (a) magnetic resonance imaging
   (b) karyotyping
   (c) electroencephalography
   (d) videofluoroscopy
   (e) echocardiography

(5) Neonatal infections were not a cause of this boy's difficulties. Which test was used to exclude these infections? What infections are excluded by this test?

Cognitive and language profile

At 4 years of age, the boy underwent a cognitive assessment. It revealed that he had borderline mental retardation (intellectual disability). His verbal IQ was 65 and his performance IQ was 80. His full IQ was 70. It was judged that receptive linguistic difficulties and a short attention span impaired the result of the test. A further cognitive assessment was undertaken at 6 years of age. Rehabilitation was already underway at this stage. Pantomime was used to measure his non-verbal reasoning abilities independently of language skills. This assessment revealed that he had a non-verbal IQ of 90, which is a low average IQ.

Expressive and receptive language was also assessed at 4 years of age (48 months). The comprehension of words and particularly sentences was delayed. His language age for word and sentence comprehension was 36 to 41 months and 30 to 35 months, respectively. He understood only a few body parts, common objects and adjectives and was not able to recognise colours. The comprehension of actions and spatio-temporal concepts in sentences was severely impaired. His sentence repetition ability was also impaired, with a language age of 30 to 35 months. Only sentences of two or three words were repeated correctly. When asked to repeat longer sentences, the boy omitted words and exhibited speech sound disorders. Naming, sentence production, and phonological and morphosyntactic skills were most impaired. In all four of these areas, the boy had a language age of fewer than 30 months. He was able to name only a few body parts and common objects. He produced only single-word sentences and used mimicry and gestures to communicate. His intelligibility was poor.

Unit 17.2 Cognitive and language profile

(1) During cognitive assessment the boy consistently displayed better non-verbal (performance) IQ than verbal IQ. Is there any evidence that the boy is using his stronger non-verbal cognitive capacities to facilitate communication?

(2) The comprehension of sentences involving spatio-temporal concepts is delayed in this boy. Which of the following sentences require a mastery of these concepts?

(a) She has a black dog.
(b) The car is in the garage.
(c) The boys are playing football.
(d) The book is on the table.
(e) The girl sleeps during the day.

(3) Why might this boy have difficulty understanding the following sentences?
The woman has a red bag.
The flower is yellow.

(4) The boy's performance during language evaluation reveals an interesting interaction between syntax and phonology. What is that interaction?

(5) The boy's morphosyntactic skills are among a number of expressive language skills which are particularly impaired. How might this affect the boy's production of the following sentence: *The boys are running?*

Speech evaluation

A wide-ranging assessment of the boy's speech function was also undertaken at 4 years of age. This included voice, oromotor function, and articulatory and phonological skills. A perceptual and acoustic analysis of voice was performed. A perceptual rating indicated that voice quality was normal. Jitter and shimmer values, which were based on sustained phonation of [a], were also within the normal range. Fundamental frequency was normal. A nasolaryngoscopic evaluation failed to reveal any organic or functional disorder. An evaluation of oromotor function revealed a number of significant findings. They included an open bite malocclusion, slow oral motor speed, poor coordination and hypomobility of the palate, and moderate nasal emission on pressure sounds.

A picture naming test was used to assess articulatory and phonological skills. Only 20% of the words in this test were correctly pronounced. A further 33.6% of words were simplified, while 46.4% of words were unintelligible. All seven Italian vowels were produced correctly. The consonant inventory was very limited. The only sounds that the boy could produce were the plosives /t/ and /p/, the nasals /m/ and /n/, and the affricate /ʧ/ in word-initial and word-medial positions. The lateral /l/ was correctly produced only in word-medial position. This limited inventory found 76% of consonants missing in word-initial position, and 71% of consonants missing in word-medial position. No consonant clusters were produced.

Unit 17.3 Speech evaluation

(1) During the boy's speech evaluation, the following assessment was used: the Grade, Roughness, Breathiness, Asthenia and Strain (GRBAS) scale (Hirano, 1981). Which specific speech function was assessed through the use of the GRBAS scale?

(2) Which of the following are *true* statements about the voice assessment that the boy underwent?
(a) Fundamental frequency is the physical correlate of pitch.
(b) Jitter and shimmer values are obtained by means of an acoustic analysis of the voice.

(c) Lesions of the vocal cords were not excluded during the voice assessment.

(d) During nasolaryngoscopy, a flexible scope is passed into the oral cavity.

(e) Jitter and shimmer are measures of the cycle-to-cycle variations of fundamental frequency and amplitude, respectively.

(3) How would you characterise the function of this boy's velopharyngeal port?

(4) Which specific speech feature suggests that a diagnosis of childhood apraxia of speech would not be appropriate in this case?

(5) This boy is unable to produce any fricative sounds. Describe *two* factors which may contribute to this boy's difficulty in producing fricative sounds.

Speech and language intervention

The boy received speech and language intervention as part of a wide-ranging programme of rehabilitation that involved a number of different professionals. The rehabilitation team included a child neuropsychiatrist, audiologist and phoniatrist, clinical psychologist, sociologist, speech and language therapist, and neuropsychomotor therapist. The boy received four individual speech and language therapy sessions per week. Each session was 45 minutes in duration, with the last 15 minutes reserved for the clinician to discuss progress and homework with the boy's parent.

The boy's cognitive functions were targeted in intervention through the use of computerised cognitive programmes. These functions included attention, memory, information processing, logical reasoning and problem-solving. Activities that involved crumpling, drawing, the use of scissors and cubes, threading and plugging were used to improve eye-to-hand coordination and fine motor functions. Hyperkinetic conduct was targeted through the use of behavioural modification strategies. These same strategies were used to improve attention span, mood control and personal and social functions.

Language training programs were used to improve receptive and expressive language. These involved naming, speech organisation, event description, storytelling and play. To improve speech intelligibility and articulation, speech training programmes involving auditory discrimination, phonological intervention, phonetic training, oral motor coordination and biofeedback were used. The boy's limited consonant inventory and systematic consonant substitutions made his phonology a priority for intervention. Lists of non-words were used to resolve structure processes such as consonant harmony. The non-words each had a plosive phoneme in word-initial position and a fricative phoneme in the intervocalic position. A picture character was associated with each non-word. Non-words were used initially as minimal pairs and then in picture stories. Phonetic training was used to improve the articulation of affricates and of trill /r/. Minimal pairs were also used to improve cluster reduction. Alongside phonological and phonetic intervention, oral motor exercises were used to strengthen the oral muscles and improve their coordination. Writing and reading were areas of difficulty for the boy when he commenced primary school. During the first two years of primary school, he was assigned an auxiliary teacher to assist with the development of these areas.

Unit 17.4 Speech and language intervention

(1) The speech and language therapist is a key member of the multidisciplinary team that is treating this boy. Describe *three* advantages of a multidisciplinary approach to intervention.

(2) Several cognitive functions including attention, memory and problem-solving were addressed during intervention. What umbrella term is used to capture these functions?

(3) Among the tasks used to treat language were event description and storytelling. These tasks address language skills above the level of individual sentences. Which of the following language levels is best addressed by these tasks?
(a) phonology
(b) morphology
(c) syntax
(d) semantics
(e) discourse

(4) Biofeedback was used during the boy's speech training. Which of the following techniques can provide biofeedback for speech production?
(a) videofluoroscopy
(b) nasolaryngoscopy
(c) electropalatograpy
(d) audiometry
(e) nasometry

(5) One of the processes that was targeted during phonological intervention was consonant harmony. Using examples, describe this phonological process.

Outcome of intervention

The child's language skills continued to be tested up to 89 months. His receptive language skills were age-appropriate at 71 months. All expressive language functions continued to improve also. He could speak in longer sentences at 89 months and had an adequate vocabulary at 77 months. By 84 months, his phonological and articulation disorders had disappeared. There was also improvement in his tongue and palate movement. His nasal emission disappeared. Oral motor speed and coordination also improved. Other remediated areas including eye-to-hand coordination, fine motor functions, attention span, mood and hyperactivity control had also improved. By 8 years of age, the boy was in a mainstream class. His linguistic abilities were adequate and he was able to follow the class programme. There were no particular difficulties in learning.

Unit 17.5 Outcome of intervention

(1) The boy received a course of speech and language therapy that lasted 48 months. The authors contend that many of the boy's improvements can be attributed to this intervention. What other factor may also contribute to these improvements?

(2) Nasal emission eventually disappeared from this boy's speech. What *two* factors may have contributed to its disappearance?

(3) The boy's fine motor functions improved as a result of intervention. Name *two* skills that involve these functions.

(4) An early assessment of the boy's intellectual functioning was compromised by two factors. What were these factors? Would they still have an adverse impact on an assessment of intellectual function by the end of intervention?

(5) By the end of intervention, the boy had sufficient language skills to access the school curriculum. What two linguistic skills are particularly important in terms of achieving this access?

Case study 18

Woman aged 28 years with autism

Introduction

The following exercise is a case study of a woman ('Mary') of 28 years of age who was studied by Dobbinson et al. (1998). Mary has autism, a neurodevelopmental disorder which has significant implications for all aspects of an individual's functioning. A clinical description of autism was first given in 1943 by Leo Kanner. Today, a diagnosis of autism is based on criteria that are contained in the Diagnostic and Statistical Manual of Mental Disorders (DSM). For a diagnosis of autism spectrum disorder to be made, the fifth edition of DSM states than an individual must display persistent deficits in social communication and social interaction, and restricted, repetitive patterns of behaviour, interests or activities. Moreover, these symptoms must be present in the early developmental period (American Psychiatric Association, 2013). The case study is presented in five sections: primer on autism spectrum disorder; client history and cognitive-communication status; focus on topic management; focus on conversational overlaps; and focus on conversational pauses.

Primer on autism spectrum disorder

Autism spectrum disorder (ASD) is a common neurodevelopmental disorder which is found in all countries and cultures. In a recent study of the epidemiology of ASD, it was estimated that in 2010 there were an estimated 52 million cases of ASD worldwide (Baxter et al., 2014). This equates to a prevalence of 7.6 per 1,000 population or 1 in 132 persons. Alongside the high prevalence of ASD, there is also evidence that the disorder has a large and increasing incidence, and that there is a significant difference in the number of males and females who develop ASD. Hinkka-Yli-Salomäki et al. (2014) calculated the annual incidence rate in the Finnish population to be 53.7 per 100,000. Also, there was an eightfold increase in the incidence rates of ASD in children born between 1987 and 1992. This study also obtained a sex ratio (boys:girls) of 3.5:1. ASD has a complex, heterogeneous, multifactorial aetiology which involves genetic and neurobiological factors (Parellada et al., 2014). Many individuals with ASD have comorbid conditions such as intellectual disability, epileptic disorders and attention deficit hyperactivity disorder (ADHD) (Memari et al., 2012).

There is a broad spectrum of communicative disability in children and adults with ASD. Approximately 50% of individuals with autistic disorder do not develop functional speech (O'Brien and Pearson, 2004). For those individuals who do become verbal communicators, early vocal anomalies (atypical non-speech vocalisations) as well as receptive and expressive prosodic impairments have been identified (Peppé et al., 2007; Schoen et al., 2011). In terms of phonology, developmental phonological processes (e.g. cluster reduction) and non-developmental errors (e.g. phoneme-specific nasal emission) have been identified in the speech of children with ASD (Cleland et al., 2010). Studies of syntax in ASD have produced conflicting findings. Although some studies have failed to find syntactic deficits in ASD (Allen et al., 2011; Naigles et al., 2011), there is evidence that aspects of complex syntax such as the comprehension of subject and object relative clauses are disrupted (Durrleman et al., 2015). In terms of lexical semantics, word learning in children with ASD is compromised, with impairment related to these children's reduced sensitivity to the social informativeness of gaze cues (Norbury et al., 2010). By far the most significant language deficits in ASD are found in pragmatics. The understanding of figurative utterances, the comprehension of inferred meaning and the appreciation of humour have all been reported to be impaired in ASD (Lewis et al., 2008; MacKay and Shaw, 2004). Children with ASD also have difficulty drawing inferences that are needed to understand metaphor and produce speech acts (Dennis et al., 2001). Not all aspects of pragmatics are impaired in ASD. There is evidence, for example, that scalar inferences are intact in individuals with ASD (Chevallier et al., 2010; Pijnacker et al., 2009).

Unit 18.1 Primer on autism spectrum disorder

(1) Speech-language pathologists have to have basic knowledge of the epidemiology of the disorders they assess and treat. Part of that knowledge involves an understanding of the terms 'prevalence' and 'incidence'. Give a definition of each of these terms.

(2) Why do you think the incidence of ASD is increasing?

(3) Why is the presence of comorbid conditions in ASD of relevance to speech-language pathologists?

(4) According to the above account of language and communication in ASD, the comprehension of each of the following utterances is problematic for individuals with ASD. For each utterance, explain why this is the case.
(a) This is the driver who caused the accident.
(b) Jack left Spain with a heavy heart.
(c) This is the house that the auctioneer sold.
(d) The children were little demons as soon as their parents left.
(e) Pippa had her heart in her mouth on the day of the exam results.

(5) Explain how reduced sensitivity to the social informativeness of gaze cues can compromise word learning.

Client history and cognitive-communication status

Mary is 28 years old. She was diagnosed at 6 years of age with autism. At the time of study, Mary was a resident in a community in Yorkshire, England, for people with autism. The principal caregiver at her residential centre and Mary's parents provided background information for the study. Mary attended playschool and mainstream school despite her mother's concerns that she was experiencing psychological problems. From around the time of her third year, Mary's mother reported that she had concerns about her daughter. Mary exhibited late global development in these early years including delayed walking and spoken language development. Mary's mother recalls her as an anxious child who cried excessively. Mary exhibited no spontaneous play. Instead, she perseveratively waggled objects such as tissues. She did not display ordering or spinning behaviours. Mary preferred to sit on her potty rather than approach her mother for comfort when she was overcome with anxiety. She displayed a lack of interest in her peers and elder sibling. As a child, Mary had imaginary friends. However, these did not assume the role of a passive interlocutor.

Mary is considered by those involved in her care to be a talkative individual. Her talk mostly takes the form of lengthy monologues on her favourite topics. These topics, several of which she pursues obsessively, include the dates of birthdays of her acquaintances, the British royal family and politics. Over time, Mary's obsessive interests can decrease. Mary keeps a diary which she uses to express her anxieties and troubles. She enjoys music and sometimes sings in a monotonous fashion. There is restricted use of tone and pitch movement in her spoken language. Mary can read with comprehension. Her mother taught her to write before beginning school using a system in which specific letters were associated with colours. On the Wechsler Adult Intelligence Scale – Revised (WAIS-R; Wechsler, 1981), Mary had a full scale IQ of 66. There was a slight disparity between her verbal and performance subscale scores which were 70 and 65, respectively. Mary displayed fairly even performance on the verbal tests. Subtest analysis revealed that she had relatively good short-term memory skills for number sequences.

Unit 18.2 Client history and cognitive-communication status

(1) Which aspect of Mary's behaviour in the developmental period reveals a deficit of imagination?

(2) Which aspect of Mary's behaviour in the developmental period reveals a deficit of empathy?

(3) Mary is described as making restricted use of tone and pitch movement in her spoken language. Which of the following aspects of language is disrupted in Mary's case?
   (a) expressive syntax
   (b) receptive prosody
   (c) receptive semantics
   (d) expressive prosody
   (e) expressive phonology

(4) Mary produces lengthy monologues on her favourite topics. Which of the following statements characterise these behaviours?
   (a) Mary is not well oriented to the dyadic structure of conversation.
   (b) Mary selects topics in accordance with the interests of her interlocutor.
   (c) Mary is well oriented to the dyadic structure of conversation.
   (d) Mary contributes irrelevant utterances to conversation.
   (e) Mary does not select topics in accordance with the interests of her interlocutor.

(5) Mary achieved a full-scale IQ of 66 on the WAIS-R. What can be concluded from this result?

Focus on topic management

During a series of visits to Mary's residential centre, conversational data were collected. Audio-recordings were transcribed using the notation shown below. Some sessions were also video-recorded. The conversations were informal in nature, with topics arising naturally between Mary (M) and the researcher (R). Occasionally, other participants were also present. The specific setting of these conversational exchanges varied between rooms in the centre that were used for structured activities, and the living room and kitchen of Mary's satellite house. In extract 1, the conversation opens with Mary and the researcher discussing Mary's participation in the mini-olympics. In extract 2, Mary and the researcher are continuing their conversation from extract 1 with a discussion of Amy's birthday cake. In extract 3, Mary is discussing the topic of housework.

Transcription notation

kind	emphasis
ca::ke	prolongation of sounds
da-	cut-off sounds
(1.3)	timed pause
(.)	micro-pause
[ ]	overlapped speech
=	no interval between speakers
?	rising intonation
.	falling intonation
↑up↑	marked rising tone
↓down↓	marked falling tone
YES	loud volume
°yes°	softness
hhh	out breath
.hhh	in breath
(hhh)	laughter or crying

Extract 1

1   R: what happens at ↑tho::se↑ then.
2   what will happen at them? (.)
3   M: we- well (.) you choose the:: errr (3.66)
4   you choose the:: errr (.) the event that you want to go in (1.87)
5   the eve- it depe- pending on what you're good enough (.)
6   but I want t- to learn how .hhh to get better at badminton so I can play with Amy (.)
7   R: ↑aaa::h↑ does Amy play badminton. =
8   M: = yes she does (1.23)
9   R: is she good at it. (.)
10 M: .hh yes but I've got to get a lot a got to (.) get a lot better (.) a lot better .hhh
11   and last night they went to the er speak up advocacy group .hhh
12   and err (3.28) we signed (.) a birthday card f for Amy from the speak up .hhh
13   advocacy speak up grou::p. .hh and e- (.) and e- (.) Amy was (2.9) cutting her cake
14   cutting her birthday cake .hh and we sang (.) and we all sang happy birthday to
15   Amy (.)
16 R: ↑o:::h↑ that's lovely. (.)
17   how ↑old↑ was she. (.)

18 M: she was twenty ni:ne. (.)
19   she'll be <u>thirty</u> next year (.)
20 R: she <u>wi::ll</u>. (.)
21   is she ↑old↑er than you. (.)
22 M: yes she is (.)
23 R: how [<u>old</u> are] you.
24 M: [two year]
25   two years old (.) she's two years older than me (.)
26   I'm twenty six (.)
27   I'll be twenty <u>seven</u> in er (.) September.
28 R: aa:::h ri::ght (1.12)
29   so- (.) you had a ↑<u>birthday</u>↑ party then. (1.26)
30 M: .hh we sa- (.) we sang (.) Amy took her birthday cake to the sp- (.) advocacy speak up
31   group for everybody to have. (1.24)
32 R: w- who made her ↑<u>birthday</u>↑ cake for her.

Extract 2

1   M: errrr (.) Juliette went down to the (1.05) cake shop to order it for her
2   and Patty (.) brought it up to the erm (.) the <u>day</u> centre for her. (1.69)
3   R: that's <u>lovely</u>
4   that was <u>kind</u> of them. wasn't it. (.)
5   M: yes (.)
6   R: and was it a sur↑<u>prise</u>↑. (.)
7   M: it was a surprise yes .hhhh
8   it was a (.) it was a very nice birthday ca:ke. (.)
9   R: what was it li:ke. (1.27)
10 M: I had a look at it (.) and it was <u>pink</u> and it was very nice (.)
11   and Gloria (1.19) wh gl- gl- Gloria came down .hhhh to the day centre she says to me
12   <u>what's that</u> (.)
13   she says to Amy wh- what's that is that- is that a- (1.01) is that a <u>cake</u>
14   or- (.) is that a pi- (.) is
15   that (.) <u>cake</u> or piece of or or is it a <u>rabbit</u>. (1.03)
16 R: (hhhhhhhhh) .hhh
17   why was it- why did she say <u>that</u>. (.)
18 M: just a joke. (.)
19 R: why- (.) what was (.) why =
20 M: = when I was walking up with <u>Katy Post</u>. (2.09)
21 R: aa:::h right
22   <u>why</u> did she make a joke like <u>that</u>
23   why [was that]
24 M: [she was just] saying it (1.72)
25 R: what did the cake <u>look</u> like. (.)
26 M: it looked <u>very</u> ni::ce. (1.10)
27 R: wh- what <u>shape</u> was it. (1.13)
28 M: it's like a <u>hea:rt</u> shape. (.) but she still got some left for toni::ght. (.)
29 R: ↑aa↑:::::h. (1.37)
30   what [<u>colour</u>]

31 M: [en we-] en we had that (.)
32   its <u>pink</u> (.)
33   en we had that errr- (.) <u>choc</u>olate gateau for- (1.08) that we we
34   bought with Kirsty (1.07) .hhh
35   l- (.) last ni::ght (.) with <u>Katy Post</u> that we bought with <u>Kirsty Barker</u>
36   the day .hh from the
37   <u>Lo</u>-Cost. (.) the errr the <u>night</u> before .hhh for <u>Amy</u>'s <u>birth</u>day. (1.39)
38   that we had it after tea last ni::ght (.)
39 R: chocolate ↑<u>gat</u>↑eau. (.)
40 M: ye:s (.)
41 R: was it <u>ni::ce</u>.

Extract 3

M: .hh I'd made ss- (1.64) ev <u>yesterday</u>::y (.) I made some errrr (4.71) apple (.) fr- <u>fruit</u>
crumble with er- <u>Anita</u> (.) then err (.) Matt Lewis hoovered the the the landing downstairs
.hhh I hoovered the hallway (1.26) downstairs (.) I hoovered the <u>stairs</u> and hoovered the
<u>land</u>ing upstairs. .hhh and then errr (.) then I hoovered (.) the the <u>lounge</u> room and I
dusted and <u>polished</u> (.) the <u>lounge</u> room. (.) then I hoovered th (.) the dining room then
er (.) then helped <u>Anita Sales</u> to err (.) to mow the back (.) back <u>lawn</u> with a <u>lawn</u>mower
(.) at Bankfield yesterda::y (1.27)

Unit 18.3 Focus on topic management

(1) In extract 1, several topics feature in the exchange between Mary and the researcher.
     The conversation begins with a discussion of the mini-olympics, moves onto Amy
     playing badminton, then addresses Amy's birthday, then moves to Amy's and Mary's
     respective ages before returning to the topic of Amy's birthday. How are these topics
     introduced and managed by Mary and the researcher?

(2) Cohesive devices also play a role in topic management in conversation. Using data in
     extract 1, give *one* example of each of the following types of cohesion:
     (a) personal reference
     (b) demonstrative reference
     (c) ellipsis
     (d) conjunctions
     (e) lexical reiteration

(3) In extract 2, Mary is able to contribute to the topic of the birthday cake at the outset
     of the exchange. However, between lines 17 and 32 there is a noticeable decrease in
     Mary's ability to contribute to the topic. How is this manifested by Mary and how does
     the researcher maintain the conversational exchange in the face of it?

(4) Topics can be developed in ways which may be more or less successful in engaging the
     interest of an interlocutor in conversation. Several devices may be used to this end. In
     extract 2, Mary uses one such device between lines 11 and 15. Describe the device in
     question.

(5) In extract 3, Mary is discussing the topic of housework. How does she manage to
     maintain this topic over a single, extended turn?

Focus on conversational overlaps

When speech takes place simultaneously between the participants in a conversational exchange, overlaps arise. Overlaps can occur for a number of reasons including a desire to take the turn from the current speaker and to support a speaker in his or her turn (e.g. the use of backchannel behaviours such as 'uh-huh'). The management of overlapping talk requires conversational skills which may not be present in individuals with autism spectrum disorder. It is interesting to consider if Mary, who makes extensive use of overlapping talk, exhibits the skills that are needed to manage this talk. To this end, consider the following conversational extracts between Mary and the researcher:

Extract 1

1 M: it's like a <u>hea:rt</u> shape. (.) but she still got some left for
toni::ght. (.)
2 R: ↑aa↑:::::h. (1.37)
3   what [<u>colour</u>]
4 M: [en we-] en we had that (.)

Extract 2

1 R: ↑mmm↑hm. (2.09)
2   why –why do you <u>fee::l</u> like you don't want to go
↑swim↑ming sometimes. (.)
3 M: I just ↑<u>do</u>↑ someti:mes (.)
4 R: don't you want to get <u>wet</u>. (2.97)
5   does it- does it <u>not</u> [feel]
6 M: [because] I want to do the same things as what
7   Matt Lewis and Peter Smith do. (.)

Extract 3

1 R: ↑aa↑ah::. (.)
2   is that (.) one of those pools that's got (.) <u>slides</u> [and] things.
3 M: [yes] (.)
4   slides and things (.)

Extract 4

1 R: but Ella and Haley didn't. (.)
2 M: no she just saw Elly and she (.) [told (1.00) told] Ella (.)
3 R: [oh she told Ella]
4   yeah (1.34)
5   that's ↑<u>bril</u>↑liant

Unit 18.4 Focus on conversational overlaps

(1) In line 4 in extract 1, Mary overlaps with the researcher. What function is served by Mary's overlapped talk in this exchange?

(2) Mary engages in further overlapped talk in extract 2. Why does this overlap occur? How does this overlap differ from the overlap in extract 1?

(3) By way of explanation of the overlaps in extracts 1 and 2, the authors of the study consider the possibility that they reveal slowed cognitive processing on Mary's part. What features of these overlaps support this explanation?

(4) A further overlap occurs in extract 3. Is slowed cognitive processing on Mary's part a likely explanation of the overlap in this exchange?

(5) In extract 4, the researcher produces overlapped talk. The researcher's overlapped talk appears to have a quite different purpose to those seen in the overlapped sequences in extracts 1 to 3. How would you characterise that purpose?

Focus on conversational pauses

Mary's conversational data contains many pauses, a substantial number of which are of long duration (they exceed 1 second). Pauses are often revealing of the cognitive processes that attend conversation, with both their location and duration conveying important information about their function. Several of Mary's long pauses are shown below:

Extract 1

M: we- well (.) you choose the:: errr (3.66) you choose the:: errr (.) the _event_ that you want to go in (1.87) the eve- it depe- pending on what you're good enough (.)

Extract 2

M: and last night they went to the er speak up advocacy group .hhh and err (3.28) we signed (.) a birthday card f for Amy from the speak up .hhh advocacy speak up grou::p. .hh and e- (.) and e- (.) Amy was (2.9) cutting her cake cutting her birthday cake .hh and we sang (.) and we all sang happy birthday to Amy (.)

Extract 3

M: I'd made ss- (1.64) ev _yesterday_::y (.) I made some errr (4.71) apple (.) fr- _fruit_ crumble

Extract 4

R: (1.7) can you _na:me_ a prime minister of _great_ Britain during the second world war.
M: (7.0) was it John Astley.
R: (3.4) °that's a good answer° (2.4) right (0.7) okay (.) who wrote _Ham_let.
M: (2.8) I don't know

Extract 5

R: ↑ye↑a::h. (2.45) what does everybody _else_ do at the swimming pool (.) do they a:ll =

M: = just have a swim abo- (.) bou::t (.) Elly Grey (2.15) guess what (.) Elly Grey came came back to Bankfield once. and she told (1.14) whoever was on that she she'd done (1.05) <u>thirty</u> lengths (.) across the swimming pool

Unit 18.5 Focus on conversational pauses

(1) Two long pauses occur in extract 1. Why do you think these pauses have arisen? Support your explanation with evidence.

(2) Two long pauses also occur in extract 2. One is a grammatical pause and the other is a non-grammatical pause. State which term applies to each of these pauses.

(3) In extract 3, Mary uses two long pauses which appear to be related to a word search. Describe *three* features of this extract which suggest that these pauses are related to a word search.

(4) In extract 4, Mary is responding to questions in the information subtest of the WAIS-R. Although long pauses precede each of her answers, the first of her pauses is significantly longer than the second pause. How would you explain the difference in the duration of these pauses?

(5) The long pauses in extracts 1 to 4 all appear to be related to aspects of cognitive processing such as lexical retrieval. Does the pause of 2.15 seconds in extract 5 also appear to be related to cognitive processing? Provide evidence to support your answer.

Case study 19

Girl with Sturge–Weber syndrome

Introduction

The following exercise is a case study of a girl ('CA') who was studied between 7;11 and 13;01 years by Lovett et al. (1986) and Dennis and Whitaker (1976). CA has Sturge–Weber syndrome (SWS). This is a rare, congenital neurocutaneous condition which has an incidence of approximately 1 in 20,000 to 50,000 infants (Garro and Bradshaw, 2014). It is characterised by capillary malformation of the face (port-wine birthmark), a capillary-venous malformation in the eye, and a capillary-venous malformation in the brain known as a leptomeningeal angioma (Comi, 2011). Seizures are a common feature of SWS. Sujansky and Conradi (1995) reported seizures in 80% of a sample of 171 individuals with SWS. In CA's case, seizures were controlled by a left hemispherectomy which was performed when she was 28 days old. The case study is presented in five sections: primer on epilepsy in Sturge–Weber syndrome; medical history; language and cognitive assessment; language and cognitive profile; and focus on narrative discourse production.

Primer on epilepsy in Sturge–Weber syndrome

Although SWS is a congenital condition, its early diagnosis is impaired by the poor sensitivity of imaging in the neonatal period and infancy (Comi, 2007). The presence at birth of a facial angioma in the trigeminal nerve area raises a suspicion of SWS (Nabbout and Juhász, 2013). However, there are rare cases of the syndrome in the absence of a port-wine stain (Shekhtman et al., 2013). Most individuals with SWS survive into adulthood with varying degrees of neurological impairment. This includes epilepsy, hemiparesis, visual field deficits and cognitive impairments that range from mild learning disabilities to severe deficits (Comi, 2011). It has been suggested that epileptogenesis is caused by chronic ischaemia in cortical areas that are affected by leptomeningeal angioma or by ischaemia-related cortical malformations (Murakami et al., 2012). In one clinical sample, the age of seizure onset ranged from birth to 23 years, with 75% of individuals experiencing the onset of seizures before 1 year of age (Sujansky and Conradi, 1995). Parents can be trained to use benzodiazepines to treat seizures. However, in patients with intractable epilepsy, surgery may be considered (Nabbout and Juhász, 2013).

SWS and related epilepsy have adverse implications for the language, cognitive and academic skills of children with the disorder. Suskauer et al. (2010) reported expressive language delays in 9 of 14 infants aged 0 to 3 years with SWS. None of these children had receptive language problems. Raches et al. (2012) found that a group of SWS children with seizures were more impaired than seizure-free children with SWS on 9 of 15 measures of behavioural and academic functioning. Moreover, children with seizures were more than 10 times as likely as seizure-free children to have received special education services.

Treatment of intractable epilepsy in the form of hemispherectomy also has implications for language and cognitive skills. Mariotti et al. (1998) examined language and visuospatial abilities in a patient who underwent early removal of the left hemisphere on account of SWS. This patient's language skills were mildly impaired but equivalent to those of IQ controls. Non-literal language comprehension was intact. However, visuospatial skills were worse than those of IQ controls. Vargha-Khadem et al. (1997) reported the case of a boy with SWS whose comprehension of single words and simple commands did not progress beyond an age equivalent of 3 to 4 years. Following left hemidecortication performed at 8.5 years, there was a rapid improvement in his speech and language skills, with receptive and expressive language on testing at the end of the period of study (15 years) placing him at an age equivalent of 8 to 10 years.

Unit 19.1 Primer on epilepsy in Sturge–Weber syndrome

(1) Which of the following structures are compromised by a leptomeningeal angioma?
   (a) basal ganglia
   (b) pia mater
   (c) brainstem
   (d) arachnoid membrane
   (e) internal carotid artery

(2) Which of the following cerebral abnormalities occur in SWS?
   (a) cerebral calcification
   (b) hydrocephalus
   (c) agenesis of the corpus callosum
   (d) cerebral atrophy
   (e) white matter abnormalities

(3) The boy studied by Vargha-Khadem et al. (1997) experienced a protracted period of mutism prior to hemispherectomy. The use of augmentative and alternative communication (AAC) may be warranted in such a case. Which *three* neurological deficits in SWS must be considered within the selection of an appropriate form of AAC?

(4) Which of the following aspects of language is intact in the case studied by Mariotti et al. (1998)?
   (a) phonology
   (b) morphology
   (c) syntax
   (d) semantics
   (e) pragmatics

(5) The cases studied by Mariotti et al. (1998) and Vargha-Khadem et al. (1997) both had unexpected language outcomes following a left hemispherectomy. In what respect were these clients' language outcomes unexpected?

Medical history

When CA was born, she had a marked port-wine stain on the left side of her face and over the distribution of the trigeminal nerve on the right. Immediately after birth, there was twitching of the right arm and leg which soon progressed to right-sided seizures. At 6 days of age, CA was admitted to hospital with twitching of her right arm. An X-ray revealed her skull to be within normal limits in size and contour and there was no evidence of increased intracranial pressure. An EEG showed a significant asymmetry, with a depression of voltage over the left hemisphere. At 28 days of age, CA underwent a left hemispherectomy. During surgery, the exposed cortex was plum-coloured over its surface and the arachnoid was dense purple in some areas. On gross examination, the brain tissue was softer than normal. The complete left hemisphere was removed in stages. The basal ganglia were spared. Pathological examination revealed a haemangioma of the meninges and calcification and gliosis of the sub-adjacent cortex. Focal areas of calcification were found in all lobes of the cortex. For the most part, it was confined to the white matter, although it was also scattered throughout the grey matter as well. There was some alteration of cortical grey matter in the parieto-temporal lobe. Following surgery, CA displayed some questionable right-sided twitching for which she received anticonvulsive medication. After 10 days, this medication was discontinued. An EEG performed after surgery revealed no evidence of right-sided seizures. At the time of study, CA has a spastic hemiplegia. However, she has remained free of seizures in the nine-year period following surgery.

Unit 19.2 Medical history

(1) Clinical descriptions of SWS refer to the presence of a port-wine birthmark in the distribution of the trigeminal nerve. What is the trigeminal nerve? What is the function of this nerve in speech and hearing?

(2) What is the significance of the colouring of the cortex and arachnoid during surgery?

(3) Which of the following brain structures was *not* removed during CA's hemispherectomy?
   (a) right parietal lobe
   (b) left temporal lobe
   (c) right putamen
   (d) left frontal lobe
   (e) left caudate nucleus

(4) A hemispherectomy was performed on CA just days after birth. Apart from achieving seizure control, describe *one* advantage of undertaking this procedure early.

(5) CA exhibits a cortical grey matter anomaly in the parieto-temporal lobe. Which of the following neuroanatomical structures are likely to be compromised as a result?
   (a) Broca's area
   (b) brainstem
   (c) Wernicke's area
   (d) cerebellar vermis
   (e) corpus callosum

Language and cognitive assessment

CA's language and cognitive skills were extensively examined between 7;11 and 9;7 years. The content of the standardised assessments only will be examined in this unit. The results of these tests will be discussed in unit 19.4. At 9;5 years, CA's language skills were tested on the Illinois Test of Psycholinguistic Abilities (ITPA; Kirk et al., 1968). This wide-ranging assessment employs 10 subtests to examine comprehension, association and expression across auditory, visual and manual modalities. For example, the subtest on grammatic closure measures a subject's ability to use proper grammatical forms to complete a statement (e.g. 'Here is a dog. Here are two _____'). The manual expression subtest measures a subject's ability to express an idea with gestures (e.g. 'Show me what to do with a hammer'). The scores on each subtest are expressed as age equivalences. Phoneme discrimination was assessed using the Auditory Discrimination Test (Wepman, 1958) and the Goldman–Fristoe-Woodstock Test of Auditory Discrimination (Goldman et al., 1970). In the former test, subjects are presented with word pairs and asked to determine if they are the same words or different words. In word pairs which are different, phonemes from the category of stops, for example, will be replaced by other stops. In the latter assessment, a word is read to subjects who then select a picture from a set of four pictures that corresponds to it. Phoneme production was assessed using the Goldman–Fristoe Test of Articulation (Goldman and Fristoe, 1969). Subjects are shown pictures of familiar objects which they are required to name.

Word comprehension was tested using the Peabody Picture Vocabulary Test (PPVT; Dunn, 1965) and the Word Discrimination Test (WDT; Goodglass and Kaplan, 1972a). In the PPVT, subjects select a picture from a set of four that corresponds to a spoken word. The WDT assesses comprehension of words in six semantic categories: objects; geometric forms; activities; letters; colours; and numbers. Word production was assessed by means of Visual Confrontation Naming (Goodglass and Kaplan, 1972a), Responsive Naming (Goodglass and Kaplan, 1972a) and Naming Fluency (Goodglass and Kaplan, 1972a). The first of these assessments examines production of words in the same six semantic categories used in the WDT. Auditorily cued word retrieval is assessed in Responsive Naming. In Naming Fluency, subjects have to name as many animals as possible in 90 seconds. The word 'dog' is given to initiate a response. The Test of Syntactic Comprehension (Parisi and Pizzamiglio, 1970) was used to assess the comprehension of a range of simple and complex syntactic contrasts (e.g. direct–indirect object). Comprehension of affirmative and negative active and passive sentences was tested using the Active–Passive Test (Dennis and Kohn, 1975). The Story Completion Test (Goodglass et al., 1972) examines subjects' productive control of syntactic forms. Sentences are presented orally to subjects who must complete them with a highly predictable final sentence or phrase, e.g. 'I sold her a small car. The car was red. In other words I sold her _____' (response: a small red car). The Token Test (De Renzi and Vignolo, 1962) was used to assess comprehension of commands which vary in information and syntactic complexity. The commands presented in the five parts of this test are:

Part 1: 'Touch the red circle'
Part 2: 'Touch the small red circle'
Part 3: 'Touch the yellow circle and the red rectangle'
Part 4: 'Touch the small blue circle and the large green circle'
Part 5: 'Touch the yellow circle with the blue rectangle'

Finally, intellectual functioning was assessed using the Wechsler Intelligence Scale for Children (WISC; Wechsler, 1976). The WISC is used to obtain a verbal and performance IQ as well as a full-scale IQ.

Unit 19.3 Language and cognitive assessment

(1) CA has a spastic hemiplegia. Other children with SWS can have visual field deficits. How might these difficulties compromise the aforementioned assessments?

(2) The following item is taken from the grammatic closure subtest of the ITPA: 'Here is a dog. Here are two _____'. This item is assessing the use of a specific linguistic structure. What is that structure?

(3) The Naming Fluency test asks subjects to name as many animals as possible within 90 seconds. Which of the following cognitive skills is assessed by this test?
    (a) phonological memory
    (b) cognitive flexibility
    (c) inhibition of prepotent responses
    (d) semantic memory
    (e) attention

(4) The Active–Passive Test assesses comprehension of the following types of sentence. Using the labels *active, passive, affirmative* and *negative*, characterise the syntactic structure of each of these sentences:
    (a) The girls were not attacked by the dog.
    (b) She slammed the gate behind her.
    (c) Fran did not lock the car.
    (d) The confidential papers were shredded by the secretary.
    (e) Mark and John were not pursued by the gang.

(5) In which two parts of the Token Test is (a) the informational load of commands increased, and (b) the syntactic complexity of commands increased?

Language and cognitive profile

On the ITPA, CA had a composite psycholinguistic age of 7;3 years which was well below her CA of 9;5 years. Her best performances were on the auditory reception, visual reception and visual memory subtests (age equivalents of 8;4, 8;10 and 8;4 years, respectively), while her worst performances were on the visual association, verbal expression and visual closure subtests (age equivalents of 6;6, 6;0 and 6;6 years, respectively). Phoneme discrimination and production were areas of relative strength, with the percentage of correct responses on the Auditory Discrimination Test, the Goldman–Fristoe-Woodstock Test of Auditory Discrimination, and the Goldman–Fristoe Test of Articulation 97.5%, 87.0% and 100%, respectively. The PPVT was performed at 7;11 years. CA's mental age on this test was 7;5 years and her IQ was 95. The percentage of correct responses on Word Discrimination, Visual Confrontation Naming and Responsive Naming was 98.6%, 99.0% and 90.0%, respectively. CA was able to name 10 animals in the most fluent 60-second period during Naming Fluency. Children of a similar age to CA typically produce 12 animal names in 60 seconds. The Test of Syntactic Comprehension was performed at 9;6 years, with CA achieving 93.4% correct responses. The Active–Passive Test was also performed at 9;6 years. Although CA displayed relatively good comprehension of active sentences (active affirmatives: 90.6%; active negatives: 84.4%), comprehension of passives was considerably poorer (passive affirmatives: 50.0%; passive negatives: 71.9%). The large majority of CA's responses on the Story Completion Test (78.2%) showed that she had productive control of grammatical constructions. The Token Test was performed at 8;0 years. On the first four parts of this test, CA achieved 100% correct responses. However, this dropped to 77.3% on part 5. Finally, on the WISC, CA's verbal IQ was 91, her performance IQ was 108 and her full-scale IQ was 99.

Unit 19.4 Language and cognitive profile

(1) Is there any evidence of a dissociation of auditory and visual modalities in CA's comprehension of language?

(2) Respond with *true* or *false* to each of the following statements:
   (a) CA has a reduced system of phonological contrasts.
   (b) CA's receptive vocabulary is within the normal range.
   (c) CA has intact category fluency.
   (d) CA displays superior naming in response to auditory over visual cues.
   (e) CA displays superior confrontation naming for animate over inanimate items.

(3) On the Active–Passive Test, CA's performance on active sentences is relatively strong but is little more than at chance levels on passive sentences. Why do you think this is the case?

(4) Which factor – informational load or syntactic complexity – best explains CA's performance on the Token Test?

(5) On the basis of CA's performance across these different language tests, which of the following aspects of language appears to be most disrupted by the surgical removal of the left hemisphere?
   (a) phoneme production
   (b) word comprehension
   (c) phoneme discrimination
   (d) syntactic comprehension
   (e) word production

Focus on narrative discourse production

At 13;01 years, CA's narrative discourse skills were examined. Four narrative texts were used to investigate narrative production: 'Little Red Riding Hood'; 'The Frog Prince'; 'The Practical Princess'; and 'Goldilocks'. Only two of these texts – 'Little Red Riding Hood' and 'Goldilocks' – will be discussed in this unit. Each text was read to CA by the examiner. At the same time, puppets were used to perform the roles of the main protagonists. After hearing each narrative, CA retold the story to the examiner, using the puppets as and when required. The narratives were audio-recorded and transcribed.

'Little Red Riding Hood' text related to CA

The wolf got there first. He knocked at the door. "Who's there?" said Grandmother. "Little Red Riding Hood", said the wolf. "Oh, come in", said Grandmother. And the wolf came in, locked Grandmother in a cupboard and put on all her clothes. Then Little Red Riding Hood came to the house and knocked on the door. "Who's there?" said the wolf. Little Red Riding Hood thought her grandmother sounded funny and she wondered if she had a cold. "It's Little Red Riding Hood", she said. "Come in", said the wolf.

CA's retelling

And then when the wolf got there she knocked on the door and- um- the Grandmother came and she answered the door and she said, "Um- hello-" No- he said, "Who's there?" And the wolf said, "Little Red Riding Hood". So she opened the door. Then- uh- the wolf grabbed her and he locked her up into the closet. And then she put on all her clothes and everything like that. And then later on Little Red Riding Hood came to the door and then she knocked on the door. And then the wolf said, "Who is it?" And the Little Red Riding Hood said, "It's Little Red Riding Hood". So she came in. So when she- when she came in.

'Goldilocks' text related to CA

They went into the bedroom. Now Goldilocks had pulled the pillow on Father Bear's bed. He cried out, "Someone's been sleeping in my bed!" in his big rough voice. And Goldilocks had messed up the sheets in Mother Bear's bed. She said, "Who's been sleeping in my bed?" And when Baby Bear came to look at his bed, there was a big lump in the bed. He cried out, "Someone's been sleeping in my bed, and SHE'S STILL THERE!!" Goldilocks woke up suddenly. When she saw the bears she was quite frightened. They said angrily, "Why do you come into our house and eat our porridge and break our chairs and sleep in our beds?" And they chased Goldilocks out of the house and into the woods. And the three bears never saw anything more of her.

CA's retelling

And then they went – they went to their beds. And then Father Bear said, "Who's been sleeping in my bed because my little pillows gone-been-loose?" And Mother Bear says, "Who's been sleeping in my bed?" because the sheets were all crimpled-like. And then Baby Bear said, "Who's been sleeping in my bed because she's still here!" And then Gol- then they went to Baby Bear's bed and then they saw Goldilocks. And then Goldilocks woke up and she was surpri- she was astoniged then she ran out the door. They never saw her again.

Unit 19.5 Focus on narrative discourse production

(1) In CA's retelling of 'Little Red Riding Hood', there are a number of noteworthy linguistic and discourse features. Several of these are listed below. Give *one* example of each feature:
  (a) CA uses an incorrect subject pronoun.
  (b) CA displays self-initiated repair.
  (c) CA reports events in the wrong order.
  (d) CA uses non-specific language.
  (e) CA uses direct reported speech.

(2) Does CA omit any story elements during her retelling of 'Little Red Riding Hood'? If an omission does occur, how might it be explained?

(3) In 'Goldilocks', CA misrepresents the order in which events took place. Where does this occur? What linguistic device is CA not using correctly for this misrepresentation to occur?

(4) When Goldilocks is discovered by the bears, she is portrayed as having a certain affective mental state. What is that state, and does CA succeed in representing it?

(5) Across both narratives, CA tends to overuse a somewhat immature linguistic device to link clauses and events in her stories. What is this device, and what semantic meaning does it express?

Case study 20

Man aged 47 years with temporal lobe epilepsy

Introduction

The following exercise is a case study of a man ('DL') aged 47 years who was studied by Smith Doody et al. (1992). DL developed temporal lobe epilepsy subsequent to encephalitis. He exhibited recurrent fluent aphasia in association with his temporal lobe seizure activity. Post-encephalitic epilepsy is a relatively common neurological disorder which has implications for speech and language. It is thus a disorder which falls within the professional remit of speech-language pathologists. The case study is presented in five sections: primer on post-encephalitic epilepsy; medical history; cognitive assessment; language assessment; and focus on expressive language.

Primer on post-encephalitic epilepsy

Adult-onset epilepsies can be caused by a number of diseases and injuries. These epilepsies may arise on account of cerebral infections like viral encephalitis and bacterial meningitis. They may also be caused by cerebrovascular disease, tumours, neurosurgical procedures and traumatic brain injuries. Epilepsy is a relatively common neurological sequela in adults who develop encephalitis. Singh et al. (2015) examined 198 adults aged 41 to 69 years with acute encephalitis. These investigators reported post-encephalitic epilepsy in 29.9% of patients. Seizures were most commonly found in adults with auto-immune encephalitis (54.5%). However, viral encephalitis (24.2%) and encephalitis of unknown or other aetiology (33.9%) were also associated with seizure activity. Encephalitis is increasingly being linked to adult-onset temporal lobe epilepsy. Bien et al. (2007) examined 38 patients with temporal lobe epilepsy whose median age at onset was 37.8 years. Nine patients (24%) had a diagnosis of definite auto-immune encephalitis, and a further 11 patients (29%) had a diagnosis of possible auto-immune encephalitis. In a study of 74 adults who underwent temporal lobectomy, Uesugi et al. (1998) related the onset of temporal lobe epilepsy to undiagnosed episodes of mild encephalitis/meningitis in childhood.

Post-encephalitic epilepsy is associated with a range of language and cognitive problems. Kishi et al. (2010) reported the case of a 59-year-old woman with limbic encephalitis who presented with severe anterograde and retrograde memory impairment and transient fluent, phonemic paraphasia. Bianchi et al. (2009) examined five patients with adult-onset, medically intractable, post-encephalitic epilepsy. These patients experienced auditory auras which ranged from unformed buzzing to structured language. Okuda et al. (2001) reported the case of a 25-year-old woman who developed pure anomic aphasia following encephalitis. The patient's naming difficulty persisted during a two-year follow-up period in the absence of any other language or memory dysfunction.

Unit 20.1 Primer on post-encephalitic epilepsy

(1) Which of the following pathogens is a cause of viral encephalitis?
   (a) streptococcus
   (b) varicella zoster
   (c) candida albicans
   (d) herpes simplex
   (e) E. coli

(2) *True* or *false*: Limbic encephalitis may have an infectious or autoimmune aetiology.

(3) *True* or *false*: Word-finding difficulties are rarely found in temporal lobe epilepsy.

(4) *True* or *false*: An individual with anterograde amnesia following encephalitis is unable to form new memories.

(5) Okuda et al.'s subject developed anomic aphasia following encephalitis. Which of the following linguistic deficits occurs in anomic aphasia?
   (a) jargon output
   (b) verbal perseveration
   (c) word-finding difficulty
   (d) agrammatism
   (e) dyslexia

Medical history

DL is a 47-year-old, right-handed, Hispanic man. In March 1988, he experienced a headache. This was followed by fever and a right focal seizure which then generalised. He was admitted to hospital with a diagnosis of encephalitis. After discharge, he did well for a 2-month period but was then readmitted for the sudden onset of confusion. A left frontal brain biopsy was performed, but it was non-diagnostic. DL was discharged on Dilantin and phenobarbital. He was admitted again seven months later for worsening mental status and received a 10-day course of acyclovir. Over time, DL improved to a baseline of good functioning but he was unable to return to work. His family reported that he understood all but the most difficult discussions and continued to read. Apart from his finances, which he was not able to handle without assistance, DL was able to take care of his usual activities. His medication at this stage was 200 mg Dilantin by mouth twice a day. Phenobarbital was being tapered.

On 23 September 1989, DL was admitted to the Houston Veterans Affairs Medical Center for the sudden onset of altered mental status. That morning, he had been feeling well and was talking to his family about job prospects. They left him and returned half an hour later to find him crying and confused. He was unable to explain what was wrong. An examination of his mental status in hospital revealed him to be alert but disoriented to person, place, time and situation. He displayed a receptive aphasia. A general physical examination was normal. A general neurological examination revealed only a slight circumduction of the right lower extremity. CBC (complete blood count) and

SMAC (a broad screening tool to evaluate organ function) were normal. Thyroid function tests, vasculitis screen and cerebrospinal fluid examination were also normal. An MRI showed a slight, generalised increase in ventricular size but no other focal abnormalities since his post-craniotomy study performed 16 months earlier. An EEG was conducted the morning after admission. There was recurrent moderate to high voltage spike, and slow and sharp and slow wave activity in the left temporal region which occurred every 1 to 3 seconds. Two episodes of staring with unresponsiveness occurred on the second hospital day. These correlated with continuous spike and wave discharges in the left temporo-occipital region on EEG. DL was given 10 mg of Valium without clinical effect. He was loaded with 500 mg Dilantin and 60 mg phenobarbital. In a follow-up EEG, there was a left temporal slow wave focus with frequent spikes and sharp waves and a normal background.

Unit 20.2 Medical history

(1) On his third admission to hospital, DL received a 10-day course of acyclovir. What type of encephalitis is suggested by the administration of this drug?

(2) What may have compromised the assessment of DL's orientation to person, place, time and situation?

(3) Are DL's neurological problems likely to be caused by (a) bacterial meningitis, (b) a metabolic disorder or (c) cerebrovascular disease? Provide evidence to support your answer.

(4) An EEG revealed abnormal electrical activity in the left temporal region. The function of which language centre is likely to be disrupted by this activity?

(5) On the basis of the above information, is DL's receptive aphasia mild, moderate or severe? Provide evidence to support your answer.

Cognitive assessment

Early on the fifth day of hospitalisation, DL's cognitive skills were assessed using the Mini-Mental State Examination (MMSE; Folstein et al., 1975). This assessment contains five subtests: orientation; registration; attention and calculation; recall; and language. DL spelled the word 'world' backwards quickly and without errors, but made two errors when he attempted to state the months of the year backwards. When questioned in writing, he was fully oriented (he scored 9/10 correct). However, he did not comprehend the orientation questions when orally questioned. He was able to copy the drawing on the MMSE correctly. Comprehension difficulties precluded an assessment of visual memory and verbal memory. He was accurate on the Digit–Symbol substitution subtest of the Wechsler Adult Intelligence Scale-Revised (WAIS-R; Wechsler, 1981). DL was unable to complete the sequence 1–A, 2–B, 3–C, and so on. He made three omission errors on the 'A's test' of vigilance. DL displayed inconsistent insight into his situation.

Unit 20.3 Cognitive assessment

(1) Assign each of the following tasks to one of the five subtests of the Mini-Mental State Examination:

(a) Subject is asked to spell 'world' backwards.

(b) Subject is asked to follow a three-stage command.

(c) Subject is asked what hospital he is in.

(d) Subject is asked for the names of three objects repeated earlier in the examination.

(e) Subject is asked to read and obey the following: CLOSE YOUR EYES.

(2) During testing on MMSE, DL displayed superiority of one language modality over another language modality. Which modality is strongest in DL's case?

(3) DL displayed accurate performance on the Digit–Symbol substitution subtest of the WAIS-R. Which of the following are *true* statements about this subtest?

(a) Digit–symbol scores are highly correlated with chronological age.

(b) Subjects must use a code table to assign a symbol to a digit.

(c) This subtest assesses lexical retrieval abilities.

(d) Subjects must use a code table to assign a symbol to a colour.

(e) Digital–symbol scores are not highly correlated with measures of intelligence.

(4) DL was unable to complete the sequence 1–A, 2–B, 3–C. Which of the following cognitive skills are assessed by means of this task?

(a) visual tracking

(b) inhibition of prepotent responses

(c) set-shifting

(d) working memory

(e) sequencing ability

(5) DL did not appear to realise when he was not making sense, but expressed his difficulty understanding others. How is this behaviour characterised above?

Language assessment

DL's language skills were also extensively examined. On the Boston Diagnostic Aphasia Examination (Goodglass and Kaplan, 1983b), DL displayed moderate auditory comprehension deficits. He was able to understand simple one- and two-step commands and displayed intact comprehension of 2 of 5 sentences. Repetition was very impaired – he was not able to repeat any sentences presented to him. DL was able to read aloud 5 of 7 sentences, with evidence of mild, occasional paraphasias. His reading comprehension was mildly impaired – he was able to understand 5 of 7 commands. On the Boston Naming Test (Kaplan et al., 1983), DL named only 18 of 60 items. DL's spontaneous language production is examined in unit 20.5.

At the end of testing, DL laughed suddenly, stood up, stared and exhibited motor automatisms (eye blinking, picking movements with his fingers). He could only respond to questions with 'yes' or 'si'. He was led back to his bed. When this period of staring and reduced responsiveness had passed, DL's aphasia was much worse. He was alert and was attempting to communicate. He used gestures to express his frustration. Orientation and memory testing were not possible as he did not appear to understand what was required of him. His speech, which had been previously fluent, was almost completely neologistic and unintelligible. His verbal comprehension was markedly decreased, and he understood no verbal commands. During reading aloud, he produced neologistic jargon. He was still able to copy a drawing. On occasion, he stopped talking and blinked for a few seconds. During this period, a bedside EEG revealed seizure activity in the left temporal region.

Unit 20.4 Language assessment

(1) The Boston Diagnostic Aphasia Examination (BDAE) was used to assess DL's language skills. Which of the following are *true* statements about the BDAE?
   (a) The BDAE assesses language through spoken and written modalities.
   (b) The BDAE is not a standardised language assessment.
   (c) The BDAE is an assessment of pragmatic language in adults.
   (d) The BDAE can be used to diagnose aphasia syndromes in clients.
   (e) The BDAE contains the cookie theft picture description.

(2) DL was diagnosed with fluent, jargon aphasia. Identify *five* linguistic features of this type of aphasia.

(3) DL's speech is described as paraphasic. What *three* types of paraphasic errors is DL likely to produce?

(4) DL's communication skills altered quite markedly with the onset of seizure activity. Describe three changes in these skills.

(5) Even after the onset of seizure activity, DL was still able to copy a drawing. Explain why this is the case.

Focus on expressive language

This unit contains three extracts of expressive language produced by DL. These extracts are taken from: (1) the session during which DL's history was taken; (2) the session during which language testing was performed; and (3) DL's attempt to describe the cookie theft picture. Although these extracts are short, they are nonetheless revealing of DL's language problems.

History

I've been disabled all this (*incomprehensible neologisms*), last week I lost a lot of (*incomprehensible neologisms*), I lost my concern I'm just now concentrated went to the hospital about an hour on my brain.

Language testing

I lost my language – I'm just kind of waking up – I lost my concen – I'm just now concentrating – Everybody that's talking to me I don't understand them (*spoken rapidly*).

Cookie theft picture description

O.K. cookie jar, cookin-fallin' water trees. To interpret what he's doing? He's falling . . . to get the cookies I don't know if he's trying to say and ofring? The water the sink. I told you about the she's claimin? the glass. I don't know if he's asking him to drink or what the girl I don't know if I can figure out if he's a girl I mean a boy that's about all the wh . . . outside.

Unit 20.5 Focus on expressive language

(1) A particular theme dominates DL's spontaneous language in the first two extracts. What is that theme?

(2) Is there any evidence of perseveration in the data? Provide support for your answer.

(3) Is there any evidence that DL is able to monitor and initiate repair of his verbal output?

(4) DL's picture description is difficult to follow on account of pronoun anomalies. Give *three* examples of where these anomalies occur.

(5) From DL's own verbal report and the results of neuropsychological assessment, it is clear that he is experiencing a range of cognitive difficulties. Is impaired theory of mind likely to be one of those difficulties? Provide evidence to support your answer.

Case study 21

Girl aged 10 years with traumatic brain injury

Introduction

The following exercise is a case study of a 10-year-old girl ('DG') who was studied by Oelschlaeger and Scarborough (1976). DG developed a language disorder following a traumatic brain injury. She was assessed before and after a 6-month period of intensive speech and language therapy. The case study is presented in five sections: primer on paediatric traumatic brain injury; client history; speech, language and hearing assessment; therapeutic programme; and post-intervention language skills.

Primer on paediatric traumatic brain injury

Traumatic brain injury (TBI) is a leading cause of death and disability in children. In a review of research conducted since 1990, Thurman (2015) obtained the following median estimates of the annual incidence of brain injuries in children and young people aged 0–20 years: 691 per 100,000 population treated in emergency departments, 74 per 100,000 population treated in hospital, and 9 per 100,000 population deaths from TBI. Among children less than 10 years, the risk of head injury is 1.4 times higher in males than in females. Among children over 10 years, the risk is 2.2 times higher in males than in females. Falls are the leading cause of TBI in children less than 5 years, while road traffic accidents are the leading cause of injury in adolescents aged 15 years and older. Thurman estimated that the prevalence of disability among children who were hospitalised with TBI could approximate 20%.

The sequelae of TBI in children are wide-ranging in nature. They include motor problems, cognitive deficits, communication disorders, sensory impairments, epilepsy, behavioural difficulties and swallowing problems. Often, these sequelae persist over many years and adversely affect functioning in adulthood. In a study of 25 children (mean age: 13.7 years) with severe TBI, Emanuelson et al. (1996) reported motor problems, epilepsy and speech impairment in 88%, 28% and 56% of children, respectively. Of 23 survivors who were followed up at 2 to 6 years post-injury, all had at least one sequela and 21 survivors had multiple sequelae. Morgan et al. (2010) examined 1,895 children with TBI who were consecutively referred to a tertiary paediatric hospital over an eight-year period. The incidence of dysarthria and dysphagia in these children was 1.2% and 3.8%, respectively. Among children with severe TBI, the incidence of dysphagia was 76%. In a study of 100 subjects who sustained a TBI prior to 12 years of age, Penn et al. (2009) found that 31% had reported hearing loss. This was confirmed audiologically in 14% of subjects. Barlow et al. (2005) reported visual deficits in 48% of 25 children who sustained an inflicted TBI. Gerrard-Morris et al. (2010) examined 87 children who sustained a TBI between 3 and 6 years of age. Children with severe TBI had generalised cognitive deficits, while those with less severe TBI had problems with visual memory and executive function. Behaviour and personality can be markedly disrupted following TBI in children. Neuropsychiatric disorders include personality change, secondary attention deficit hyperactivity disorder, other disruptive behaviour disorders and internalising disorders (Max, 2014).

Speech-language pathologists assess and treat the significant speech and language disorders that attend TBI in children. In children with dysarthria, speech deficits are found across respiration, prosody, resonance, articulation and phonation (Morgan et al., 2010). Perceptual, instrumental and physiological assessments are used to examine these speech production subsystems. Cahill et al. (2005) used perceptual and instrumental assessments to examine speech production in 24 children with TBI. Perceptual assessment revealed consonant and vowel imprecision, increased length of phonemes and an overall reduction in speech intelligibility. There was significant impairment in lip and tongue function during an instrumental assessment, with rate and pressure in repetitive lip and tongue tasks particularly impaired. Language disorders also occur in paediatric TBI and are often related to the presence of cognitive deficits. Beauchamp and Anderson (2013) state that although there have been some isolated reports of aphasia following childhood TBI, these cases are rare and tend to recover with time following injury (915). Pragmatic and discourse skills are frequently disrupted in children who sustain TBI. Walz et al. (2012) examined narrative discourse skills in 43 children with moderate TBI and 19 children with severe TBI who were between 3 years and 6 years 11 months at the time of injury. Children with TBI performed worse than an orthopaedic control group on most discourse indices. Children with severe TBI were less proficient than children with moderate TBI at identifying unimportant story information. Age and pragmatic skills were predictors of these children's discourse performance.

Unit 21.1 Primer on paediatric traumatic brain injury

(1) Which of the following are *true* statements about TBI in children?
- (a) In a child with closed head injury, the brain is damaged in the presence of a skull fracture.
- (b) Children who sustain TBI under 10 years of age experience full language recovery.
- (c) Intracranial haemorrhage and cerebral contusion can occur in pediatric TBI.
- (d) In a child with open head injury, the brain is damaged in the presence of a skull fracture.
- (e) Non-accidental injury is the most common cause of TBI in children.

(2) Children with TBI can experience multiple sequelae. Classify the following conditions as sensory, motor, swallowing or communication sequelae of TBI:
- (a) sialorrhoea
- (b) mutism
- (c) hemiplegia

(d) dysarthria

(e) hemianopia

(3) What type of instrumental assessment can be used to measure lip and tongue function in dysarthria?

(4) Each of the following difficulties can be found in children who develop dysarthria following TBI. Classify each difficulty according to one of these speech production subsystems: *phonation; respiration; articulation; prosody;* and *resonation*.

(a) The child has a breathy voice.

(b) The child exhibits hypernasal speech.

(c) The child places stress on the wrong syllables in words.

(d) The child cannot achieve lip closure for the production of bilabial sounds.

(e) The child displays marked clavicular breathing during speech production.

(5) Discourse skills are often abnormal in children who sustain TBI. Are discourse deficits in this clinical population related to cognitive deficits? Provide support for your answer.

Client history

DG sustained a head injury in May 1974 when she fell off her horse onto the pavement. As a result of her fall, she was unconscious and bled from her left ear. She was taken to hospital where a left hemicraniectomy was performed three hours later. DG's postoperative diagnosis was 'left subdural haematoma, epidural haematoma and brain laceration'. When DG was discharged from hospital, she had a right hemiplegia and severe traumatic aphasia. There was no involvement of the right cerebral hemisphere. Prior to DG's head injury, she was a healthy, 'normal', active 10-year-old girl. She was in the fourth grade at school and was performing well academically, obtaining all As in the past academic year.

Unit 21.2 Client history

(1) DG underwent a left hemicraniectomy. What is this surgical procedure? What does it aim to achieve?

(2) DG sustained a subdural haematoma and an epidural haematoma. Describe these cerebral injuries.

(3) When DG was discharged from hospital, she had a right hemiplegia. Describe *two* ways in which a right hemiplegia might compromise the communication skills of this client.

(4) A right hemiplegia also has implications for the SLT management of DG. Describe *two* ways in which a right hemiplegia must be considered in the SLT management of this client.

(5) There was no evidence of right cerebral hemisphere involvement in DG's case. Which of the following disorders are associated with right hemisphere damage?

(a) left hemiplegia

    (b) conduction aphasia

    (c) anosognosia

    (d) apraxia of speech

    (e) left-sided neglect

Speech, language and hearing assessment

DG underwent a comprehensive assessment of speech, language and hearing. Pure-tone audiometry was unsuccessful as DG could not be conditioned to the task. However, when free-field, pure tones were presented at 15 dB, DG did display orienting responses. DG was also able to attend to environmental sounds such as the voice of a speaker and the sound of a door opening. DG displayed no response to simple questions or commands to identify pictures, objects and body parts. On the Peabody Picture Vocabulary Test (Dunn, 1959), DG was unable to make even one correct response. This test demands a pointing response, which could only be elicited in DG with gestural stimulation – DG did not comprehend verbal instruction. However, DG pointed randomly to one or sometimes to all pictured items. DG was unable to produce almost any spontaneous language. The only verbal output was iteration of the syllable 'na' which was uttered without meaning. DG was unable to engage in imitative verbalisation. She was, however, able to protrude, elevate and lateralise her tongue in imitation of the examiner. DG could not match written words to either pictures or objects. She was able to visually match geometric objects, numbers and pictures. Through the use of her left, non-dominant hand, DG was able to copy words of four or five letters. However, writing was limited to copying (i.e. it was never spontaneous), and could not be elicited through any other type of stimulus presentation.

Unit 21.3 Speech, language and hearing assessment

(1) DG could not comply with the assessment requirements of pure-tone audiometry. However, is there any evidence that DG's language difficulties are related to hearing loss?

(2) Which of the following aspects of language is assessed by the Peabody Picture Vocabulary Test?

    (a) expressive syntax

    (b) receptive semantics

    (c) receptive syntax

    (d) expressive semantics

    (e) receptive vocabulary

(3) Which of the following statements characterise DG's communicative status?

    (a) DG displays impairment of more than one language modality.

    (b) DG displays neuromuscular weakness of the articulators.

    (c) DG displays post-traumatic mutism.

    (d) DG has mild auditory verbal comprehension impairment.

    (e) DG exhibits hypernasal speech.

(4) Does DG have an oral apraxia? Provide support for your answer.

(5) DG has intact visual perceptual skills. What evidence is there that this is the case? Why do you think these skills are intact?

Therapeutic programme

Five principles were integral to the therapy that DG received. These principles were (1) the use of intensive auditory stimulation, (2) the requirement that a response is made to each stimulus presentation, (3) the use of meaningful language units, (4) the use of controlled stimulus presentations, and (5) the use of all language modalities. Stimulus items were restricted to just four categories: *food* (bread, milk); *clothing* (coat, shoes); *place setting* (knife, fork); and *grooming articles* (brush, comb). Activities were designed to stimulate all language modalities and were sequentially introduced on the basis of their presumed difficulty. The same three activities were used at the start of each therapy session. These were matching like pictures or objects, graphic imitation of printed word and matching graphic imitation with printed word. The next tasks in the order of difficulty involved matching picture or object to word and matching word to picture or object. The next activity in the hierarchy of difficulty involved matching auditory stimuli to printed words, pictures or objects. A decrease in the amount and type of information that was available for correct responding varied the difficulty level of this task. An activity which aimed to elicit spontaneous verbal production followed successful auditory comprehension. Stimuli such as printed words, objects or pictures were used to elicit the desired response. A spontaneous writing task was the last activity to be used. The same stimuli that were used in previous tasks were also used to elicit writing in this activity.

Unit 21.4 Therapeutic programme

(1) Give *three* reasons why the use of all language modalities might be advantageous as a principle of language intervention in general.

(2) Fill in the blank space in this statement: *The stimulus items used in DG's intervention all belonged to one of four semantic* _____.

(3) The same three activities were used at the start of each therapy session. The activities in question were all tasks that DG was known to perform well. Give *one* reason why such activities may be used at the start of a session.

(4) One of the activities DG performed involved matching auditory stimuli to printed words. For some words, this can be achieved through the application of sound-to-letter rules. What is this class of words called?

(5) In which set of tasks does DG need to access her semantic system?

Post-intervention language skills

DG was still successfully matching pictures and objects and graphic imitation to printed words at the end of therapy. However, where therapeutic progress was clearly made was in the matching of words with pictures or objects, or matching pictures or objects with words. These tasks were performed with 90% and 95% accuracy, respectively. DG could not perform either of these tasks at the outset of therapy. By the end of therapy, DG's auditory comprehension exhibited 61.24% accuracy. In effect, DG was now identifying pictures, words or objects correctly when given an auditory stimulus nearly two-thirds of the time. Although this still represented an impairment of auditory comprehension, it was nevertheless a significant improvement. DG's spontaneous verbal production also improved considerably. Prior to therapy, DG did not use language spontaneously. By the end of therapy, she displayed a mean spontaneous verbal production of 20.5%. In terms of spontaneous writing, DG was able to write the stimulus word 'egg' on two separate occasions when provided with auditory cues. The words 'spoon', 'comb' and 'brush' were written during one of the final sessions without any cues. DG was also able to print the first three or four letters of a word when shown an object but she could not complete it. An auditory cue frequently elicited the final letter of the word.

Unit 21.5 Post-intervention language skills

(1) What evidence is there that DG's word semantics had improved by the end of therapy?

(2) DG's auditory comprehension and spontaneous verbal production both improved as a result of therapy but not to the same extent. Is the gap between DG's receptive and expressive language skills also a feature of language in normally developing children?

(3) By the end of therapy there was also an improvement in DG's spontaneous writing. What type of words (regular/irregular) was DG able to write?

(4) What type of cuing (phonemic/semantic) is effective at eliciting target letters in DG?

(5) Murdoch (2010) states that 'ten years of age is considered by many authors the upper limit for complete language recovery' (341). Does the case of DG provide support for or against this statement?

Case study 22

Girl aged 9;11 years with right cerebellar tumour

Introduction

The following exercise is a case study of a girl who was studied longitudinally between 9;11 and 11;9 years by Docking et al. (2007). At 9;11 years, the girl was diagnosed with an ependymoma of the right cerebellar hemisphere. Long-term speech, language and cognitive deficits have been reported in children following polytherapy (surgery, radiotherapy and/or chemotherapy) of cerebellar tumours (De Smet et al., 2012; Hoang et al., 2014; Levisohn et al., 2000). The case study is presented in five sections: diagnosis and medical intervention; assessment battery; language evaluation at 10;9 years; language evaluation at 11;9 years; and cognitive functions of the cerebellum.

Diagnosis and medical intervention

The girl presented with a three-month history of poor balance, nausea, intermittent vomiting and dizziness. A MRI scan was performed at 9;11 years. It revealed a 2-cm mass in the anterior cerebellum, just to the right of the midline and adjacent to the right posterior aspect of the fourth ventricle. The mass was a low-grade ependymoma. Treatment was initiated. It consisted of total surgical removal of the mass and an eight-week course of radiotherapy. Radiotherapy involved the administration of 54 Gy (Gray) to the cranial posterior fossa in 30 fractions using 6-MV photons via the right and left posterior oblique fields.

Unit 22.1 Diagnosis and medical intervention

(1) The girl was diagnosed with a low-grade ependymoma. Which of the following are *true* statements about this type of tumour?
   (a) Ependymomas arise from the ependymal cells that line the ventricles of the brain.
   (b) Low-grade ependymomas tend to be slow growing and are often amenable to surgical excision.
   (c) Ependymomas are the most common childhood brain tumour.
   (d) Ependymomas are rarely found in the fourth ventricle.
   (e) Low-grade ependymomas have a high proliferative rate and tend to infiltrate surrounding brain.
(2) Which of this girl's presenting symptoms suggests the presence of cerebellar dysfunction?

(3) Which of the following is associated with cranial irradiation?
   (a) radionecrosis
   (b) reduced intellectual function
   (c) agenesis of the corpus callosum
   (d) intracerebral calcification
   (e) cerebral atrophy

(4) Which of the following are *true* statements about the cerebellum?
   (a) Damage to the cerebellum causes ataxic dysarthria.
   (b) The cerebellum has two hemispheres which are separated by the vermis.
   (c) The cerebellum is not involved in motor coordination.
   (d) The cerebellum is located in the posterior fossa of the skull, dorsal to the pons and medulla.
   (e) The cerebellum has no role in cognitive functions.

(5) The cerebellum is compromised in this case by a tumour. Name *two* other causes of cerebellar pathology.

Assessment battery

The girl underwent a wide-ranging assessment of her general and high-level language skills. Several tests were used for this purpose. The Clinical Evaluation of Language Fundamentals (CELF3; Semel et al., 1995) tests a child's syntax/morphology, semantics and pragmatics through a series of expressive and receptive language subtests. For example, a child may be asked to point to one of four pictures in response to an orally presented stimulus to test comprehension of sentence structure, and to list as many words as possible within a given category in 1 minute. The Hundred Pictures Naming Test (Fisher and Glenister, 1992) is a confrontation naming test that is designed to evaluate rapid naming ability. One hundred line drawings of noun objects which are familiar to both children and adults are used. The Peabody Picture Vocabulary Test (PPVT-III; Dunn and Dunn, 1997) is one of the most commonly used, standardised tests of receptive vocabulary. Test items, each of which has four corresponding black-and-white illustrations, are arranged in 17 sets of 12 in order of increasing difficulty. The examiner says a word and the examinee must select the picture that best illustrates the meaning of the stimulus word. The Test of Language Competence – Expanded Edition (TLC; Wiig and Secord, 1989) is used to diagnose disorders of higher-level language function. Subtests examine a range of pragmatic language skills: Ambiguous Sentences; Listening Comprehension: Making Inferences; Oral Expression: Recreating Speech Acts; and Figurative Language. There is also a supplemental memory subtest. The Test of Word Knowledge (TOWK; Wiig and Secord, 1992) identifies students who lack the semantic skills that are the foundation of mature language use in thinking, learning and communication. The test contains a series of subtests that assess various aspects of semantic development and lexical knowledge: Knowledge of Figurative Language; Multiple Meanings; Conjunctions and Transition Words; and Receptive and Expressive Vocabulary. The Test of Problem-Solving – Elementary, Revised (Bowers et al., 1994) is a diagnostic test of problem-solving and critical thinking. It assesses an individual's language-based thinking abilities and strategies using logic and experience.

Due to the holistic nature of critical thinking and problem-solving, the test is not divided into subtests. Responses to tasks reveal skills in problem-solving, determining solutions, drawing inferences, empathising, predicting outcomes, using context cues and vocabulary comprehension.

Unit 22.2 Assessment battery

(1) At least two of these assessments examine figurative language. Each of the following utterances is an example of figurative language. State what type of figurative language is used in each of these utterances.
   (a) A stitch in time saves nine.
   (b) Fred kicked the bucket.
   (c) The children were angels for their grandmother.
   (d) Sally hit the sack quite early.
   (e) The rugby players were lions on the pitch.

(2) One of the CELF-3 subtests asks a child to list as many words as possible within a given category in one minute. Which of the following skills is assessed by this subtest?
   (a) phonological memory
   (b) inhibition of prepotent responses
   (c) semantic memory
   (d) oromotor skills
   (e) cognitive flexibility

(3) At least two of these assessments examine an individual's ability to draw inferences. Some inferences are based on word meanings (semantic inferences). Other inferences draw heavily on one's knowledge of the world (elaborative inferences). Still other inferences are based on one's knowledge of conversational maxims and rules (pragmatic inferences). Classify each of the inferences on the right below as one of these three types of inference:
   (a) Jack is a bachelor → Jack is an unmarried man
   (b) Bill is meeting a woman this evening → The woman is not Bill's sister
   (c) The karate champion hit the block → The karate champion broke the block
   (d) Jack kissed Jill → Jack touched Jill
   (e) The chemist had acid on his coat → The chemist spilled acid on his coat

(4) The Test of Language Competence contains a subtest that examines ambiguous sentences. Sentences may be ambiguous on account of (a) lexical ambiguity, (b) structural ambiguity and (c) lexical and structural ambiguity. Give *one* example of each of these types of ambiguous sentence.

(5) The Test of Language Competence also contains a subtest that examines the use of speech acts. Name *three* different speech acts and give *one* example of each.

Language evaluation at 10;9 years

At 10;9 years the girl underwent extensive testing of her language skills. Six weeks prior to testing, the girl had an MRI scan which revealed no evidence of recurrent tumour. Standard scores on the receptive language, expressive language and total language components of the CELF-3 were above the normal range. All CELF-3 subtest standard scores were either within or above the normal range. The standard score on the PPVT-III was also above the normal range. The girl named 93 of 100 objects correctly on the Hundred Pictures Naming Test. Standard scores on the receptive and expressive composites of the Test of Word Knowledge were also within the normal range. The performance on subtests that examined the reception of synonyms, word opposites, figurative language and vocabulary was within the normal range. Performance on expressive subtests of word definitions and vocabulary was also within the normal range. On the Test of Language Competence the girl did not exhibit difficulty drawing inferences during listening comprehension or interpreting figurative language. Her performance on expressive subtests of the TLC was also within the normal range. The one assessment where the girl's performance was judged to be poor was the Test of Problem Solving. Her standard score of 78 on this test placed her outside the normal range of 85 to 115.

Unit 22.3 Language evaluation at 10;9 years

(1) The results of language testing at 10;9 years revealed the girl to have a number of intact structural language skills. Five of these skills are listed below. Give *one* test result which supports each of these skills:
   (a) expressive syntax
   (b) receptive vocabulary
   (c) receptive syntax
   (d) expressive vocabulary
   (e) receptive semantics

(2) Which test result(s) indicate(s) that it is too simplistic to characterise the girl's language in terms of intact structural language and impaired pragmatic language?

(3) The girl's performance on a TOWK subtest that examines the reception of word opposites (antonyms) fell within the normal range. Give *one* example of each of the following types of antonyms:
   (a) gradable antonyms
   (b) converse antonyms
   (c) reverse antonyms
   (d) binary antonyms

(4) Given the nature of this girl's language problems, it is likely that they would not be detected during a routine language evaluation. Explain why this is likely to be the case.

(5) Respond with *true* or *false* to each of the following statements:
   (a) The girl's high-level language deficits are secondary to structural language impairments.
   (b) The girl's high-level language deficits are caused by tumour recurrence.
   (c) The girl's high-level language deficits reflect a significant impairment of pragmatics.
   (d) The girl's high-level language deficits reflect an impairment of cognitive function.
   (e) The girl's high-level language deficits will have few, if any, implications for communication.

Language evaluation at 11;9 years

At 11;9 years the girl underwent follow-up language evaluation. This was 12 months after the first language evaluation, and nearly two years after the MRI scan which resulted in the diagnosis of her tumour. Her standard scores on the CELF-3, the PPVT-III, the TOWK and the TLC were still within the normal range or exceeded the normal range (receptive language on the CELF-3). Her naming performance on the Hundred Pictures Naming Test was almost unchanged at 95 objects out of 100 named correctly. However, there was a significant deterioration on the Test of Problem Solving (TOPS). Although her TOPS standard score was previously also outside of the normal range, it was now more than 2 standard deviations below the normal range.

Unit 22.4 Language evaluation at 11;9 years

(1) This girl's high-level language skills displayed a marked decline in the 12-month period since her last language evaluation. What factor is likely to have made the single, biggest contribution to this decline in skills?

(2) What implications does this case have for speech-language pathologists who must assess and treat children with cerebellar tumours?

(3) Why might high-level language skills be considered a priority for intervention in a girl of 11;9 years?

(4) The language-based skills examined by the Test of Problem Solving sit at the intersection of a number of cognitive areas, not all of which are familiar to speech-language pathologists. For example, empathy requires the cognitive capacity to attribute affective mental states such as sadness to the minds of others. What is the name of this cognitive capacity?

(5) The persistence of high-level language deficits into adolescence and beyond is likely to compound the significant, adverse psychosocial effects of brain tumour for this girl. Using research findings, state what those effects are.

Cognitive functions of the cerebellum

The authors of this study argue that their findings contribute to a growing body of evidence which suggests a role for the cerebellum in language and cognition. Alongside the high-level language deficits of this girl, studies have demonstrated a range of cognitive-language disorders in children who have received treatment for cerebellar tumours. De Smet et al. (2009) reported language and cognitive deficits in five of eight children following posterior fossa tumour resection. Language deficits included agrammatism, anomia, impaired verbal fluency and comprehension deficits. Neurocognitive deficits included executive dysfunctions, concentration deficits and visuo-spatial disorders. All children presented with behavioural and affective disturbances. Aarsen et al. (2009) found that children with cerebellar pilocytic astrocytoma had significantly lower scores than the normal population on tests of sustained attention and speed, long-term visual–spatial memory, executive functioning and naming. In an earlier investigation (Aarsen et al., 2006), children with infratentorial cerebellar tumours were also shown to have long-term social and behavioural problems. The cluster of disturbances of executive function, impaired spatial cognition, linguistic difficulties and personality changes is, these authors report, referred to as the cerebellar cognitive affective syndrome.

Unit 22.5 Cognitive functions of the cerebellum

(1) The language deficits displayed by De Smet et al.'s subjects differ from those of the girl in this case study. These subjects exhibit symptoms which are found in the classical aphasia syndromes. Name *two* such symptoms.

(2) De Smet et al.'s subjects also displayed impaired verbal fluency. Was verbal fluency impaired in the girl in this case study? Support your answer with evidence.

(3) How might differences in the linguistic performance of the girl in this case study and the subjects reported in this unit be explained?

(4) Affective disturbances are a consistent finding in the subjects reported in this unit. How did the authors of this case study test the affective functioning of the girl at the centre of the study?

(5) The presence of language disorders alongside cognitive, affective and other deficits in children with cerebellar tumours has an important implication for the management of these clients. What is this implication?

Case study 23

Woman with post-irradiation speech and language disorder

Introduction

The following exercise is a case study of a 39-year-old woman who was studied by Murdoch and Chenery (1990). This woman presented with the features of a latent aphasia and flaccid dysarthria 20 years after receiving a course of radiotherapy following surgical excision of a pituitary fossa tumour. Speech, language, hearing and swallowing disorders are common sequelae of cranial irradiation for the treatment of brain tumours. Gonçalves et al. (2008) found speech, language and hearing symptoms in 42% of a sample of 190 children and adolescents with brain tumours. Mei and Morgan (2011) reported dysarthria and dysphagia to affect around one in three children who underwent surgery for posterior fossa tumour. Ribi et al. (2005) reported language deficits in 56% of their sample of 26 survivors of paediatric medulloblastoma. The case study is presented in five sections: history and referral; neurological and neuroradiological evaluation; neuropsychological evaluation; speech evaluation; and language evaluation.

History and referral

The client is a 39-year-old, right-handed woman who underwent intracranial surgery at 16 years of age for the removal of a posterior fossa tumour. Following surgery, the client received radiotherapy which involved the administration of 6,000 rads of radiation to the tumour site. Twenty years post-surgery, the client's family reported deterioration in her speech. Prior to that time, her speech had been normal. Speech intelligibility was noted to be impaired by increasing hypernasality. The use of a palatal lift prosthesis was unsuccessful in addressing the client's hypernasality. The woman was referred for investigation of her hypernasal speech three years after the onset of her speech disorder.

Unit 23.1 History and referral

(1) The client underwent surgery for the removal of a posterior fossa tumour. Which of the following are *true* statements about this type of tumour?
   (a) The posterior fossa houses the brainstem and cerebellum.
   (b) The posterior fossa does not contain cranial nerves.
   (c) Tumours are the most common pathology to affect the posterior fossa.
   (d) The foramen magnum is the smallest opening of the posterior fossa.
   (e) Posterior fossa tumours account for up to two-thirds of brain tumours in children.

(2) Many individuals who undergo surgical excision of a posterior fossa tumour develop posterior fossa syndrome. Which of the following are signs and symptoms of this syndrome?
(a) mutism or speech disturbance
(b) dysphagia
(c) hemianopia
(d) emotional lability
(e) hemiplegia

(3) Name *three* structural changes that can occur in the brain following radiotherapy for the treatment of CNS malignancies.

(4) The client presented with hypernasal speech 20 years post-surgery. Which speech production mechanism is malfunctioning to cause the client's hypernasality? Is a structural or neurogenic aetiology the basis of this malfunction?

(5) A prosthetic intervention – the use of a palatal lift device – proved to be unsuccessful in addressing the client's hypernasal speech. Describe how such a device may be used to treat hypernasal speech, and explain why it was unsuccessful in this case.

Neurological and neuroradiological evaluation

Two months prior to referral for speech and language evaluation, the client underwent a neurological examination. This revealed a malfunction of the Xth cranial nerve bilaterally. There was no hemiplegia or hemisensory loss, and deep tendon reflexes were mildly hyperactive on the right. No visual field defect was demonstrated by confrontation, and no Babinski sign was evident. Other general examination revealed no abnormality. A CT scan was also conducted prior to referral. It revealed central focal calcification at the pontomesencephalic junction and scattered throughout the pons and medulla. Both thalami and the anterior limb of the left internal capsule also exhibited calcification. The lenticular nucleus was involved in the calcification of the anterior limb of the left internal capsule, while the ventrolateral nucleus was the most significant area of calcification in the left thalamus. The CT scan further revealed dilation of both lateral ventricles. The frontal horn and body of the right lateral ventricle were particularly enlarged. The third ventricle was also dilated.

Unit 23.2 Neurological and neuroradiological evaluation

(1) The neurological examination revealed an impairment of the Xth cranial nerve. What is the name of this nerve? Which three branches of this nerve are vital for motor speech production? Which branch is compromised in this client in producing hypernasal speech?

(2) The client did not exhibit a visual field defect. Which of the following terms describes such a defect?
(a) visual agnosia
(b) nystagmus
(c) hemianopia

     (d) cortical blindness

     (e) glaucoma

(3) No Babinski sign was evident during the neurological examination. What is this sign and what does its presence reveal?

(4) The CT scan revealed that two nuclei – the lenticular nucleus and the ventrolateral nucleus – were in areas of considerable calcification in the brain. What are these nuclei?

(5) Certain ventricles of the brain were observed to be enlarged on the CT scan. Give a brief description of the structure and function of the ventricles.

Neuropsychological evaluation

To establish the extent of any memory impairment or other cognitive dysfunction, a neuropsychological assessment was conducted. Four tests were used for this purpose: the Wechsler Adult Intelligence Scale – Revised (WAIS-R; Wechsler, 1981); the Wechsler Memory Scale (Wechsler, 1945); the Rey Auditory Verbal Learning Test (Rey, 1964); and the Rey Figure (Rey, 1941). On the WAIS-R, the client was identified as having difficulty in learning and utilising novel visual and verbal stimuli or information. She was also found to have problems in abstracting 'general' from 'specific' information in order to gain an understanding of the wider meaning of language, pictorial material and cause-effect relationships. The client displayed literal interpretation. Both performance and verbal IQ were within the low average range. The client's long-term memory and immediate memory were intact. In particular, she displayed learning and encoding of verbal material. Performance decrements were related to retrieval problems. The client scored below the 10th percentile on the Rey Figure test. Her copy was carried out in a relatively unsystematic fashion. There were no obvious difficulties with angles, orientation or neglect. Her recall of the figure revealed a profound retention deficit for complex material.

Unit 23.3 Neuropsychological evaluation

(1) The WAIS-R was one of four cognitive assessments used to test the client. Which of the following are *true* statements about this test?

     (a) The WAIS-R is designed specifically for adults who have neurogenic communication disorders.

     (b) The WAIS-R is a standardised test of intellectual ability.

     (c) The WAIS-R contains a subtest called Pragmatic Language.

     (d) The WAIS-R can be used to derive full scale, verbal and performance IQs.

     (e) The WAIS-R contains subtests called Block Design and Vocabulary.

(2) The results of the cognitive assessments indicate that the client may have difficulties with one or more of the following aspects of language. Indicate the level(s) concerned, and give *one* example of how the level(s) in question may be compromised.

     (a) phonology

     (b) morphology

     (c) syntax

     (d) pragmatics

     (e) discourse

(3) Which cognitive finding suggests the client may have difficulty with establishing the gist of a story?

(4) The client scored below the 10th percentile on the Rey Figure test. What does this result mean?

(5) The client did not appear to have difficulties with angles, orientation or neglect. Which lobes of the brain which are responsible for these functions would seem to be intact?

Speech evaluation

The client's speech production skills were assessed by means of the Frenchay Dysarthria Assessment (Enderby, 1983). It revealed that the client had a flaccid dysarthria which was associated with pharyngolaryngeal palsy. The client displayed considerable difficulty with eating and drinking. Frequent coughing and choking were noted, and there was occasional nasal regurgitation of fluid. Eating was very slow and the client's diet required modification. There was also some dribbling particularly when the client was not concentrating. There were no lip or jaw abnormalities. The tongue also appeared normal in appearance and function and there was normal lingual contribution to consonant articulation. However, the tongue was slow in performing alternating movements. Other speech production abnormalities were also observed. The client spoke quickly, with noticeable breaks in fluency and short phrase length. Her speech was severely hypernasal with noticeable nasal emission. The soft palate showed no elevation on phonation. There was a marked reduction in the length of phonation, poor control of volume and reduced pitch. Phonation was also husky. In terms of intelligibility, the client's speech was severely distorted, and she needed to repeat herself frequently. Fast rate, severe hypernasality and consequent consonant imprecision contributed to reduced intelligibility. Listeners relied on contextual and referential cues during conversation to comprehend the client.

Unit 23.4 Speech evaluation

(1) The client was assessed to have a flaccid dysarthria associated with a pharyngolaryngeal palsy. Which of the following are *true* statements about a flaccid dysarthria?
   (a) Flaccid dysarthria results from damage to the upper motor neurones involved in speech production.
   (b) Muscles affected by flaccid paralysis may begin to atrophy over time.
   (c) Lack of innervation can cause fasciculations which may be especially visible in the tongue.
   (d) Pharyngolaryngeal palsy results from damage to CN X (vagus nerve).
   (e) There is increased muscle tone (hypertonia) in flaccid dysarthria.

(2) The client's tongue was observed to be slow in performing alternating movements. What test is standardly used by speech-language pathologists to assess an individual's ability to perform alternating articulatory movements?

(3) Respond with *true* or *false* to each of the following statements:
   (a) The client is at risk of aspiration pneumonia.
   (b) The client's drooling is related to excessive saliva production.

    (c) Nasal regurgitation is related to velopharyngeal incompetence.

    (d) The client has iatrogenic dysphagia.

    (e) The client has psychogenic dysphagia.

(4) What evidence is there that the client is experiencing respiratory problems during speech production?

(5) The client experienced a number of phonatory disturbances. Which of these disturbances is related to reduced respiratory support for speech?

Language evaluation

A wide-ranging language evaluation of the client was conducted. It revealed that she had a severe impairment in word fluency and sentence construction, with test scores in these areas placing her below the 20th percentile for normal subjects. On visual naming and the auditory comprehension of long and complex sentences, the client's scores placed her at the 40th and 32nd percentile, respectively. On tasks of sentence repetition, digit repetition forwards and digit repetition backwards, the client displayed well-preserved repetitional abilities. On the Boston Naming Test (BNT; Kaplan et al., 1983), the client achieved a score of 29 out of 60. This score placed her more than two standard deviations below the score for normal subjects. Her naming errors included the following: 'tomb' for *pyramid*; 'almond' for *acorn*; 'snake' for *pretzel*; and 'pen' for *dart*. The remaining naming errors on the BNT were no responses. During naming, the client benefited from the use of phonemic cues and there were no phonemic paraphasias. There were also problems at the level of connected speech. The client exhibited reduced efficiency of information transfer as well as a reduction in the amount of information transferred. The client's language problems did not amount to an overt aphasia, and it was not possible to classify them as one of the classical cortical aphasia syndromes.

Unit 23.5 Language evaluation

(1) What evidence is there that the client's phonological level of language is intact?

(2) What type of error occurs during the naming of *pyramid* and *acorn*? What level of language is disrupted to produce these errors? Is there any further evidence of disruption to this language level?

(3) How might the errors produced during the naming of *pretzel* and *dart* be explained?

(4) The client clearly benefited from the use of phonemic cues during naming. Do you think semantic cues might facilitate this client's naming? Provide evidence to support your answer.

(5) Is this client likely to be an informative communicator? Provide evidence to support your answer.

Case study 24

Woman aged 66 years with Wernicke's aphasia

Introduction

The following exercise is a case study of a woman ('RC') aged 66 years who was studied by Hough (1993). RC developed Wernicke's aphasia which was characterised by neologistic jargon and a severe auditory comprehension deficit following two left-hemisphere strokes. For eight months post-stroke, an intervention which was aimed at managing RC's rambling communicative style and improving auditory comprehension met with no communicative or linguistic improvements. A new treatment regimen which emphasised reading was subsequently introduced. The case study is presented in five sections: primer on Wernicke's aphasia; client history and presentation; pre-intervention language assessment; new language intervention; and post-intervention language assessment.

Primer on Wernicke's aphasia

Aphasia is a common symptom in stroke patients. However, Wernicke's aphasia affects fewer stroke clients in comparison to other aphasia syndromes. Hoffmann and Chen (2013) found aphasia in 625 (34.8%) of 1,796 stroke patients. Only 10 patients (1.6%) had Wernicke's aphasia which was principally caused by cardioembolism or a haemorrhage. Broca's, global, anomic and subcortical aphasias were all more common than Wernicke's aphasia. Yang et al. (2008) reported Wernicke's aphasia in 14.8% of aphasic patients, with Broca's, global and anomic aphasia all accounting for more cases of the disorder. Wernicke's aphasia is typically caused by stroke-induced damage of the language comprehension regions in the left temporoparietal cortex (Robson et al., 2014). However, this form of aphasia has also been found in patients with damage in other neuroanatomical areas (Jodzio et al., 2003), and some individuals with lesions in Wernicke's area on MRI display no language symptoms at all (Yang et al., 2008).

Individuals with Wernicke's aphasia display impaired auditory comprehension and produce fluent, well-articulated speech. Spoken output may contain so many neologistic, phonological and/or verbal paraphasias that it is no longer understandable (so-called 'jargon aphasia'). There is poor awareness of communication difficulties. In less severe cases, only the comprehension of complex sentences and low frequency and abstract words may be impaired, and there may only be occasional use of paraphasias. Although individuals with aphasia can produce long, complex sentences, these are often ungrammatical on account of incompleteness and erroneous grammatical constructions ('paragrammatism'). The repetition of words and sentences, naming of objects and actions, silent reading and writing are usually severely affected. However, reading aloud can be more or less normal (Bastiaanse and Prins, 2014).

Unit 24.1 Primer on Wernicke's aphasia

(1) Which of the following conditions is *not* in the aetiology of Wernicke's aphasia?
   (a) cerebrovascular accident
   (b) Alzheimer's disease
   (c) traumatic brain injury
   (d) encephalitis
   (e) brain tumour

(2) Which of the following is a *true* statement about the epidemiology of Wernicke's aphasia?
   (a) Wernicke's aphasia has a higher prevalence than Broca's aphasia.
   (b) Wernicke's aphasia is more common in women than in men.
   (c) The incidence of Wernicke's aphasia increases with age.
   (d) Wernicke's aphasia has a lower prevalence than anomic aphasia.
   (e) The incidence of Wernicke's aphasia decreases after 65 years of age.

(3) What is the neuroanatomical location of Wernicke's area? Is a lesion of this area always associated with Wernicke's aphasia?

(4) A speaker with jargon aphasia produces the following utterance: 'We have to go to the pargoney'. What type of error has this speaker produced?

(5) An adult with Wernicke's aphasia is shown a picture of a bike and is asked to name it. The response is: 'I used to run one. Oh, I used to love to ride it!'. What type of error has this adult committed?

Client history and presentation

RC is a left-handed woman who sustained two strokes of the left cerebral hemisphere which were confirmed by CT scan and neurological examination. The CT scan after the first stroke revealed a lesion of the posterior portion of the first temporal gyrus, and RC was diagnosed as having Wernicke's aphasia. One month after the first stroke occurred, RC sustained a second cerebrovascular accident. On this occasion, the CT scan revealed the original lesion as well as an extension into the anterior portion of the supramarginal gyrus. A diagnosis of Wernicke's aphasia with jargon was made. Hough's first contact with RC took place seven months after the second stroke. To this point, RC had been receiving twice weekly speech therapy. Notwithstanding this intervention, she displayed differentiated, rambling, neologistic jargon. She was unable to repeat language, had poor auditory comprehension, and exhibited a lack of intrapersonal and interpersonal monitoring. RC's incessant verbalisations appeared to limit her ability to detect conversational cues from her environment. The interpretation of her messages was compromised by the fact that she frequently used prosodic patterns which were not appropriate to her communicative intentions.

Unit 24.2 Client history and presentation

(1) Why is there an increased likelihood that RC may have right-hemisphere language dominance? Is this subsequently borne out by the results of brain imaging?

(2) There is evidence that the anterior temporal lobes can support comprehension of visually presented material (written words and pictures) in individuals with Wernicke's aphasia (Robson et al., 2014). Is this neuroanatomical area intact in RC?

(3) RC exhibits a number of linguistic impairments. Which *four* impairments are typical of Wernicke's aphasia?

(4) RC's incessant verbalisations were described as limiting her ability to detect conversational cues from her environment. Give *one* example of a cue that RC is unlikely to detect, and explain how this is likely to compromise communication.

(5) RC is described as having difficulty in the use of prosodic patterns that are appropriate to her communicative intentions. Give *one* example of this type of prosodic difficulty.

Pre-intervention language assessment

At the onset of RC's second stroke and at seven months post-onset, RC's language skills were assessed using the Boston Naming Test (BNT; Kaplan et al., 1983) and the Boston Diagnostic Aphasia Examination (BDAE; Goodglass and Kaplan, 1983a). The second testing session occurred just before the introduction of a new therapy programme. RC's performance on both assessments was almost unchanged between onset and seven months post-onset. There was no change on the Boston Naming Test and the following subtests of the BDAE, all of which were rated '0': word discrimination; complex ideational material; automatised sequences; repetition of words; repetition of phrases; word reading; responsive naming; animal naming; and oral sentence reading. There were negligible increases or decreases in the following BDAE subtests (scores at onset and at seven months post-onset are given in parentheses): body part identification (1;0); oral commands (0;1); visual confrontation naming (1;2); and reading comprehension of sentences and paragraphs (0;1). A score of '3' was obtained on both sittings of the BDAE picture-word match subtest. The Aphasia Severity Rating remained unchanged at '0' (no usable speech or auditory comprehension). Within the Rating Scale Profile, which scores items from 1 (severe impairment) to 7 (no impairment), articulatory agility (5;5) and melodic line (4;4) were areas of relative strength, with phrase length (3;4), grammatical form (2;3) and paraphasia (1;1) lagging behind. The results of these language assessments were confirmed by the report of RC's previous clinician. She reported that neither she nor RC's family had observed any improvement in RC's communicative interactions with others or in her ability to monitor her errors.

Unit 24.3 Pre-intervention language assessment

(1) The following items are taken from the Boston Diagnostic Aphasia Examination. Match each of these items to one of the BDAE subtests described above.
   (a) The client is asked: 'Point to the ceiling, then to the floor'.
   (b) The client is asked to recite the days of the week.
   (c) The client is asked: 'What do you do with a razor?'.
   (d) The client is asked: 'Can you use a hammer to pound nails?'.
   (e) The client is asked to read and complete the following sentence with one of the words in parenthesis: A dog can . . . (talk bark sing cat).

(2) Which of the BDAE results relates to the use of prosody by RC?

(3) None of RC's subtest scores are particularly good. However, there is one subtest score which suggests that the visual modality may prove to be a promising avenue in terms of intervention. What is this subtest?

(4) What cognitive process known to be disrupted by lesions in the left temporoparietal cortex is likely to play a role in RC's impaired repetition?

(5) RC's performance on the Boston Naming Test was very poor on each occasion of testing. The following items are taken from this test. Devise *three* lexical and/or conceptual distinctions along which these items may be categorised: *camel, wheelchair, house, volcano, octopus, dart, comb, pelican, bed, toothbrush, cactus, sphinx.*

New language intervention

Until seven months post-onset, RC's language intervention included the use of picture categorisation tasks, auditory comprehension tasks, a communicative-oriented strategy similar to Promoting Aphasics' Communicative Effectiveness (PACE; Davis and Wilcox, 1981, 1985) and attempts to manage RC's rambling communicative style. These were discontinued at eight months post-onset because they had resulted in no general communicative or linguistic improvement in any modality. At this stage, a new language intervention was introduced. This emphasised the visual modality and in particular the use of visual comprehension tasks. All auditory and verbal stimuli and communicative interaction were withdrawn. This visual modality therapy emphasised written word and sentence comprehension tasks. RC was encouraged to match written words and sentences to pictures. She was presented with two words and asked if they matched each other along the following parameters: same/different (e.g. boy vs. boy), familiarity (e.g. fellow vs. yellow), same category (e.g. pants vs. dress; pants vs. apple), word class (e.g. pen vs. write), synonym (e.g. couch vs. sofa) and association (e.g. books/bookcase vs. books/rodeo). RC was also encouraged to follow instructions and answer questions. These varied in terms of length, structural complexity (e.g. active vs. passive), semantic plausibility (e.g. eat your lunch vs. eat your shoes) and contextual and linguistic redundancy (semantically supportive words within and outside the sentence boundary). Success in these tasks was defined as 90% accuracy over two consecutive sessions with a large number and variety of stimulus materials.

Unit 24.4 New language intervention

(1) One of the activities used in therapy until seven months post-onset was picture categorisation tasks. Describe these tasks, and explain what aspect of language they are aimed at remediating.

(2) An intervention similar to PACE was used to treat RC in the seven months following stroke onset. Which of the following is a *true* statement about PACE intervention?
   (a) PACE is a conversational treatment in which any modality can be used to communicate ideas.
   (b) PACE can be used to treat clients with different types and severities of aphasia.

(c) PACE is not appropriate for users of augmentative and alternative communication.

(d) Only the client assumes the role of message sender in PACE.

(e) In PACE the client must convey a message which is not already known by the clinician.

(3) Using your knowledge of RC's lesion sites, explain why a therapy which emphasises visual comprehension is rationally motivated.

(4) The word–word matching tasks that were used in the new language intervention are targeting different aspects of word knowledge. Describe *three* such aspects.

(5) Some of the sentence comprehension tasks presented to RC varied in contextual and linguistic redundancy. Explain how increasing this redundancy might affect RC's comprehension.

Post-intervention language assessment

After two months of the new language intervention, the Boston Naming Test and the Boston Diagnostic Aphasia Examination were repeated. There was some improvement in visual comprehension skills and verbal output in the form of naming ability. However, results on the BDAE revealed that there had been no improvement in auditory comprehension. Nevertheless, RC was observed and reported to respond more accurately in simple conversational situations with the examiner and her family. There was a decrease in neologistic jargon and corresponding increase in semantic jargon. Some of RC's responses on the BNT and the visual confrontation naming subtest of the BDAE are shown in the table below. At 10 months post-onset, RC's performance on comprehension tasks which required her to match written sentences to pictures ranged from 56% to 73% accuracy. Her performance was highest on 5-word and 7-word active sentences (73% and 62%, respectively), and lowest on 7-word reversible and non-reversible passive sentences (57% and 56%, respectively). In terms of following instructions, RC's best performance of 79% was recorded on 4-word instructions (e.g. Pick up the cup), with performances of 60% and 53%, respectively, obtained on 7-word, 2-item instructions (e.g. Point to the pencil and the cup) and 6-word instructions that used prepositions (e.g. Tap the spoon with the pencil). Finally, RC was able to answer 4–5 word yes–no questions with 82% accuracy. Four-to-six word what-, who-, when- and where-questions were answered with 59%, 51%, 50% and 54% accuracy, respectively.

	8 months post-onset	10 months post-onset
BNT		
'scissors'	/saɪbwɚ/	/kʌtmæn/
'flower'	/fenhɑl/	/blumpat/
'pencil'	/gɪfku/	/pɛnres/
BDAE		
'drinking'	/nodɪk/	/kʌpʌp/
'cactus'	/sʌtʌs/	/prɪkəl/

Unit 24.5 Post-intervention language assessment

(1) RC's auditory comprehension on the BDAE did not improve as a result of the new language intervention. Yet, her ability to respond with accuracy in simple conversational interactions with her family did improve. How would you account for this difference?

(2) At 10 months post-onset RC's use of semantic jargon had increased while her use of neologistic jargon had decreased. Give *five* examples of RC's use of semantic jargon. For each example, indicate how RC's response during naming is related semantically to the target word.

(3) Explain why RC performs better on the comprehension of active sentences than passive sentences. Why might we have expected RC to display better comprehension of non-reversible passive sentences than reversible passive sentences?

(4) Which *two* factors account for the performance exhibited by RC in the comprehension of the following instructions? Which of these factors appears to be most influential in RC's comprehension?

> *Pick up the cup.*
> *Point to the pencil and the cup.*
> *Tap the spoon with the pencil.*

(5) Aside from syntactic complexity, what factor do you think might account for RC's greater difficulty understanding wh-interrogatives than understanding yes–no interrogatives?

Case study 25

Woman aged 41 years with Broca's aphasia

Introduction

The following exercise is a case study of a woman ('HW') who was studied by Bastiaanse (1995). HW developed Broca's aphasia following a cerebrovascular accident (stroke) in August 1986. Aphasia is a common post-stroke sequela, which has been reported to occur in 30% of patients with first-ever ischaemic stroke (Engelter et al., 2006) and 34.8% of sub-acute stroke patients (Hoffmann and Chen, 2013). Broca's aphasia is the most common subtype, accounting for 27.2% of all aphasias in a large, sub-acute stroke population (Hoffmann and Chen, 2013). The case study is presented in five sections: history and initial assessment; assessment 15 months post-onset: part 1; assessment 15 months post-onset: part 2; focus on spontaneous speech: part 1; and focus on spontaneous speech: part 2.

History and initial assessment

HW is a right-handed woman and native speaker of Dutch. She is married and has two children, a 15-year-old son and a 12-year-old daughter. Prior to her stroke, HW did cleaning two mornings a week and was a 'reading mother' at a primary school. Her hobbies were reading, needlework and fishing. With the exception of a hearing impairment on the left side, HW was healthy prior to her stroke.

In August 1986, HW experienced sudden paralysis on the right side. She was aphasic and was hospitalised in an unconscious state. Upon regaining consciousness, HW was unable to speak. Her right limbs were paralysed and her vision was also impaired. A CT scan was conducted two weeks post-onset. It revealed an ischaemic infarct in parts of the temporal and frontal lobes, with damage extending to the left parietal lobe. At one month post-onset, HW was discharged from hospital and admitted to a rehabilitation centre. Her right arm was still not functional. However, the paresis of her right leg had decreased with the result that she was able to walk using a delta-stick.

At four months post-onset, HW underwent linguistic and neuropsychological assessment as an inpatient of the rehabilitation centre. It revealed that HW was suffering from a typical Broca's aphasia. HW displayed relatively intact comprehension of spoken language – her score on the Token Test was 56/61. Neuropsychological assessment revealed that HW had poor verbal memory due to retrieval deficiencies – she had a percentile score of 50 compared to aphasics. HW scored in the 7th decile compared to other aphasics on the Raven Coloured Progressive Matrices. No other neuropsychological deficits were found. In an attempt to improve HW's language abilities and help both her and her family cope with her aphasia, HW received speech therapy five times a week. Her language therapy focused on sentence construction, writing and text comprehension, using a programme for training sentence construction. HW also received physiotherapy, occupational therapy and the assistance of a social worker.

Unit 25.1 History and initial assessment

(1) HW sustained an ischaemic stroke. Which of the following are *true* claims about ischaemic stroke?
  (a) Ischaemic stroke includes thrombotic and embolic subtypes.
  (b) Atherosclerosis is a risk factor for ischaemic stroke.
  (c) Ischaemic stroke is the leading cause of death in the US.
  (d) Seizures are a neurological complication of ischaemic stroke.
  (e) Ischaemic stroke is not a cause of dysphagia.

(2) HW experienced an unspecified visual impairment following her stroke. Which CT finding might account for this impairment?

(3) HW's linguistic assessment revealed that she had a typical Broca's aphasia. Which of the following are features of this type of aphasia?
  (a) relatively intact auditory verbal comprehension
  (b) use of jargon output
  (c) agrammatism
  (d) fluent verbal output
  (e) poor sentence repetition

(4) Which of the features identified in (3) above is explained by the neuropsychological finding that HW has poor verbal memory?

(5) HW received speech therapy not only to improve her language skills but also to help her and her family cope with aphasia. Today, the management of aphasia places considerable emphasis on the psychosocial aspects of the condition. Describe in brief the psychosocial implications of aphasia.

Assessment 15 months post-onset: part 1

At 15 months post-onset, a further assessment of HW's linguistic and neuropsychological abilities was performed. A percentile score of 100 was obtained on a verbal memory test. HW had a score comparable to an IQ of 110 on the Raven Standard matrix. Comprehension of nouns was intact at the previous assessment and was not examined again. Comprehension of verbs was assessed using a test in which HW had to select one of four action pictures. Alongside the correct picture, there are three semantically related distractors. HW displayed 100% correct performance on this assessment. A Dutch version of the Test for Reception of Grammar (TROG; Bishop, 1983) was used to assess HW's auditory comprehension of sentences. There were only two errors committed on this test. One error concerned the single–plural distinction of nouns, while the other error involved an embedded sentence. HW got 28 of the 30 items on the Token Test correct. Spontaneous speech was analysed and will be considered in units 25.4 and 25.5. HW named all 40 items correctly on the Dutch version of the Boston Naming Test (Kaplan et al., 1983). HW's ability to retrieve low-frequency words was assessed using the Graded Naming Test (McKenna and Warrington, 1983). HW named 15 of 30 items correctly, a score which is comparable to that of normal controls. Errors included circumlocutions and wrong interpretations of the picture. In a test of naming actions, HW named 37 out of 40 actions correctly. She used the infinitive form of verbs to name the actions. The three verbs which she could not name were: to carpenter (HW: to strike the nail into the plank), to moor (HW: to hang the boat on the hook) and to dig (HW: the man polders, the man shovels out the land, shovels hole).

Unit 25.2 Assessment 15 months post-onset: part 1

(1) How would you characterise HW's single-word and sentence-level comprehension? Provide evidence to support your answer.

(2) HW was unable to name items like *pagoda* and *centaur* on the Graded Naming Test. Is this likely to be on account of a word-finding difficulty? Justify your response.

(3) One of the items that HW failed on the TROG involved an embedded sentence. Which of the following items from the TROG was in error for HW?
   (a) The cup is in the box.
   (b) The girl is pushing the horse.
   (c) The shoe the comb is on is blue.
   (d) The book is on the box that is red.
   (e) Not only the bird but also the flower is blue.

(4) HW was unable to produce the names of the actions *to carpenter*, *to moor* and *to dig*. What type of linguistic behaviour occurs during HW's response to these actions?

(5) During the Graded Naming Test, HW produced the response 'soldier in former days' for the test item *yashmak* (the name of the face veil worn by Muslim women in public). This error may simply reflect the fact that *yashmak* was not part of HW's pre-morbid vocabulary. However, there is another possible explanation of this error. What is this explanation?

Assessment 15 months post-onset: part 2

The repetition of single words and sentences was also assessed at 15 months post-onset. HW's repetition of words was intact. There was a slight impairment of sentence repetition, particularly in longer sentences. For example, when asked to repeat *In the classroom all children were talking aloud*, HW said 'In the classroom all children talk loud'. To test sentence construction, a sentence anagram test and a subtest of the Aachen Aphasie Test (Graetz et al., 1992) were used. The anagram test was performed with little difficulty. In the Aachen Aphasie Test, the items used and HW's responses were as follows:

The man is begging for money.
The old man the old man is begging for money.

The woman is cleaning the coffeepot.
The woman is cleaning the teapot.

The boy is playing with the dog.
The boy the boy the boy feeds the dog.

The man fishes a boot out of the water.
The man fishes in the wat no the man has a boot on the hook.

The boy breaks a glass.
The boy the boy drops a vase cries.

Father and son are playing Indians.
The indian the indian buttons up the indian fastens the man on the tree.

The policeman arrests the thief.
Policeman the policeman fastens handcuffs.

Two men are having an argument.
Two people are talking to each other.

The teacher writes something on the blackboard for the girl.
The teacher writes word on the blackboard.

The man is lying on the couch, smoking a pipe and reading the newspaper.
The man is lying on the couch to he is smoking a pipe he is reading the newspaper.

Unit 25.3 Assessment 15 months post-onset: part 2

(1) HW's word and sentence repetition skills are much stronger at 15 months post-onset than they were when HW was first tested. What aspect of HW's neuropsychological performance at 15 months post-onset might account for this improvement?

(2) What class of words (open- or closed-class) are most compromised during sentence repetition for HW? Provide evidence to support your answer.

(3) During sentence construction, repetition occurs frequently. Which grammatical structure within the sentence appears to be vulnerable to repetition? Is there any evidence that HW may be using repetition to correct her output?

(4) A number of other anomalies occur during sentence construction. These are listed below. Give *one* example of each anomaly in the data:
 (a) omission of article in the noun phrase
 (b) use of word semantically related to the target word
 (c) omission of coordinating conjunction
 (d) failure to use ellipsis
 (e) use of word visually related to the target word

(5) Is there any evidence of the use of circumlocution during HW's sentence construction?

Focus on spontaneous speech: part 1

At 15 months post-onset, an assessment of HW's spontaneous speech was also conducted. Extracts of HW's spontaneous speech will be examined in detail in units 25.4 and

25.5. In the extract below, the interviewer (INT) and HW are discussing HW's language problems

INT: Can you tell me what are your problems?

HW: Er talking problem yes but forming difficult sentences easy when no easy when first not er difficult words er to think yes doesn't soon occur to me

INT: You have problems finding the words?

HW: Yes yes

INT: But, as I understand, you also encounter problems when making a sentence?

HW: Yes it doesn't come at moment when I write er goes that er slow er no

INT: When you are writing?

HW: Yes before the time I did know writing down er I write down nothing remembers me

INT: Yes, but when you really want to, can you speak in correct sentences?

HW: Yes

INT: Why don't you do that?

HW: Er too fast to talk

INT: What do you mean, too fast?

HW: Er I too fast to talk er I cannot er search for words

INT: Yes, when you talk in sentences, you can't look for words?

HW: No

INT: And looking for words, is that difficult too?

HW: Yes

INT: That's why you talk in short sentences?

HW: Yes the a and I leave out I just leave er

INT: Do you do that on purpose?

HW: No on God no

INT: That happens automatically?

HW: Yes I hear always what I says sentences quick I hear er and the I hear er always er what I says wrongly

INT: You do hear that?

HW: Yes yes

Unit 25.4 Focus on spontaneous speech: part 1

(1) Notwithstanding her expressive difficulties, HW is able to comprehend a range of the interviewer's utterances. Several of these utterances are described below. Provide *one* example of each of the following in the extract:
   (a) HW is able to comprehend prosodic questions.
   (b) HW is able to comprehend requests for clarification.
   (c) HW is able to comprehend yes–no interrogatives.
   (d) HW is able to comprehend wh-interrogatives.
   (e) HW is able to comprehend indirect speech acts.

(2) The interviewer uses several utterances that contain demonstrative pronouns. Is HW able to establish the referents of these pronouns? Provide *five* examples to support your response.

(3) When HW describes her language problems to the interviewer, she makes extensive use of mental state language. Give *three* examples of the use of mental state language in HW's expressive output. The use of this language suggests that a certain cognitive capacity is intact in HW. What is the name of this capacity?

(4) Apart from HW's admission that she has word-finding problems, what other evidence is there that HW has difficulties with this aspect of language?

(5) Provide *one* example of each of the following linguistic errors in HW's turns in the above extract:

(a) incorrect verb morphology

(b) omission of *be* as a main verb

(c) omission of object noun or pronoun

(d) omission of subject noun or pronoun

(e) omission of subject pronoun and *be* as a main verb

Focus on spontaneous speech: part 2

In this lengthier extract, also recorded at 15 months post-onset, the interviewer and HW are discussing Christmas and HW's new house.

INT: Okay, something else, it will soon be Sinterklaas and Christmas

HW: Yes yes

INT: Do you have any plans?

HW: Yes no plans not not Sinterklaas shopsbusiness me purse always empty future no past er

INT: Won't you celebrate Sinterklaas?

HW: No absolutely

INT: Don't you do anything?

HW: In the pan tasty things snacks tasty

INT: But no presents?

HW: No no

INT: And at Christmas and New Year's Eve, are you going to do something?

HW: Er eat tasty things presents Christmas draw numbers all er get presents ten guilders ten guilders each

INT: You are not going out?

HW: I don't know

INT: You don't know

HW: No we sold house our house new about March er er we saving pennies

INT: Yes, I can imagine. Where did you buy a house?

HW: In G. M-straat centre of G. the middle in G. ah beautiful place puh

INT: Where do you live now?

HW: G.

INT: You live in G. already?

HW: Yes outskirts of G. near D.

INT: The house you bought, what does it look like?

HW: New building subsidised beautiful house oh dear

INT: Tell me

HW: Yes beautiful house magnificent from the outside windows extremely beautiful house

INT: And what size is it?

HW: Er room er ninety meters no

INT: No, that seems very large

HW: No nine meters all thresholds gone oh nice

INT: And how many floors does it have?

HW: Er three ground floor first bed-rooms two shower

INT: Three floors, upstairs two bedrooms

HW: Yes and an attic a bed-room Reinier row about I want in the attic Renate no I want in the attic

INT: And who is going to the attic?

HW: Reinier

INT: That is the oldest one, isn't it?

HW: Yes yes

INT: Do you have a bedroom downstairs yourself?

HW: No upstairs I can walk on the stairs

INT: Is there also a garden?

HW: Ah big one big one behind the house fifteen meters width seventeen no seven meters

INT: That's nice

HW: Yes nice

INT: Is it brand new?

HW: Yes built now

INT: So there is nothing in the garden yet?

HW: No now tiles on roof

INT: So you will have a bare garden

HW: Yes er ah future eh trees apple-trees ah delicious pear-trees pears

INT: Yes, you want to plant trees

HW: Yes blossoms beautifully oh magnificent new trees small trees

INT: You are going to move in May?

HW: No er about March new house delivered extremely beautiful

INT: You are glad with it, aren't you?

HW: Oh beautiful

INT: Were you eager to move?

HW: Yes

INT: What kind of house did you have?

HW: Old house about after the no war built block

Unit 25.5 Focus on spontaneous speech: part 2

(1) In this extract, HW provides the interviewer with some contradictory information. Identify *two* instances where this occurs.

(2) Substitution confers cohesion on conversation and other forms of discourse. Can HW comprehend the use of substitution by the interviewer? Can HW use substitution appropriately in her own utterances? Provide evidence to support your answers.

(3) At one point in this extract, HW uses direct reported speech. Where does this occur, and why is it used?

(4) Can HW engage in self-initiated and other-initiated repair of utterances? Provide evidence to support your answer.

(5) Provide *one* example of each of the following linguistic errors in HW's turns in the above exchange:
  (a) omission of *be* as an auxiliary verb
  (b) use of non-specific vocabulary
  (c) utterance abandoned mid-stream
  (d) omission of determiner in noun phrase
  (e) incomplete verb phrase

Case study 26

Man with stroke-induced Broca's aphasia

Introduction

The following exercise is a case study of a man ('Roy') with agrammatic aphasia who was studied by Beeke et al. (2007). Seven years prior to this study, Roy sustained a left-hemisphere cerebrovascular accident (CVA). Among other problems, his CVA caused Broca's-type aphasia. The principal language feature of his aphasia was a severe, chronic agrammatism. Aphasia is a common sequela of stroke-induced brain damage. Godefroy et al. (2002) reported aphasia in 207 (67.2%) of 308 patients admitted to a stroke unit. Some aphasia subtypes are more common than others. Non-fluent aphasia – of which Broca's aphasia is one type – is less common than fluent aphasia, accounting for 34.2% and 65.8% of cases in one clinical sample (Laska et al., 2001). The case study is presented in five sections: history and communication status; assessment battery; focus on agrammatism; discourse production; and conversational data.

History and communication status

At the time of study, Roy was in his mid-to-late forties – his exact age was unknown. Seven years earlier, he sustained a left-hemisphere cerebrovascular accident while waterskiing. Also unknown are the aetiology, size and location of the lesion in this CVA. Roy is fully mobile. However, his CVA caused a dense hemiplegia that affected his right arm, and he has little useful movement of this limb. His hearing and vision are normal. Roy lives with his wife. He is an active member of his local stroke group and attends an exercise group.

Roy's CVA caused Broca's-type aphasia. He also has a mild articulatory dyspraxia and mild-to-moderate word-finding difficulties. He has severe agrammatism and non-fluent spoken output. His spoken language contains few identifiable syntactic structures and few, if any, verbs. There is a high frequency of adverbs, nouns and phrases such as *I think* and *you know*. Pronouns, articles and prepositions are largely absent. These language features are evident in the description that Roy gives of events around his stroke below. Notwithstanding his severe expressive difficulties, Roy's comprehension of language in conversational situations appears very good. Roy reported having speech and language therapy (SLT) both as an in- and out-patient in the months following his stroke. However, he has not had any SLT for some years. The content and duration of earlier SLT are unknown.

'um . . . so s- er skiing . . . er waterskiing . . . yeh uh Greenbridge . . . yeah? uh Kent . . . uh . . . uh . . . four of them . . . uuuhh . . . blokes y'know . . . uh . . . uhhh . . . boat . . . and . . . anyway . . . sort of . . . waterskiing . . . and strange! . . . sort of . . . and then . . . ur . . . bang! [*mimes falling over*] . . . funny . . . and all of a sudden . . . bang.'

Unit 26.1 History and communication status

(1) Using your knowledge of neuroanatomy, explain why adults like Roy who sustain a left-hemisphere stroke may have Broca's aphasia *and* a right hemiplegia affecting the arm.

(2) Roy is reported to have word-finding difficulties. What evidence is there of these difficulties in the description he gives of the events surrounding his stroke?

(3) Explain why Roy can still communicate effectively even in the presence of severe agrammatic language.

(4) Although Roy's comprehension of language appears extremely good in conversational situations, it may not necessarily be so during language testing. Explain why this might be the case.

(5) How does Roy attempt to compensate for his limited expressive language skills during the description of events surrounding his stroke?

Assessment battery

Roy's language and communication skills underwent a wide-ranging assessment by a speech and language therapist. The assessments were intended to elicit quantitative and qualitative data at the word, sentence and narrative levels. The Psycholinguistic Assessments of Language Processing in Aphasia (PALPA; Kay et al., 1992) contains 60 subtests that assess all components of language structure such as orthography and phonology, word and picture semantics, and morphology and syntax. Spoken and written input and output modalities are assessed through tasks that require subjects to make lexical decisions, and undertake repetition and picture naming. One PALPA subtest in particular – Spoken Picture Naming – was used to assess Roy's naming abilities. An assessment known as Thematic Roles in Production (TRIP; Whitworth, 1996) was used to assess Roy's retrieval of the same item in single word and sentence contexts. A series of 80 picture cards is used to explore words that are assigned different thematic roles in sentences of varying argument structure. The examiner models all target responses at the outset of the test as the subject views the picture stimuli. Like PALPA, TRIP draws on the cognitive neuropsychological literature for its theoretical base. The Verb and Sentence Test (VAST; Bastiaanse et al., 2002) assesses the production and comprehension of verbs and sentences. The test is theoretically motivated and can be used as a basis for treatment. Subjects are required to undertake a series of tasks with a single practice item rehearsed at the outset of each task. The tasks are: verb comprehension; sentence comprehension; grammaticality judgement; action naming; filling in finite verbs and infinitives in sentences; sentence construction; sentence anagrams with pictures; sentence anagrams without pictures; and wh-anagrams. The cookie theft picture description (Goodglass and Kaplan, 1983a) was also part of the assessment battery. In this picture, a woman is standing at the kitchen sink drying a plate, while the sink is overflowing with water. Meanwhile, a boy (presumably, the woman's son) has climbed a stool which is rocking precariously and is taking cookies from a jar in the cupboard. A girl (presumably, the boy's sister) has her hand raised upwards to receive the cookies that her brother is taking. A cartoon description task, adapted from Fletcher and

Birt (1983) and featuring a dinner party, was also included in the assessment battery. Narrative production was examined through 'Cinderella' storytelling. Finally, a video-recorded sample of conversation between Roy and his daughter Di was also collected and analysed. The sample was 23 minutes in duration and was recorded at home.

Unit 26.2 Assessment battery

(1) Both PALPA and TRIP are based on a cognitive neuropsychological (CNP) model of human cognition. Which of the following are *true* statements about this model?
  (a) The CNP model has its roots in linguistics and neurology.
  (b) The CNP model assumes that some of the components of the cognitive system are modular in that they operate independently of other components.
  (c) The CNP model assumes that cortical lesions can cause modules and mappings between modules to be selectively damaged or lost.
  (d) The CNP model is based on data from individuals who have developmental and acquired disorders of cognition.
  (e) The CNP model is designed only to explain language processing.

(2) The TRIP is used to examine words that are assigned different thematic roles in sentences of varying argument structure. For each of the following sentences, indicate if the verb has a one-, two-, or three-argument structure. Also, identify the participant or thematic roles in each sentence.
  The boy runs.
  The woman cooks the meal.
  The man put the book on the shelf.

(3) One of the VAST subtests examines the ability of subjects to comprehend single verbs. The subject is presented with four pictures. The examiner reads a verb aloud and the subject points to one of these pictures. One of the verbs used in this subtest is 'biting'. Describe the relation of each of the following distractor pictures to this target: *teeth*; *scratching*; *nails*.

(4) Two picture description tasks were part of the assessment battery: the cookie theft picture and the dinner party cartoon strip. There is a significant difference in the type of descriptions that these tasks are intended to elicit. What is that difference?

(5) Picture description tasks elicit monological discourse while conversation is a type of dialogical discourse. Why is it important to have samples of both types of discourse within an assessment of language and communication in aphasia?

Focus on agrammatism

The results of the assessment battery reveal the nature and extent of Roy's agrammatism. On the subtest of the PALPA that examines spoken picture naming, Roy named 33 of 40 items correctly. Of the seven errors produced, five were similar in nature to the following: 'water' for *glass* and 'giraffe' for *elephant*. Roy's production of verbs of varying argument structure was impaired. His production of one-, two- and three-argument verbs on the TRIP was 80%, 30% and 0%, respectively. At sentence level on the TRIP, Roy produced a sentence for 47% of constructions with a one-argument verb and 15% of constructions with a two-argument verb. Examples of his productions are shown below. Level and falling intonation are indicated by a comma and full stop, respectively:

The girl is skipping.
'Girl, (2.8) she, (4.2) skipping'

The girl is kicking the snake.
'um right (1.7) girl, (3.4) girl, (11.6) kick, (1.7) snake'

No sentences were produced that contained a three-argument verb. None of Roy's sentences were structurally or morphologically well formed. Determiners and verb tense morphology were omitted. The progressive *–ing* ending was used on 72% of all verbs, while the remaining 28% of verbs were uninflected. On the VAST, Roy produced only 8 of 40 verbs correctly as single words. When asked to produce verbs within a sentence, Roy used single words for 16 of 40 items and produced no response at all for the remaining 24 items. The single words were mostly isolated verbs. However, if a verb proved difficult to produce, he named an object in the picture (30% of his responses were nouns). Of all verbs elicited, 71% contained the progressive *–ing* form, 9% were uninflected, and 20% were indistinguishable from nouns because of the lack of sentence structure.

Unit 26.3 Focus on agrammatism

(1) During the spoken picture naming subtest of PALPA, Roy produced a predominance of one type of error. What is that error?

(2) On the TRIP, how many sentences of the following type was Roy able to produce? *Jill gave the book to the woman.*

(3) Using the examples of Roy's productions during the TRIP, describe *three* ways in which his expressive language is compromised by agrammatism.

(4) During the VAST, Roy is not able to produce any sentences at all. However, he was able to produce seven sentences with one-argument verbs and three sentences with two-argument verbs during the TRIP. How might this difference be accounted for?

(5) Roy produced the following responses during the VAST: 'scissors' when shown a picture of a woman cutting paper, and 'hoe' when shown a picture of a man raking the lawn. How would you characterise these responses?

Discourse production

Roy's impaired sentence production during language testing deteriorates yet further on the picture description and storytelling tasks. Roy produces only two phrases and one sentence, all within the dinner party cartoon strip description. These phrases and sentence were 'large trout', 'four people' and 'man washing up'. However, Roy still manages to achieve communicative success through the use of a number of strategies that compensate for the absence of verbs and arguments. These strategies are illustrated by the discourse data shown below.

Extract A 'Cinderella' storytelling

R: (0.6) so, (0.2) then, (.) all of a sudden, (1.3) uh (2.9) spell

T: mhm

R: (1.7) and (0.4) ur (1.4) ah (0.7) twenty or something, (.) hh and (0.2) uh uh (0.5) suddenly, (1.5) uh (0.4) rich.

T: mhm

Extract B Cookie theft picture description

R: um (2.8) wu- (0.5) er (1.0) tuh ach! (3.8) plate, (2.2) [*sits upright, gazes to middle distance, enacts the woman wiping a plate*]

T: [*nods*]

Extract C Dinner party cartoon strip description

(Roy is describing a scene in which the pet cat has eaten the fish intended for the meal. Earlier in the strip, the cat was shown disappearing under the dining table.)

R: (0.2) uh uhu- ur (0.4) cat. (1.6) yeah. (0.2) actually I thought, (0.3) dog, but no, um yeah exactly yeah

T: mm

Extract D Dinner party cartoon strip description

(Roy is describing a scene in which the host of the dinner party runs out of the house in order to buy fish and chips to replace the ruined meal. The hostess is crying over the stolen fish and is being comforted by the female guest.)

R: um (1.3) tuh (0.9) ar (0.7) quick, I know. (2.0) and (1.8) oooooh, (0.6) eh (0.4) crying, and, (0.5) er (3.7) never mind. ehh heh heh

T: hm hehm

Unit 26.4 Discourse production

(1) In extract A, Roy succeeds in describing an event in the 'Cinderella' story in the absence of any verb production. Describe how he achieves this.

(2) A quite different, but equally effective, strategy is used by Roy in extract B to communicate that the woman is drying the plate in the cookie theft picture. What is that strategy?

(3) In extract C, Roy successfully communicates that he was mistaken in thinking that the tail disappearing under the dining table belonged to the dog. Explain how he achieves this, notwithstanding the severely agrammatic nature of his output at the beginning of this extract.

(4) In extracts A to C, Roy succeeds in communicating via the juxtaposition of certain elements. He does so again in extract D. What are those elements in this extract?

(5) Which of the following statements best characterises the communicative strategies that Roy uses to overcome his agrammatism?

(a) Roy makes extensive use of circumlocution and semantic paraphasias.
(b) Roy builds his message incrementally through the juxtaposition of elements such as reported speech, adverbs, nouns and set phrases.
(c) Roy augments his spoken utterances with mime.
(d) Roy is passive in communication and defers to his partner.
(e) Roy uses one- and two-argument verbs extensively.

Conversational data

An examination of Roy's communication skills during conversation with his daughter Di reveals other strategies that he uses to address his agrammatic output. Also, conversation analysis exposes how Di has successfully accommodated to her father's severe impairment of expressive language in conversation. Several extracts from the conversational exchange between Roy and Di are presented below.

Extract A The topic of conversation is racing

R: u- ur (0.1) you know, (0.1) u- uh- ur racing,
D: mm
R: (0.2) ur- (0.3) Newmarket, (0.2) Epsom,
D: yeah
R: anywhere, (0.2) but (0.5) me, (0.5) u- ur (0.2) Ascot, no.
D: you've never been have you
R: no no
D: perhaps you can go next year

Extract B The topic of conversation is Di's job as a nursery nurse

R: uh- u e interesting actually, (0.3) uh- bu- bi- because- (2.4) er now, (2.1) me,
D: m
R: (0.3) I (0.9) think no, (0.5) er er- (0.7) u- special. (0.3) honestly.
D: what working with children
R: yeah, definitely.
D: yeah not everyone can do it can they

Extract C The topic of conversation is Di's upcoming 21st birthday party

D: it'll be a good night though
R: oh uh- uh- tu- i- really. (0.3) yeah
D: mmm
R: u- u- and now, (0.6) o- two weeks innit
D: (1.3) not this weekend (0.4) not the weekend after, the weekend after
R: eh- yeah

D: two weeks this Saturday

R: yeah (0.7) I know and suddenly [*clicks fingers*]

D: I know.

Unit 26.5 Conversational data

(1) Describe the communicative strategy that Roy uses in extract A to convey to Di that he has attended racing at Newmarket and Epsom but not at Ascot. What is Di's contribution to the conversational exchange?

(2) A different, but equally effective, communicative strategy is employed by Roy in extract B. How would you characterise this strategy, and Di's contribution to this exchange?

(3) Even aside from the communicative strategies that Roy uses, there is evidence that he is also able to employ a range of other features of language. Several of these features are listed below. Give *one* example of each feature in extract C:
   (a) Roy is able to use phrases.
   (b) Roy is able to establish the referents of pronouns.
   (c) Roy is able to comprehend temporally deictic expressions.
   (d) Roy is able to use mental state language.
   (e) Roy is able to use tag questions.

(4) Respond with *true* or *false* to each of the following statements:
   (a) Roy struggles with aspects of topic management.
   (b) Roy contributes overly informative utterances to conversation.
   (c) Roy makes appropriate use of turn-taking in conversation.
   (d) Roy is unable to establish Di's communicative intentions.
   (e) Roy is able to use intonation to signal the completion of his turn.

(5) Notwithstanding his limited expressive language, Roy is able to use language to fulfil a number of functions and purposes. Several of these are described below. Give *one* example of each use in extracts A to C:
   (a) Roy is able to use language to describe past events.
   (b) Roy is able to use language to express an opinion.
   (c) Roy is able to use language to confirm facts.
   (d) Roy is able to use language to convey an evaluation.
   (e) Roy is able to use language to support his partner's conversational turn.

Case study 27

Man aged 41 years with non-fluent aphasia

Introduction

The following exercise is a case study of a man ('BB') of 41 years of age who was studied by Jones (1986). In November 1978, BB suffered a left cerebral embolus that resulted in a right hemiplegia and Broca's type aphasia. Despite long-standing and intensive speech and language therapy, BB's single-word output had remained unchanged for six years. A new therapy programme was commenced in December 1984 which resulted in a significant improvement in BB's expressive language. The case study is presented in five sections: medical and communication history; assessment battery; assessment findings; language intervention; and language performance during therapy.

Medical and communication history

In November 1978, BB experienced a left cerebral embolus which resulted in a right hemiplegia and Broca's-type aphasia. Prior to his cerebrovascular accident, BB had been a wholesale greengrocer. A CAT scan revealed extensive damage in the territory of the left middle cerebral artery. This damage involved the frontal, temporal and parietal lobes and extended vertically to a depth of 6mm. Following his CVA, BB's comprehension of auditory and visual material was severely affected but superior to his expressive language. BB could only produce a few common words (e.g. 'yes', 'no', 'hello'), which were awkwardly articulated. His articulatory difficulties were diagnosed as articulatory apraxia. BB's written output was limited to copying using the non-preferred left hand. For the next three years, BB received individual therapy three times a week and group therapy twice a week. Individual therapy was terminated when it was felt that BB had reached his maximum potential. At this stage, BB had improved auditory comprehension although his comprehension of visual material was still severely affected. Spoken output was limited to nouns and the occasional well-learnt phrase (e.g. 'are you well?'). Twice weekly group therapy continued for another three years. This therapy was supervised by speech and language therapists but was conducted by volunteers. Volunteers also provided twice weekly therapy on a domiciliary basis when BB was the subject of a number of research studies. These studies examined his problems with reading (he was diagnosed as having deep dyslexia), writing (particularly spelling) and his severe word-finding difficulties.

The author of the study first met BB in November 1984. By that stage, BB had not received individual therapy for three years, with the exception of work on his spelling problems. Comprehension was functional in everyday situations. It was heavily reliant on pragmatic and contextual cues. BB could read simple written material but could not decode more complex and less redundant material. There had been almost no change in

BB's spoken output in over three years. BB could still only produce single words (nouns) and had a severe word-finding deficit. No verb production was evident. Articulatory fluency varied, with well-learnt phrases produced fluently and with stereotyped prosody. BB was embarrassed about his communication problems and rarely initiated conversation. When he did attempt to communicate, there was an increased burden on his listener. Written output had improved in terms of spelling but, like spoken output, it was limited to the single-word level. In November 1984, BB's expressive language during picture description and narrative production appeared as below.

Cookie theft picture description

Girl, boy . . . eh . . . don't know . . . um . . . water . . . don't know *(Can you tell me anything else – what about this? – pointing to mother)* . . . um . . . man . . . no . . . woman . . . window . . . oh . . . eh . . . /k/ . . . /k/ . . . tea . . . eh . . . don't know.

Narrative production about previous work

eh . . . eh . . . oh . . . no . . . um . . . eh . . . don't know . . . no . . . eh . . . potatoes . . . um . . . no.

Unit 27.1 Medical and communication history

(1) BB suffered a left middle cerebral artery (MCA) stroke. Strokes of the MCA territory are common – accounting for 50.8% of all strokes in a recent, large clinical sample – and are associated with poor functional outcomes (Ng et al., 2007). Explain why this is the case.

(2) Apraxia of speech and Broca's aphasia often occur together, as they do for this client. Using your knowledge of neuroanatomy, explain why this is the case.

(3) BB was diagnosed as having Broca's-type aphasia. Describe *five* features of BB's clinical presentation which are consistent with this type of aphasia.

(4) Using the language data presented above, characterise BB's agrammatic verbal output.

(5) BB was diagnosed as having deep dyslexia. Which of the following are *true* statements about this type of dyslexia?
   (a) Deep dyslexia is a developmental reading disorder.
   (b) Semantic errors occur in deep dyslexia (e.g. reading RIVER as 'ocean').
   (c) There is an advantage for reading abstract over concrete words.
   (d) Visual errors occur in deep dyslexia (e.g. reading SCANDAL as 'sandals').
   (e) Morphological errors are not found in deep dyslexia (e.g. reading FACT as 'facts').

Assessment battery

Prior to embarking on a new therapy programme, the author of the study conducted a wide-ranging assessment of BB's expressive and receptive language skills. Several tests and tasks were used for this purpose. Alongside the cookie theft picture description and an account of his prior work (see above), BB's sentence production abilities were examined in other ways. BB was presented with 24 verb pictures, and was asked to describe the actions that people were performing. He was explicitly instructed to produce just a 'doing' word. BB was also asked to describe what was happening in 10 subject–verb–object-type pictures. The pictures depicted only animate actors and inanimate patients. The same 10 verbs that were depicted in these pictures were then given to BB in infinitive form. BB was asked to generate a sentence around each verb. To decrease his processing load and help him concentrate on sentence construction, BB was given access to the pictures if he requested them. During the Word Order Test (Jones, 1984), BB was given a series of individual pictures. For each picture, the three elements of the target sentence depicted in the picture were given to BB on separate pieces of paper (e.g. the fireman/the policeman/follows). BB was required to place the elements in the order that matched the scene depicted in the picture.

To test receptive language, several tests and tasks were also used. The Test for Reception of Grammar (TROG; Bishop, 1983) was completed to obtain a comprehensive picture of BB's comprehension skills. In the picture selection comprehension task of the Word Order Test, BB was presented auditorily with a sentence which he was then required to match to one of three pictures. The sentences were simple active reversible declaratives which contained three types of verbs (non-motion verbs, non-directional-motion verbs, directional-motion verbs). The three pictures represented the target sentence, the same sentence with the arguments reversed, and the same noun arguments in the same order as the target sentence but with a different verb. In a test of recognition of sentence patterns, BB was presented with a number of written sentences which varied in complexity. He was asked to 'block off' words in the sentence which he believed 'belonged together'. He was also asked to re-assemble the sentences using the 'blocked off' words that he had generated.

Unit 27.2 Assessment battery

(1) When BB was presented with verb pictures, he was explicitly instructed to produce just a 'doing' word. Why do you think BB was given this instruction?

(2) BB was asked to describe what was happening in subject–verb–object-type pictures. The pictures depicted only animate actors and inanimate patients. What type of sentence did this feature force BB to produce?

(3) BB was given the infinitive form of a verb and asked to generate a sentence around it. What specific aspect of production is this task attempting to assess?

(4) During the Word Order Test, BB was required to match an auditorily presented sentence to one of three pictures. The presented sentences were simple active reversible declaratives. Give *one* example of this type of sentence.

(5) BB was presented with written sentences and was asked to 'block off' words which he believed 'belonged together'. What do you think this task is attempting to assess?

Assessment findings

When presented with verb pictures, and asked to produce a 'doing' word, BB achieved a score of 20/24. All 'doing' words were gerunds. When asked to describe 10 subject–verb–object pictures, the following responses were produced:

The boy is kicking the ball: eh . . . um . . . push . . . push . . . no . . . ball . . . no
The boy is riding the bike: girl . . . no boy . . . bike . . . well . . . um . . . boy . . . um

The girl is writing a letter: writing . . . /r/ . . . /r/ . . . read . . . girl
The boy is painting a picture: eh . . . boy . . . no girl? . . . um . . . don't know
The boy is digging the garden: /g/ . . . /g/ . . . don't know . . . (cued 1st syllable) gar-den . . . boy . . . is . . . no
The boy is reading a book: oh . . . /k/ . . . /k/ . . . /k/ . . . don't know
The girl is brushing her hair: eh . . . um . . . /k/ . . . don't know
The boy is eating an apple: boy . . . no (pointing to apple) drink? . . . no
The boy is climbing a ladder: me! (indicating boy) no . . . boy /k/ . . . climb up . . . yes!
The boy is drinking orange: /b/ . . . boy . . . ah! . . . boy is . . . /i/ . . . eat . . . no . . . um

When given the infinitive form of verbs and asked to generate a sentence around each verb, the following responses were produced:

Kick: /k/ . . . kick . . . no . . . football . . . don't know
Ride: ride a . . . ride a . . . um . . . no
Write: write . . . eh . . . pen . . . um . . . letter
Paint: paintbrush! . . . paint . . . oh . . . brush house . . . Good!
Dig: dig . . . garden . . . yes!
Read: read . . . letter . . . um . . . write . . . no . . . read . . . no!
Brush: brush . . . um . . . yes . . . hair? . . . no . . . comb
Eat: eat . . . food! . . . me! . . . eat . . . eh . . . Barbara (his wife) . . . no
Climb: /k/ . . . climb up . . . eh . . . climb? . . . don't know
Drink: beer! . . . drinking . . . no

When asked to rearrange sentence elements in the Word Order Test, BB produced a total of 29/60 (48%) errors. His errors primarily took the form of object–verb–subject constructions. However, there were also a number of verb–subject–object and verb–object–subject constructions.

On the TROG, BB passed 12/20 blocks in the auditory version and 8/20 blocks in the visual (reading) version. Items which produced errors in both versions were singular/plural, simple active reversible, comparatives, monosyllabic prepositions and postmodified subjects. When presented with a spoken sentence and asked to match it to one of three pictures, the total number of errors produced was 36/60 (60%). For all three types of verbs included in these sentences, the errors were the same – BB chose the picture in which the arguments were reversed. When asked to 'block off' elements within sentences, BB displayed intact performance. However, when he was given the same elements that he had 'blocked off' and was asked to form sentences, he had considerable difficulty. Several of his attempts at this task were:

For a new spanner/£2/paid/John.
Sarah and Tom/in Bath/lived/in a house.
His dinner/Tom/ate.
Ann/a new red bike/got/for her birthday.

Unit 27.3 Assessment findings

(1) When asked to produce 'doing' words in response to verb pictures, BB displayed relatively good performance (a score of 20/24). How can BB's performance in this task be explained? Give an example of the form that his 'doing' words took.

(2) The following statements capture the results of the task in which BB describes subject–verb–object pictures. Use BB's responses in this task to support each of these statements:
   (a) BB produces five verb structures.
   (b) BB produces semantic paraphasic errors on three verbs.
   (c) BB produces only one inflected verb.
   (d) BB produces the actor argument on three occasions.
   (e) BB produces the actor and patient arguments on two occasions.

(3) Compare BB's performance on SVO picture description to his performance on the sentence construction task in which he is given the infinitive form of the verb. Across both tasks, is there evidence that BB can consistently access and produce verb argument structure?

(4) On both versions of the TROG, BB was unable to understand simple active reversible sentences. Give an example of this type of sentence. Why do you think sentences of this type are difficult for BB to comprehend?

(5) BB was able to 'block off' words which 'belong together' in sentences. However, when he was given these same 'blocked off' elements and asked to form sentences, he was unable to do so. How do you explain these findings?

Language intervention

Given BB's lack of progress after several years of therapy, it was decided that a new approach to therapy was needed. This was instituted in December 1984 when BB started to receive therapy three times a week. Intervention followed seven stages:

(1) BB was required to 'block off' elements within written sentences. The verb was the focus of attention. BB was required to label the verb, and there was discussion of its role in signalling the state or activity undertaken in the sentence. Although the use of correct inflections of the verb was not the aim of this stage, several different verb forms were used but not discussed.

(2) The concept of the actor was introduced in this stage. It was explained that the actor answers to the question 'who' or 'what' undertakes the activity expressed by the verb. Initially, verbs were used which take a human subject to convey 'who', and an animal or inanimate subject to convey 'what'. Verbs were also chosen for their intransitive structure and high imageability.

(3) The concept of the theme (or object) argument was introduced. Verbs were used which have an obligatory theme. The question words 'who' and 'what' were used again. To avoid confusion with the use of these same question words in relation to the actor, verbs were chosen which had an obligatory human actor and an inanimate theme, or a non-human animate actor and an inanimate theme.

(4) Verbs were introduced which have an obligatory argument that answers to the question 'where' in a prepositional phrase (e.g. put). The prepositional phrase was presented in both initial and final positions in the sentence. Some verbs were also used where the prepositional phrase could be used in the absence of a theme (e.g. 'He ate in the kitchen').

(5) Further sentence elements were introduced which answered to the questions 'when', 'why' and 'how'. The need for these elements was discussed in terms of how much information the listener wants to be given. BB was given a chart of all the question words which had been introduced and their relationship to verbs in sentences.

(6) At this stage, BB performed tasks which were intended to reinforce the skills acquired to date. Written sentences were presented in which obligatory arguments occurred in the wrong location and BB was required to judge their acceptability. In other sentences, obligatory arguments were omitted and BB was required to supply them, along with the relevant question word. BB was also presented auditorily with an actor and a transitive verb and was required to supply the question word that would achieve completion of the sentence.

(7) Passive voice sentences were introduced at this stage. To ease their introduction, irreversible sentences such as 'The ball was kicked by the boy' were first to be used. Embedded and subordinate clauses were then introduced. To ease their introduction, the same actor was used of both verbs, with the second use taking the form of a pronoun (e.g. 'Bob ate the bun because he was hungry'). It was also emphasised to BB that the subordinate clause in sentences of this type answered to the question 'why'. Two different actors were then introduced in sentences that contained subordinate clauses. BB struggled with embedded clauses in reversible sentences, but had little difficulty with embedded clauses in irreversible sentences. To overcome these difficulties, it was emphasised to BB that in sentences such as 'The cat chasing the dog is black', 'the dog' is the argument of 'chase' and not 'is'.

Unit 27.4 Language intervention

(1) Why were intransitive verbs used to introduce the concept of actor? Give examples of the types of sentence that fulfil the requirements on the two kinds of actor introduced in stage (2).

(2) In stage (3), verbs were used which have an obligatory theme. What types of verbs have an obligatory theme? Because the same question words (who? what?) can be used of both the actor and theme in a sentence, the therapist used initially sentences that had an obligatory human actor and an inanimate theme. Give an example of such a sentence, indicating the question words to which the arguments answer.

(3) At stage (4), verbs like 'put' were introduced to demonstrate that verbs can have an argument that answers to the question 'where?' in a prepositional phrase (e.g. Jack put the juice *in the fridge*). Are verbs like 'put' one-, two-, or three-argument verbs? Why do you think the therapist used sentences in which the prepositional phrase appears at the beginning and end?

(4) At stage (5), BB is introduced to sentences which contain elements that answer to the questions 'when', 'why' and 'how'. Devise sentences which contain each of these elements. Also, a pragmatic constraint on the production of these sentences is addressed at this stage. What is that constraint?

(5) Another pragmatic consideration motivates the therapist's decision to introduce irreversible passive voice sentences first to BB in the final stage of therapy. What is that consideration?

Language performance during therapy

In March 1985, three months into the new therapy program, BB underwent further assessment. He repeated the cookie theft picture description and the narrative production task in which he was asked to describe his previous work. The language that was elicited in these tasks is shown below.

Cookie theft picture description

Girl and boy and woman . . . and . . . /kikiz/ . . . /kikiz/ . . . and near the . . . /a/ . . . no . . . near the . . . don't know . . . no . . . and . . . eh . . . woman . . . drying the washing up. Filled the water . . . /s/ . . . falling to the floor. The window is open and flowers and trees and . . . footpath . . . the . . . no . . . oh . . . no . . . yes alright. Girl wants one.

Narrative production about previous work

eh . . . eh . . . sold . . . potatoes . . . um . . . drive van . . . to Cambridge . . . restaurant . . . chips . . . no . . . um . . . don't know . . . sorry . . . pack the van . . . and . . . no . . . um . . . don't know.

The subject–verb–object picture description task was also repeated in March 1985. His responses on this task are shown below:

The boy is kicking the ball: eh . . . kick the ball . . . boy is kicking the ball.
The boy is riding the bike: The girl . . . is riding . . . a bike.
The girl is writing a letter: Letter! eh . . . the girl . . . is writing . . . a letter . . . to . . . eh . . . friend.
The boy is painting a picture: The boy is . . . painting . . . eh . . . a picture . . . a house. Good!
The boy is digging the garden: The boy . . . is digging . . . his garden.
The boy is reading a book: eh . . . The boy is reading a . . . /k/ comic.
The girl is brushing her hair: The girl is . . . comb . . . her hair.
The boy is eating an apple: Eating an apple . . . eh . . . the girl . . . no boy . . . is eating an apple.
The boy is climbing a ladder: The boy is . . . eh . . . um . . . oh . . . a ladder no!
The boy is drinking orange: The boy is drinking . . . orange squash.

In July 1985, the TROG (auditory version) was repeated, with BB passing 17/20 blocks. When asked to rearrange sentence elements in the Word Order Test, BB produced a total of 7/60 (11.6%) errors (his previous error rate was 48%). The seven errors which occurred all took the form of object–verb–subject constructions. Previously, his errors (29 in total) had also involved verb–subject–object and verb–object–subject constructions. Also on the Word Order Test, when presented with a spoken sentence and asked to match it to one of three pictures, the total number of errors produced was 14/60 (23%) (BB's previous error rate was 60%). The errors still all involved the reversal of the arguments in the sentence. In September 1985, the cookie theft picture description and the narrative production task were undertaken for a third time. The language that was elicited in these tasks is shown below.

Cookie theft picture description

The woman is washing up . . . and water is flowing over the bowl . . . on concrete floor and the boy is reaching for cookies and the stool falling down. And the girl is reaching up for the cookies. The window is opened and through the window . . . see trees and the grass . . . and trees and the pebbles. And the two cups on top of the . . . table and the . . . one bowl is . . . there.

Narrative production about previous work

I have a van and drove to the . . . Cambridge and . . . chips in the restaurant . . . shop . . . sold chips. I was a vegetable salesman *(The patient then volunteered the following information about his CVA)* I was in bed in October 1978. Well . . . I don't know! . . . woke up and I was lifeless. I was in bed at home. Drove to Cambridge . . . sold chips . . . then we went through to the hospital. *(What happened there?)* Don't know . . . upstairs . . . lie down on the bed . . . arm, leg and couldn't talk!

By April 1985, BB was reported by his wife and others to have become much more confident in communicating. There were also reports that sentence structure was beginning to appear in BB's spontaneous output.

Unit 27.5 Language performance during therapy

(1) In March 1985, BB displayed improved verb production in both the cookie theft picture description and the narrative production task. Across these two tasks, give *seven* examples of BB's use of verbs along with their arguments. For the examples you give, indicate if any obligatory arguments are missing.

(2) Also in March 1985, BB displayed improved performance on the subject–verb–object picture description task. Give *one* example of each of the following features using the picture description data presented above:
(a) BB produces a sentence with complete argument structure.
(b) BB produces a semantic paraphasic error.
(c) BB initiates repair of an utterance.
(d) BB produces arguments in the absence of a verb.
(e) BB produces an optional argument.

(3) Notwithstanding BB's improved verb production, there is evidence in July 1985 that BB's knowledge of verb argument structure is still not fully recovered. What is that evidence?

(4) By September 1985, the agrammatic character of BB's earlier expressive language has considerably reduced. Describe *five* features of the language used by BB during the cookie theft picture description task which were either sparsely used or absent altogether in BB's earlier verbal output.

(5) BB's narrative production in September 1985 contains a number of discourse anomalies. Give *three* examples of such anomalies.

Case study 28

Man aged 60 years with right hemisphere damage

Introduction

The following exercise is a case study of a man ('OP') with right hemisphere damage (RHD) who was studied by Abusamra et al. (2009). OP is 60 years old. Following a stroke three years earlier, OP displays many of the pragmatic and discourse deficits that are found in clients with right hemisphere language disorder. These deficits were revealed during assessment of his language skills using the MEC protocol (Joanette et al., 2004). The case study is presented in five sections: primer on right-hemisphere language disorder; right-hemisphere language assessment; client history and assessment; focus on metaphor; and focus on narrative discourse.

Primer on right-hemisphere language disorder

Historically, the right cerebral hemisphere has been somewhat neglected by investigators as a seat of significant language and communication disorder. This is on account of the fact that the right hemisphere is not typically associated with aphasic language disturbances. (Crossed aphasia – aphasia following a right-hemisphere lesion in right-handed individuals – is an obvious, but relatively uncommon exception.) Also, the pragmatic and discourse deficits that arise in RHD are not addressed by the types of language batteries that are used to assess aphasia, and have often evaded characterisation for this reason. Today, there is widespread acknowledgement among speech-language pathologists that clients who sustain RHD can experience significant communication problems. So-called right-hemisphere language disorder (RHLD) is a unique clinical syndrome which can be distinguished from the aphasias and from the types of language impairments that are associated with the dementias. However, like language in the dementias, RHLD is associated with cognitive deficits, earning it the name of a cognitive-communication disorder. The linguistic and cognitive features of RHLD are examined in this unit.

Focal damage to the right cerebral hemisphere can result in pragmatic and discourse deficits. In clients who sustain RHD, there may be an impairment of the comprehension of non-literal language including implicatures (Kasher et al., 1999), metaphors (Rinaldi et al., 2004), idioms (Papagno et al., 2006), sarcasm (Giora et al., 2000; Shamay-Tsoory et al., 2005) and indirect speech acts (Hatta et al., 2004). Although errors of interpretation vary, there is a general tendency towards literal interpretation of these utterances. Tompkins (2012) remarks how adults with RHD may comprehend expressions such as metaphors better when they are preceded by moderately to strongly biased linguistic context (e.g. the first two utterances in 'The man is stubborn. He never quits. The man is a mule'). Problems with the interpretation of non-literal language have been attributed to theory of mind deficits (Winner et al., 1998) and visuo-perceptual and visuo-spatial deficits (McDonald, 2000; Papagno et al., 2006). To the extent that affective prosody also plays a role in utterance interpretation, the well-recognised prosodic deficits of this population of clients may also compromise the understanding of figurative and other non-literal language (Yuvaraj et al., 2013).

Discourse deficits have been extensively documented in clients with RHD. These deficits include the production of narratives which contain tangential errors and conceptually incongruent utterances (Marini, 2012). The picture descriptions of clients with RHD have poor information content, cohesion and coherence (Marini et al., 2005). Lehman Blake (2006) reported that discourse produced by adults with RHD during a thinking-out-loud task was rated as more tangential and egocentric than the discourse of healthy older adults. RHD discourse also contained extremes of quantity (i.e. extreme verbosity or paucity of speech). Alongside expressive discourse deficits, clients with RHD also have well-documented problems comprehending narrative discourse. Jerônimo et al. (2011) examined narrative discourse comprehension in a 53-year-old man with RHD. This client was able to comprehend narratives at the micro-propositional level. However, he had significant difficulty in processing narrative macro-structure and situational model, especially in comprehending the main idea of narratives. Adults with RHD have been found to have difficulty drawing high-level inferences about the motives of characters in narratives (Tompkins et al., 2009). The suppression of inappropriate inferences is a significant predictor of narrative discourse comprehension in adults with RHD (Tompkins et al., 2000, 2001).

Unit 28.1 Primer on right-hemisphere language disorder

(1) Which of the following is in the aetiology of right hemisphere damage?
   (a) cerebrovascular accident
   (b) cerebral tumour
   (c) HIV infection
   (d) Creutzfeldt–Jakob disease
   (e) traumatic brain injury

(2) Why might a client with RHD have difficulty understanding the following utterances?
   (a) The ship ploughed through the sea.
   (b) Mary promised not to spill the beans.
   (c) Jack is overweight but healthy.
   (d) Please keep your adorable child from kicking me!
   (e) Can you tell me the time?

(3) An inability to decode prosody can compromise utterance interpretation in clients with RHD. However, these clients can also have difficulty with productive aspects of prosody. Describe *one* way in which this may compromise communication for clients with RHD.

(4) Clients with RHD display a number of linguistic strengths as well as weaknesses. Describe *three* aspects of language which are well preserved in RHD. The preservation of these aspects sets RHLD apart from another acquired language disorder. What is that disorder?

(5) Respond with *true* or *false* to each of the following statements about discourse in RHD:
  (a) Clients with RHD have difficulty observing maxims of relation and quantity during discourse production.
  (b) Clients with RHD struggle to comprehend the propositional content of narratives.
  (c) Clients with RHD can have difficulty establishing the gist of stories.
  (d) Clients with RHD produce many cohesive links between utterances.
  (e) Clients with RHD display discourse problems which are related to cognitive deficits.

Right-hemisphere language assessment

Speech-language pathologists have recognised for some time that RHD disrupts language in ways that are inadequately assessed by aphasia batteries. When Penelope Myers undertook the first formal study of communication impairments in adults with RHD, it was a discourse task – the cookie theft picture description from the Boston Diagnostic Aphasia Examination (Goodglass and Kaplan, 1972b) – that was used to characterise these impairments. These adults, Myers remarked, produced 'irrelevant and often excessive information' and seemed 'to miss the implication of [a] question and to respond in a most literal and concrete way' (Myers, 1979: 38). When attempting to respond to open-ended questions, these patients 'wended their way through a maze of disassociated detail, seemingly incapable of filtering out unnecessary information' (38). The components of a narrative, although available to these patients, could not be assembled into a narrative. There was difficulty 'in extracting critical bits of information, in seeing the relationships among them, and in reaching conclusions or drawing inferences based on those relationships' (39). Although the detail provided by these patients was related to the general topic, its appearance seemed irrelevant because it had not been 'integrated into a whole' (39).

It was nearly 10 years after Myers' study that Bryan (1988) confirmed what many clinicians had long suspected was the case: adults with RHD communicate inadequately even as they have no identifiable language disorder on aphasia batteries. Bryan devised a set of tests which included metaphorical comprehension and the understanding of inferred meaning and humour. Along with the Western Aphasia Battery (Kertesz, 1982), these tests were administered to adults with left and right cerebral hemisphere damage and to normal control subjects. A discourse analysis was also undertaken. While the subjects with RHD were not significantly different from controls on the aphasia test, their performance was impaired compared to control subjects on the metaphor and other tests. Bryan (1995) subsequently went on to develop the Right Hemisphere Language Battery. The seven tests in this battery include tests of spoken and written metaphor appreciation, verbal humour appreciation, comprehension of inference, production of emphatic stress and lexical semantic comprehension. There is also a comprehensive discourse analysis. The battery has been translated into other languages including Polish and Italian (Jodzio et al., 2005; Zanini et al., 2005), and has been used in subjects with RHD caused by cerebrovascular accidents and brain tumours (Bryan and Hale, 2001; Thomson et al., 1997).

The patient with RHD in this case study was assessed using the Protocole Montréal d'Évaluation de la Communication (MEC; Joanette et al., 2004). This standardised test was designed primarily for clients with RHD, although the authors also recommend its use in the assessment of clients with aphasia, traumatic brain injury and dementia. Verbal communication skills are assessed by means of 14 subtests. These tests examine conversational discourse, the comprehension and recall of narrative discourse, semantic judgement, repetition and understanding of emotional and linguistic prosody, and understanding of metaphors and indirect speech acts. The MEC is standardised on a sample of 180 non-brain-damaged control subjects who range in age from 30 to 85 years. Participants with RHD are also included in the psychometric data. Although the original MEC was in French, there are now versions available in Brazilian Portuguese and Spanish (Ferreres et al., 2007; Fonseca et al., 2008).

Unit 28.2 Right-hemisphere language assessment

(1) Myers' description of the discourse problems of adults with RHD is particularly vivid and is as relevant today as it was in 1979. Which part of her description corresponds to the finding that adults with RHD have difficulty understanding indirect speech acts?

(2) Adults with RHD can display weak central coherence (Martin and McDonald, 2003). This is a type of processing in which there is a preference for parts over wholes. Which aspect of Myers' description suggests a tendency on the part of her subjects for weak central coherence?

(3) Why do you think humour is assessed in the Right Hemisphere Language Battery?

(4) Emotional prosody and linguistic prosody are examined in the MEC. Explain the difference between these two types of prosody within the context of utterance interpretation.

(5) In which subtest of the MEC would the understanding of the utterances *This homework is a nightmare* and *The stressed lawyer was a steam kettle* be assessed?

Client history and assessment

OP is a 60-year-old lawyer. He has 18 years of formal education. OP first attended the aphasiology service at the hospital, where the lead author of the study, Valeria Abusamra, works, when he was three years post-onset a cerebrovascular accident (personal communication, August 2015). At that time, he had a single, right-sided brain lesion. However, his neurological condition was subsequently complicated by the onset of epilepsy, and he exhibited bilateral brain lesions. At that point, it was decided that OP should be excluded from further investigation. The MEC protocol was used to assess OP. He performed very poorly in the tasks that assessed narrative, metaphors and speech acts. OP's responses on a task in which an examiner (EX) asked him to explain the meaning of indirect speech acts are shown below.

Indirect speech act 1

EX: Louise sees her dirty Ford parked on the street and asks her husband: "Don't you think it's a bit too dirty?" What do you think Louise means by that?

OP: That it would be convenient to wash the car. The Ford or any other car.

EX: Very good. Which of these options explains it best? Is she trying to tell her husband that the Ford is not clean, or does she want her husband to wash the Ford?

OP: No, I'd probably go with option A. I mean, because . . . if not, it's another . . . she's superimposing, imposing an assigned chore, regarding the husband [*sic*]. Because in theory, although the car can be washed in a car wash, the husband usually washes it, but the wife could just as easily wash it.

Indirect speech act 2

EX: Mr Martinez is busy in his living room when the phone starts ringing. He tells his spouse: "The phone is ringing". What do you think Mr Martinez means by that?

OP: He's busy.

EX: (Rereads)

OP: That . . . well, it's assumed that he wants his wife – it isn't known what she's up to, it doesn't say that it isn't known if she's also busy or not. What is stated is that Mr Martinez is busy, but nothing is known about what the wife is doing, which could be in another task [*sic*] just as or more urgent or more of a different urgency [*sic*]. But with the information as stated here what's suggested is that she should answer the phone.

EX: And from the following options you have, is he trying to say that he hears the phone ring, or does he want his spouse to answer?

OP: Well, yes, he's says both things.

EX: Together.

OP: Right, because he hears the phone ring, yes. Which he's listening to, he's . . . now, in theory, along with that there's a request.

EX: Good.

OP: There should be a request.

EX: Right, in this given situation? When he says "the phone is ringing"?

OP: If he assumes . . . If he assumes that the wife, wife or spouse, already knows he's busy, then he's referring to the latter. But she does not know the former, you have to see whether the wife knows or not. Normally, in theory, living together makes . . . makes B work, but within a context, a specific context.

Indirect speech act 3

EX: Martin sits down in his living room to watch television. He tells his wife who's in the kitchen: "My glasses are on the table". What do you think Martin means by that?

OP: Well, what he actually means – he's manifesting the difficulty he's having to watch television, which insofar that in theory, it's assumed that he needs glasses to watch television. He also could be requesting his partner, who's his actually his wife, partner, which is not legally correct . . . that he doesn't necessarily want them, well let's see . . .

EX: Let's see, from the following options, does he want to tell her where his glasses are, or does he want her to bring his glasses over to the living room?

OP: Well, he's obviously telling her where his glasses are, but in theory he's requesting that she bring him his glasses to the living room, where he's trying to watch television.

Indirect speech act 4

EX: Last one. The last one of this task. Peter works in an office and needs to print a document. Therefore, he tells his secretary: "There's no more paper". What do you think Peter means by that?

OP: Well, here according to the guidelines that are followed within work relationships, in effect, insofar that she is his secretary [*sic*]. The word "his" is there, which is important to notice. He's requesting something, insofar that in theory she has a work obligation . . . of complying with her boss's requests.

EX: Very good. So what does it mean when he says there's no more paper, or does he want his secretary to put more paper in the printer?

OP: Well, it means both things. He explicitly says it, because you can't say there's no . . .

EX: But, in this case, which one do you think is best? If you had to choose one of the two for this situation.

OP: In theory, the second one, because let me say, the topic of . . . of the connection with "her" is important.

Unit 28.3 Client history and assessment

(1) OP first participated in Abusamra et al.'s study three years after suffering a stroke. However, he was later excluded from the study. Why do you think the decision was taken to exclude OP from further investigation?

(2) How would you characterise OP's understanding of indirect speech act 1?

(3) In indirect speech act 2, what evidence is there that more than one interpretation of the speech act is salient for OP?

(4) OP also entertains more than one interpretation of indirect speech act 3. But what other inference does he draw in this exchange? What is the significance of this inference for the speech act in the exchange?

(5) OP is eventually able to indicate to the examiner that indirect speech act 4 is a request for the secretary to put more paper in the printer. However, before he arrives at this interpretation of the speech act, OP appears to dwell on one aspect of the scenario that is presented to him. What is that aspect?

Focus on metaphor

In the following exchange, an examiner has asked OP to explain the meaning of one of the metaphors from the MEC protocol. The metaphor is 'My friend's mother-in-law is a witch':

EX: What does this phrase mean: My friend's mother-in-law is a witch?

OP: Let's change also one word: My son-in-law's mother-in-law is a witch?

EX: And so what does it mean?

OP: I know she is a person who hasn't had a pleasant life, throughout her marriage. That . . . that she's about to be separated from her husband; I'm referring to the mother-in-law of my son-in-law (ha, ha, ha)

EX: OK it's not important – it's the same.

OP: Certainly! The mother-in-law of my son-in-law. The mother-in-law of my son-in-law is a witch!

EX: What does being a witch mean?

OP: Because the woman is separated, because all her life she has criticized her husband for the way he is; only seen in his defects, who has kept his daughter all her life under a glass bell and she's now a poor lady because she can't find the fiancé her mother would like.

EX: So what does witch mean, then?

OP: What does it specifically mean? It means being tied down to religious sects, to religions, to umbanda . . . who knows, there are so many.

EX: So therefore, "The mother-in-law of my son-in-law is a witch". Does it mean the mother-in-law of my friend practices black magic? And the mother-in-law of my friend has many brooms and she is also a bad person and rude?

OP: It's absolutely clear. My friend's mother-in-law has many brooms . . . no! My friend's mother-in-law practises black magic.

Unit 28.4 Focus on metaphor

(1) OP is clearly having difficulty explaining the meaning of this particular metaphor. How would you characterise his understanding?

(2) Is there awareness on OP's part that his interpretation of the metaphor may not be accurate?

(3) Egocentric discourse is a feature of right hemisphere language disorder. Is there any evidence that OP makes use of egocentric discourse in the above exchange?

(4) The appreciation of humour is often impaired in clients with RHD. Is there any evidence that OP makes appropriate use of humour in this exchange with the examiner? Provide support for your answer.

(5) To what extent is OP's use of referring expressions contributing to his discourse difficulties? Support your response with evidence from the above exchange.

Focus on narrative discourse

OP was also read a narrative text from the MEC Protocol and was asked to retell the story. The original narrative text and OP's retelling are shown below.

Original text

John is a farmer from the north. He has been busy for several days digging a well on his land. The work is almost over. This morning John has arrived to finish his work and sees that during the night the well has collapsed and half of it is filled with earth. He's very upset about this. He thinks for some minutes and says to himself, "I have an idea." He leaves his shirt and cap on the edge of the well, hides the pick and pail, and climbs up a tree to hide himself. Later, a neighbour passes by and approaches John to talk to him a little. When he sees his shirt and cap he thinks John is working at the bottom of the well. The fellow passes nearby, bends down a little, and sees the well half-filled with dirt and starts to desperately cry out, "Help! Help! Friends! Come immediately! John is buried under the well!" The neighbours run towards the well and start digging to save poor John. When the neighbours stop taking away the earth, John comes down the tree, approaches them and says, "Thanks a lot, you've been a great help."

OP's retelling

There was a farmer who was digging a hole uh uh uh uh well he was digging a hole until at a certain depth . . . uh uh uh uh . . . er. who was digging a well eh eh eh so he was digging with a shovel and a pick . . . uh uh uh . . . objects that don't look like what we call shovel and pick I mean they have really something to do with the ground . . . not only uh uh uh . . . generally a wine . . . the farmer moves the it it it more with shovel than pick or at least like a pick. And so he went down to a certain depth and he was, was tired, it was night and so and the next day . . . he sees the well has collapsed I mean collapsed from a part of of of of You don't remind me any more . . .

Unit 28.5 Focus on narrative discourse

(1) OP really only gets his narrative properly underway when he utters 'And so he went down . . . '. How would you characterise OP's narrative prior to this point?

(2) Does OP succeed in narrating the main events in the story? Provide support for your answer.

(3) Is there any evidence from OP's retelling of the story that he may be experiencing visuo-perceptual deficits?

(4) OP only introduces one character, the farmer, into his narrative. Is this introduction skilfully achieved?

(5) Respond with *true* or *false* to each of the following statements about OP's narrative:
   (a) OP produces an informative narrative.
   (b) OP relates events in the correct temporal order.
   (c) OP succeeds in capturing the motivations of the farmer.
   (d) OP selects the wrong lexemes to describe objects.
   (e) OP produces a fluent narrative.

Case study 29

Man aged 24 years with closed head injury

Introduction

The following exercise is a case study of a 24-year-old man who was studied by Mentis and Prutting (1991). This man was diagnosed by a neurologist as having sustained a closed head injury (CHI). A CHI is a type of traumatic brain injury in which the brain sustains damage in the absence of a skull fracture. It is a relatively common condition in children and adults which can have implications for language and other cognitive skills for many years post-injury. The case study is presented in five sections: primer on traumatic brain injury; client history and cognitive-communication status; pragmatic and discourse assessment; focus on conversation: part 1; and focus on conversation: part 2.

Primer on traumatic brain injury

A traumatic brain injury (TBI) occurs when a traumatic force damages the brain. This force may be a missile which penetrates the skull and damages the brain (open or penetrating head injury). Alternatively, the brain may be damaged in a road traffic accident while the skull remains intact (closed head injury). TBI is a relatively common condition and significant cause of death and disability. In a study of the epidemiology of TBI, Corrigan et al. (2010) reported that each year 235,000 Americans are hospitalised for non-fatal TBI, 1.1 million are treated in emergency rooms and 50,000 die of the injury. These investigators also report that an estimated 43.3% of Americans have residual disability 1 year after hospitalisation with TBI, and that the prevalence of US civilian residents living with TBI-related disability is 3.2 million. Falls and road traffic accidents are the most common causes of TBI, accounting for 52.6% and 31.6% of trauma mechanisms, respectively, in a sample of 921 patients with TBI (Walder et al., 2013). Intracranial damage in TBI can be focal or diffuse in nature, and includes epidural and subdural haematomas, cerebral contusions, traumatic axonal injury and cerebral oedema (Andriessen et al., 2010). Most TBIs are mild in severity. In a review of European studies of TBI epidemiology, the ratio of mild vs. moderate vs. severe cases was 22:1.5:1 (Tagliaferri et al., 2006).

Speech, language, hearing and swallowing disorders are among the sequelae of TBI. In a study of 116 persons with TBI, Safaz et al. (2008) reported aphasia, dysarthria and dysphagia in 19.0%, 30.2% and 17.2%, respectively. In a paediatric TBI population of 100 subjects, 14% had audiologically confirmed hearing loss (Penn et al., 2009). Even in the absence of aphasia, clients with TBI can have significant pragmatic and discourse deficits (Rousseaux et al., 2010). These deficits not only compromise communication, but have also been found to correlate significantly with social integration and quality of life in clients with TBI (Galski et al., 1998). Notwithstanding the importance of pragmatic and discourse skills to the functioning of clients with TBI, a recent survey of 265 speech-language pathologists revealed that less than half of them (44.3%) routinely assessed domains such as discourse (Frith et al., 2014). Less than 10% used tools that assessed functional performance, discourse and pragmatic skills. Alongside language problems, clients with TBI often exhibit significant cognitive deficits, even those with mild TBI (Rabinowitz and Levin, 2014). These deficits most often involve executive functions, a group of cognitive skills which is integral to the planning, execution and regulation of goal-directed behaviour. However, there is also evidence that clients with TBI can experience deficits in theory of mind (Henry et al., 2006). Both types of cognitive deficits are implicated in the language and pragmatic problems of clients with TBI (see Cummings (2009, 2014a, 2014b) for further discussion).

Unit 29.1 Primer on traumatic brain injury

(1) Falls and road traffic accidents are the most common causes of TBI. But they are certainly not the only causes of TBI. State *five* other causes of TBI in children and adults.

(2) Epidural and subdural haematomas are one of the pathophysiological features of TBI. What are epidural and subdural haematomas?

(3) Hearing loss is one of the sequelae of TBI. What type of hearing loss (conductive/sensorineural) is associated with (a) a blunt head trauma and (b) a blast-related brain injury?

(4) Why do you think speech-language pathologists do not routinely assess domains like discourse in clients with TBI? Give *three* reasons.

(5) Rabinowitz and Levin (2014) report that 65% of patients with moderate to severe TBI report long-term problems with cognitive functioning, mostly relating to executive functions. Why are executive function deficits so common in individuals who sustain TBI?

Client history and cognitive-communication status

The subject is a 24-year-old man who has been diagnosed by a neurologist as having a closed head injury. He is a native speaker of General American English. He left high school during the 11th grade (16–17 years) and was employed inconsistently as a dishwasher and short order cook. He also worked for a roofing company. At the time of his accident he was unemployed. When the subject was tested 4;10 years post-injury, he was not receiving any type of rehabilitation. However, subsequent to his accident, he had received speech, physical and occupational therapy. The subject was living alone and was unemployed at the time of study.

The subject displayed mild symptoms of dysarthria on the Motor Speech Evaluation (Wertz et al., 1981) and the oral portion of the Western Aphasia Battery (WAB; Kertesz, 1982). On a severity rating from 1 to 7, where '7' indicates severe impairment, the subject obtained scores of 1 and 2 for single-word and single-sentence repetition, respectively. In connected speech, a score of 2 was obtained. On the WAB, the subject achieved an aphasia quotient of 92.3. (Language is classified as normal on the WAB if an aphasia quotient of 93.8 or above is achieved.) He was classified as having anomic aphasia. On the praxis, reading, drawing and calculation subtests of the WAB, the subject achieved scores above the mean of a normal control group. His performance on the writing subtest was within one standard deviation below the mean of the normal control group. He obtained a cortical quotient of 92.9 on the WAB (the maximum score is 100). The cortical quotient score is a more general measure of cortical functioning than the aphasia quotient. On the Raven's Colored Progressive Matrices, the subject was above the mean of the normal control group.

Unit 29.2 Client history and cognitive-communication status

(1) Respond with *true* or *false* to each of the following statements:
   (a) The subject's employment status at the time of study is typical of many individuals who sustain a severe TBI.
   (b) The subject is still likely to be experiencing significant spontaneous recovery at the time of study.
   (c) The subject's employment status at the time of study can only be partially explained by his TBI.
   (d) Independent living is a key indicator of functional outcome in clients with TBI.
   (e) Most individuals with moderate or severe TBI are able to live independently.

(2) The subject was considered to have mild dysarthria based on a motor speech evaluation. What other motor speech disorder will have been considered within this evaluation?

(3) One of the subtests on the Motor Speech Evaluation requires the examinee to take a medium-sized breath and prolong the vowel 'ah' as long as possible. Which of the following speech production subsystems is assessed by means of this subtest?
   (a) prosody
   (b) articulation
   (c) phonation
   (d) resonation
   (e) respiration

(4) The subject was diagnosed on the WAB as having anomic aphasia. Which of the following features is typical of this form of aphasia?
   (a) good comprehension
   (b) agrammatism
   (c) word-finding difficulty
   (d) good word and sentence repetition
   (e) jargon output

(5) What can we say about the subject's intellectual functioning? Which assessment was used to examine the subject's intellectual level?

Pragmatic and discourse assessment

Ten language samples were collected in order to assess the subject's pragmatic and discourse skills. Video-recordings of six conversations between the subject and a familiar partner (his speech-language pathologist) were made and transcribed into standard orthography. Four monologue discourse samples were also collected and transcribed. Conversations took place under three conditions: topic unspecified (unstructured conversational discourse), concrete (e.g. television, sports) and abstract (e.g. poverty, religion). Monologues were recorded under two conditions: topic concrete (e.g. a visit to the dentist) and abstract (e.g. talking about 'truth'). The six conversational samples were rated using the Pragmatic Protocol (Prutting and Kirchner, 1987). The percentage of appropriate pragmatic parameters ranged from 73.3% (abstract condition) to 76.7% (unspecified and concrete conditions). The following pragmatic parameters were rated as inappropriate across all three conditions: topic maintenance; turn-taking pause time; turn-taking quantity/conciseness; specificity/accuracy; cohesion; vocal quality; and prosody. In the abstract condition, a further pragmatic parameter – topic change – was rated inappropriate.

The monologue samples were analysed using intonation units. An intonation unit is a sequence of words combined under a single, coherent intonation contour and (usually) preceded by a pause. Intonation units were further categorised as ideational, textual or interpersonal in nature, following the analysis of Halliday. For Halliday, ideational meaning is the representation of experience or meaning in the sense of 'content'. Ideational units were further analysed according to whether or not they contained new information, no new information, or were problematic in other ways (e.g. ambiguous or incomplete). A further measure was the number of issues that were introduced by the subject in relation to the monologue topic. This was a measure of how comprehensively each monologue topic was discussed. Issues were classified as new, unrelated (independent concepts not related to the topic), and reintroduced issues. Some results from the analysis of the monologue samples are shown below for the concrete and abstract conditions. The results of a normal control (NC) subject are included for comparison:

Total intonation units

CHI subject: 906 (concrete); 1233 (abstract)
NC subject: 1722 (concrete); 1123 (abstract)

Total ideational units

CHI subject: 488 (concrete); 646 (abstract)
NC subject: 1090 (concrete): 669 (abstract)

Percentage of ideational units which contain:

New information

CHI subject: 48.8% (concrete); 56.0% (abstract)
NC subject: 83.9% (concrete); 79.4% (abstract)

No new information

CHI subject: 12.7% (concrete); 12.0% (abstract)
NC subject: 9.7% (concrete); 16.6% (abstract)

Problematic in other ways

CHI subject: 37.9% (concrete); 32.0% (abstract)
NC subject: 3.7% (concrete); 3.6% (abstract)

Total issues introduced

CHI subject: 74 (concrete); 66 (abstract)
NC subject: 116 (concrete); 99 (abstract)

Percentage of issues which are:

New

CHI subject: 77.1% (concrete); 74.1% (abstract)
NC subject: 94.6% (concrete); 97.6% (abstract)

Reintroduced

CHI subject: 11.4% (concrete); 12.1% (abstract)
NC subject: 5.4% (concrete); 2.4% (abstract)

Unrelated

CHI subject: 11.4% (concrete); 13.8% (abstract)
NC subject: 0% (concrete); 0% (abstract)

Unit 29.3 Pragmatic and discourse assessment

(1) Which of the following statements best characterises the Pragmatic Protocol?
   (a) It is a standardised assessment of receptive language.
   (b) It is a checklist of verbal pragmatic parameters.
   (c) It is a standardised assessment of expressive syntax.
   (d) It is a checklist of structural language skills used in conversation.
   (e) It is a checklist of verbal, non-verbal and paralinguistic pragmatic parameters.

(2) The findings obtained on the Pragmatic Protocol revealed that the subject with CHI has problems with specificity and accuracy. Which of this subject's language deficits might account for the poor rating on this item?

(3) Explain why prosody is included in an assessment of pragmatic parameters in the Pragmatic Protocol.

(4) Using your knowledge of cognitive deficits in TBI, explain why the inclusion of a concrete–abstract condition in this study is warranted.

(5) Clients with TBI have often been described as being tangential, repetitive and uninformative in conversation and other forms of discourse. Which of the findings from the analysis of the monologue samples supports this clinical impression?

Focus on conversation: part 1

The subject in this study has conversational and discourse difficulties which are most evident during an examination of actual conversational data. To assess these difficulties and residual conversational skills, two short extracts of conversation will be examined in units 29.4 and 29.5. In these extracts, the subject with CHI is speaking to his speech-language pathologist (SLP). The questions posed at the end of units 29.4 and 29.5 will address conversational skills *and* deficits, and encourage the reader to think more widely about communication in clients with TBI.

Transcription notation

. . . =   pause less than 2 seconds
(2.0) =   pause of 2 seconds' duration
. =   falling intonation
? =   rising intonation
, =   continuing intonation

Each line is a separate intonation unit.

SLP: . . . have you ever been to a Halloween party, um where there were like really outrageous
     costumes?
CHI: . . . uh,
SLP: . . . you know . . . when people just went . . . all out, and rented costumes, and stuff like that.
CHI: . . . no.
     . . . no I haven't.
     . . . I've seen-
     . . . no . . . I've seen people,
     . . . who things,
     . . . like go somewhere and,
     you go and coming through and keep going.
     . . . oh well that's . . . good looking costume.
SLP: uh huh.

Unit 29.4 Focus on conversation: part 1

(1) This subject has word-finding difficulty as part of an anomic aphasia. This difficulty leads him to use a number of non-specific lexemes. Give *three* examples of such lexemes in the above conversational exchange.

(2) A discourse feature that this subject is able to use is grammatical ellipsis. Give an example of the use of this type of ellipsis in the conversational data presented above.

(3) The analysis of the monologue samples in unit 29.3 revealed that this subject produced incomplete utterances. Give *three* examples of incomplete utterances in the conversational data.

(4) At the start of the exchange, the speech-language pathologist asks a question which she expands in her second turn. Why does this expansion occur? Is there an alternative interpretation of the behaviour which appears to trigger this expansion?

(5) Can referents be assigned to the pronouns that the subject uses? Provide evidence to support your answer.

Focus on conversation: part 2

This exchange between the subject with CHI and the speech-language pathologist further exemplifies some of the client's difficulties with spoken discourse. It also illustrates the types of strategies that the communicative partners of clients with TBI can use to adapt to these difficulties. The exchange begins with the speech-language pathologist asking the subject what he has been working on.

SLP: . . . so . . . what is this thing,
　　　that you've been . . . kinda working on.
CHI: . . . well it's like . . . art . . . you know,
SLP: . . . art?
CHI: . . . yeah.
SLP: . . . uh huh,
CHI: . . . you jus' sit down . . . and you really concentrate.
SLP: . . . um hm,
CHI: . . . and it . . . seems . . . like . . . that's-
　　　. . . a big circle,
　　　. . . gets down to a,
　　　. . . little circle,
　　　. . . and that's what you're doing . . . you know,
SLP: . . . um hm,
CHI: . . . and . . . it seemed to ah,
　　　(2.0) over,
　　　. . . kinda go over . . . to I do other things,
SLP: . . . um hm,
CHI: . . . you know I really get into it.
SLP: . . . so are you talking about trying to focus your attention,
　　　. . . toward doing a . . . really . . . superior job on one thing,
　　　. . . but not being . . . kind scattered,
　　　. . . is that what you're saying?
CHI: . . . yeah.

Unit 29.5 Focus on conversation: part 2

(1) Give *one* example of each of the following linguistic features in the above exchange:
　　(a) The subject uses a filler in front of a pause to retain his turn.
　　(b) The subject uses an incomplete prepositional phrase.
　　(c) The subject uses a personal pronoun in the absence of a referent.
　　(d) The subject uses an adverb as a premodifier in a verb phrase.
　　(e) The subject uses a demonstrative pronoun in the absence of a referent.
(2) The subject with CHI uses the discourse marker *well* at the start of his first turn in this exchange. Jucker (1997) states that this discourse marker has five distinct uses in

Modern English. These uses are listed below. Which one best describes the use of *well* by the subject with CHI?

    (a) *Well* can be used to introduce a new topic.
    (b) *Well* can be used to preface direct reported speech.
    (c) *Well* can be used to preface a reply which is only a partial answer to a question.
    (d) *Well* can be used to preface a disagreement.
    (e) *Well* can be used to bridge interactional silence.

(3) The subject with CHI uses a number of markers of sympathetic circularity. These are expressions like 'sort of' and 'ain't it' which invite the listener to assume the speaker's point of view, and which allow speakers a degree of imprecision or inexplicitness on the grounds that not everything should be, or can be, explicitly stated. Identify *three* such markers in the utterances of the subject in the above exchange.

(4) The subject with CHI displays a restricted pattern of grammatical cohesion in his use of conjunctions. What is that pattern?

(5) What is the function of the speech-language pathologist's final turn in the exchange?

Case study 30

Woman aged 87 years with early-stage Alzheimer's disease

Introduction

The following exercise is a case study of a woman ('Martha') aged 87 years who was studied by Hydén and Örulv (2009). At the time of study, Martha had had a diagnosis of Alzheimer's disease for four or five years and was living in a residential care unit. The case study is presented in five sections: primer on Alzheimer's disease; language in Alzheimer's disease; focus on language in Alzheimer's disease; discourse in Alzheimer's disease; and focus on discourse in Alzheimer's disease.

Primer on Alzheimer's disease

Alzheimer's disease (AD) is the foremost cause of dementia worldwide, accounting for up to 75% of all dementia cases (Qiu et al., 2009). This neurodegenerative disorder manifests as progressive memory impairment followed by a gradual decline in other cognitive abilities which lead to complete functional dependency (Rafii and Aisen, 2015). In a systematic review of data from Europe and the US published between January 2002 and December 2012, Takizawa et al. (2015) reported that the prevalence of AD ranged between 3% and 7%. The annual incidence of AD is increasing, with an incidence of 377,000 new cases in the US in 1995 expected to increase to 959,000 cases in 2050 (Hebert et al., 2001). There are two different forms of AD based on age of onset and genetic pre-disposition. Sporadic or late-onset AD accounts for over 95% of cases and begins after the age of 65 years. Early-onset or familial AD is rare and usually manifests before 60 years of age (Bali et al., 2012). The two primary lesions associated with AD are neurofibrillary tangles and amyloid plaques. These are abnormal proteins which accumulate inside neurones in the case of neurofibrillary tangles and in the spaces between nerve cells in the case of amyloid plaques. A further morphological alteration in AD is the loss of synaptic components (Perl, 2010).

Alzheimer's disease is an underlying pathology in many of the clients who are assessed and treated by speech-language pathologists. This is because these clients can present with considerable speech, language, cognitive and swallowing problems. The motor speech disorders apraxia of speech and dysarthria are a feature of AD. Cera et al. (2013) reported significantly lower scores for speech and orofacial praxis in 90 individuals at different stages of AD than in normal controls. Spastic dysarthria has been reported in two children and their mother, all of whom experienced early-onset familial AD in their 30s (Rudzinski et al., 2008). Aphasic and non-aphasic language impairments are present in AD. Ahmed et al. (2013) analysed connected speech samples from 15 patients with autopsy-confirmed AD using measures of syntactic complexity, lexical content, speech production, fluency and semantic content. Subtle language changes were evident during the prodromal stages of AD. There were significant linear trends in syntactic complexity and semantic and lexical content over the prodromal, mild and moderate stages of disease. Cognitive deficits in clients with AD range from mild cognitive impairment in the prodromal stage of disease to increasingly severe forms of dementia with disease progression (Ward et al., 2013). Swallowing is problematic for individuals with AD and not just for those with late-stage disease. Priefer and Robbins (1997) reported significantly increased oral transit duration, pharyngeal response duration and total swallow duration in individuals with mild-stage AD relative to healthy, elderly controls.

Unit 30.1 Primer on Alzheimer's disease

(1) Which of the following are *true* statements about Alzheimer's disease?
  (a) Individuals with AD have an impairment of episodic memory.
  (b) Amnestic mild cognitive impairment is a feature of late-stage AD.
  (c) There is no genetic basis to sporadic AD.
  (d) Sensory impairments (e.g. hearing loss) are a significant feature of AD.
  (e) AD is a significant cause of death and disability in developed countries with aging populations.

(2) The language impairment in AD is described as a 'cognitive-communication disorder'. Explain why this is the case.

(3) Which of the following is a communication feature of late-stage Alzheimer's disease?
  (a) executive dysfunction
  (b) glossomania
  (c) mutism
  (d) egocentric discourse
  (e) flight of ideas

(4) *True* or *False*: Augmentative and alternative communication is not an appropriate intervention for clients with Alzheimer's disease.

(5) Which of the following is the client with AD and dysphagia at risk of developing?
  (a) loss of gag reflex
  (b) malnutrition
  (c) periodontal disease
  (d) dehydration
  (e) aspiration pneumonia

Language in Alzheimer's disease

Alongside other cognitive functions, language is disrupted with the onset and progression of Alzheimer's disease. Language impairments in AD are wide-ranging in nature, and can take the form of an aphasia syndrome or a non-aphasic language disorder. Cummings et al. (1985) examined 30 patients with dementia of the Alzheimer type, and found aphasia in all patients. The language disorder resembled a transcortical sensory aphasia. Murdoch et al. (1987) examined the language profile of 18 patients with Alzheimer's disease. On a standard aphasia test battery, these patients scored significantly lower than non-neurologically impaired control subjects in the areas of verbal expression, auditory comprehension, repetition, reading and writing. The language disorder of these patients resembled a transcortical sensory aphasia. Semantic abilities were impaired while syntax and phonology were relatively intact. That language subsystems deteriorate at different stages in AD is confirmed in a review of studies of language impairment by Emery (2000). Emery reported a negative relation between sequence in language development and language decline. Specifically, language forms which are learned last in the sequence of language development and are most complex are the first to deteriorate in AD.

Alzheimer's disease pathology is also associated with primary progressive aphasia (PPA), a neurodegenerative disorder in which language impairment is the primary feature. A form of PPA called logopenic/phonological aphasia is most often related to AD pathology. Rohrer et al. (2012) examined the language features of 14 patients with PPA and confirmed AD. These patients exhibited relatively non-fluent spontaneous speech, phonemic errors and reduced digit span. Verbal episodic memory was also impaired in most patients.

Unit 30.2 Language in Alzheimer's disease

(1) Respond with *true* or *false* to each of the following statements about language in AD:
   (a) Receptive language and expressive language are impaired in AD.
   (b) Phonology is disrupted in early-stage AD.
   (c) Language is disrupted in spoken and written modalities in AD.
   (d) Semantics is relatively intact until late-stage AD.
   (e) Language impairments in AD are always a classic aphasia syndrome.

(2) Di Giacomo et al. (2012) examined semantic associative relations in patients with mild Alzheimer's dementia. Subjects were asked to match a target word with one of three noun choices. For the target word 'guitar', the following words were shown together with distractor words:
   (a) *instrument* (superordinate)
   (b) *piano* (contiguity)
   (c) *chord* (part/whole)
   (d) *loud* (attribute)
   (e) *to play* (function)
   The results of the study showed that semantic associative relations acquired in later developmental stages are less preserved in persons with AD. Which *two* of these relations do you think were most impaired in the subjects with AD in this study? (*Clue*: Think about the abstractness of these relations.)

(3) Complete the blank spaces in the following sentences:

   Language decline is usually the fastest and predominant change in _____. In Alzheimer's disease, language decline is usually associated with global _____ deficits.

(4) Which of the following is *not* a feature of language impairment in AD?
   (a) verbal perseveration
   (b) echolalia
   (c) circumlocution
   (d) pronoun reversal
   (e) word-finding difficulty

(5) A standard aphasia test battery was used to examine the language skills of the patients with AD in Murdoch et al.'s study. Give the name of *one* such battery. Why should these batteries be supplemented with other forms of assessment when examining the language skills of clients with AD?

Focus on language in Alzheimer's disease

To illustrate some of the language problems that occur in Alzheimer's disease, this unit will examine the conversational discourse of a woman called Martha. Martha had had a diagnosis of AD for four or five years at the time of study. She is still in a relatively early stage of the disease. Martha has word-finding problems and some difficulty tracking the referents of terms, particularly pronouns. However, she is able to handle these problems by using circumlocutions and semantically related words as well as some formulaic language. She rarely uses neologisms. Martha is telling Catherine, an 88-year-old resident of the care unit, about her former experience of learning to drive, purchasing a car and taking the family on a long car journey one summer. Catherine has had a diagnosis of AD for seven or eight years. Her role in the storytelling is largely that of a confidante to Martha.

Transcription notation

((*italic text*))	non-verbal actions and clarifications
[text]	brackets indicate the start and end points of overlapping
=	following previous utterance in immediate succession
:	elongated syllable
•hh	audible inhalation
"text"	reported speech, marked explicitly or with paralinguistic measures such as change in voice quality
—	interrupted speech
(xx xx)	inaudible speech
•yeah	inhalation speech
?	question intonation
speech	(numbered within double parentheses when two such instances occur next to each other)
(text)	unclear speech
underlining	emphasis

Extract 1

(1)	MARTHA:	((*looks down*))
(2)		Yes
(3)		But I have been driving too of course
(4)		When I should ((*looks up again*)) have ((*nods at Catherine*))
(5)		So I have [taken my driving test so I had my license]
(6)	CATHERINE:	[I see:]
(7)		mm
(8)		((*smacking sound*)) well
(9)		That was a good invention

(10)		A little car
(11)		((*turns an imaginary steering wheel with both hands in the air*))
(12)	MARTHA:	Yes
(13)	CATHERINE:	= that wasn't a bad thing
(14)	MARTHA:	And you know it wasn't that small beetle
(15)		((*turns her hand back and forth*))
(16)	CATHERINE:	[no no]
(17)	MARTHA:	[that small] e:h
(18)		Volkswagen
(19)		No it was the newest one ((*forms a shape in the air in front of her with a gentle stroke*)) that we [took]
(20)	CATHERINE:	[God]
(21)	MARTHA:	Came home with
(22)	CATHERINE:	That's swell
(23)		((*claps her hand against Martha's knee and then again takes hold of the imaginary steering wheel with a satisfied smile*))
(24)	MARTHA:	Yes
(25)		And then I said to the driving teacher •hh
(26)		"but you see
(27)		I don't have any mon–
(28)		I cannot afford a
(29)		A completely new one" I said
(30)	CATHERINE:	Hnn

Extract 2

(1)	MARTHA:	And then we drove up to eh
(2)		X-county an' an' an' [further up] ((1))
(3)	CATHERINE:	[X-county?] ((1)) [(xx xx)] ((2))
(4)	MARTHA:	[to X-county and further up] ((2))
(5)		I drove 700 kilometers then
(6)		[(xx xx)]
(7)	ASS. NURSE:	[wow]
(8)	MARTHA:	I was so afraid Edward ((*her husband*)) would get ahead of me to
(9)		The wheel so I eh
(10)		Was in an awful hurry whenever we were to drive off ((*laughter in her voice at the end of this line*))
(11)		((*laughter*))
(12)	ASS. NURSE:	But did you drive all the way by yourself?
(13)	MARTHA:	= yes I did
(14)	ASS. NURSE:	= wow
(15)	CATHERINE:	= you were stubborn
(16)	ASS. NURSE:	•yeah
(17)	CATHERINE:	But then you manage [that]
(18)	ASS. NURSE:	[but] then you had many rests?
(19)		Did you stop ma-?
(20)	MARTHA:	= well we stopped here and there and had (wild strawberries) and had berries an'
(21)		And there were lingonberries and bilberries too
(22)	ASS. NURSE:	= ye:ah

(23) Martha: •yeah
(24) And then we had relatives along the route too
(25) Ass. nurse: Yes, okay ((nodding))

Unit 30.3 Focus on language in Alzheimer's disease

(1) Give *one* example of each of the following linguistic features in these extracts:
   (a) Martha is able to use grammatical ellipsis.
   (b) Martha is able to comprehend yes–no interrogatives.
   (c) Martha uses vague language.
   (d) Martha abandons utterances.
   (e) Martha uses mental state language.

(2) What evidence is there that Martha is experiencing some word-finding problems? Refer to *two* linguistic features in your answer.

(3) As is typical of patients with early-stage AD, Martha has relatively intact syntax. Give *one* example of each of the following syntactic features in Martha's expressive language:
   (a) Martha is able to use prepositional phrases.
   (b) Martha is able to use superlative adjectives.
   (c) Martha is able to link clauses with conjunctions.
   (d) Martha is able to use relative clauses.
   (e) Martha is able to use verbs which have a present perfect progressive aspect.

(4) Alongside evidence of word-finding problems, Martha still also displays considerable lexical diversity. Give *one* example of this diversity in these extracts.

(5) Martha's conversational partner, Catherine, also has AD. However, Catherine is nevertheless skilled in supporting Martha in the construction of her story. Describe *two* ways in which she achieves this support.

Discourse in Alzheimer's disease

Aside from structural language problems in Alzheimer's disease, clients with AD can also experience considerable pragmatic and discourse deficits. Often, these deficits emerge earlier than structural language impairments. Their combined effect is to reduce the communicative effectiveness of the speaker with AD. In terms of pragmatics, clients with AD exhibit deficits in the comprehension of all forms of non-literal language. This includes the comprehension of metaphors (Roncero and de Almeida, 2014), idioms (Rassiga et al., 2009), proverbs (Leyhe et al., 2011) and sarcasm (Maki et al., 2013). Impaired understanding of non-literal language explains the evident difficulties with humour appreciation and social communication in individuals with AD. Aspects of politeness facework are disrupted in clients with AD (Rhys and Schmidt-Renfree, 2000). Individuals with AD also have difficulty contributing relevant, informative utterances to conversation and other forms of discourse (Dijkstra et el., 2004; St-Pierre et al., 2005).

Among discourse deficits in AD are referential disturbances. Clients with AD are unable to ground reference in the shared knowledge and experience of their communicative partners (Feyereisen et al., 2007). This makes narrative and other forms of discourse particularly difficult to follow as expressions such as demonstratives can lack clear referents.

Topic management is also compromised in AD, with clients displaying a reduced ability to change topics whilst maintaining discourse flow and difficulty in contributing to the propositional development of a topic (Mentis et al., 1995). Discourse cohesion and coherence are impaired in AD. Ripich et al. (2000) reported a significant decline in the use of ellipses and conjunctions in 23 subjects with early to mid-stage AD over time. Pragmatic and discourse deficits in AD have been related to theory of mind impairments and executive dysfunction (see chapter 3 in Cummings (2014b) for discussion of the cognitive basis of these deficits).

Unit 30.4 Discourse in Alzheimer's disease

(1) During a language assessment, a client with AD displays poor understanding of the following utterances. For each utterance, explain why this is the case.
  (a) She left the movie with a heavy heart.
  (b) The lawyers were sharks in court.
  (c) John decided to hit the sack.
  (d) One swallow doesn't make a summer.
  (e) The children were angels for their grandparents.

(2) A client with AD is asked by a speech-language pathologist to describe a recent visit to the hospital. The client states that an ambulance took her home, that she had a chest X-ray and that her daughter will travel to Spain next week. Which of the following maxims are problematic in the response of this client?
  (a) relation
  (b) manner
  (c) quantity
  (d) quality
  (e) both (a) and (d) above

(3) Topic management is a complex cognitive-linguistic skill which is disrupted in clients with AD. Which of the following stages of topic management is compromised in the client with AD who produces uninformative utterances in conversation? *topic selection; topic introduction; topic development; topic termination.*

(4) One of the reasons that the discourse of clients with AD is so difficult to follow is that the use of cohesive devices is disrupted. What types of cohesion are disrupted in the following examples? The underlined words will give you a clue.
  (a) A: Would you like a coffee or a tea? B: I would like a coffee.
  (b) She did not want the blouse or the cardigan, but it was the last one in the shop.
  (c) It was the city's main attraction. The cathedral and the castle had considerable historic significance.
  (d) A: Will you take the dog for a walk or will you wash the car? B: I will.
  (e) Sally bought a blue dress and a pink hat. Her mother adored it.

(5) Explain how a theory of mind impairment might compromise the interpretation of sarcastic utterances by clients with AD.

Focus on discourse in Alzheimer's disease

To illustrate some of the discourse deficits (and strengths) that are found in clients with AD, it is useful to return to Martha's narrative about learning to drive a car. The extract that follows is preceded by Martha describing her husband's doubts about her driving and his questioning of her ability to drive. Before the extract begins, Martha relates how she told her husband and her children that she was to take the driving test the following day. On this occasion, Martha and Catherine are joined by a nurse at the care unit as well as another resident called Niels.

(1)	MARTHA:	He said "you were eas-"
(2)		"You you took the driving test easily" he said
(3)	NURSE:	Uh-huh
(4)	MARTHA:	"You have studied I guess you have studied enough to make it then" he said
(5)	NURSE:	Uh-huh [(((*laughs*))]
(6)	MARTHA:	[(((*laughs*))]
(7)	NIELS:	[(((*laughs*))]
(8)	CATHERINE:	[some people are lucky] ((*turning to Niels, then forward again*))
(9)		I never dare think about that
(10)	MARTHA:	((*turns towards Catherine*)) come again?
(11)	CATHERINE:	You're so lucky ((*pointing at Martha*))
(12)		And f f s: ((*making a gesture throwing her arms about*))
(13)		Can just s s–
(14)		Say "I'll have a new car" or huh-huh ((*making a similar gesture*))
(15)		Like nothing
(16)		I don't dare do that ((*shakes her head*))
(17)	MARTHA:	And then we drove up to eh
(18)		X-county an' an' an' [further up]
(19)	CATHERINE:	[X-county?]

Unit 30.5 Focus on discourse in Alzheimer's disease

(1) Both Martha and Catherine use pronouns in the absence of clear referents. Identify *two* instances where this occurs in the extract.

(2) Martha has a number of pragmatic and discourse skills at her disposal. One of these is the ability to make requests for clarification. Give *one* example of where this occurs in the above extract. What cognitive and linguistic skills must Martha possess in order to make such requests?

(3) Notwithstanding difficulties in some aspects of discourse, Martha is an engaging narrator for the most part. Which discourse device does she (and Catherine) employ to good effect in the above extract to engage the narrator in the unfolding story?

(4) Is Martha able to reflect the temporal order of the events in her story through the use of conjunctions? Provide support for your answer.

(5) Catherine makes more extensive use of gesture than Martha. However, only some of her gestures facilitate the communication of her message, while others are too vague to have much communicative value. Give *one* example of each type of gesture.

Case study 31

Man aged 36 years with AIDS dementia complex

Introduction

The following exercise is a case study of a 36-year-old man with AIDS dementia complex (ADC) who was investigated by McCabe et al. (2008). AIDS dementia complex is a subcortical dementia which occurs in advanced HIV disease. It is an AIDS-defining complication with a complex of signs and symptoms (Brew, 1999). ADC has been reported to occur in 3% and 4.5% of a recent South American sample and an earlier European sample, respectively (Chiesi et al., 1996; Ramírez-Crescencio and Velásquez-Pérez, 2013). The case study is presented in five sections: personal and medical history; cognitive and psychological profile; language and communication profile; focus on conversation; and impact of AIDS dementia complex on communicative competence.

Personal and medical history

The client, who is referred to by the pseudonym 'Warren', is a 36-year-old, right-handed man. Warren contracted HIV 14 years earlier as a result of male-to-male sexual activity. He has been diagnosed as having AIDS dementia complex by an AIDS specialising neurologist. Warren lives alone. He has a wide-ranging employment history which includes work as a nursing assistant, a personal carer, a cook, a housekeeper and various handyman jobs. Warren has spent 13 years in education, and has a general nurses' aide certificate. He stopped working in the 12-month period before his first assessment on account of a peripheral neuropathy and AIDS dementia complex. However, he frequently talks about returning to the workforce and would like to undertake an occupational therapy degree. A guardian has been appointed by the courts to manage Warren's finances. Warren would like to move to a rural area, but is not permitted to do so by his guardian. There is a positive history of recreational drug use, and Warren was regularly smoking marijuana during the research study.

Warren has experienced a number of opportunistic infections including oral and anal *candida* (thrush), pneumonia and systemic *Cytomegalovirus* infection. He uses a cane to walk on account of his peripheral neuropathy. Previously, he has been prescribed antiviral drugs but has reported poor compliance with these treatment regimes. Warren does not report any change in his communication skills since HIV infection. He does not have a family history of speech or language impairment, and there was no cognitive or language impairment, psychiatric illness or neurological disorder prior to his diagnosis of dementia.

Unit 31.1 Personal and medical history

(1) Which of the following is a *true* statement about dementia in adults with HIV infection?
    (a) Dementia is seen in approximately 3% of adults with HIV.
    (b) Dementia is seen in approximately 23% of adults with HIV.
    (c) Dementia is seen in approximately 43% of adults with HIV.
    (d) Dementia is seen in approximately 63% of adults with HIV.
    (e) Dementia is seen in approximately 83% of adults with HIV.

(2) Which of the following is associated with HIV infection in adults?
    (a) sensorineural hearing loss
    (b) stuttering
    (c) apraxia of speech
    (d) cognitive-communication problems
    (e) conductive hearing loss

(3) Which features of Warren's medical history suggest that dysphagia may be an issue for him?

(4) Which of Warren's opportunistic infections may have contributed to the development of his peripheral neuropathy?

(5) Apart from HIV infection, is there any other feature of Warren's personal history which may be contributing to his cognitive problems?

Cognitive and psychological profile

Warren underwent neuropsychological testing at his second assessment, which took place six months after his first assessment in the study. Warren was reported by the neuropsychologist to have an average estimated premorbid IQ. The results of neuropsychological tests showed that Warren had average working memory, psychomotor speed, visuo-construction and verbal fluency performance. As part of his neuropsychological assessment, the Stroop Colour and Word Test (Trenerry et al., 1989) and the Symbol Digit Modalities Test (SDMT; Smith, 1982) were conducted. These tests revealed significant impairments. Warren's Stroop score placed him at 2.53 standard deviations from the mean and his SDMT score placed him at 2.18 (written) and 1.70 (oral) standard deviations below the mean. On other tests, Warren's performance in verbal learning, recall of verbal information, information processing speed and fine motor (right hand) function was between 1 and 1.5 standard deviations below the mean. This was not statistically significant. The Beck Depression Inventory-II (Beck et al., 1996), a norm-referenced, self-completed questionnaire, showed that Warren had average anxiety and depression. Information about Warren's premorbid functioning and emotional state was not available.

Unit 31.2 Cognitive and psychological profile

(1) Respond with *true* or *false* to each of the following statements:
    (a) Tests revealed that Warren has deficits in affective theory of mind.
    (b) Tests revealed that Warren has psychomotor slowing.

(c) Tests revealed that Warren has difficulty suppressing a habitual response.

(d) Tests revealed that Warren has deficits in cognitive theory of mind.

(e) Tests revealed that Warren has impaired information retrieval from memory.

(2) Warren had average verbal fluency performance. Verbal fluency can be assessed in different ways. Which of the following are *true* statements about the assessment of verbal fluency?

(a) Subjects generate words that belong to a certain semantic category.

(b) Category fluency is an assessment of phonological memory.

(c) Subjects establish the mental states of characters in a story.

(d) Subjects generate words that begin with a certain letter.

(e) Category fluency is an assessment of semantic memory.

(3) Warren clearly has executive function deficits. From your knowledge of these deficits, which of the following aspects of language are most likely to be compromised for Warren?

(a) use of inflectional suffixes such as *–ed* and *–ing*

(b) use of consonant clusters in word-initial position

(c) production of well-organised narratives

(d) topic management in conversation

(e) comprehension of yes–no interrogatives

(4) Why is it important for the speech-language pathologist to know that Warren has depression?

(5) A speech-language pathologist will undertake a comprehensive assessment of Warren's communication skills. However, based on these cognitive findings, which of the following is/are likely to feature prominently in such an assessment?

(a) assessment of diadochokinetic rates

(b) assessment of figurative language

(c) assessment of phonetic inventory

(d) assessment of causal and temporal relations between narrative events

(e) assessment of intonation

Language and communication profile

Several standardised tests and other assessments of Warren's language and communication skills were undertaken. Warren was not aphasic on the Western Aphasia Battery (Kertesz, 1982). His performance on the Boston Naming Test (Kaplan et al., 1983) was above the norm. On the Right Hemisphere Language Battery (Bryan, 1988) Warren had significant difficulty with metaphor comprehension. At the second of three assessments conducted over 13 months, Warren achieved a score of 5 out of 10 metaphor items correct. His performance at the first and third assessments was worse still, with a score of zero achieved on both occasions. Warren's performance on word fluency generation by initial letter varied between 9 and 15 words, which was lower than a score of 22 achieved by a HIV negative control, but higher than a score of 8 achieved by an AIDS control with no dementia. Warren's conversational skills were judged to be inappropriate on the Pragmatic Protocol (Prutting and Kirchner, 1987). As an indication of the extent of his inappropriateness, Warren's performance was worse than that of the AIDS control, whose performance was worse in turn than that of the normal control. Areas which were inappropriate at all three assessments were topic selection, topic maintenance, style variability, prosody and eye gaze. It is worth noting that at the third assessment, which was conducted 13 months into the study, Warren's total number of inappropriate items exceeded that at the previous two assessments. Warren's conversational skills were also analysed using Clinical Discourse Analysis (CDA; Damico, 1985). The CDA assessment was based on a 15-minute extract from the first interview with Warren. In that time, Warren produced no fewer than 109 pragmatically inappropriate behaviours. Only 33 were produced by the AIDS control during the same period of time. The percentage of Warren's utterances with pragmatically inappropriate behaviours was 62%. This compared with only 24% in the AIDS control. The three areas of greatest difficulty for Warren were the use of non-specific vocabulary, informational redundancy and poor topic maintenance.

Unit 31.3 Language and communication profile

(1) Based on Warren's language profile, which of the following aspects of linguistic performance are likely to be compromised? State why in each case.
   (a) The production of subordinate clauses.
   (b) The comprehension of utterances like *The children were angels all day.*
   (c) The comprehension of locative prepositions.
   (d) The naming of pictures and objects.
   (e) The comprehension of utterances like *The soldiers were lions in battle.*

(2) Warren's performance on word fluency generation by initial letter was impaired relative to a HIV negative control. Which of the following statements is supported by this finding?
   (a) Warren has a deficit in first-order theory of mind.
   (b) Warren has executive dysfunction as indexed by phonemic fluency.
   (c) Warren has a deficit in second-order theory of mind.
   (d) Warren has executive dysfunction as indexed by semantic fluency.
   (e) Warren has a deficit which is specific to affective theory of mind.

(3) On the basis of the results of the Pragmatic Protocol, which of the following conversational skills are likely to be problematic for Warren?
   (a) the use of turn-taking in conversation
   (b) the introduction of an appropriate topic into a conversation
   (c) the production of speech acts such as directives
   (d) the use of adjacency pairs such as question and response
   (e) the inability to develop a topic introduced by a conversational partner

(4) When Warren was first interviewed, it was observed that he was verbose, unable to maintain topic, self-focused, unaware of the needs of his listener, and had word-finding problems. Which aspect of these clinical impressions might explain the finding from the Clinical Discourse Analysis that Warren makes use of non-specific vocabulary?

(5) Clinical Discourse Analysis also revealed that informational redundancy is an area of difficulty for Warren. According to CDA, informational redundancy 'involves the continued and inappropriate fixation on a proposition. The speaker will continue to stress a point or relate a fact even when the listener has acknowledged its reception and tried to proceed.' How might informational redundancy manifest itself in conversation?

(a) use of repetitive utterances
(b) use of tangential utterances
(c) use of egocentric utterances
(d) use of impolite utterances
(e) use of echolalic utterances

Focus on conversation

The following conversational extract is taken from the initial interview between Warren (W) and the researcher (R). The semi-structured interview, which took place in Warren's own home, focused on his AIDS and life in general.

R: So you'd be 34 then?

W: I've been 34 for the last 3 years

R: Ah, OK so you're actually?

W: Oh what happened was I added a year and a year at my birthday, didn't celebrate it so therefore I forgot about it. In September as a halfway between two ages I start saying what the next one is

R: Uh huh?

W: So I've added there as well and the years come along and I didn't remember doing either of the first two so I did it again when I was 32

R: Oh dear

W: Someone pointed out that I was 34 last year and 33 last year and I went "no, I'm not I'm 34", I'm gonna get me a calculator and a new set of batteries that were still in the package so that guaranteed the calculator was working properly 'cause it kept telling me I was 33 and I could'a swore it was lying to me

R: What year were you born in?

W: '64

R: '64

W: The odd thing was, was I was filling out doctors' forms and hospital forms and all sort of things, putting down the date of birth as xxth of xxxx of '64 and my age was 34 but a diversional therapist in a nursing home was the only person who actually noticed that there was something wrong with this picture. I thought "well, it's fairly obvious I'm in it" so there's your problem

Unit 31.4 Focus on conversation

(1) The researcher is clearly finding it difficult to follow what Warren is saying. To what extent are referential anomalies contributing to this difficulty? You should include examples of referential anomalies and aspects of intact use of reference within your response.

(2) Where referential anomalies occur, they confirm the clinical impression that Warren is unaware of the informational needs of his listener. This might suggest some difficulty on Warren's part in attributing knowledge and other mental states to the mind of his listener. If it is the case that Warren has difficulty attributing mental states to the minds of others, the same cannot be said of the attribution of mental states to his own mind. What aspect of Warren's use of verbs suggest that the attribution of mental states to his own mind is largely intact?

(3) Give *one* example of each of the following linguistic behaviours in the above exchange:
  (a) Warren uses non-specific vocabulary.
  (b) Warren uses substitution as a form of grammatical cohesion.
  (c) Warren produces irrelevant information.
  (d) Warren uses direct reported speech.
  (e) Warren produces contradictory information.

(4) There is evidence that Warren is able to introduce new people and objects appropriately into his conversational discourse. Explain how he achieves this.

(5) Which of the following are *true* statements about Warren's conversational skills?
  (a) Warren does not appreciate the dyadic structure of conversation.
  (b) Warren is a verbose conversational partner.
  (c) Warren can produce an appropriately informative response on occasion.
  (d) Warren's conversational difficulties are related to syntactic deficits.
  (e) Warren's conversational difficulties are related to executive function deficits.

Impact of ADC on communicative competence

To evaluate the impact of AIDS dementia complex (ADC) on communicative competence, it is helpful to compare Warren's conversational performance with the performance of a non-ADC AIDS control. In the following extracts, Warren (W) and a non-ADC AIDS control (C) are discussing their employment history with the researcher (R).

Non-ADC AIDS control

R: What did you do?
C: I'm a public service, left last year but I'm looking for another job
R: Uh huh, what sort of work did you do in the public service?
C: Worked at X consulate
R: Oh, OK, was that . . .
C: Foreign service
R: OK, that must've been very interesting
C: Issuing visas 'n stuff and then 'cause X um and Australia are connected now with visas they don't need uh like people to issue them
R: uh huh
C: and plus I was sick 'n should've just took holidays but I left
R: uh huh, OK. Alright, did you like that job?
C: Yeah, it was good.

Warren

R: What would be the longest job you had?
W: Oh when I had the business, cleaning the building
R: mm and that was for how many years?
W: 8 years, like I said I was spoiled
R: And that was when you were in your twenties?

W: Twenty two. (Name) was the only person who had total faith in me. There was an intelligent person in there that, um, he said I've got more common sense. I like that idea 'cause there's nothing common about this little black duck and if I am on my way to prove that I'm not. My great grandmother was born into a family that was indentured to a castle near Salisbury, Newcastle. Well she was supposed to be a house servant. She sort of looked at then at the age of 17 and said "Do I look like a peasant girl to you? I don't think so, I'm jumping on a boat and going to Australia . . . " (continued in same vein for 6 more utterances)

Unit 31.5 Impact of ADC on communicative competence

(1) There are considerable differences in how Warren and the AIDS control respond to questions. Describe these differences.

(2) In these extracts, Warren and the AIDS control are largely responding to questions. How does the AIDS control additionally deal with the comments of the researcher?

(3) Respond with *true* or *false* to each of the following statements. Provide evidence for each of your responses:
   (a) Warren is able to address grammatical and prosodic questions.
   (b) Warren cannot use anaphoric reference.
   (c) The AIDS control exhibits some lexical errors.
   (d) The AIDS control cannot use anaphoric reference.
   (e) Warren exhibits some play on the meaning of words.

(4) Both Warren and the AIDS control exhibit some wider semantic activation of words related to target words. Where does this occur in each case?

(5) Which of the following statements best captures the impact of ADC on communicative competence?
   (a) ADC disrupts structural levels of language only.
   (b) Clients with AIDS in the absence of ADC do not experience communicative difficulties.
   (c) ADC disrupts high-level aspects of language that are sensitive to cognitive deficits.
   (d) Clients with AIDS in the absence of ADC are verbose communicators.
   (e) ADC disrupts receptive language skills only.

Case study 32

Man aged 76 years with Parkinson's disease

Introduction

The following exercise is a case study of a man ('Robert') of 76 years of age who was studied by Saldert et al. (2014). Thirteen years prior to this study, Robert received a diagnosis of Parkinson's disease (PD). PD is a neurodegenerative disorder which is characterised clinically by resting tremor, bradykinesia, rigidity and postural instability. The condition is caused by a loss of neurones in the substantia nigra of the brain (Nussbaum and Ellis, 2003). A recent meta-analysis of worldwide data shows a rising prevalence of the disorder with age: a prevalence of 41 cases per 100,000 population rises to 1,903 cases per 100,000 in individuals over 80 years (Pringsheim et al., 2014). The main communication disorder associated with Parkinson's disease is dysarthria. However, individuals with the disease can also experience swallowing, language and cognitive problems, even in the absence of dementia. The case study is presented in five sections: primer on Parkinson's disease; client history and communication status; focus on word-finding difficulties; focus on conversational repair; and the role of the conversation partner.

Primer on Parkinson's disease

Parkinson's disease is a progressive, neurological disorder which has significant implications for a client's motor, cognitive and language functions. The cardinal signs of PD are the motor symptoms of rest tremor, bradykinesia, rigidity and loss of postural reflexes. However, there are also significant secondary motor symptoms such as dysarthria, dysphagia, sialorrhoea, micrographia and festination, and non-motor symptoms including cognitive deficits, sleep disorders and sensory problems (Jankovic, 2008). Although the risk of PD is greater in older subjects, 5.4% of patients in one community-based prevalence study were found to have disease onset below the age of 50 years (Wickremaratchi et al., 2009). The main histopathological finding in PD is the loss of dopaminergic neurones from the substantia nigra associated with the presence of Lewy bodies (an abnormal aggregate of a protein called alpha-synuclein). For symptoms to occur, it is estimated that at least 50% of these nigral neurones must degenerate, although in most cases there is more than 80% reduction of these cells at autopsy (Mackenzie, 2001).

Parkinson's disease is a significant condition for the speech-language pathologist who must assess and treat the speech, language and swallowing problems associated with the disorder. Dysarthria, sialorrhoea and dysphagia have been reported in 51%, 37% and 18% of a sample of 419 patients with moderate PD, respectively (Perez-Lloret et al., 2012). The most common form of dysarthria in patients with PD is hypokinetic dysarthria.

The features of this dysarthria are hypophonia, reduced stress and intonation patterns, abnormal voice qualities, distorted consonantal sounds, and abnormally rapid or slow speaking rates (Adams and Dykstra, 2009). Alongside dysarthria, there are also language impairments in PD, particularly in the domain of pragmatics. Reported pragmatic deficits include impairments of the comprehension of speech acts, irony and metaphor (Holtgraves and McNamara, 2010; Monetta and Pell, 2007; Monetta et al., 2009). At least some of these impairments appear to be related to cognitive deficits in PD in areas such as theory of mind and verbal working memory (Monetta and Pell, 2007; Monetta et al., 2009).

Unit 32.1 Primer on Parkinson's disease

(1) Each of the following statements is a description of one of the terms used above. Match each statement to the term to which it relates:
 (a) A term used to describe reduced vocal intensity.
 (b) A term used to describe slowness of movement.
 (c) A term used to describe a progressive reduction in amplitude during writing.
 (d) A term used to describe a brainstem nucleus in the extrapyramidal system.
 (e) A term used to describe the ability to attribute mental states to other minds.

(2) The substantia nigra contains dopaminergic neurones, i.e. neurones that produce dopamine. State what dopamine is, and describe its function in the central nervous system.

(3) Below is a list of features of hypokinetic dysarthria in Parkinson's disease. Assign each feature to one of the following speech production subsystems: articulation; resonation; phonation; respiration; and prosody
 (a) hypophonia
 (b) reduced stress and intonation
 (c) abnormal voice qualities
 (d) distorted consonantal sounds
 (e) aberrant speaking rate

(4) Which of the following utterances may prove to be difficult for the client with PD to understand? Justify your response(s).
 (a) Sally bought the book.
 (b) I adore noisy, disruptive children!
 (c) The boy is crossing the road.
 (d) The cruise liner ploughed through the sea.
 (e) The exam was more challenging than the students had expected.

(5) Clients with PD can have theory of mind (ToM) deficits. How might ToM deficits compromise utterance interpretation in such a client?

Client history and communication status

Robert is 76 years old and is a former medical doctor. He is a native Swedish speaker. His wife Sonja is 73 years old and is a former audiologist. It has been 13 years since Robert was diagnosed with PD. He is at Stage IV of the Hoehn and Yahr (1967) scale of clinical disability: 'Fully developed, severely disabling disease; the patient is still able to walk and stand unassisted but is markedly incapacitated' (433). Robert has not been diagnosed with dementia. However, he has dysarthria. His comprehensibility in contextual speech is 75%. Degree of comprehensibility was measured by calculating the percentage of correctly perceived words by a native rater out of 100 words which were uttered by Robert in the context of a video-recorded conversation. Both phonological and semantic aspects of word fluency were impaired in Robert. When asked to produce as many words as possible beginning with the letters F, A and S during one minute for each letter, Robert produced 28 words (norm 42.3 +/− 10.6). When asked to name as many animals and activities as possible during one minute, Robert named just 9 (norm for animals: 20.9 +/− 7.7; norm for activities 18.1 +/− 6.0). The Token Test (De Renzi and Vignolo, 1962) was used to measure auditory verbal comprehension. Robert achieved a score of 175, which was well below the cut-off point of 253/261.

Unit 32.2 Client history and communication status

(1) Given the advanced nature of Robert's neurological condition, which of the following should feature in the SLP management of the client?
   (a) muscle strengthening exercises
   (b) expressive syntax
   (c) augmentative and alternative communication
   (d) articulatory drills
   (e) receptive semantics

(2) Robert's comprehensibility was assessed. Comprehensibility is not the same as intelligibility. How might the difference between these notions be characterised?

(3) Robert's comprehensibility is likely to exceed his intelligibility. Explain why this is likely to be the case.

(4) Both phonological and semantic aspects of word fluency are impaired in Robert. Which group of cognitive skills are likely to be disrupted to produce this finding?

(5) Robert displays impaired comprehension of language on the Token Test. What does this result reveal about language in PD?

Focus on word-finding difficulties

Conversation between Robert and Sonja was video-recorded in their home. Thirty minutes of transcribed natural interaction were obtained. The transcription included non-vocal features such as gestures and body movements as well as talk. All instances of repair were recorded. There were 11 instances in total. Some were related to comprehension problems caused by Robert's dysarthria, while other instances of repair were related to the meaning of words. Although Sonja tended to dominate the interaction with Robert, there were several occasions where they both participated as listeners and speakers in the exchange. The topic of conversation in the following exchange is a visit to a church that Robert has undertaken along with other people at his day care centre. Just prior to the start of the extract shown below, Sonja has asked if there was any singing during the visit. It has been established that there were two girls singing and a man playing the organ. After a pause of 1.4 seconds, Robert continues to tell Sonja about the visit (underlining = emphasis; (xxx) = unintelligible sequence):

R: (and then it was) (0.6) it was some priest who (2.5) read a chapter from (1.2) eh the bible (1.6) and well (x) there were no (1.0) purposes or influ- or something that should be influenced fluenced or so but it was like what was part of their work (xxx) (0.8) help and encourage (1.4) be considerate to (0.9) elderly persons and such who are living on those pension schemes (1.1)

S: ((*subtle nod*)) mm

R: but it was a moment of =

S: = an ho- an hour or what?

R: yes

S: yes

R: it is a moment of (different) (1.8)

S: no but you are participating in the singing of <u>hymns</u>

R: yes

Unit 32.3 Focus on word-finding difficulties

(1) Robert makes extensive use of pauses in his initial turn in the above exchange. Describe *three* features of these pauses which indicate that they are related to a word search.

(2) Clients who have word-finding difficulties often use a preponderance of non-specific vocabulary. Are there any instances of this type of vocabulary in the above exchange?

(3) The presence of circumlocutions is often symptomatic of word-finding difficulties on the part of a speaker. Does Robert use a circumlocution at any point in the above exchange?

(4) Aside from Robert's word-finding difficulties, one other feature of his contribution to this exchange makes it difficult for his conversational partner to follow him. What is this feature?

(5) Notwithstanding the fact that Sonja does not explicitly attempt to repair Robert's turns, it is clear that she is not for the most part following his contribution to the exchange. How does she signal this towards the end of the exchange?

Focus on conversational repair

After agreeing that he participated in the singing of hymns, Robert returns to his earlier attempt to tell Sonja what happened during the church visit. In this part of the exchange, Sonja is more proactive in her efforts to understand what Robert is attempting to communicate. To this end, she initiates a conversational repair:

R: and then what you feel about that (1.6) that you don't know (2.6) but eh (2.9) yes it is (1.0) it is (x) it is good for such (it is) that you shouldn't (1.1) understand or (x) be able to (0.8) ehm (1.1) refer to certain (1.0) things in (2.1) (and) (2.1) but you eh (0.6) may speak quite (0.9) freely on such things

S: I <u>see</u> so you had some discussions after or?

R: no it is not much it is just a little

S: so there are questions put to you by the priest or?
R: yes it is it is not so much but eh (there is) a lit- a little
S: I see
R: to make the time pass
S: ok yes

Unit 32.4 Focus on conversational repair

(1) Robert also makes extensive use of non-specific vocabulary in this part of the conversational exchange. Give *three* examples of this vocabulary.

(2) It is also difficult in this part of the exchange to assign referents to many of the terms that Robert uses. Give *three* examples of where this occurs in Robert's turns.

(3) Sonja is less inclined in this part of the conversation to let her lack of understanding of Robert's turns pass unacknowledged in the exchange. Accordingly, she attempts a conversational repair. How would you characterise this repair? Is it effective in establishing common ground between Robert and Sonja?

(4) Is there another way of characterising Sonja's repair strategy which differs from the characterisation that you have given in your response to (3)?

(5) Robert uses and appears to comprehend mental state language. List the different instances of mental state language in the above exchange (there are *five* in total). What cognitive ability must be relatively intact in Robert in order for him to use and comprehend such language?

The role of the conversation partner

Speech-language pathologists attach considerable significance to the conversation partner of the person with an acquired neurogenic communication disorder. It has long been recognised that conversation partners can both facilitate and hinder communication with clients who have Parkinson's disease or other neurological disorders. To this end, considerable effort is expended in therapy in encouraging strategies which facilitate communication between clients and their partners, and in discouraging behaviours which impede effective communication. In a related study, Carlsson et al. (2014) examined the communicative strategies that are used by the partners of people with advanced Parkinson's disease to overcome their difficulties with dysarthria and anomia. Robert and Sonja were one of the dyads used in this study. Sonja was observed to use six different strategies during conversation with Robert: (1) *response token* where the partner indicates that she is taking part in the interaction but does not intend to undertake repair work (e.g. 'mm hm'); (2) *contribution for flow* where the partner contributes a comment or question in the area of the initiated topic, thereby maintaining the flow of conversation; (3) *topic shift* where the conversation partner shifts the topic from one that has caused problems for the person with a communication disorder; (4) *open-class initiation of repair* where the conversation partner does not specify which part of the client's contribution needs to be repaired (e.g. 'what do you mean?'); (5) *guess/completion/suggestion* where the partner guesses what the client is trying to express by providing a target word or specific alternatives; and

(6) *elaboration / specification* where the conversation partner attempts to narrow down, sum up or expand on the information provided by the client.

Unit 32.5 The role of the conversation partner

(1) During Robert's conversation with Sonja about his church visit, he attempts to tell her that someone played the organ. The exchange in question is shown below. Classify Sonja's contribution according to one of the six categories described above:

R: who played on eh (0.8)
S: on the organ or the piano?

(2) For the category you identified in response to (1), are there any further examples of its use in the conversational data shown in units 32.3 and 32.4?

(3) In the conversational data in units 32.3 and 32.4, are there any examples of the strategy called *response token*?

(4) In the conversational data in units 32.3 and 32.4, are there any examples of the strategy called *topic shift*?

(5) Some of these strategies are not related to the initiation of or participation in repair. Other strategies request a clarification or modification of the message by the client. Still other strategies provide the client with solutions. Classify each of the six categories above according to one of these three types of strategy.

Case study 33

Man aged 37 years with Huntington's disease

Introduction

The following exercise is a case study of a man ('ER') aged 37 years who was studied by Power et al. (2011). ER was diagnosed with Huntington's disease in 1996 when he was 26 years old. The case study is presented in five sections: primer on Huntington's disease; client history; communication status; ICF framework; and communication goal setting.

Primer on Huntington's disease

Huntington's disease (HD) is an autosomal dominant disorder that is caused by a defective gene on the short arm of chromosome 4. The condition is characterised by movement disorders, cognitive decline and behavioural changes (Cardoso, 2014). Fisher and Hayden (2014) estimated that the prevalence of HD in the general population in British Columbia, Canada is 13.7 per 100,000. These investigators argue that this figure suggests that there may be up to 4,700 individuals with HD in Canada and up to 43,000 individuals affected by the disease in the United States. On one estimate, the annual incidence of HD is 0.06 cases per 100,000 persons (Kim et al., 2015). In a large European cohort of 1,706 individuals with HD, Weydt et al. (2014) reported a balanced male-to-female ratio (1.04). Huntington's disease typically has its onset in midlife, although cases can arise as early as age 2 or 3 and as old as age 80 or more. Survival from onset to death is 17–20 years on average, with evidence that later onset is associated with slower progression (Myers, 2004).

The clinical picture in Huntington's disease is a complex one. Functional limitations arise on account of cognitive, neuropsychiatric, motor and behavioural problems. The motor disorder in HD has two major components – involuntary movement disorder (chorea) and voluntary movement impairment (incoordination and bradykinesia) (Bates et al., 2015: 8). Chorea usually begins early in the course of the disease and decreases in the late stages when parkinsonism, dystonia and rigidity dominate. It is common in adult but not juvenile patients. Impairment of voluntary movements is most prominent in early-onset disease, especially juvenile HD. It is also a feature of the late stages of adult-onset HD. In a study of 340 nursing home residents with a diagnosis of HD, depression, dementia, anxiety, psychosis and bipolar disease were present in 59.4%, 50.9%, 35.9%, 23.2% and 9.7%, respectively (Zarowitz et al., 2014). Moderate or severe cognitive impairment was found in 78% of residents, while 21% exhibited troublesome behavioural symptoms. Cognitive deficits in areas such as speed of processing, initiation and attention are more significant than memory loss in clients with HD (Peavy et al., 2010).

Clients with Huntington's disease present with a range of difficulties that require assessment and treatment by speech-language pathologists. Dysphagia is a significant cause of death and disability in HD. In a study of 224 cases of HD, Heemskerk and Roos (2012) reported that 86.8% died from aspiration pneumonia. Approximately one-half of the nursing home residents with HD studied by Zarowitz et al. (2014) exhibited communication difficulties. Chief among these difficulties in HD is the motor speech disorder dysarthria and language impairments in the presence and absence of dementia. Skodda et al. (2014) reported impaired motor speech performance in 21 patients with HD. These clients exhibited a reduction of speech rate, an increase of pauses and marked difficulties in the repetition of single syllables. Hertrich and Ackermann (1994) reported increased variability of utterance duration and/or voice onset time in 13 subjects with HD. A subgroup of these subjects had reduced speech tempo that was concomitant with over-proportional lengthening of short vowels.

In terms of language, individuals with HD have been found to use shorter and fewer grammatically complete utterances than their healthy peers (Murray and Lenz, 2001). Moreover, these aspects of productive syntax were related to neuropsychological and motor speech changes in these clients. Saldert et al. (2010) studied pragmatic and discourse skills in a group of 18 patients with Huntington's disease. These subjects were significantly less able than pair-matched controls to comprehend metaphors, explain lexical ambiguities in sentences and respond to questions about the (explicit and implicit) content of narrative discourse.

Unit 33.1 Primer on Huntington's disease

(1) Chorea is one of several motor problems that occur in Huntington's disease. Which of the following are *true* statements about chorea?
   (a) Chorea is characterised by twisting, writhing movements.
   (b) Severe choreic motions are known as ballismus.
   (c) Chorea is a motor disorder of the lower limbs only.
   (d) Chorea in Huntington's disease is related to basal ganglia dysfunction.
   (e) Chorea manifests as spontaneous, uncontrollable, irregular movements.

(2) Which of the following types of dysarthria is found in clients with Huntington's disease?
   (a) flaccid dysarthria
   (b) ataxic dysarthria
   (c) spastic dysarthria
   (d) hypokinetic dysarthria
   (e) hyperkinetic dysarthria

(3) Which motor disorder in Huntington's disease might account for the reduction of speech rate that is experienced by clients with this neurodegenerative disorder?

(4) Respond with *true* or *false* to each of the following statements about cognitive impairments in Huntington's disease:
   (a) The pattern of cognitive deficits in HD is similar to that found in Alzheimer's disease.
   (b) Aspects of language in HD are related to cognitive deficits.
   (c) Cognitive dysfunction is a late feature of HD.
   (d) Clients with HD can have executive dysfunction.

(e) Clients with pre-HD may exhibit subtle cognitive dysfunction that does not meet criteria for dementia.

(5) Clients with HD can present with neuropsychiatric disorders. What is the significance of these disorders for the SLT management of clients with HD?

Client history

ER was diagnosed by a neurologist with HD in 1996. He was 26 years old at the time. He had experienced increasing symptoms for approximately five to six years prior to diagnosis. These symptoms included dropping objects, arm and facial chorea and behaviour change. ER has a positive family history for HD. His father died of the disease when he was 33 years old. Both of ER's siblings also developed the disease. One sibling died at the age of 33 years in a residential care facility. The other sibling had the juvenile onset form of HD and died at 16 years of age. ER had obtained a mechanical trade qualification. Prior to finishing work, he had worked as a petrol station attendant. ER has two children aged between 5 and 10 years. Despite making efforts to maintain contact with them since his relationship with their mother ended in 1993, he is now estranged from them. Since 2002, ER has resided in specialised residential care which is some distance from his home. His primary familial contact is with his mother. The Unified Huntington's Disease Rating Scale (UHDRS; Huntington Study Group, 1996) was conducted on ER in order to stage the severity of disease. His scores on the motor, neuropsychiatric, functional and cognitive components of this scale indicated that he was in the advanced stages of HD. Among ER's difficulties were significant limb and truncal chorea, moderate apathy and visual gaze difficulties. ER required assistance with most activities of daily living.

Unit 33.2 Client history

(1) Use your knowledge of the genetic basis of HD to calculate the likelihood that ER's children will also develop the disease.

(2) Prior to diagnosis, ER presented with arm and facial chorea. Explain *two* ways in which this motor disturbance might have an adverse impact on ER's communication skills.

(3) On examination, ER displayed apathy and visual gaze difficulties. Which components of the UHDRS may be used to assess these impairments?

(4) Which components of the UHDRS may be used to assess dysarthria and executive function deficits in a client with HD?

(5) On the basis of ER's history, describe *two* aspects of his functioning which have been compromised by HD.

Communication status

ER underwent extensive assessment of his communication skills in early 2003. He was assessed using the Frenchay Dysarthria Assessment (FDA; Enderby, 1983), the Western

Aphasia Battery (WAB; Kertesz, 1982), the pragmatic protocol (Prutting and Kirchner, 1987) and the Communicative Effectiveness Index (CETI; Lomas et al., 1989). On the FDA, ER presented with mild hyperkinetic dysarthria. Specific speech findings were the production of imprecise consonants and intermittent strained–strangled and hoarse vocal quality. ER displayed forced inspiration-expiration and reduced respiratory control. He also had difficulty varying loudness and often used excessive loudness and pitch variations. On word- and sentence-level intelligibility testing, ER scored at ceiling level. Staff in ER's residential care setting reported that he displayed mild-moderate intelligibility problems in both one-to-one and group conversations and that he needed to repeat himself. ER's intelligibility varied with background noise and his severe truncal chorea.

On the WAB, ER was diagnosed as having a mild aphasic impairment. It took ER increased time to provide answers and follow instructions during testing. During picture description, ER produced simple utterances which had reduced grammatical complexity. He could identify objects and follow one- and two-step instructions. However, ER had difficulty understanding three-part instructions. His word fluency was reduced. He was able to read and comprehend paragraph-level material. On account of his chorea, ER found it difficult to write legibly and writing was also laborious. He produced spelling errors.

On the pragmatic protocol, ER displayed mild-moderate difficulties across a number of areas both in one-to-one and group settings. Topic selection was limited, and ER relied on his communication partner to initiate and maintain topics. ER produced a reduced quantity of output in short turns. He made use of increased pause times and a small number of interruptions and amount of overlap. He used a range of speech acts and was able to revise his utterances if there was a communication breakdown. His communicative style varied with the type of topic discussed. ER listened well to others during conversation and offered some opinions and observations. In a group situation, ER was more animated and discussed a wider range of conversational topics than in a one-to-one context. ER's body posture, and arm and leg movements were distracting. Facial and limb chorea distorted his more subtle gestures.

On the CETI, ER rated himself as mostly able or always able to participate in the CETI items. He judged the following as areas where he was rarely able or sometimes able: continue conversations and follow the topic; be part of a fast conversation with other people talking; understand complex information. ER's ratings were consistent with those of nursing staff and speech-language pathologists. Staff rated the following areas lower than ER: describe things in detail; start conversations with others. ER was reported by staff to meet most of his basic communicative needs without significant help.

Unit 33.3 Communication status

(1) ER's intelligibility varied with his severe truncal chorea. Which aspect of ER's speech production is most likely to be compromised by this motor disturbance?

(2) What environmental challenge is there to ER's intelligibility? Why might it be difficult for ER to address this challenge?

(3) Respond with *true* or *false* to each of the following statements about ER's language skills:
   (a) ER has an auditory verbal comprehension deficit.
   (b) ER has receptive language impairment only.
   (c) ER's problems with written language can be explained by motor factors alone.

(d) ER's problems with written language can be explained by linguistic factors alone.

(e) ER has a fluent aphasia.

(4) Which *two* aspects of ER's pragmatic skills may be explained by his apathy?

(5) ER's ratings of his communicative effectiveness on the CETI were consistent with those of nursing staff and speech-language pathologists. What does this indicate? What implication does this finding have for intervention?

ICF framework

The communication assessments described in unit 33.3 contributed to a wider evaluation of ER's impairments and functioning within the International Classification of Functioning, Disability and Health (ICF; World Health Organization, 2001). As defined by the World Health Organization, this framework is

a classification of health and health-related domains – domains that help us to describe changes in body function and structure, what a person with a health condition can do in a standard environment (their level of capacity), as well as what they actually do in their usual environment (their level of performance). These domains are classified from body, individual and societal perspectives by means of two lists: a list of body functions and structure, and a list of domains of activity and participation.

To examine communication-related activities and participation, semi-structured, guided interviews were conducted with ER and his mother. Open-ended questions based on the components of the ICF were used during these interviews, with focused probes used to clarify and explore information further. For example, environmental barriers to effective communication were interrogated by asking 'Tell me about things that make communication/being involved in life more difficult?' To examine this issue more fully, probes such as 'in relation to equipment or technology' or 'the environment at the residential facility' were used.

The semi-structured interviews revealed that ER's most significant activity limitation and participation restriction was his inability to interact and converse with his children, perform the role of father and be involved in his children's lives. ER and his mother were concerned at current and future lack of involvement with the children, with ER expressing 'I can't see my kids or be their dad' and 'they won't understand me later when I get worse'. Other limitations and restrictions considered by ER and his mother to be important were decreased speech intelligibility, reduced initiation and ER's maintenance of conversations with his mother and other residents. Problems with speech intelligibility were particularly acute during telephone conversations between ER and his mother. It was also noted that ER's socialising was dependent on others to provide opportunity and that he had reduced ability to initiate and maintain a relationship with his mother.

Specific contextual factors that contributed to ER's participation restriction were the lack of specialised facilities close to home, which limited the communication opportunities and quality time that ER and his mother had together, and the background noise near the nurse's station which had a negative impact on phone conversations between ER and his mother. Although the poor social relationship between ER and his children was not currently related to his speech and language problems, speech-language pathologists, nursing staff and family all reported concern that these problems would compromise ER's communication with his children in the future. A talking group in ER's residential care facility, ER's mother and his dog were all considered to be facilitators of communication. However, ER did not attend the talking group unless specifically invited to do so. Interviews also identified a number of significant personal factors in ER's case. His mother reported that he enjoyed the company of others but that he was not a man of many words. ER's extensive experience with HD in his own family had prepared him for the course that his disease would take and its implications for communication. ER had a positive attitude to communication books which he had helped prepare for one of his siblings.

Unit 33.4 ICF framework

(1) Which of the following are *true* statements about the ICF framework of the World Health Organization?
   (a) The ICF framework only conceives of disability and functioning in terms of impairment of body structures and functions.
   (b) The ICF framework has been designed specifically to address the needs of individuals with neurodegenerative diseases.
   (c) The ICF framework embodies a biopsychosocial approach to disability and functioning.
   (d) Conversational difficulties on account of reduced speech intelligibility are an activity limitation in the ICF framework.
   (e) An inability to perform social roles (e.g. father) is an impairment in the ICF framework.

(2) Prominent categories in the ICF framework are body structures and functions and activities and participation. Under which of these ICF categories are the results of ER's communication assessment recorded?

(3) Reduced initiation appears to contribute to ER's social communication problems. Explain this contribution. How should reduced initiation be classified in the ICF framework?

(4) Which of the following factors currently contribute to difficulties in ER's relationship with his children? Which factors might contribute to difficulties in this relationship in the future?
   (a) cognitive factors
   (b) social factors
   (c) speech factors
   (d) environmental factors
   (e) motivational factors

(5) Which type of communication intervention is ER already familiar with and likely to have a positive response to in his own case?

Communication goal setting

The ICF framework and its findings were discussed with ER and his mother. On the basis of this discussion, three communication intervention goals were established. These goals were (1) to develop a legacy life story book and DVD which would enable ER to communicate his love for his children and fulfil the role of father when he is no longer able to communicate or when he passes away; (2) to facilitate less effortful conversations between ER and his mother by providing a mobile phone which could be used in quieter areas, thus increasing ER's intelligibility; and (3) to maintain ER's conversational interaction with other residents by means of nursing staff and speech-language pathologists extending invitations to ER to attend the weekly talking group. These goals focused on the priority areas of communication and interactions/relationships for ER. They are also consistent with the desire of individuals with HD and their family members for greater social communication participation (Hartelius et al., 2010).

Unit 33.5 Communication goal setting

(1) The development of a legacy item is used to address a participation restriction. What is that restriction?

(2) Which of the three communication goals established for ER is intended to address environmental factors identified during interviews with ER's mother?

(3) Three themes were dominant for the individuals with HD in the study conducted by Hartelius et al. (2010). These themes were the lack of initiative in communication, the concentration that was needed to communicate, and the negative impact on individuals with HD of the speed of other people's communication. What factor is common to these themes?

(4) Which of the three communication goals established for ER is intended to address the impact of his apathy and reduced initiation on communication?

(5) One of the factors that influenced communication negatively for family members and carers in the study by Hartelius et al. was personality changes in individuals with HD. Give *one* example of how these changes compromised ER's communicative abilities.

Section C

Fluency disorders

Case study 34

Boy aged 4 years with developmental stuttering

Introduction

The following exercise is a case study of a boy ('DL') who was studied by Matthews et al. (1997). DL has a moderate to severe stutter. He attended a local clinic for 17 weeks along with his parents. The case study is presented in five sections: primer on developmental stuttering; client history; speech and language evaluation; parent–child interaction therapy; and speech outcome.

Primer on developmental stuttering

Developmental stuttering is by far the most extensively studied disorder of fluency. Notwithstanding this fact, it continues to pose a considerable assessment and treatment challenge for fluency professionals. Wingate (2002: 9) defines stuttering as a 'unique anomaly in the flow of speech characterised by iterative and/or perseverative speech elements involving word/syllable-initial position'. Although the general population prevalence of developmental stuttering is typically taken to be 1%, Yairi and Ambrose (2013) have recently argued in a review of the epidemiology of the disorder that a lifespan prevalence of 0.72% appears to be a reasonable estimate. There is evidence that the prevalence of stuttering is higher in certain special populations such as individuals with intellectual disability or genetic and chromosomal syndromes. Bloodstein and Bernstein Ratner (2008) reported that estimates of the prevalence of stuttering among individuals with Down's syndrome range from 21% to 48%. The lifespan incidence of stuttering has standardly been reported at approximately 5%. (Yairi and Ambrose (2013) have described this as a conservative figure, which should be revised upwards to approximately 8%.) There is a significant gender bias in adults who stutter, with a male:female ratio of 4:1 or larger standardly reported. However, Yairi and Ambrose (2013) reported that considerably smaller ratios are found in very young children who are near stuttering onset.

Although there is general agreement that stuttering has its onset in early childhood, there has been considerable variation between studies on the mean or median age at onset. Yairi and Ambrose (2013) state that 95% of the risk for stuttering onset is over by age 4. There is a high level of natural recovery from stuttering, that is, recovery in the absence of intervention. Using data from the Twins Early Development Study, Dworzynski et al. (2007) examined parental reports regarding stuttering at 2, 3, 4 and 7 years. Based on the number of children who were still reported to be stuttering at 7 years, these investigators calculated a 69% recovery rate for children with stuttering onset at 2 years, a 79% recovery rate for children with stuttering onset at 3 years, and a 53% recovery rate for children with stuttering onset at 4 years. Children who stutter can present with a range of other disorders including speech and language problems. In a survey-based study of 1,184 speech-language pathologists serving 2,628 children who stutter, Blood et al. (2003) reported the presence of articulation disorders in 33.5%, phonology disorders in 12.7%, learning disabilities in 15.2%, literacy disorders in 8.2% and attention deficit disorders in 5.9%.

Stuttering has adverse psychosocial implications for the person who stutters and his or her family. McAllister et al. (2013) examined the impact of parent-reported adolescent stuttering on the psychological distress of people who stutter at age 42 years. Members of a British birth cohort who were reported to stutter (217 subjects) had higher psychological distress scores than controls in the study. However, they were not found to be at an increased risk of serious mental health difficulties. Erickson and Block (2013) reported that adolescents who stutter have below average self-perceived communication competence, heightened communication apprehension and are teased and bullied more often than their fluent peers. The families of these adolescents experienced high levels of emotional strain and family conflict. There is also evidence that certain occupational roles are deemed to be unsuitable for people who stutter. Gabel et al. (2004) asked 385 university students to report their perceptions of appropriate career choices for people who stutter. These respondents considered 20 careers, including speech-language pathologist, audiologist and occupational therapist, to be unsuitable for people who stutter. The extent to which this vocational stereotyping actually influences the careers pursued by people who stutter remains unclear.

Unit 34.1 Primer on developmental stuttering

(1) Which of the following are *true* statements about the speech features of developmental stuttering?
   (a) Iterations and perseverations in stuttering are distinct from normal non-fluencies.
   (b) Iterations are most commonly found in word-final position.
   (c) Iterations typically involve full syllables.
   (d) Perseverations are the prolongation of phonemes beyond their normal duration.
   (e) Iterations and perseverations decrease in frequency when the person who stutters is made aware of speech errors.

(2) The significant gender bias in adults who stutter is less evident in very young children who are near stuttering onset. What does this tell us about the process of natural recovery?

(3) In their study of the persistence of and early recovery from stuttering, Dworzynski et al. (2007) found that concordance rates were consistently higher for monozygotic than for dizygotic twin pairs. What does this finding tell us about the aetiology of stuttering?

(4) Why do speech-language pathologists have to be attentive to comorbid conditions in stuttering?

(5) Clinicians must increasingly consider the psychosocial implications of communication disorders in their clients. Which of the following statements characterise those implications in regard to stuttering?
   (a) Psychosocial implications extend well into adulthood.
   (b) Psychosocial implications must be addressed in the management of the person who stutters.

(c) Psychosocial implications are usually time-limited in nature.

(d) Psychosocial implications are limited to the person who stutters.

(e) Psychosocial implications can have an adverse impact on the occupational domain.

Client history

DL was aged 4;2 years at the outset of the study. He was from a two-parent family and had one younger sister who was aged 1;7 years. An interview with DL's parents revealed a significant family history of stuttering. DL's father, paternal grandfather and uncle had all stuttered. DL's mother was also dysfluent as a child. The parental interview revealed a number of other noteworthy points. The information from this interview suggested that DL had immature attention and delayed speech motor processes. The interview also identified DL's birth history as a possible significant physiological factor. The family had recently undertaken a stressful move. The interview revealed that there were difficulties in managing DL's behaviour. The parents reported considerable anxiety about DL's dysfluency. DL was also described as having a sensitive and anxious nature.

Unit 34.2 Client history

(1) The onset of DL's stuttering was prior to 4 years of age. Given the information about onset in pp. 241–2, is DL's onset typical of stuttering?

(2) Which feature of DL's history indicates that he has an increased genetic risk of stuttering?

(3) The history suggests that DL is also at risk of comorbid disorders. Name *two* such disorders.

(4) Are there any environmental factors that may be contributing to DL's stutter?

(5) DL was reported to have a sensitive, anxious nature. The relationship between anxiety and stuttering is complex. Which of the following are *true* statements about anxiety in stuttering?

(a) There is a high rate of social anxiety disorder among people who stutter.

(b) Social anxiety is a psychological concomitant of stuttering.

(c) Social anxiety is typically only found in adolescents who stutter.

(d) Social anxiety causes stuttering.

(e) Collaboration between speech-language pathologists and psychologists is required in order to assess and treat social anxiety in people who stutter.

Speech and language evaluation

DL's speech and language skills were assessed. In terms of DL's dysfluencies, these were characterised by whole- and part-word repetitions, prolongations and blocking of sounds on 8.4% of words. A number of non-verbal behaviours, including hand-flapping, facial grimacing and avoidance of eye contact, were concomitant with these dysfluencies. Both content words and function words were affected. Single words could display several dysfluencies. An example of DL's spoken output is 'Its its ha-ha-haaa:vn't got got a window'.

When questioned about his speech, DL did not display any concern. However, DL's parents reported that he was frustrated about his speech at home. Combined with his concomitant behaviours, this suggested that DL was aware of his dysfluency. DL's rate of speech was 3.8 syllables per second. The Clinical Evaluation of Language Fundamentals: Pre-school (CELF-P; Wiig et al., 1992) was used to assess DL's receptive and expressive language skills. The CELF-P revealed a considerable language delay, with DL's overall age equivalent 12 months below his chronological age.

An analysis was also undertaken of parent–child interaction. Video-recordings were made of DL in play with each of his parents separately. This analysis revealed a number of behaviours which were subsequently addressed in therapy. DL's mother displayed a fast speech rate and rapid turn-taking. She often interrupted DL's attempts to communicate and failed to wait for his responses. She made excessive use of questions to initiate conversation. Eye contact with DL was rarely achieved. DL's father also used a rapid rate of speech. However, this was reduced somewhat by his dysfluency. He was highly directive in his play sessions with DL. He tended to dominate verbally the interaction through his use of many questions, imperatives and by taking lengthy turns. He used extended explanations which were too complex in terms of their syntax and semantics for DL's delayed language skills.

Unit 34.3 Speech and language evaluation

(1) Conture (1997) argues that if a child exhibits three or more within-word (stuttered) speech dysfluencies per 100 words of conversational speech, then he or she is at risk of continuing to stutter. Based on this figure, is DL at risk of continuing to stutter? Provide evidence to support your answer. The percentage of stuttered words is only one measure of stuttering frequency. What other measure do clinicians use to assess stuttering severity?

(2) How would you characterise the dysfluencies in the utterance 'Its its ha-ha-haaa:vn't got got a window'?

(3) Respond with *true* or *false* to each of the following statements:
   (a) DL exhibits secondary behaviours or accessory features.
   (b) DL does not extend sounds beyond their normal duration.
   (c) DL's language skills do not place him at risk of stuttering.
   (d) DL exhibits dysfluencies on grammatical words.
   (e) DL's speech rate is within the normal range for his age.

(4) Describe *three* verbal behaviours which suggest that DL's parents are not particularly attuned to his language difficulties.

(5) Aside from language, the style of interaction adopted by the parents in this case is likely to be challenging for certain other cognitive skills in DL. Name *two* such skills. Indicate the parental behaviours which are likely to challenge these skills.

Parent–child interaction therapy

The parent–child interaction therapy proposed by Rustin et al. (1996) was undertaken. For 17 weeks, DL attended a local clinic along with his parents. For the first six weeks, DL's parents were video-recorded as they took it in turns to play with him for 20 minutes. During recordings, the other parent and clinician remained in the room. The observed parent was told to use whatever toys in the room that he or she wanted to use. However, no advice was given on the way in which the toys should be used or on any other aspect of the session. Transcriptions of DL's utterances from the recordings were used to calculate the number of dysfluencies produced per 100 words. This figure was calculated both for the mother-led and father-led play sessions, resulting in two measures of dysfluency every week. To ensure that this measure was reliable, a speech and language therapist specialised in dysfluency viewed recordings from three of the weekly sessions. There was 95% agreement between the judges.

Therapy was delivered during the next six weeks. First, video-recordings were made of the parents playing with DL. These were then viewed by the parents and clinician. DL's parents were encouraged to identify one positive aspect of their interaction with him, and one negative aspect which they would like to change. If these identifications were difficult for the parents, the clinician guided them to parts of the recordings which they were encouraged to describe in detail. The parents were asked to consider how changes to their behaviour might be helpful to DL. They also had the opportunity to put their ideas into practice during the session. The target behaviours that were identified in the session became the focus of a home activity. This activity was a five-minute playtime which each parent agreed to undertake five days a week. DL had the choice of play during this activity. The parents recorded his choice as well as their success in implementing their target behaviours. In subsequent sessions with the clinician the parents had the opportunity to reflect on their progress during these playtimes with DL.

DL's parents were offered specific advice during this six-week period. Both parents were advised to reduce their use of questions and to replace them with comments. Additionally, DL's mother was encouraged to have eye contact with him during communication. In order to gain DL's attention, techniques such as using animation, touch and calling his name were encouraged. DL's father was advised to be less directive when playing with him, and to allow DL to lead activities, to make his own decisions and to solve his own problems. The father's use of imperatives was discouraged, and he was advised to comment on DL's play. He was also encouraged to reduce his speech rate and to use vocabulary that was appropriate for DL's language skills. In the final five-week period, measures of DL's dysfluency continued to be made. The parents also worked on their special playtimes with DL at home, and reflected on their progress each week. However, there was no new information or advice given to the parents at this stage.

Unit 34.4 Parent–child interaction therapy

(1) During the first six weeks of contact with DL and his parents, the clinician did not undertake direct therapy. What purpose within the overall intervention do you think this period served?

(2) Why do you think video-recordings were used when audio-recordings could have provided the authors of the study with the transcribed utterances that were used to measure dysfluencies?

(3) Which of the following statements best characterises parent–child interaction (PCI) therapy?
   (a) PCI therapy aims to desensitise the child to stuttered speech.

(b) PCI therapy aims to teach the child fluency-modification techniques such as smooth speech.

(c) PCI therapy aims to increase the child's fluency by modifying how parents communicate with their child.

(d) PCI therapy aims to change parental attitudes towards stuttering.

(e) PCI therapy aims to teach the child techniques for how to stutter more easily.

(4) The parents in this case received specific advice on how to modify their communication with DL. Explain how and why DL's parents were encouraged to modify their use of speech acts during communication with him.

(5) During the last five weeks of contact with DL and his parents, the clinician offered no new information or advice. What purpose within the overall intervention do you think this period served?

Speech outcome

The percentage of dysfluencies per 100 words was collected every week for both parents. These measurements are collated and tabulated below. The collated measurements also display the mean rate of dysfluency for each week of the investigation. The tabulated results are reproduced from Matthews et al. (1997: 352).

Week	Rate of dysfluency with father	Rate of dysfluency with mother	Mean rate of dysfluency
Phase A			
1	8.7	10.6	9.65
2	5.9	7.28	6.59
3	7.74	9.86	8.8
4	8.82	9.78	9.03
5	13.3	7.01	10.16
6	11.69	7.34	9.52
Phase B			
7	9.95	8.39	9.17
8	2.5	10.49	6.5
9	1.94	3.12	2.53
10	5.47	4.36	4.92
11	3.6	5.7	4.65
12	5.84	3.3	4.57
Phase C			
13	2.07	3.43	2.75
14	1.21	3.55	2.38
15	7.18	7.58	7.28
16	8.01	5.5	6.76
17	4.04	9.35	6.7

Statistical analysis of the baseline period (Phase A) revealed a non-significant result, suggesting that there was no observable trend during this time. However, analysis of Phases A and B produced a significant result. This supported the claim that there was a significant decrease in the number of dysfluencies during the treatment phase. During Phase C, there was an increase in the number of dysfluencies produced by DL. However, statistical analysis revealed that this was not a significant increase. There was no significant difference in the number of dysfluencies used by DL during mother-led and father-led sessions. Although there was no formal recording of DL's language skills during the three phases of the study, he was noted by the end of the study to be using more utterances and longer utterances.

Unit 34.5 Speech outcome

(1) Is there any evidence from this study that DL's dysfluency was improving spontaneously, i.e. without direct intervention? Provide support for your answer.

(2) There is considerable fluctuation in DL's dysfluency during Phase A of the study. How might this inconsistency pose a problem for an intervention that uses as its baseline a single measure of dysfluency that is based on a discrete point in time?

(3) Although parent–child interaction therapy is not a language intervention *per se*, is there any evidence that DL's language skills improved following this therapy?

(4) For young, dysfluent children, clinicians have found it helpful to conceive of intervention in terms of balancing the demands on and the capacities of the child. Explain how this way of conceiving of intervention can be applied to the case of DL.

(5) The authors of the study attributed the (non-significant) increase in dysfluency in Phase C to a number of 'distracting and uncontrollable variables' which may have created emotional anxieties for DL. These variables included a family holiday and the parents' marriage. What linguistic variable may have contributed to the increase in DL's dysfluency towards the end of the study?

Case study 35

Man aged 29 years with acquired stuttering

The following exercise is a case study of a 29-year-old man ('Mr A') who was studied by Leder (1996). Mr A was initially diagnosed with acquired stuttering related to a conversion reaction. However, this diagnosis was subsequently revised to acquired neurogenic stuttering in the presence of a Parkinsonian-like syndrome. The case study is presented in five sections: primer on acquired stuttering; client history and presentation; speech pathology evaluation; psychiatric and neurological evaluation; and fluency therapy.

Primer on acquired stuttering

The onset of dysfluency in adulthood is known as acquired stuttering. There are two forms of acquired stuttering in adults. In acquired *psychogenic* stuttering, the onset of dysfluency is associated with a traumatic event, psychological distress, or the presence of a psychiatric disorder. Raphael and Schoenfeld (2006) described the case of a 44-year-old woman with bipolar affective disorder and a history of childhood sexual abuse who presented with severe stuttering. A neurological evaluation of this woman was negative. In acquired *neurogenic* stuttering, the onset of dysfluency is caused by neurological injuries and disorders. Strokes or cerebrovascular accidents are the single biggest cause of neurogenic stuttering. Theys et al. (2011) reported neurogenic stuttering in 17 (5.3%) of 319 subjects who sustained a stroke. Stuttering persisted for more than six months in at least 2.5% of these subjects. Individuals with comorbid aphasia displayed a significantly higher frequency of stuttering compared to those without aphasia. Traumatic brain injury, progressive supranuclear palsy (a form of parkinsonism) and multiple sclerosis are less common causes of neurogenic stuttering (Kluin et al., 1993; Mower and Younts, 2001). Some cases of acquired stuttering have both neurological and psychological factors in their aetiology. Mattingly (2015) described the case of a service member returning from war with the comorbid diagnoses of post-traumatic stress disorder and a mild traumatic brain injury who experienced the onset of stuttering.

The speech features of acquired stuttering differ in significant ways from those of developmental stuttering. Helm-Estabrooks (1999: 260) states six features which, she claims, help to distinguish neurogenic stuttering from developmental stuttering in adults: (1) dysfluencies occur on grammatical words nearly as frequently as on substantive words; (2) the speaker may be annoyed but does not appear anxious; (3) repetitions, prolongations and blocks do not occur only on initial syllables of words and utterances; (4) secondary symptoms such as facial grimacing, eye blinking, or fist clenching are not associated with moments of dysfluency; (5) there is no adaptation effect whereby there are fewer and fewer dysfluencies on repeated readings of a passage; (6) stuttering occurs relatively consistently across various types of speech tasks. However, the results of some studies indicate that it may not always be possible to perceptually distinguish neurogenic from developmental stuttering, as these criteria would appear to suggest. Van Borsel and Taillieu (2001) presented a panel of professionals with random speech samples from four developmental and four neurogenic stutterers. The results indicated that based on verbal output alone, it is often difficult to distinguish neurogenic from developmental stuttering.

Unit 35.1 Primer on acquired stuttering

(1) The epidemiology of acquired stuttering is not as well investigated as the epidemiology of developmental stuttering. Name *one* feature of the epidemiology of developmental stuttering which does not appear to hold true of acquired stuttering.

(2) Which of the following is *not* a cause of acquired neurogenic stuttering?
   (a) cerebral infection
   (b) bipolar disorder
   (c) closed head injury
   (d) conversion reaction
   (e) multiple sclerosis

(3) Which of the following scenarios describes acquired stuttering of mixed aetiology?
   (a) A 40-year-old man exhibits stuttering following a head injury sustained in a road traffic accident.
   (b) A 30-year-old woman, who first received fluency therapy in childhood, participates in an intervention for adults who stutter.
   (c) A 55-year-old woman, who had a recent family crisis, experiences sudden onset of dysfluency.
   (d) A 40-year-old man, who has been under medical supervision for psychological distress following a head trauma sustained in a violent assault, is referred to speech-language pathology for fluency evaluation.
   (e) A 77-year-old man exhibits stuttering following an intracerebral haemorrhage.

(4) The following speech is produced by a 36-year-old man with multiple sclerosis who was studied by Mower and Younts (2001). What *two* speech features characterise this extract?

   'Well, we-we-we-we-we in-in-in port mo-most of time and-and when-when-when I got-got married, got-got-got-got-got-got an apar-par-partment.'

(5) Fill in the blank spaces in the following statement:

   Adults with acquired neurogenic stuttering fail to achieve fluency under conditions which are known to induce fluency in individuals with _____ stuttering. Two such conditions are _____ speaking and delayed _____ feedback.

Client history and presentation

Mr A is a 29-year-old white male who is a graphic designer at a university. He was referred by his primary care physician to speech pathology following the sudden onset of dysfluent speech on 21 November 1993. Mr A has no prior history of dysfluency. His only medical complaint is headaches for which he takes aspirin. He reports that for some months he has been under considerable stress at work as he prepares a museum catalogue. On the day when Mr A first experienced dysfluency, he could not say the word 'paper'. The following day Mr A's dysfluency increased during the morning and by early afternoon he was severely dysfluent. Although his vocal pitch was normal at the time, it did increase over the next three to four days. Mr A's pitch returned to normal over the next month but his severe dysfluency persisted. Writing was also disrupted. Although lower case printing and cursive writing were unimpaired, Mr A was unable to write in capital letters. Capital letters were used extensively in Mr A's work as a graphic designer. His problem with writing persisted for seven days, and then resolved spontaneously. Also in November 1993, Mr A underwent a neurological evaluation. EEG, MRI without gadolinium, CT scans and lumbar puncture were all normal. With one exception, there was no history of neurological disease in Mr A's family. Mr A's father, who was 58 years old, had suffered complex partial seizures since his early twenties.

Unit 35.2 Client history and presentation

(1) On the basis of this history and presentation, what type of acquired stuttering do you think Mr A has? Provide evidence to support your answer.

(2) On the basis of this history and presentation, which of the following might be considered a cause of Mr A's dysfluency?
   (a) cerebrovascular accident
   (b) relapse in developmental stuttering
   (c) conversion reaction
   (d) bipolar disorder
   (e) traumatic brain injury

(3) Alongside the onset of dysfluency, Mr A displayed *two* communicative features which are seldom reported in acquired stuttering. What are these features?

(4) Mr A was able to form lower case letters but was unable to write upper case or capital letters. Is this impairment suggestive of writing difficulties in a neurodegenerative disorder?

(5) Which of Mr A's neurological examinations excluded epileptic seizures as a cause of dysfluency?

Speech pathology evaluation

Mr A underwent a speech pathology evaluation on 9 December 1993. This was 19 days after the onset of stuttering. He displayed frequent syllable and word repetitions while blocks on syllables and words were infrequent. Multiple repetitions and/or blocks were present on every syllable and word. For example, during conversational speech and oral reading 20 or more repetitions per syllable were routinely noted. Mr A's stuttering pattern was unaltered during choral reading. Stuttering was also present when words were mouthed without voicing during conversational speech and reading. Mr A's vocal pitch had increased following what appeared to be tension in the shoulder and neck areas. He did not make use of starters or secondary characteristics. He exhibited no avoidances or word or situational fears (e.g. telephone use). In this early, post-onset period there were no tremors or lingual fasciculations. Tremors and fasciculations appeared in March 1994, and necessitated a referral for a further neurological evaluation. Mr A's cognitive functions and expressive and receptive language were intact. Mr A was both distressed about his stuttering and motivated to correct it.

Unit 35.3 Speech pathology evaluation

(1) Describe *two* ways in which the repetitions exhibited by Mr A differ from the iterations of developmental stuttering.

(2) Name *one* speech feature which is present in developmental stuttering but which is absent in Mr A's case.

(3) Mr A's stuttering behaviour differs in other significant respects from developmental stuttering. State *three* such respects.

(4) In the early, post-onset period, Mr A did not display lingual fasciculations, although he later went on to develop them. What are lingual fasciculations? What type of neurological damage causes fasciculations?

(5) Individuals with acquired neurogenic stuttering can sometimes exhibit comorbid aphasia. Is this true of Mr A's case?

Psychiatric and neurological evaluation

Based on an initial diagnosis of a conversion reaction, Mr A started receiving psychiatric treatment in December 1993. He was prescribed 200 mg doxepin hydrochloride at night for depression and sleep. A biweekly telephone call between the psychiatrist and speech-language pathologist was used to discuss the behavioural and psychiatric strategies that were used to address Mr A's dysfluency. However, by March 1994 there had been no improvement in dysfluency and the psychiatrist concluded that Mr A's stuttering had an organic origin.

On 23 August 1994, a second neurological evaluation of Mr A was performed. Normal proportions of dopamine were revealed by SPECT scanning. With the exception of markedly slow tongue movements Mr A's cranial nerve examination was also normal. A sensory examination was normal. During a cerebellar examination, Mr A was able to perform normal finger to nose movements in procession. However, movements were slow. A tremor, which did not increase in amplitude, persisted during these movements. There was a tremor at rest in both arms (right more than left), and a slight tremor at rest in the right leg. Mr A could stand but was unable to walk on either his heels or toes. Pushing on his chest and back produced mild instability with no reflexive compensatory movements of his arms. Mr A's face was without expression. Movements were slow to begin and to complete. He was unable to perform rapid alternating movements. Mr A was prescribed carbidopa-levodopa. An initial dose of four times a day (August 1994) was gradually reduced to once a day (May 1995) as improvements occurred in speech and motor skills. Stuttering increased in severity as the dose of drug was decreased.

Unit 35.4 Psychiatric and neurological evaluation

(1) After a period of psychiatric intervention it became clear that Mr A's dysfluency was not related to a conversion reaction. What were the *two* main features of this intervention? Did either of these features result in an improvement in speech?

(2) There are *four* cardinal signs of Parkinson's disease. What are these signs? Does Mr A exhibit each sign?

(3) In relation to the results of SPECT scanning, the author of the study concludes that there is either no biochemical basis for Mr A's symptoms or that his symptoms are the result of receptor dysfunction. Explain this conclusion.

(4) Mr A exhibited the mask-like facial expression that is characteristic of clients with Parkinson's disease. Give a description of this expression.

(5) Mr A's speech and motor symptoms displayed a good response to carbidopa-levodopa. Along with neurological findings, what does this suggest about the aetiology of Mr A's stuttering?

   (a) A psychogenic aetiology is still plausible as a cause of Mr A's stuttering.
   (b) A relapse in developmental stuttering appears to be the most likely cause of Mr A's stuttering.
   (c) The aetiology of Mr A's stuttering is likely to be neurogenic in nature.
   (d) Mr A's stuttering has no known cause and is idiopathic in nature.
   (e) Mr A's stuttering is one symptom of a wider parkinsonian syndrome.

Fluency therapy

Fluency therapy took place three times a week for a three-month period. Among the therapy techniques used were the use of soft contacts in stop and fricative phonemes and relaxation of the shoulders and neck area. Also, Mr A was encouraged to adopt a continuous breath flow as a means of promoting an open glottis. This was followed by producing a whisper and then progressing to voicing by humming vowels and nasal continuants /m, n/. Mr A was successful in using these techniques in the initial session in order to control his stuttering and increase his fluency. There followed a discussion with Mr A which focused on responsibility for and control of his stuttering. Through his use of breath flow, soft contacts and negative practice, Mr A was able to exhibit control of fluent and stuttered speech production. The following fluency-shaping goals were pursued: (1) breath flow, soft contacts and relaxation were attempted first on rote speech tasks (e.g. counting) then short, overlearned phrases (e.g. How are you?), and finally on conversational speech, while maintaining fluency; (2) the rate of speech was increased while maintaining fluency; (3) the loudness of speech was increased while maintaining fluency; and (4) appropriate vocal pitch was pursued by decreasing tension in the neck and shoulders. Daily telephone contact was used to support maintenance, carry-over and generalisation to conversational speech. With the exception of pitch, which returned to normal, Mr A did not continue to show improvement.

Unit 35.5 Fluency therapy

(1) Which of the following techniques and approaches were used in fluency therapy with Mr A?
  (a) cognitive behavioural therapy
  (b) personal construct therapy
  (c) relaxation techniques
  (d) fluency-modification techniques
  (e) avoidance reduction therapy

(2) Which of the techniques shown in question (1) was used to address Mr A's vocal pitch anomalies? These anomalies improved while other aspects of Mr A's stuttered speech did not. Why do you think this was the case?

(3) One of the fluency-shaping techniques employed with Mr A was the use of soft contacts. Describe what is involved in this technique.

(4) The techniques used in fluency therapy target different aspects of speech production. Which technique targets the respiratory–phonatory mechanism?

(5) Name *one* aspect of prosody which is targeted by Mr A's fluency intervention.

Case study 36

Boy with developmental cluttering

Introduction

The following exercise is a case study of a boy ('Michael') who was studied by Daly and Burnett (1996). Michael was first evaluated at 9;7 years of age. He subsequently received a course of therapy and was re-evaluated when he was 11;8 years of age. The case study is presented in five sections: primer on cluttering; client history; pre-intervention speech-language evaluation; cluttering therapy; and post-intervention speech-language evaluation.

Primer on cluttering

Although there is no consensus on a definition of cluttering, a widely used definition, and one that is accepted by the International Cluttering Association, states that:

cluttering is a fluency disorder characterized by a rate that is perceived to be abnormally rapid, irregular, or both for the speaker (although measured syllable rates may not exceed normal limits). These rate abnormalities further are manifest in one or more of the following symptoms: (a) an excessive number of disfluencies, the majority of which are not typical of people who stutter; (b) the frequent placement of pauses and use of prosodic patterns that do not conform to syntactic and semantic constraints; and (c) inappropriate (usually excessive) degrees of coarticulation among sounds, especially in multisyllabic words. (St. Louis et al., 2007: 299–300)

The key elements of this definition are consistent with the features of cluttering that are reported in clinical studies. In a survey of 29 clutterers in 12 articles, St Louis (1996) identified 53 symptoms that were used by the authors of these articles to characterise cluttering. The three most commonly reported symptoms were excessive dysfluencies, rate of speech too fast and rate of speech too irregular.

The epidemiology of cluttering is still a vastly under-investigated aspect of this fluency disorder. This is confirmed by the fact that there has been no study of the prevalence and incidence of cluttering in the general population since Becker and Grundmann (1970) reported the incidence of cluttering to be 1.5% in 7- and 8-year-olds in a German school. Cluttering is more common in certain special populations than in the general population. Coppens-Hofman et al. (2013) examined dysfluencies in the spontaneous speech of 28 adults with mild and moderate intellectual disabilities. Of the 22 (75%) of subjects who showed clinically significant dysfluencies, 21% were classified as cluttering, 29% as cluttering-stuttering and 25% as clear cluttering at normal articulatory rate. St. Louis et al. (2010) reported a male:female sex ratio for cluttering of 4.5:1. Genetic and neurological factors appear to be integral to the aetiology of cluttering. The presence of cluttering in children with genetic and chromosomal syndromes, including Down's syndrome and fragile X syndrome, suggests that genetic factors may play a role in developmental cluttering (Hanson et al., 1986; Van Borsel and Vandermeulen, 2008). Acquired cluttering has been reported in adults with neurodegenerative disorders including dementia and idiopathic parkinsonism, and in individuals who sustain cerebrovascular accidents (Hashimoto et al., 1999; Lebrun, 1996; Thacker and De Nil, 1996).

Unit 36.1 Primer on cluttering

(1) Which of the following are *true* statements about cluttering?
   (a) Cluttering is like stuttering in that it is more prevalent in males.
   (b) Cluttering is a specific deficit in speech prosody.
   (c) People who clutter often have intellectual disabilities.
   (d) Rate anomalies are a consistent feature of cluttering.
   (e) Cluttering is often found alongside, and can be misdiagnosed as, stuttering.

(2) The neural correlates of cluttering were investigated by Ward et al. (2015). These investigators found that the caudate nucleus and putamen were overactive in adults who clutter. Which of the following neuroanatomical structures does this study suggest is compromised in cluttering?
   (a) substantia nigra
   (b) anterior insula
   (c) basal ganglia
   (d) brainstem
   (e) primary motor cortex

(3) The epidemiology of cluttering has only rarely been investigated. Why do you think this is the case?

(4) A person who clutters says [wʌfɪl] for 'wonderful'. What term is used to describe this speech behaviour?

(5) *True* or *false:* Cluttering is often associated with poor reading skills.

Client history

Michael was first seen for evaluation in May 1993 when he was 9 years 7 months old. He was a third grade student. At school, he received the support of a learning disability teacher for a reading disorder. He also received treatment from the school speech-language pathologist. The focus of earlier SLP intervention was speech rate, 'clearness' and intelligibility of articulation. Michael was seen by the speech-language pathologist during the 1993/94 and 1994/95 school years. Additionally, he also received SLP intervention in a hospital speech programme in the spring and summer of 1994. This intervention consisted of 16 treatment sessions.

Parental report indicated that Michael was just within normal limits for motor developmental milestones. However, speech and language development was significantly delayed. The mother of Michael stated that baby talk had persisted, and that family members had increasingly experienced difficulty in understanding him. According to Michael's mother, his speech intelligibility problems were related to misarticulations, an unusually fast speech rate and the presence of repetitions, which started between 2.5 and 3 years of age. A family history of fast talking and stuttering was reported by the mother. Although Michael had received intervention for speech articulation at school for several years, his mother reported that there had only been minimal improvement.

Unit 36.2 Client history

(1) Michael was just within normal limits for motor developmental milestones. State when normally developing children should attain *three* motor milestones.

(2) Does Michael have other communication problems in addition to cluttering? If so, are these problems typical of people who clutter?

(3) What aspect of Michael's history indicates that he may have been at an elevated genetic risk of having a communication disorder?

(4) What key speech feature of cluttering is evident from parental report?

(5) Intervention for speech articulation at school had only been minimally effective. Why do you think this is the case?

Pre-intervention speech-language evaluation

The initial evaluation of Michael's speech and language skills was performed at 9 years 7 months. The report of the school psychologist indicated that Michael's IQ was within the high-to-average range. Scores on arithmetic were above average, and Michael was placed in a gifted programme for mathematics and science. Although Michael's verbal skills fell in the high-to-average range, his reading ability was below average. Also, the school psychologist remarked of Michael's conversational speech that it displayed 'excessive speed, slurred or omitted syllables and sounds, and had a low volume, especially at the ends of sentences'.

The initial evaluation revealed some noteworthy speech and language problems. The organisation and formulation of language, topic maintenance, the rate and tempo of speech, prosody and intelligibility were all judged to be problematic. Additionally, Michael appeared to be largely unaware of his difficulties and his listener's difficulty in understanding him. However, there was an improvement in his speech when a recorder was introduced. Auditory memory abilities and oral motor coordination skills were below those of Michael's peers. This profile of impairments was suggestive of cluttering and so a checklist of cluttering behaviours was performed. The overall score on the checklist confirmed the clinical impression of cluttering. The nine areas which were most characteristic of Michael's speech were rapid rate, slurred articulation, speech better under pressure, reading disorder, ability to think is faster than the ability to talk or write, above average mathematical and abstract reasoning abilities, poor rhythm, timing or musical ability, other family members with the problem and lack of self-awareness.

Unit 36.3 Pre-intervention speech-language evaluation

(1) The school psychologist reported that Michael's conversational speech exhibited slurred or omitted syllables and sounds. What speech feature of cluttering does this description capture?

(2) Michael undertook diadochokinetic speech tasks as part of his evaluation. What skills are assessed by means of these tasks?

(3) The checklist revealed that Michael's speech was better under pressure, for example, during short periods of heightened attention. What observation during the initial evaluation confirms this finding?

(4) Many individuals who clutter only seek professional help for their speech problems when they are encouraged to do so by colleagues, friends and family members. Which checklist finding might explain this?

(5) People who clutter have impaired pragmatic language skills (Teigland, 1996). Which feature of the initial evaluation suggests that Michael has some impairment in the area of pragmatics?

Cluttering therapy

The findings from the checklist were used to plan Michael's therapy. It was decided that the focus of therapy should be on oral motor coordination, speech rate, language abilities, awareness of deficits and reading difficulties. Language abilities included the formulation of stories, topic maintenance and sequencing of events. These areas were treated by school and hospital speech-language pathologists (SLP). The school SLP saw Michael twice a week. To address Michael's oral motor coordination difficulties, the Oral Motor Assessment and Treatment programme (Riley and Riley, 1985) was used. The school SLP reported that although Michael had initially found the production of three-syllable sets very difficult, all sets were produced with accuracy and an even flow by the end of the semester. Rate tapes were produced in order to facilitate reduction of speech rate and improve awareness and intelligibility. The school SLP noted significant improvements during the 1994/95 school year in rate and self-monitoring during conversational speech. The hospital SLP, who had diagnosed cluttering with central auditory processing disorder, focused on the following areas during treatment: improving concentration and memory; increasing specificity of language; language skills (thought organisation, narrative production and topic maintenance), and improving self-monitoring. Substantial improvements in all areas were reported.

Unit 36.4 Cluttering therapy

(1) Cluttering has both motoric and linguistic components. Explain how these components are reflected in the intervention that Michael received.

(2) Aside from motoric and linguistic components, it is clear that cluttering also has significant cognitive components. Describe *three* ways in which these cognitive components are reflected in therapy.

(3) Michael was treated by a school and a hospital speech-language pathologist. However, the emphases of these interventions were quite different. How would you characterise the differing emphases of these interventions?

(4) The hospital speech-language pathologist diagnosed Michael as having cluttering with central auditory processing disorder. What is a central auditory processing disorder?

(5) Narrative production or the formulation of stories was an area of focus in Michael's therapy. Name *two* problematic skills in cluttering which can be effectively targeted by narrative production.

Post-intervention speech-language evaluation

More than two years after the initial evaluation, Michael was assessed for a second time. He was 11 years 8 months old at this time. The cluttering checklist was re-administered. Michael's overall score had significantly improved. Areas of improvement were rate, articulation, rhythm and awareness. These areas were all directly targeted in therapy. Michael's mean speaking rate had decreased from 126 words per minute to 116 words per minute. Where Michael had previously achieved 70% accuracy on the articulation of multisyllabic words, he now had 85% accuracy on these words. He undertook self-correction of his errors and had a positive response to minimal cuing. Michael displayed auditory memory for 23 syllables (the 12-year-old mean for auditory memory is 26 syllables). His oral motor skills for single syllables, double syllables and tri-syllables were largely consistent with 12-year norms. The one exception was single syllables, with Michael achieving times between 3.3 to 3.9 seconds (4.0 to 4.5 seconds is the 12-year norm).

Michael's language skills also showed improvement. At the initial evaluation, Michael had deviated from the topic three times in a 60-second sample. However, no topic deviations in a 60-second sample were noted at his re-evaluation. His language was no longer disorganised with multiple revisions and he was able to sequence events. It was observed during the evaluation session that Michael displayed more reserved behaviour and used a generally low volume. Michael's low volume did reduce his intelligibility to a degree. However, volume did not diminish at the end of sentences, as had been noted by the school psychologist. Michael was also observed to keep his hands in front of his mouth. He used very brief responses and only improved his eye contact upon cuing. In association with linguistic revisions and other speech production difficulties, Michael also displayed instances of blinking his eyes in a rapid, repetitive fashion. The authors of the study recommended that these behaviours should continue to be monitored.

Unit 36.5 Post-intervention speech-language evaluation

(1) At Michael's re-evaluation, there was a mixed set of prosodic findings. Identify *one* prosodic aspect which had clearly improved following therapy, and *one* prosodic aspect where improvement was not so evident.

(2) Was there any improvement in Michael's pragmatic language skills as a result of intervention? Provide support for your answer.

(3) Identify *two* cognitive skills which improved or were at least age-appropriate following therapy.

(4) Is there any aspect of Michael's presentation at his re-evaluation which is suggestive of stuttering? Provide support for your answer.

(5) Michael displayed non-verbal behaviours at re-evaluation which were not present at his initial assessment. What are these behaviours? How might the emergence of these behaviours be explained?

Section D

Voice disorders

Case study 37

Man aged 51 years with contact granuloma

Introduction

The following exercise is a case study of a 51-year-old man ('PT') with contact granuloma who was studied by Patel et al. (2012). PT is a college professor and speech-language pathologist who had a history of hoarseness and other vocal symptoms. The case study is presented in five sections: primer on organic dysphonia; client history; voice evaluation; voice therapy; and post-intervention vocal function.

Primer on organic dysphonia

An organic dysphonia is a voice disorder which is caused by disease, illness or injury. An organic voice disorder may be structural in nature. Examples include a range of benign and malignant growths which can degrade laryngeal structures or compromise their function. An organic voice disorder may be related to neurological damage such as when a laryngeal nerve is severed during surgery (e.g. thyroidectomy), leading to vocal fold paralysis and paresis. Alternatively, neurodegenerative diseases (e.g. Parkinson's disease) and events such as cerebrovascular accidents (strokes) can give rise to an organic voice disorder. Other causes of organic dysphonias include laryngeal trauma, endocrine disorders, infectious diseases, gastroesophageal reflux, auto-immune diseases (e.g. rheumatoid arthritis), age-related degeneration and pharmacological agents. Any of these conditions and agents can impair the structure and function of the larynx, resulting in organic voice disorders of varying severity.

Organic dysphonias have a high prevalence in the general population and are a significant economic burden to individuals and society. Bhattacharyya (2014) reported that 17.9 million adults in the US have a voice problem, a figure which yields a population prevalence of 7.6%. Voice problems resulted in 7.4 lost workdays in a 12-month period. Infectious laryngitis and gastroesophageal reflux disease were present in 17.8% and 8.0% of adults with voice disorders, respectively. Stein and Noordzij (2013) reported a yearly incidence of 3.47 cases of chronic laryngitis per 1,000 people in a population of 40,317 people who were seen at an urban academic medical centre from 2009 to 2010. The prevalence of voice disorders is higher in certain occupations and age groups in comparison to the general population. In a national survey of 1,879 teachers in New Zealand, Leão et al. (2015) found the prevalence of self-reported vocal problems on the day of the survey was 13.2%. The prevalence was higher still during the teachers' careers and over the course of the teaching year (33.2% and 24.7%, respectively). In a systematic review of studies, de Araújo Pernambuco et al. (2015) reported the prevalence of vocal disorders in persons aged 60 years or more to range from 4.8% to 29.1%.

A contact granuloma is one type of benign growth that can cause an organic voice disorder. Other terms for this disorder in the literature are laryngeal contact ulcer, vocal fold granuloma, post-intubation granuloma and arytenoid granuloma. A contact granuloma typically occurs on the posterior third of the true vocal fold, usually in the area of the vocal process of the arytenoid cartilage. The ulceration may be unilateral or bilateral and may present a 'cup and saucer' appearance, with a protuberance on one side and a crater or concavity on the other side (Colton et al., 2006: 180). Several factors are associated with the development of contact granulomas including vocal abuse, habitual throat clearing, laryngopharyngeal reflux and intubation. Few studies have examined the prevalence of contact granuloma. The prevalence of intubation granuloma is low, in one study accounting for only 2 of 167 (1.2%) adult patients whose tracheas were intubated during surgery (Jones et al., 1992). Contact granulomas may be treated by surgery, voice therapy and the pharmacological management of laryngopharyngeal reflux. Recurrence rates following surgical excision have been reported to approach 92% (Carroll et al., 2009).

Unit 37.1 Primer on organic dysphonia

(1) The following conditions are all causes of organic voice disorders. For each condition, indicate if the aetiology is an infectious disease, a neurodegenerative disorder, or a laryngeal trauma:
  (a) human papilloma virus
  (b) intubation
  (c) multiple sclerosis
  (d) tuberculosis
  (e) Huntington's disease

(2) The following scenarios describe clients who have organic voice disorders. For each scenario, indicate if the aetiology is an endocrine disorder, an autoimmune disease or a pharmacological agent:
  (a) A 51-year-old woman develops vocal symptoms during the menopause.
  (b) A 65-year-old man, who takes aspirin, reports voice problems to his doctor.
  (c) A 55-year-old woman with Sjögren's syndrome reports poor voice-related quality of life to her speech pathologist.
  (d) A 60-year-old woman with hypothyroidism experiences hoarseness.
  (e) A 30-year-old bodybuilder, who uses anabolic steroids regularly, develops vocal symptoms.

(3) Which of the following are *true* statements about contact granulomas:
  (a) Contact granulomas develop at the middle of the vocal folds.
  (b) Contact granulomas respond to treatment using proton pump inhibitors.
  (c) Contact granulomas are more prevalent in children than in adults.
  (d) Contact granulomas are more prevalent in men than in women.
  (e) Contact granulomas are an age-related laryngeal pathology.

(4) There is a higher prevalence of voice disorders in people aged over 60 years. State *one* organic voice disorder that is associated with advancing years.

(5) There is also a higher prevalence of voice disorders in certain occupational groups. State *three* such groups. What laryngeal pathology is often associated with these groups?

Client history

PT is a 51-year-old college professor and speech-language pathologist. An otolaryngological examination conducted four months before the start of the study revealed a contact granuloma on the left vocal process. PT has a history of laryngopharyngeal reflux. PT reported a number of vocal symptoms including vocal fatigue, hoarseness after teaching a long class and the occasional sensation of a lump in the throat in the morning. PT was also diagnosed with sulcus vocalis along the anterior one-third margin of the right vocal fold. Following diagnosis, PT was prescribed a proton pump inhibitor which he took once daily. He also adhered to anti-reflux dietary and behavioural precautions. However, a monthly stroboscopic examination of the vocal folds revealed that there was little change in the lesion size and voice quality did not improve significantly. Given the heavy professional demands on PT's voice and the persistence of his hoarseness, PT was recommended to receive voice therapy.

Unit 37.2 Client history

(1) PT has a history of laryngopharyngeal reflux (LPR). The prevalence of voice disorders in individuals with LPR is considerably higher than in the general population (Spantideas et al., 2015). Explain how LPR causes laryngeal damage. State *one* laryngeal pathology that has been linked to LPR (do not include contact granuloma in your response).

(2) PT reported a number of vocal symptoms. Which of these symptoms is likely to be related to vocal hyperfunction? Which of these symptoms is related to PT's laryngopharyngeal reflux?

(3) PT was also diagnosed with sulcus vocalis. Which of the following are *true* statements about sulcus vocalis?
  (a) Sulcus vocalis is characterised by a loss of the lamina propria, resulting in a deep, linear furrow along the free edge of the vocal fold.
  (b) Sulcus vocalis is not associated with phonotraumatic behaviour.
  (c) Sulcus vocalis may be treated by a vocal fold augmentation procedure.
  (d) Glottic insufficiency is generally not a feature of sulcus vocalis.
  (e) A thin band of mucosa (mucosal bridge) can run parallel to the vocal fold in sulcus vocalis.

(4) Respond with *true* or *false* to each of the following statements:
  (a) PT exhibits odynophagia.
  (b) Management of PT's reflux does not result in vocal improvements.
  (c) PT exhibits globus pharyngeus.
  (d) PT belongs to an occupational group which is at high risk of voice disorder.
  (e) PT belongs to an age group which is at high risk of presbylarynx.

(5) Which of the following statements best characterises the aetiology of PT's voice disorder?

(a) PT's voice disorder has a psychogenic aetiology.

(b) PT's voice disorder has a neurogenic aetiology.

(c) PT's voice disorder has a hyperfunctional aetiology.

(d) PT's voice disorder has a structural-neurogenic aetiology.

(e) PT's voice disorder has a structural-hyperfunctional aetiology.

Voice evaluation

PT's voice was evaluated pre- and post-therapy using high-speed digital imaging, stroboscopy, acoustic analysis, aerodynamic analysis and perceptual assessments of voice quality.

High-speed digital imaging: A KayPentax high-speed system model 9710 was used to make these recordings. PT was required to sustain phonation of the vowel /i/ at typical pitch and loudness. He also completed a laryngeal diadochokinetic task of repeating /hi/ four times with short breaths between syllables. The following measurements were made pre- and post-therapy: voice onset time; open quotient; maximum amplitude; speed quotient (duration of lateral movement divided by the duration of medial movement); relative peak closing velocity; peak-to-average opening velocity; and peak-to-average closing velocity.

Stroboscopy: A stroboscopic assessment was performed using the KayPentax Digital Stroboscopy system RLS 9100b. Three speech-language pathologists undertook pre- and post-therapy ratings of stroboscopic imaging. These ratings were based on a visual perceptual assessment of glottal closure configuration and phase closure during sustained phonation of the vowel /i/ at comfortable pitch and loudness.

Acoustic analysis: The KayPentax Computerized Speech Laboratory was used to make pre- and post-therapy acoustic measurements of sustained phonation on the vowel /a/. The following measurements were made: maximum phonation time (in seconds); average fundamental frequency (hertz); jitter (%); low fundamental frequency (hertz); high fundamental frequency (hertz); shimmer (decibels); and noise-to-harmonic ratio.

Aerodynamic analysis: Expiratory volumes (millilitre) and mean expiratory airflow (litres per second) were measured using the KayPentax Phonatory Aerodynamic System no. 6600.

Perceptual assessment: The Consensus Auditory–Perceptual Evaluation of Voice (CAPE-V; Kempster et al., 2009) was used by three speech-language pathologists to make a pre- and post-therapy perceptual assessment of PT's voice.

Unit 37.3 Voice evaluation

(1) High-speed digital imaging enables clinicians to perform accurate measurements of spatiotemporal vibratory features for the entire vocal fold image. Which of these measurements corresponds to the following descriptions?

Description 1: Duration of the cycle during which the vocal folds remain open divided by the duration of the entire cycle.

Description 2: Duration from initial vocal fold edge motion after complete abduction to the first vocal fold contact which is followed by steady-state cyclic oscillations.

(2) PT underwent a stroboscopic examination of the vocal folds. Explain how this instrumental assessment is conducted.

(3) Jitter and shimmer were two acoustic measurements recorded during voice evaluation. Which of the following statements captures these measurements?

    (a) Jitter and shimmer describe the cycle-to-cycle stability of fundamental frequency and amplitude, respectively.

    (b) Jitter and shimmer are the difference between the low and high fundamental frequency.

    (c) Jitter and shimmer are the difference between the maximum phonation time and the average fundamental frequency.

    (d) Jitter and shimmer are calculated by adding the noise-to-harmonic ratio to the maximum phonation time.

    (e) Jitter and shimmer describe the cycle-to-cycle stability of amplitude and fundamental frequency, respectively.

(4) Mean expiratory airflow was one of two aerodynamic measurements taken during PT's voice evaluation. How might the presence of a contact granuloma be expected to affect this measurement? How might a successful voice intervention affect this particular measurement?

(5) The CAPE-V was used to perform an auditory perceptual assessment of PT's voice. Which of the following are *true* statements about the CAPE-V?

    (a) The CAPE-V assesses voice across six parameters: overall severity; breathiness; roughness; strain; pitch; and loudness.

    (b) The CAPE-V is not suitable for use with paediatric voice patients.

    (c) The CAPE-V examines vocal performance during the production of sustained vowels, sentences and conversational speech.

    (d) The CAPE-V is not suitable for use with clients who have a neurogenic voice disorder.

    (e) The CAPE-V was developed from a consensus meeting sponsored by the American Speech-Language-Hearing Association.

Voice therapy

Over a period of six weeks, PT undertook vocal function exercises (VFEs) twice daily, once in the morning and once in the evening. The VFE approach (Stemple et al., 2000) is a type of physiological voice therapy which aims to improve: (1) the balance among the subsystems for voice production; (2) laryngeal muscle strength; (3) voice control and stamina; and (4) supraglottic modification of laryngeal tone. The exercises involve four steps: (1) warm-up; (2) stretching – gliding from the lowest note to the highest note; (3) contracting – gliding from the highest note to the lowest note; and (4) adductory power.

The latter is achieved by sustaining five musical notes (C–D–E–F–G) for as long as possible on the vowel "o" while pursing to lips to partially occlude the vocal tract.

Unit 37.4 Voice therapy

(1) Vocal function exercises are a type of physiological voice therapy. What is the emphasis of this type of voice therapy?

(2) Stemple et al. (2000) state that 'when any one or more of the voice subsystems is affected by pathology, the remaining subsystems must adjust to accommodate the change of the affected part' (331). Which of the above aims of VFE attempts to address this accommodation?

(3) Before therapy, PT had an incomplete glottal closure along the entire membranous part of the vocal fold with complete closure of the posterior glottis. How might vocal function exercises be expected to improve this glottal closure pattern?

(4) VFEs are intended to exercise specific muscles used in voice production. One such exercise involves gliding from a low pitch to a high pitch. Which laryngeal muscle is this VFE intended to strengthen?

(5) Increasingly, clinicians must consider the efficacy of the voice interventions that they offer to clients. What evidence is there of the efficacy of vocal function exercises in clients with voice disorders?

Post-intervention vocal function

Post-therapy, PT's performance on all the vocal measurements discussed in unit 37.3 was recorded. These measurements are detailed below.

High-speed digital imaging: Voice onset time was reduced from 140 to 77 milliseconds post-therapy. The mean maximum amplitude of vibration increased from 7.8% to 10%. The open quotient post-therapy was 0.674. Open quotient calculations were not applicable for the pre-therapy recordings. The mean speed quotient was also reduced for the right vocal fold (0.90–0.48) and left vocal fold (0.58–0.53). The mean peak closing velocity, measured in glottal lengths per second, increased for both folds as the vocal folds were moving greater distances over a shorter period of time. There was a decrease in the mean peak-to-average velocity during opening and closing phases following treatment.

Stroboscopy: Pre-therapy, glottis closure had a small anterior glottal gap and a complete posterior closure. Following therapy, there was a small posterior glottal gap and improved closure of the membranous vocal folds.

Acoustic analysis: Following VFEs, there was a 26.7% increase in mean intensity level. The following measures were all within normal limits pre- and post-therapy: average fundamental frequency; jitter; low and high extent of fundamental frequency; and noise-to-harmonic ratio.

Aerodynamic analysis: Following VFEs, PT demonstrated a 4.07% increase in respiratory volume and a 54.16% decrease in mean expiratory airflow.

Perceptual assessment: Before VFEs, PT had a mean overall severity rating on the CAPE-V of 18.33/100mm (a mildly deviant voice quality). Following VFEs, the mean overall severity rating on the CAPE-V was 0/100mm (a normal voice quality).

Unit 37.5 Post-intervention vocal function

(1) Why do you think open quotient calculations were not applicable for the pre-therapy recordings?

(2) Stroboscopic findings revealed a small anterior glottal gap and complete posterior closure before treatment, and a small posterior glottal gap and improved closure of the folds following therapy. Which of the following images[1] corresponds to the pre-therapy description and which corresponds to the post-therapy description?

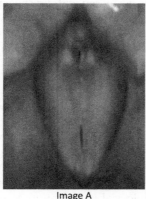 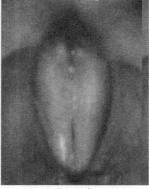

Image A   Image B

(3) Most acoustic measurements showed no change following VFEs. Moreover, these measurements were within normal limits even before treatment when PT complained of rough voice and vocal fatigue. Describe *one* implication of these findings.

(4) Is there any evidence that VFEs were successful in training PT how to breathe to his maximum capacity for the production of voice?

(5) Before treatment, PT had a mildly deviant voice quality. After treatment, he had a normal voice quality. Imagine that you are a speech-language pathologist who is defending the cost-effectiveness of voice therapy in PT's case. How might that argument proceed?

---

[1] Reprinted from *Journal of Voice*, 26:6, Rita R. Patel, Jack Pickering, Joseph Stemple and Kevin D. Donohue, A Case Report in Changes in Phonatory Physiology Following Voice Therapy: Application of High-Speed Imaging/734–741, copyright (2012), with permission from Elsevier.

Case study 38

Woman aged 50 years with psychogenic dysphonia

Introduction

The following exercise is a case study of a 50-year-old woman ('Ms S') who was studied by Sudhir et al. (2009). This client was diagnosed with psychogenic dysphonia. Detailed case history and assessment revealed significant marital difficulties and other psychological stressors in this woman's life. The case study is presented in five sections: primer on psychogenic dysphonia; client history; voice assessment; psychological assessment; and therapeutic programme.

Primer on psychogenic dysphonia

Within the nosology of voice disorder, psychogenic dysphonia is a *functional* voice disorder alongside muscle tension dysphonia and voice disorders that result from phonotrauma (Connor and Bless, 2014). Psychogenic dysphonia is defined as the 'loss of voice where there is insufficient structural or neurological pathology to account for the nature and severity of the dysphonia, and where loss of volitional control over phonation seems to be related to psychological processes such as anxiety, depression, conversion reaction, or personality disorder' (Baker, 2003: 308). An organic pathology is typically excluded as a cause of the voice disorder by means of a comprehensive laryngological examination. An equally comprehensive psychological examination is needed to reveal the complex psychological processes which may play a causative role in the onset of the voice disorder. Regardless of the triggers for psychogenic dysphonia, this voice disorder is known to have a significant adverse impact on an individual's quality of life and occupational and social functioning (Merrill et al., 2011). It is for these reasons that psychogenic dysphonia is assessed and treated by speech and language therapists among other voice professionals.

Little is known about the prevalence and incidence of psychogenic dysphonia. Kollbrunner et al. (2010) reported that psychogenic aphonia, a so-called conversion disorder, is a rare condition which has a point prevalence of 0.4%. The category of functional voice disorders, to which psychogenic dysphonia belongs, is altogether more prevalent, and accounts for the majority of cases of dysphonia in many clinical samples. In a study of 882 patients attending the ENT Department at the University Hospital in Ghent, Belgium between 2004 and 2008, Van Houtte et al. (2010) found functional voice disorders in 30% of their clinical sample. Psychogenic dysphonia is considerably more common in women than in men. Martins et al. (2014) examined 28 adult patients with psychogenic dysphonia, 26 of whom were women. Between February 2000 and May 2006, Kollbrunner et al.

(2010) identified 22 patients with psychogenic aphonia in the Department of Otorhino-laryngology, Head and Neck Surgery at Bern University Hospital. Of these patients, 19 were female. The mean ages of clients in Martins et al.'s study and Kollbrunner et al.'s investigations were 47.3 years and 40.3 years, respectively. Voice disorders are more common in certain occupational groups including teachers and professional voice users such as singers (Cantor Cutiva et al., 2013; Fortes et al., 2007). Psychogenic dysphonia is no exception in this regard, with teachers and sales clerks accounting for nine of 11 adults with psychogenic dysphonia who were in employment in Martins et al.'s study.

The onset of psychogenic dysphonia in clients is often preceded by upper respiratory tract infections and/or asthma or allergy-like symptoms. Schalén and Andersson (1992) examined 40 consecutive patients with psychogenic voice disorder. An upper respiratory tract infection prior to the onset of dysphonia was identified in 25% of patients, with as many as 40% of clients treated with antibiotics on one or more occasions. Asthma and allergy-like symptoms were reported in 37.5% of patients, a level which exceeded the incidence of asthma/allergy in the Swedish adult population. Combined with the fact that a perceptual analysis of voice profiles in psychogenic dysphonia and acute laryngitis has been shown to reveal similar aberrations (Schalén et al., 1992), the presence of these other conditions can complicate a differential diagnosis of psychogenic dysphonia and lead to misdiagnosis of the voice disorder.

Unit 38.1 Primer on psychogenic dysphonia

(1) Which of the following is a *true* statement about psychogenic dysphonia?
   (a) Psychogenic dysphonia is a hyperfunctional voice disorder.
   (b) Psychogenic dysphonia can manifest in some cases as complete aphonia.
   (c) The vegetative functions of the larynx are compromised in psychogenic dysphonia.
   (d) Psychogenic dysphonia can arise following a stressful or traumatic event.
   (e) Vocal nodules are a common pathological finding in psychogenic dysphonia.

(2) Name *three* medical and health professionals who are involved in the assessment and treatment of clients with psychogenic dysphonia.

(3) In the nosology of voice disorders, psychogenic dysphonia is a functional voice disorder. Which of the following voice disorders is a functional dysphonia?
   (a) puberphonia
   (b) presbylarynx
   (c) conversion aphonia
   (d) spasmodic dysphonia
   (e) muscle tension dysphonia

(4) Give *two* reasons why psychogenic dysphonia is frequently misdiagnosed.

(5) Which of the following is a *true* statement about the epidemiology of psychogenic dysphonia?
   (a) Psychogenic dysphonia has a similar prevalence in children and adults.
   (b) Psychogenic dysphonia is more common in women than in men.
   (c) Psychogenic dysphonia is more common in certain ethnic groups.
   (d) Psychogenic dysphonia has a peak incidence in adolescence.
   (e) Psychogenic dysphonia is a common voice disorder in the elderly population.

Client history

Ms S reported to the authors' hospital with complaints of a hoarse voice and intermittent aphonia which had lasted 5 months. Ms S's vocal symptoms had started abruptly with fluctuations in voice quality. She reported that while she was visiting her cousins on holiday in her home country of Asian origin, there had been complete restoration of her voice. She did not experience throat pain. Her complaints included low mood, feelings of anxiety and sleeping problems. Ms S had been employed as a teaching assistant at a local school for over 10 years. Her occupational functioning had been affected by her voice problems, as she was unable to take classes. Also, much of her work had to be delegated to colleagues, as she was only able to undertake tasks that did not require her to talk for long periods of time.

Ms S is married to a business man and is a university graduate. She left her home country and migrated to a European country following her marriage. Her husband is also from her country of origin, but migrated with his family when he was an adolescent. At the time of her referral, Ms S was living with her spouse, two daughters and a son. She reported significant difficulties in her marriage to her spouse. There were frequent disagreements and anger over the children's futures and the relationship between Ms S and her mother-in-law. This was not Ms S's first attempt to seek help. She had attended several centres previously with little reported success.

Unit 38.2 Client history

(1) Which of the following statements characterise the onset of Ms S's voice disorder?
    (a) Her vocal symptoms had an insidious onset.
    (b) Her vocal symptoms were accompanied by odynophagia.
    (c) Her vocal symptoms were intermittent and varied with context.
    (d) Her vocal symptoms included a breathy voice.
    (e) Her vocal symptoms included a lack of phonation.

(2) Which *two* features of Ms S's self-report suggest that she is at risk of psychogenic dysphonia?

(3) Which aspect of Ms S's functioning is most compromised by her voice disorder?

(4) Why should an organic disorder not be rejected as a cause of Ms S's voice disorder at this stage?

(5) Ms S had previously attempted to have her voice disorder addressed but with limited success. Name *one* factor which may account for the lack of success of these earlier interventions.

Voice assessment

Ms S underwent a laryngeal examination by an otolaryngologist which revealed no organic abnormality. She reported that she used her voice for singing hymns as an amateur and for formal teaching as well as for everyday speech. Perceptual and acoustic analyses of

Ms S's voice were undertaken. The GRBAS scale (Hirano, 1981) was used to perform a perceptual assessment. This scale assigns ratings of 0 (normal) to 3 (extreme degree of impairment) to a number of parameters: grade (G), roughness (R), breathy (B), asthenia (A) and strained (S). Ms S obtained scores of G_1, R_1, B_0, A_1, S_1 during sustained phonation. On a speech task, her scores were G_3, R_1, B_3, A_3, S_3. Ms S's volitional cough was good. An acoustic analysis was conducted using a speech software system. Sustained phonation of the vowel [a] had a mean habitual frequency of 220 Hz. Ms S's speaking range was from a minimum of 197.53 Hz to a maximum of 266.66 Hz. The maximum phonation duration at the mean habitual frequency was only 4 seconds. However, this was well sustained. At other frequencies – 212 Hz, 241 Hz, 271.03 Hz and 328 Hz – phonation was also well sustained, and the transition between frequencies as Ms S went up the modal register was smooth. At 359.75 Hz, the quality of the voice became strained-hoarse and Ms S was advised not to go higher in the pitch scale.

Unit 38.3 Voice assessment

(1) Which of the following procedures might an otolaryngologist use to exclude the presence of an organic laryngeal abnormality in Ms S's case?
   (a) videofluoroscopy
   (b) stroboscopy
   (c) nasometry
   (d) electropalatography
   (e) tympanometry

(2) Ms S had a good volitional cough. What does this indicate?

(3) The GRBAS scale indicates that Ms S has more pronounced vocal abnormalities during a speech task than during sustained phonation. What does this suggest about the aetiology of Ms S's voice disorder?

(4) The fundamental frequency of Ms S's speaking voice ranged from 197.53 Hz to 266.66 Hz, while her mean frequency for sustained phonation of [a] was 220 Hz. Are these values within the normal range?

(5) Ms S's maximum phonation duration was 4 seconds. Is this within the normal range for a woman of Ms S's age?

Psychological assessment

Ms S was assessed by a clinical psychologist. The assessment revealed that there were significant interpersonal difficulties between Ms S and her spouse and mother-in-law. Issues concerning communication patterns, decision-making in the marriage, child rearing and Ms S's ability to express her feelings and thoughts about the marriage tended to dominate. Ms S experienced feelings of alienation and distance from her spouse's family whom she perceived to be demanding. The early years of the marriage were described as difficult. Ms S felt she was criticised by her spouse over trivial matters. This caused her anxiety which led her to be somewhat disorganised in her daily activities. Her spouse was characterised as a perfectionist who was critical and demeaning about Ms S's style of functioning. In a separate interview, the spouse was found to be domineering in the relationship and particular about being on time and organised. Ms S had steadily decreased her contribution to family discussions as she had felt her ideas were criticised and dismissed as being worthless. She described how she felt 'silenced' by her spouse and stated that she was never 'heard'. Both Ms S and her spouse expressed anger by not talking to each other for days. The couple did not have a healthy sexual relationship. During joint sessions with her spouse, Ms S was noted to have considerable variation in her voice. This ranged from hoarseness to aphonia, which corresponded with Ms S and her spouse having an argument.

Alongside these difficulties with her spouse Ms S had additional problems in the relationship with her mother-in-law. As the eldest son, Ms S's spouse had a duty to look after his mother. This required Ms S to spend considerable time with her spouse's family, including many family gatherings which she did not enjoy. As the eldest and only daughter-in-law of domiciliary origin, Ms S was expected to conform to family expectations and tradition, even though she and her husband now lived in a foreign culture. Ms S exhibited further anxieties about her three children growing up in western culture. Her son had failed to establish a career and had not yet moved out of the parental home. Ms S and her spouse had had several discussions about their son's career. Her daughters were both young adults. They felt restricted by their mother's expectations and value system. One of the daughters had moved to a nearby university. The other daughter had looked for a part-time job to fund herself. Ms S's children, and especially her daughters, had initially expressed concerns about her voice problems.

Three assessments of Ms S were conducted: Beck's Depression Inventory (BDI; Beck et al., 1961); Dysfunctional Attitudes Scale (DAS; Weissman and Beck, 1978); and Sentence Completion Test (SCT; Sacks and Levy, 1959). The BDI is a 21-item, self-report measure of clinically derived categories of depression. Ms S obtained a score of 15 on this assessment, indicating the presence of depression of mild severity. The DAS is a 40-item, self-report measure which assesses an individual's attitudes across several domains. Ms S displayed problems in the approval–rejection domain of DAS and imperative assumptions. She had difficulty endorsing items on autonomy. She endorsed views that others did not like her if they disagreed with her, and that she was worthless if someone she loved did not reciprocate. Ms S's responses on the SCT indicated significant difficulties in the area of marriage and heterosexual relations. However, she recalled a happy childhood.

Unit 38.4 Psychological assessment

(1) Issues around speaking out and having one's voice heard are often revealed in a psychological assessment of the client with psychogenic dysphonia. Is that true of the present case?

(2) Communication is a dominant theme in Ms S's personal psychology. But there is another way in which communication issues manifest themselves in the present case. What is that way?

(3) Are fluctuations in Ms S's vocal symptoms reflective of her emotional state? Provide support for your answer.

(4) Primary and secondary gains are thought to play an important role in maintaining and reinforcing certain psychogenic voice disorders (Roy, 2004: 28). A primary gain describes the avoidance of anxiety that is made possible when a psychological conflict

does not enter one's conscious awareness. A secondary gain is the avoidance of an undesirable responsibility or activity and the extra attention that is conferred on the patient who has a voice disorder. Is there any secondary gain for Ms S in having a voice disorder?

(5) Clearly, a psychological assessment of the voice client is only of clinical value to the extent that its findings can be successfully addressed in therapy. Is there any evidence that a combined treatment involving speech therapy and psychotherapy is more effective than speech therapy alone?

Therapeutic programme

Ms S received a programme of therapy which was jointly delivered by a clinical psychologist and speech pathologist. During a three-week period, Ms S received a total of 15 sessions of cognitive behavioural therapy. These sessions attempted to restore voice and improve the client's ability to cope with emotional problems. The possible meaning of Ms S's symptoms was addressed in the sessions. To assist Ms S in reducing the physiological arousal that was related to her anger and anxiety, and associated sleep problems, training in deep muscle relaxation was adopted. Dysfunctional assumptions were identified and clarified through Socratic questioning with the aim of cognitively restructuring them. Negative cognitions in the domains of Ms S's children's future and her relationship to her spouse and his family were the focus of sessions. Ms S was encouraged to adopt more neutral alternative interpretations during interactions. Sessions also aimed to increase Ms S's problem-solving skills, decision-making and organisation of tasks. During sessions with the couple, tasks and goals were identified which were intended to help improve communication and resolve conflicts about child rearing and sexual interactions. The critical attitudes and expectations of Ms S's spouse were addressed in these sessions, although he appeared reluctant to modify them.

In each session of voice therapy, Ms S received direct voice therapy and counselling. Direct therapy began with the non-phonatory task of cough which was immediately followed by sustained production of [a]. From cough and phonation, Ms S progressed to phonation with soft contact. Gradually, phonation was extended to other speech sounds (e.g. [u] and [i]). Reassurance and encouragement was provided to maintain a good quality of voice production. Other tasks included sustained humming and the matching of pitch patterns. During counselling the abuse of Ms S's voice in the context of her family problems were subjected to psychotherapeutic examination. Efforts were made to reduce her psychosocial stress. Vocal hygiene and the effects of voice misuse were also addressed. When Ms S could sustain voice for a longer duration in the clinic, she was encouraged to generate words from lexical categories in a prolonged manner. She was eventually able to engage in sustained conversation for a period of 15 minutes. After approximately six 1-hour sessions Ms S was able to sustain voicing even in the presence of her spouse. Although Ms S experienced intermittent dysphonia during this period, she was able to regain her voice with humming and she was encouraged to sing hymns as she had done previously. After sustained voice was achieved over several days, voice therapy was terminated. By this stage, Ms S had a mean habitual frequency for [a] of 207.79 Hz. Her GRBAS scale scores were zero across all parameters.

Unit 38.5 Therapeutic programme

(1) Ms S received cognitive behavioural therapy (CBT). Which of the following are *true* statements about CBT as applied to clients with dysphonia?

    (a) CBT is the only psychological intervention used by voice therapists.

    (b) Stress management is a part of CBT for clients with dysphonia.

    (c) CBT is most effective in the absence of voice therapy.

    (d) CBT is only used when dysphonia has persisted for six months.

    (e) Assertiveness training is a part of CBT for clients with dysphonia.

(2) During direct voice therapy Ms S progressed to using phonation with soft contact. Explain what 'soft contact' means in this context.

(3) Vocal hygiene was addressed during Ms S's treatment. Describe some of the issues which are brought to the client's awareness during a discussion of vocal hygiene.

(4) Ms S was also educated about voice misuse. Why are clients with psychogenic dysphonia at risk of voice misuse?

(5) What do GRBAS scale scores of zero across all parameters indicate?

Case study 39

Man aged 62 years with laryngeal carcinoma

Introduction

The following exercise is a case study of a man ('MT') who was studied by Burkart et al. (2010). MT presented with a late-stage supraglottic carcinoma. He was treated with open supraglottic laryngectomy and postoperative radiation therapy. The case study is presented in five sections: primer on laryngeal carcinoma; client history; medical evaluation and diagnosis; medical and surgical management; focus on post-laryngectomy communication.

Primer on laryngeal carcinoma

Laryngeal cancer is a life-threatening disease which also causes significant disability in the individuals who develop it. The epidemiology of laryngeal cancer is monitored through the Surveillance, Epidemiology, and End Results (SEER) Program of the National Cancer Institute in the United States. According to SEER statistics, there were an estimated 88,852 people living with laryngeal cancer in the US in 2012. There were 13,560 estimated new cases in 2015 and 3,640 deaths in the same year. Between 2008 and 2012, most new laryngeal cancers (31.2%) occurred in the age group 55 to 64 years (National Cancer Institute, 2015). Historically, more men than women have developed laryngeal cancer. This is still the case today. However, there is evidence that women are representing an increasing proportion of cases over time (Brandstorp-Boesen et al., 2014). MacNeil et al. (2015) reported a five-year survival rate of 57.4% in a study of 4,298 patients who were diagnosed with laryngeal cancer in Ontario between 1995 and 2007. This was lower still (45.4%) for laryngectomy-free survival. This study also showed that overall and laryngectomy-free survival had remained unchanged since the mid-1990s.

Laryngeal carcinoma has a multifactorial aetiology. Among the factors linked to the development of the disease are smoking and alcohol consumption, gastroesophageal reflux disease (GERD), immunosuppression (in HIV/AIDS and transplant recipients), infection with human papillomavirus and helicobacter pylori, and a history of head and neck cancer in first-degree relatives. Laskaris et al. (2014) examined HPV infection in 54 patients with squamous cell carcinoma of the larynx. HPV DNA was present in 18.5% (10/54) laryngeal squamous cell carcinomas. HPV 16, which was the most common type, was detected in 7.5% of patients. Zhang et al. (2014) conducted a systematic review of studies published up to November 2013 that examined the prevalence of GERD in laryngeal or pharyngeal cancer. In a meta-analysis of 10 studies, GERD was found to be significantly associated with laryngeal cancer, but not pharyngeal carcinoma. Piselli et al. (2015) reported a particularly elevated standardised incidence ratio for cancer of the larynx in liver transplant recipients with alcoholic liver disease.

Treatment for laryngeal cancer involves surgery, radiotherapy and chemotherapy. Today, protocols emphasise organ- and function-preserving interventions as a primary treatment method. When a laryngectomy is performed, it is often undertaken as a salvage procedure when radiation or chemoradiation has failed. The result has been a decrease in the number of laryngectomies that are performed (Grau et al., 2003). When surgery is adopted as the primary modality, conservative procedures (partial laryngectomy) are pursued whenever possible. The choice of total versus partial laryngectomy as well as type of partial laryngectomy is determined by a range of factors including the location of a tumour. For example, a supraglottic laryngectomy is performed if there is a tumour of the false vocal fold. However, if a supraglottic lesion extends to the glottis, a supracricoid laryngectomy is performed. These procedures have different implications for voice and swallowing function. A supraglottic laryngectomy can leave an individual with relatively good voice quality but often causes serious swallowing difficulties. When a carcinoma of the tongue or oesophagus invades laryngeal tissues, the larynx may also need to be removed. In this case, laryngectomy is performed alongside glossectomy or oesophagectomy.

Unit 39.1 Primer on laryngeal carcinoma

(1) The epidemiology of laryngeal cancer has revealed that women are representing an increasing proportion of cases over time. Why do you think this is the case?

(2) The subjects studied by Piselli et al. (2015) had a particularly elevated standardised incidence ratio for cancer of the larynx. Which *two* risk factors for laryngeal cancer do these subjects exhibit?

(3) Gastroesophageal reflux disease (GERD) is now recognised as a significant risk factor for laryngeal cancer. Explain how GERD is associated with the development of laryngeal cancer.

(4) Which of the following procedures may be used to treat a tumour of the epiglottis and false vocal folds?
   (a) total laryngectomy
   (b) vertical partial laryngectomy
   (c) supraglottic laryngectomy
   (d) supracricoid laryngectomy
   (e) hemilaryngectomy

(5) Respond with *true* or *false* to each of the following statements about swallowing after laryngectomy:
   (a) Aspiration is a significant risk after total laryngectomy.
   (b) There is a high incidence of dysphagia after supracricoid laryngectomy.
   (c) Videofluoroscopy can be used to evaluate swallowing after laryngectomy.
   (d) Dysphagia normally resolves within 6 months after laryngectomy.
   (e) Manometry can be used to evaluate swallowing after laryngectomy.

Client history

MT is a 62-year-old man who is a construction worker. He presented for assessment because of hoarseness which had lasted for three months. He reported mild dysphagia and odynophagia. He exhibited no weight loss or otalgia and is otherwise healthy. MT has smoked one pack of cigarettes per day for 40 years and has consumed alcohol socially.

Unit 39.2 Client history

(1) MT conforms to the demographic profile of individuals who are most likely to develop laryngeal cancer. In what *two* respects is this the case?

(2) Which *two* lifestyle risk factors for laryngeal cancer does MT have?

(3) MT presented for assessment on account of persistent hoarseness. Depending on the location of a laryngeal tumour, hoarseness can be an early symptom of disease or a sign of a more advanced tumour. Explain.

(4) Among the symptoms that MT exhibited were odynophagia and otalgia. Describe these symptoms.

(5) Apart from the symptoms described above, list *three* other symptoms associated with laryngeal cancer.

Medical evaluation and diagnosis

MT underwent an extensive medical evaluation. His larynx was mobile on physical examination. Flexible fibreoptic laryngoscopy was performed. It revealed a friable, ulcerated mass on the laryngeal surface of the infrahyoid epiglottis and the left false vocal fold. The true vocal folds were crisp and appeared to be clear of tumour. There was no involvement of the anterior and posterior commissures and the arytenoids. The right vocal fold was fully mobile and was effectively compensating for mildly impaired mobility of the left vocal fold. MT had a left, firm, palpable, enlarged, upper jugular node which was less than 3 cm in diameter. There were no other signs of adenopathy or other masses in the head and neck region on examination. MT had poor dentition.

Other medical investigations were performed. MT had a CT scan of the head and neck. This revealed a $2.5 \times 2.3 \times 1.9$ cm left supraglottic tumour that involved the epiglottis and left false vocal fold but not the laryngeal cartilages. The scan also showed a single 2.5 cm ipsilateral level 2 lymph node with central necrosis but no other adenopathy. Panendoscopy was performed and revealed no second primary tumour. The base of the tongue had normal consistency during bimanual palpation. There was fullness in the pre-epiglottic space. The laryngeal tumour biopsy that was performed during direct laryngoscopy revealed a moderately differentiated keratinising squamous cell carcinoma. Squamous cell carcinoma clusters were obtained from a fine-needle aspiration of the cervical lymph node. A chest radiograph was negative for metastatic foci. On the basis of these investigations, a diagnosis was made: MT had a stage III (T2N1M0) squamous cell carcinoma of the supraglottic larynx.

Unit 39.3 Medical evaluation and diagnosis

(1) During a visual examination of the larynx, MT's tumour was found to involve certain laryngeal structures while other structures appeared to be free of disease. The diagram

below is a coronal section of the larynx viewed from the back. Place an **X** on the structures that are compromised by MT's tumour.

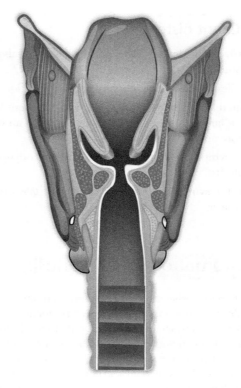

(2) What type of laryngectomy is warranted in MT's case? Provide support for your answer. Is any additional surgical procedure necessary?

(3) What significance does the poor condition of MT's dentition have for any post-surgical rehabilitation?

(4) One of the medical investigations that were undertaken was a panendoscopy. What is panendoscopy? Give *two* reasons why this procedure is performed.

(5) Speech-language pathologists who work with cancer patients must understand the TNM staging system. On the basis of this system, MT was diagnosed as having a T2N1M0 squamous cell carcinoma of the supraglottic larynx. Explain what T2N1M0 means.

Medical and surgical management

MT was treated with open supraglottic laryngectomy. He also underwent left modified radical neck dissection and right selective neck dissection. The neck specimen revealed extracapsular spread, for which MT received postoperative radiation therapy.

Unit 39.4 Medical and surgical management

(1) MT was treated with open supraglottic laryngectomy. Which aspect of this client's post-surgical rehabilitation will be of most concern to the speech-language pathologist?

(2) Which of the following stages of swallowing is most compromised in clients with supraglottic laryngectomy? *oral preparatory; oral propulsive; pharyngeal; oesophageal*. Explain why the stage you have selected is most compromised.

(3) Which other aspect of MT's management is likely to contribute to any swallowing problems?

(4) MT was treated with an open supraglottic laryngectomy. What other type of supraglottic laryngectomy can be performed? Do these different procedures have the same voice and swallowing outcomes?

(5) Which histological finding is a poor prognostic indicator for MT?

Focus on post-laryngectomy communication

MT underwent an open supraglottic laryngectomy in which his vocal function was preserved. Such a procedure can establish safe short-term swallow function. However, clients who have a partial laryngectomy may subsequently require completion laryngectomy because of late dysphagia and chronic aspiration (Bagwell et al., 2015). After completion laryngectomy, clients face a new challenge of alaryngeal communication. In this unit, different methods of post-laryngectomy voice production will be examined. These methods are as relevant to clients who require completion laryngectomy as they are to clients who have total laryngectomy as a primary treatment modality.

The three methods of communication that are available to clients after total laryngectomy are (i) the use of an artificial or electronic larynx, (ii) the use of oesophageal voice and (iii) the use of a tracheoesophageal voice prosthesis. There are different types of commercially available artificial or electronic larynxes. The electronic neck-type and electronic mouth-type artificial larynxes are the most common of these devices (Benninger et al., 2007). In the neck-type device, a battery-produced sound is conducted through the neck into the oral cavity where the articulators proceed to produce speech sounds as normal. The head of the device is placed against the neck. For effective sound conduction to occur, neck tissue must be supple. Post-operative swelling of the neck tissue and changes to neck tissue related to radiotherapy may make this device difficult to use initially. In the electronic mouth-type device, battery produced sound is carried via a mouth tube into the oral cavity. Because these devices produce continuous sound at the push of a button, clients must be taught strategies for normal phrasing and dealing with the inability to produce contrasts between voiced and voiceless sounds (Benninger et al., 2007). An electronic neck-type device is shown in Figure 39.1.

In the second method of alaryngeal communication after laryngectomy – oesophageal voice production – air is either inhaled or injected into the hypopharynx. The inhaled or injected air is then quickly expelled through the pharyngoesophageal (PE) segment, a narrow sphincter of muscle fibres at the juncture of the hypopharynx and the oesophagus (Benninger et al., 2007). Because this method only has access to air in the hypopharynx,

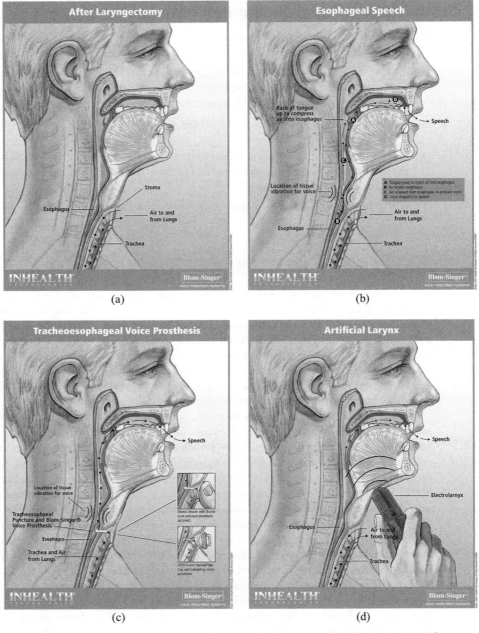

Figure 39.1(a)–(d) Diagrams showing: (a) anatomical structures after laryngectomy and various methods of alaryngeal communication; (b) oesophageal voice; (c) tracheoesophageal voice prosthesis; (d) artificial larynx. Source: images courtesy of InHealth Technologies (www.inhealth .com).

there are reduced air volumes for speech. Accordingly, oesophageal voice users need to frequently insufflate the PE segment during continuous speech. In rehabilitation, clients can be taught different methods of optimal air intake and how to achieve appropriate phrase lengths during speech. They can also be advised on how to avoid stoma and air injection noise (Benninger et al., 2007). The quality of oesophageal voice is associated with the vibratory function of the PE segment. Van Weissenbruch et al. (2000) found that hypertonicity, spasm, strictures, and hypotonicity of the PE segment were correlated significantly with poor or moderate alaryngeal speech in 60 post-laryngectomy patients. The use of oesophageal voice is also illustrated in Figure 39.1.

The third method of alaryngeal communication is the use of a tracheoesophageal voice prosthesis (TEVP). TEVP has become the gold standard in the management of clients who undergo total laryngectomy (Kapila et al., 2011). A fistula is surgically created in the common wall of the posterior trachea and the anterior oesophagus. A voice prosthesis is fitted into this fistula, with the proximal end in the stoma and the distal end in the lumen of the oesophagus (Benninger et al., 2007). The prosthesis is a one-way valve. As such, it permits air to enter the oesophagus but prevents food and secretions in the oesophagus from entering the trachea. When the stoma is manually occluded, pulmonary air is directed through the valve into the oesophagus where it travels superiorly to vibrate the PE segment. An adjustable tracheostoma valve obviates the need to manually block the stoma. A TEVP may be fitted at the time that a total laryngectomy is performed (primary TE puncture). Alternatively, it may be fitted some weeks after total laryngectomy (secondary TE puncture). Because a pulmonary airstream is used to vibrate the PE segment in this form of alaryngeal communication, it is easier for clients to produce continuous speech using a TEVP than standard oesophageal voice. The use of a TEVP is also illustrated in Figure 39.1.

Unit 39.5 Focus on post-laryngectomy communication

(1) Respond with *true* or *false* to each of the following statements about alaryngeal communication:
    (a) Blom-Singer is one type of voice prosthesis.
    (b) Clients can use more than one method of alaryngeal communication.
    (c) There are four different methods of oesophageal insufflation.
    (d) Voice prostheses cannot prevent aspiration into the airway.
    (e) Irradiated tissue presents challenges for alaryngeal communication.

(2) Effective alaryngeal communication is integral to the quality of life of clients who have a laryngectomy. Describe *three* ways in which alaryngeal communication can contribute to quality of life in laryngectomy clients.

(3) All three methods of alaryngeal communication have drawbacks as well as advantages. Five of these drawbacks are listed below. Identify the form of alaryngeal communication to which each of these drawbacks relates:
    (a) Volume and pitch alterations can be achieved but are compromised.
    (b) Regular equipment maintenance is required.
    (c) A limited air source results in reduced continuous speech.
    (d) Management of secretions is required.
    (e) Enlargement of the tracheoesophageal puncture can occur along with periprosthetic leakage.

(4) The use of external beam radiation therapy and chemotherapy to treat upper aerodigestive tract malignancy can result in radiation-induced pharyngoesophageal stenosis (Urben et al., 2012). Which method(s) of alaryngeal communication are compromised by PE stenosis? What other function is compromised by PE stenosis?

(5) Some voice prostheses require daily or weekly cleaning. What *two* skills must a client have to be considered a candidate for TEVP?

Case study 40

Male-to-female transgender adolescent aged 15 years

Introduction

The following exercise is a case study of a male-to-female transgender adolescent ('LA') aged 15 years who was studied by Hancock and Helenius (2012). LA was diagnosed at 14 years of age with gender dysphoria by a neuropsychologist. The case study is presented in five sections: primer on gender dysphoria and transsexual voice; client history; voice evaluation; voice and communication therapy; and communication outcomes.

Primer on gender dysphoria and transsexual voice

The Royal College of Psychiatrists (2013) states that '[g]ender dysphoria is the distress associated with the experience of one's personal gender identity being inconsistent with the phenotype or the gender role typically associated with that phenotype' (12). Several recent epidemiological studies have estimated the prevalence of gender dysphoria in a number of European countries. Judge et al. (2014) estimated the prevalence of gender dysphoria in the Irish population to be 1:10,154 (male:female) and 1:27,668 (female:male). Kuyper and Wijsen (2014) used three measures to estimate the prevalence of gender dysphoria in the Dutch population. The measures were gender identity, dislike of the natal female/male body, and wish to obtain hormones/sex reassignment surgery. These measures combined resulted in figures of 0.6% and 0.2% for the prevalence of gender dysphoria in males and females, respectively. De Cuypere et al. (2007) reported an overall prevalence of 1:12,900 for male-to-female transsexuals and 1:33,800 for female-to-male transsexuals in Belgium. These investigators calculated the male:female sex ratio in the total Belgian population to be 2.43:1.

Management of the transsexual client by speech-language pathologists has focused for the most part on the assessment and treatment of voice. The pitch of the speaking voice is the main area of concern, particularly for male-to-female transsexuals. However, there is increasing recognition that areas such as resonance and articulation also make an important contribution to the perception of the speaker as female (Dacakis et al., 2012). In male-to-female transsexuals, voice therapy is the primary means of achieving pitch elevation, with a range of surgical procedures offered if the client's desired voice quality is not achieved. These procedures work by altering one of the physiological parameters that are known to control pitch: vocal fold tension, length and mass (Anderson, 2014). The vocal attributes of female-to-male transsexuals is still a relatively under-investigated area (Azul, 2015). This is despite the fact that pitch-lowering difficulties have been identified in approximately 10% of female-to-male transsexuals (Cosyns et al., 2014). One reason for this neglect is the mistaken assumption that testosterone-induced voice changes are sufficient in themselves to achieve the type of vocal result that female-to-male transsexuals desire.

Unit 40.1 Primer on gender dysphoria and transsexual voice

(1) It is difficult for epidemiological studies to obtain accurate estimates of the prevalence of gender dysphoria. Some of these studies have based their findings on the number of individuals attending gender clinics (e.g. Judge et al., 2014). Are these studies likely to be overestimating or underestimating the true prevalence of gender dysphoria in the general population? Provide support for your answer.

(2) Respond with *true* or *false* to each of the following statements about gender dysphoria:
   (a) 'Gender dysphoria' is a diagnostic term in the fifth edition of the Diagnostic and Statistical Manual of Mental Disorders (DSM-5).
   (b) A diagnosis of gender dysphoria is made by speech-language pathologists.
   (c) The individual with gender dysphoria must experience clinically significant distress.
   (d) Speech-language pathologists are an integral part of the multidisciplinary team which assesses and treats clients with gender dysphoria.
   (e) Typically, there is no impairment in social, occupational or other areas of functioning in clients with gender dysphoria.

(3) Pitch elevation is the primary aim of voice therapy in male-to-female transsexuals. Which physical attribute of the speaking voice must be modified in order to make pitch elevation possible?

(4) Which of the following types of phonosurgery are used in transsexual clients?
   (a) laryngeal microsurgery
   (b) cricothyroid approximation
   (c) medialisation surgery
   (d) anterior commissure advancement
   (e) glottic widening

(5) For a number of female-to-male transsexuals, pitch-lowering poses significant difficulties. Which of the following factors best explains these difficulties?
   (a) Pitch-lowering difficulties are the result of poor compliance on the part of clients with voice therapy techniques.
   (b) Pitch-lowering difficulties are the result of diminished androgen sensitivity on the part of some female-to-male transsexual clients.
   (c) Pitch-lowering difficulties are the result of low frequency voice therapy.
   (d) Pitch-lowering difficulties are related to structural anomalies of the larynx.
   (e) Pitch-lowering difficulties are related to the use of inappropriate behavioural techniques in voice therapy.

Client history

LA is a healthy teenager with an unremarkable medical history. She is 5 feet 9 inches tall and weighs 140 lbs. English is her first language and she speaks Standard American English dialect. LA has had no prior contact with speech-language pathology.

A neuropsychologist diagnosed LA with gender dysphoria at 14 years of age. LA first told her friends that she was a girl followed by her family. She then began a month-long transition from living as a male to living as a female. At first, she presented as gender-neutral at school and as female at home. After one month, when school had ended, she presented as female 100% of the time. Two months after beginning to live as female, LA started hormone therapy (1mg oestradiol and 15mg spironolactone, each twice daily). At this stage, she was post-puberty, Tanner Stage 4.

At 15;3 years of age, LA started voice and communication therapy. LA's clinical social worker referred her for voice assessment and voice feminisation therapy to the Speech and Hearing Center at George Washington University. According to LA, her voice embarrassed her, made her feel less feminine, and got in the way of her living as a female. At her initial voice evaluation, LA estimated that she used her male birth voice approximately 85% of the time even though she was living as female 100% of the time. The remaining 15% of the time, LA used what she described as a 'higher-pitched female voice'. LA's ability to pass as female on the phone was assessed by clinicians to be approximately 50%, while the ability to pass as female in face-to-face interaction was approximately 70%. LA reported no significant abusive vocal behaviours, and did not have a history of acid reflux or alcohol and tobacco use.

LA was well supported by family members and friends. A member of her family always accompanied her to weekly voice therapy sessions. LA also received the full support of her high school. Despite this, she chose to be home schooled for the autumn semester in her tenth grade year, and also for half of her courses in the spring semester of the same year.

Unit 40.2 Client history

(1) LA's hormone therapy included oestradiol (an oestrogen) and spironolactone (an anti-androgen). Respond with *true* or *false* to each of the following statements about the effect of hormone therapies on the voice in transsexual clients:

(a) Oestrogen and anti-androgen therapy cannot reverse pubertal changes in the voice in the male-to-female transsexuals.

(b) Laryngeal tissues are largely insensitive to androgen therapy.

(c) Androgen therapy in female-to-male transsexuals causes the vocal folds to become thicker and heavier.

(d) Laryngeal tissues are more sensitive to oestrogen therapy than other tissues in the body.

(e) Androgen therapy can achieve acceptable pitch-lowering in most female-to-male transsexuals.

(2) LA is at Tanner Stage 4 in pubertal maturation. What is the significance of this stage for the characteristics of the voice?

(3) How would you characterise LA's voice-related quality of life at the point of referral to a university voice clinic?

(4) What evidence is there that the auditory–perceptual characteristics of LA's voice resulted in listener misidentification of her gender?

(5) LA reported no significant abusive vocal behaviours, and did not have a history of acid reflux or alcohol and tobacco use. Why is it important for LA's voice clinicians to know about abusive vocal behaviours on the one hand, and acid reflux and alcohol and tobacco use on the other hand?

Voice evaluation

LA's voice was evaluated on a weekly basis prior to a therapy session. Visi-Pitch™ software was used to analyse her voice during three speech tasks – reading, picture description and monologue. She received instructions to speak at a comfortable volume and pitch into a microphone that was placed approximately 4 inches in front of her mouth. Several acoustic measures were recorded for each speech task in order to chart LA's progress in therapy. These measures included: total frequency range; mean speaking fundamental frequency; minimum and maximum speaking frequencies with range in Hertz and semitones; and loudness in decibels. LA's speaking rate, calculated as the number of words produced per minute, was also recorded on a weekly basis.

Unit 40.3 Voice evaluation

(1) Visi-Pitch software was used to analyse LA's voice. Which of the following are *true* statements about this software?
  (a) Voice parameters are displayed in real-time to help clients achieve therapy goals with visual feedback.
  (b) Visi-Pitch is only suitable for use with clients who have voice disorders.
  (c) Split screens allow a client's attempts to be compared to a target vocalisation along a number of parameters.
  (d) Visi-Pitch can be used to display fundamental frequency, amplitude and spectral characteristics.
  (e) Visi-Pitch can provide clients with auditory feedback.

(2) LA's voice was assessed during three different speech tasks: reading, picture description and monologue. Why is it important to include different speech tasks in a voice assessment?

(3) Mean speaking fundamental frequency was one of the acoustic measures recorded during LA's voice assessment. Why is fundamental frequency an important measure to record in LA's case?

(4) The mean fundamental frequency of the male speaking voice is 125 Hz (range 107–146 Hz), while the mean fundamental frequency of the female speaking voice is 212 Hz (range 197–227 Hz).[1] For the male-to-female transsexual to be perceived as female, the fundamental frequency of the speaking voice must approximate that of natal females. Which of the following figures reflects the minimum speaking fundamental frequency that must be achieved by the male-to-female transsexual in order to be perceived as female?
  (a) 150–155 Hz
  (b) 160–165 Hz
  (c) 175–1880 Hz
  (d) 190–195 Hz
  (e) 205–210 Hz

---

[1] These figures are based on a review of 15 studies of mean fundamental frequency in males and seven studies of mean fundamental frequency in females conducted by Aronson and Bless (2009).

(5) LA's speaking rate and loudness were also recorded on a weekly basis. Why is it important for LA's speech-language pathologist to monitor speaking rate and loudness?

Voice and communication therapy

Over a period of seven months, LA received a total of 15 sessions of voice therapy. Therapy was conducted by a certified speech-language pathologist with expertise in transgender communication and a master's-level speech-language pathology student clinician. There were a number of elements to LA's therapy. These included education, posture, relaxation and breathing; oral resonance; intonation; pitch; voice quality; and rate. Generalisation and stabilisation were also addressed in therapy. These various components are addressed below.

Education, posture, relaxation and breathing: During education and counselling, LA was informed about abusive vocal behaviours. Anatomy and physiology of voice production were also described and the goals and objectives of therapy were discussed. LA was instructed in how to achieve aligned and relaxed posture. Mind and body meditation were used during relaxation and were followed by neck stretches and shoulder rolls. A weekly massage of the suprahyoid space and laryngeal musculature was performed by the clinician. The clinician also modelled and explained diaphragmatic–abdominal breathing.

Oral resonance: Feminine oral resonance was modelled by the clinician. LA was encouraged to feel the 'buzz' that was created by resonance in her oral cavity and to project her voice to the back of the room using a smooth, full sound. A resonant sound was attempted first at a single-sound utterance level (i.e. sustained /ah/, gradual increase in volume on /ah/, gradual increase in pitch on /ah/). This same technique was then implemented on single words, and longer and more complex utterances until resonance could be achieved in connected speech.

Intonation: Female and male intonation patterns were compared. The clinician modelled female intonation. Female intonation was first used by LA in single words, then longer and more complex utterances and eventually in connected speech.

Pitch: When more efficient breathing, resonance, relaxation and intonation had been achieved by LA, attention turned to the fundamental frequency of her voice. A speech sample which had been recorded at the beginning of the session was played to LA. The Visi-Pitch program display was used to show LA the acoustic measure of fundamental frequency. LA was then encouraged to read brief sentences at a pitch which was slightly higher than the one she had just heard. Acoustic measures were again shown to LA. Through the use of auditory and visual feedback, LA was able to gauge whether her vocal adjustments were successful.

Voice quality: LA's female voice had a breathy quality that was 'wispy' or weak especially as pitch increased. She was instructed in how to produce a 'soft, gentle' voice that was strong rather than weak. A feminine vocal quality was achieved after one treatment session.

Rate: At the beginning of therapy, LA's speaking rate when reading the Rainbow Passage was approximately 260–80 words per minute (wpm). LA was able to gradually decrease her speaking rate to 190–200 wpm by means of her clinician giving her a verbal cue to 'slow' and using a gesture of slow arm movement as in conducting an orchestra.

Generalisation and stabilisation: LA was encouraged to use her new voice in more challenging situations such as asking strangers for directions and ordering quickly in a fast food line. When speaking to her parents and brother, some aspects of LA's new voice lapsed. For example, she spoke with a lower pitch and increased rate to her brother than when she was with the clinician. Around the university campus she simulated more challenging situations with the clinician. Follow-up at two months revealed that LA was pleased with her voice and communication. Her new voice no longer required her conscious attention in order to be used.

Unit 40.4 Voice and communication therapy

(1) During therapy the use of diaphragmatic–abdominal breathing was encouraged. This type of breathing provides optimal respiratory support for voice production. Which respiratory pattern will LA's clinician be aiming to avoid?

(2) Oral resonance was targeted during LA's voice therapy. Can modifications of oral resonance in male-to-female transsexuals increase perception of the speaker as female? Provide evidence to support your answer.

(3) Intonation was also considered to be an important aspect of LA's voice feminisation. Respond with *true* or *false* to each of the following statements about intonation in male-to-female transsexuals:

    (a) Male-to-female transsexuals who are not perceived as female use less upward and more downward intonations than those who pass as female.

    (b) Intonation does not influence gender perception in male-to-female transsexuals.

    (c) Male-to-female transsexuals who are not perceived as female use more upward and less downward intonations than those who pass as female.

    (d) Intonation in male-to-female transsexuals is resistant to therapeutic intervention.

    (e) Intonation makes a less significant contribution to gender perception in male-to-female transsexuals than speaking fundamental frequency and resonance.

(4) In a retrospective chart review of 25 male-to-female transsexuals, Hancock and Garabedian (2013) reported that 28% presented with a voice disorder that was separate from gender presentation concerns. Why are these clients at an increased risk of voice disorder? Which aspect of LA's intervention is intended to reduce this risk?

(5) Palmer et al. (2012) found that male-to-female transsexuals who reported passing as females had incomplete glottal closure (a posterior glottal gap) and phase closure ratios which were skewed towards more open time. Which aspect of LA's voice quality might be explained by these endoscopic and stroboscopic findings?

Communication outcomes

LA reported a positive change in attitude and self-perception following therapy. She completed the Transgender Self-Evaluation Questionnaire (TSEQ; Dacakis, 2006) at three points in time. At her initial evaluation, LA scored 106/120 on the TSEQ, which indicated that her voice negatively affected her life to a severe degree. Six months later, her score had dropped to 79/120 (moderate degree). Four months later – two months after therapy had been terminated – LA scored 53/120.

The Consensus Auditory–Perceptual Evaluation of Voice (CAPE-V; American Speech-Language-Hearing Association, 2002) was used to describe the auditory–perceptual attributes of LA's voice before and after therapy. At initial evaluation, roughness, strain and loudness were judged to be within normal limits. Breathiness was mild and pitch was assessed to be mildly low. It was also observed at initial evaluation that LA used imprecise articulation, had a voice tone that resonated in the laryngeal area rather than forward in the oral cavity, displayed limited intonation and had an excessive speech rate (282 wpm). LA's posture was mildly slouched and she used thoracic breathing. There was also mild suprahyoid and laryngeal tension. After eight therapy sessions, LA's mild breathiness and low pitch had improved. Also, LA had forward-focused resonance in the oral cavity, demonstrated relaxed and aligned posture, and used diaphragmatic–abdominal breathing at follow-up two months after the termination of treatment.

At the initial evaluation, LA's male voice during monologue had a mean speaking fundamental frequency of 136 Hz. During production of a sustained vowel, perturbation measures for her male voice were within normal limits. The speaking fundamental frequency of LA's female voice was 151 Hz during conversation, 141 Hz during picture description and 158 Hz when reading. LA's female voice was excessively breathy and sounded unnatural. Shimmer (%) values were high, but noise-to-harmonic ratio values were not excessive. At discharge, LA's mean fundamental frequency was near 200 Hz when reading or describing a picture and was 172 Hz during monologue. Stable pitch levels near 200 Hz for sustained /a/, reading and picture description were maintained at two-month follow-up. Pitch during monologue was slightly lower at 169 Hz. Jitter was above normal limits at follow-up. The total range of frequency had reduced from discharge but was still within normal limits at 30 semitones.

LA's resonance was assessed during treatment. The first formants (F1) and second formants (F2) of the four corner vowels in /hVd/ context were measured. These formants correspond to tongue height and tongue fronting, respectively. F1 and F2 values are higher in females because of the different sizes of the male and female vocal tracts, and the more open oral cavity and anterior oral resonance in females. With the exception of the back vowel /u/, LA's formant frequencies moved towards average female values during treatment. LA's speaking rate gradually decreased to near 200 wpm. Listener perceptions of LA's voice were also recorded. For picture description and monologue, ratings of femininity increased from 27 to 79 (a 192% increase) and from 31 to 72 (a 132% increase), respectively. Ratings of the softness of LA's voice displayed similar increases. These ratings were stable two months after discharge.

Unit 40.5 Communication outcomes

(1) Voice therapy in male-to-female transsexuals is judged to be effective if it achieves an improvement in the voice-related quality of life of these clients. How would you characterise the effectiveness of the therapy that LA has received?

(2) Before therapy, LA displayed mild suprahyoid and laryngeal tension which improved after treatment. What type of voice disorder might LA have been at risk of developing if this tension had been allowed to persist?

(3) At initial evaluation, LA's female voice was perceived to be mildly breathy. However, after eight therapy sessions, her breathiness had improved. Which acoustic measure confirms the impression of breathiness?

(4) At discharge, LA's mean fundamental frequency was near 200 Hz when reading or describing a picture. How would you characterise LA's mean fundamental frequency upon completion of treatment?

(5) LA also achieved a more female type of resonance as a result of treatment. Which other speech modification that occurred during therapy might have facilitated LA in making resonatory changes?

Section E

Hearing disorders

Case study 41

Boy aged 19 months with Goldenhar syndrome

Introduction

The following exercise is a case study of a 19-month-old boy ('George') who was studied by Belenchia and McCardle (1985). George has oculo-auriculo-vertebral spectrum (OAVS) or Goldenhar syndrome. He has extensive physical anomalies, a number of which have implications for speech, language and hearing. The case study is presented in five sections: primer on Goldenhar syndrome; client history; clinical presentation; speech, language and hearing assessment; and post-therapy communication status.

Primer on Goldenhar syndrome

Goldenhar syndrome or OAVS is a complex developmental disorder which is typically characterised by ear anomalies, hemifacial microsomia (underdevelopment of one side of the face), and defects of the vertebral column. The disorder results from abnormalities of the first and second pharyngeal arches during embryogenesis (Beleza-Meireles et al., 2014). Although the aetiology of OAVS is largely unknown, twinning, assisted reproductive techniques and maternal pre-pregnancy diabetes have been confirmed as risk factors (Barisic et al., 2014). In a large European epidemiological study of 355 infants diagnosed with OAVS between 1990 and 2009, Barisic et al. (2014) reported the prevalence of the disorder to be 3.8 per 100,000 births. The male-to-female sex ratio is approximately 3:2 (Wenger et al., 2014). The most common anomalies among infants with OAVS are microtia (88.8%), hemifacial microsomia (49.0%) and ear tags (44.4%). Other anomalies include congenital heart defects (27.8%), atresia/stenosis of the external auditory canal (25.1%), eye defects (24.3%) and vertebral abnormalities (24.3%) (Barisic et al., 2014).

OAVS has significant implications for speech, hearing, language and feeding. Strömland et al. (2007) examined 18 patients with OAVS who were aged 8 months to 17 years. Ear abnormalities and hearing impairment were present in 100% and 83% of patients, respectively. Difficulties in feeding and eating were identified in 50% of patients, while 53% exhibited speech problems. Intellectual disability (39%) and severe autistic symptoms (11%) were also identified in these subjects. Of all these deficits, ear abnormalities and hearing loss have been most extensively investigated in OAVS. Scholtz et al. (2001) reported ear deformities in a 10-day-old deceased infant with OAVS. These deformities included deformity of the auricle, atresia of the external auditory canal, and malformation of the tympanic cavity and ossicles. There were also abnormalities of the stria vascularis and semicircular canals. Hennersdorf et al. (2014) examined otological abnormalities in 21 patients with Goldenhar syndrome. Of these patients, 19 exhibited external and middle ear problems, and seven had inner ear abnormalities. The inner ear problems of these patients included vestibular enlargement, cochlear hypoplasia and common cavity (a condition in which there is no differentiation between the cochlea and the vestibule, both forming a cystic cavity).

Unit 41.1 Primer on Goldenhar syndrome

(1) State *one* middle ear abnormality that occurs in OAVS. What type of hearing loss is associated with this abnormality?

(2) Children with OAVS can have expressive and receptive language disorder (Cohen et al., 1995). Describe *two* factors which may contribute to the development of language disorder in these children.

(3) Abnormalities of the semicircular canals and cochlear hypoplasia are two inner ear problems in OAVS. Which of these abnormalities gives rise to a disturbance of balance?

(4) Name *two* outer ear abnormalities that occur in OAVS. Which of these abnormalities is associated with conductive hearing loss?

(5) State *one* inner ear abnormality in OAVS which is associated with sensorineural hearing loss.

Client history

George is an ambulatory 19-month-old boy. He is the second child of triplets. The other siblings did not survive the postnatal period. One sibling died at 17 days as a result of aspiration pneumonia. The other sibling died at 3 months of sudden infant death syndrome. Since this time George has been on an apnoea monitor at home. George was delivered by caesarean section at eight months' gestation. He weighed 4lb 1oz. His mother was 22 years old when she gave birth to him. From the seventh month of pregnancy, she had received ritodrine in order to inhibit premature labour. She was also under medical supervision for anaemia and toxaemia during pregnancy. There was no history of either multiple births or congenital anomalies in George's family.

Unit 41.2 Client history

(1) Does George's history contain any risk factors for Goldenhar syndrome or OAVS?

(2) What is aspiration pneumonia? What is its relevance to the speech-language pathologist?

(3) George's mother was administered ritodrine from the seventh month of pregnancy. This drug is not known to have teratogenic effects in humans, although there is evidence of such effects in other animal species (Little, 2006: 283). Even if this drug were shown to be a teratogen in humans, why could it not be a cause of Goldenhar syndrome in George?

(4) At 4lb 1oz, George had a low birth weight. Name *three* developmental areas which are compromised in low birth weight babies.

(5) George's mother experienced anaemia and toxaemia during pregnancy. Which of the following are *true* statements about these conditions?
  (a) Toxaemia is a disease of the first trimester of pregnancy.
  (b) Anaemia is a condition in which blood calcium is elevated.
  (c) Toxaemia is characterised by raised blood pressure, the presence of the protein albumin in the urine and oedema.
  (d) In anaemia, the number of red blood cells or their oxygen-carrying capacity is insufficient to meet physiological needs.
  (e) Toxaemia is a common parasitic infection of pregnancy.

Clinical presentation

George was diagnosed with Goldenhar's syndrome at a children's hospital in Tennessee. His clinical presentation included microtia, mild hemifacial microsomia, cleft lip and submucous cleft, vertebral anomalies and anal stenosis. His vertebral anomalies included butterfly vertebral body in the mid-thoracic area with some cervical ribs. George was hospitalised for one month after birth. His discharge diagnosis included dysplasia of the right ear, right ear atresia, bilateral vesicoureteral reflux, and focal interventricular and periventricular haemorrhages. At 5 months of age, George was observed to have hydrocephalus. He was re-admitted to hospital at 8 months of age for fever, rash and an evaluation of hydrocephalus. A CT scan revealed cranial and facial asymmetry, and right frontal and temporal cortical atrophy. His hydrocephalus was felt to have arrested at this stage.

Unit 41.3 Clinical presentation

(1) George had a cleft lip and submucous cleft. Explain why clefts of the lip and palate are often found in OAVS.

(2) George exhibited a number of cerebral anomalies. Name *three* such anomalies.

(3) Hydrocephalus was diagnosed in George when he was 5 months old. Complete the blank spaces in the following definition of hydrocephalus:

Hydrocephalus is an active distension of the ventricular system of the brain resulting from inadequate passage of _____ from its point of production within the cerebral _____ to its point of absorption into the systemic circulation.

(4) George exhibited microtia. Which of the following are *true* statements about this otological abnormality?
  (a) Microtia is frequently associated with failure of development of the external auditory canal (aural atresia).
  (b) Middle ear structures, including the tympanic membrane and ear ossicles, are intact in children with microtia.
  (c) Aural atresia is associated with severe conductive hearing loss.
  (d) Microtia results from abnormal development of the first and second branchial arches and the first branchial cleft.
  (e) Children with microtia have inner ear deformities and sensorineural hearing loss.

(5) George displayed a mild hemifacial microsomia. Which of the following is *not* associated with this craniofacial defect?
   (a) otosclerosis
   (b) velar paralysis or paresis
   (c) mandibular deformity
   (d) cholesteatoma
   (e) transverse oral cleft or macrostomia

Speech, language and hearing assessment

In September 1983, when George was one year old, he underwent an evaluation of his speech, language and hearing. His overall language development was significantly delayed. On the Receptive–Expressive Emergent Language Scale (REEL; Bzoch and League, 1970), George's performance was at the 4–5 month age level, with his receptive language age at 6–7 months and his expressive language age at 2–3 months. George performed at the 8-month level for receptive language and the 6-month level for expressive language on the Wisconsin Behavior Rating Scale (WBRS; Song and Jones, 1979). George was reported to respond to 'no'. He also seemed to recognise a few familiar words (e.g. mama, daddy, ball, bottle, bye-bye). When accompanied by gestural or physical promptings, he followed simple verbal commands.

Audiological testing was conducted in a controlled sound field. George responded to his name at 15 dB HL, a 1,500-Hz warbled tone at 20 dB HL and a bell at 30 dB HL. George's mother reported that he turned his head towards voices at 8 months. He consistently responded to speech during the evaluation by turning his head towards the speaker. George vocalised randomly and in response to verbal stimulation. His vocalisations consisted of /ʌ/ produced with varied loudness, repetitive productions of /ŋʌ/, and occasional production of /m/. During vocal play with his mother or the examiner, George did not imitate specific vowels or consonants. George's mother reported that his vocalisations had increased since his lip repair which was conducted at 10 months of age. His voice was hypernasal with audible nasal emission.

Unit 41.4 Speech, language and hearing assessment

(1) George's receptive language skills are consistently superior to his expressive language skills. Explain why this receptive–expressive gap is present.

(2) Although they are superior to his expressive language skills, George's receptive language skills are still not age-appropriate. How does George facilitate his impaired comprehension of language?

(3) George's responses on audiological testing were assumed to be representative of the left ear. Why do you think this is the case?

(4) George has a highly restricted speech sound repertoire. What *two* factors are likely to contribute to his limited phonetic inventory?

(5) George's voice was hypernasal with audible nasal emission. What is the likely articulatory basis of these speech anomalies?

Post-therapy communication status

In January 1984, George enrolled in an early intervention programme at a centre in Mississippi. After he had received four months of language therapy, his speech and language skills were re-evaluated. On the REEL, he achieved an overall language age of 20 months, which was one month above his chronological age. George had a receptive language age of 26 months and an expressive language age of 21 months on the WBRS. His behavioural age was 22.4 months. The Preschool Language Scale (Zimmerman et al., 1979) was also administered. George had an auditory comprehension age of 30 months and a verbal ability age of 20 months on this assessment. Approximations of words were accepted for expressive language. George used language appropriately. He was able to make requests, produce comments and initiate communicative interactions. George displayed significant phonological progress over his earlier assessment. He produced a range of vowels and consonants – /k, g, ŋ, n, b, m, w/. It is difficult for the uninitiated listener to understand George on account of his hypernasal speech and nasal emission. The intelligibility of his speech is expected to improve with surgical intervention for velopharyngeal incompetence and submucous cleft.

Unit 41.5 Post-therapy communication status

(1) George exhibited significant language gains after just four months of therapy. What factor unrelated to the intervention itself may account for these gains?

(2) How would you characterise George's pragmatic language skills at his second evaluation?

(3) At his second evaluation, George displayed use of a greater range of consonant sounds than he did at his first evaluation. Describe how his consonant repertoire has expanded following therapy.

(4) The intelligibility of George's speech is expected to improve following surgical intervention for his velopharyngeal incompetence and submucous cleft. Name *one* surgical intervention and *one* prosthetic intervention for velopharyngeal incompetence.

(5) In unit 41.1, it was stated that children with Goldenhar syndrome can have severe autistic symptoms. Which assessment finding suggests that George does not have autism?

Case study 42

Woman aged 49 years with congenital sensorineural hearing loss

Introduction

The following exercise is a case study of a woman ('Chelsea') aged 49 years who was studied by Dronkers et al. (1998). Chelsea was born with severe-to-profound sensorineural hearing loss but did not receive speech, language or hearing services until adulthood. The lack of exposure to linguistic data during development has severely compromised Chelsea's language skills, with some aspects of language more impaired than others. The case study is presented in five sections: primer on congenital sensorineural hearing loss; client history; cognitive and language assessment; pragmatic assessment; and focus on conversational speech.

Primer on congenital sensorineural hearing loss

Sensorineural hearing loss (SNHL) in newborns can arise on account of a number of factors. These factors include in utero infections (cytomegalovirus, rubella, syphilis, herpes, toxoplasmosis), craniofacial anomalies (e.g. Goldenhar syndrome), syndromes associated with SNHL (e.g. Pendred syndrome), ototoxic medication (e.g. neomycin) and hyperbilirubinaemia (i.e. elevated blood bilirubin concentration). Speleman et al. (2012) reported unilateral or bilateral SNHL in 4.1% of 615 neonates, with *in utero* infections (especially cytomegalovirus), craniofacial anomalies and syndromes associated with SNHL the most significant risk factors. Ohl et al. (2009) examined 1,461 infants at risk of hearing impairment at the French University Hospital of Besançon from 2001 to 2007. SNHL was found in 3.1% of these infants. The risk factors for SNHL were, in order of statistical significance, severe birth asphyxia, neurological disorder, syndromes associated with hearing loss, infections (toxoplasmosis, rubella, cytomegalovirus, herpes), family history of deafness, age at the time of screening, and the association of two or more risk factors.

Increasingly, congenital SNHL is managed through the use of cochlear implantation. However, even in children who receive cochlear implants, language development deviates from that of normal hearing children. Children with cochlear implants display impaired non-word repetition in relation to normal hearing children, a finding explained by their reduced sensitivity to phonological structure (Nittrouer et al., 2014a). Nittrouer et al. (2014b) used a range of measures to examine language skills in normal hearing children and children with cochlear implants: mean length of utterance in morphemes; number of conjunctions excluding 'and'; number of personal pronouns; number of bound morphemes; and number of different words. Phonological awareness and lexical knowledge were also assessed. On all language measures including lexical knowledge, the mean scores of children with cochlear implants were approximately one standard deviation below those of children with normal hearing. On two of three measures of phonological awareness, the mean scores of children with cochlear implants were nearly two standard deviations below those of normal hearing children. Age at cochlear implantation is a significant factor in language outcome. Murri et al. (2015) examined oral narrative ability in 30 children with congenital, bilateral, severe-to-profound SNHL. The mean age at cochlear implant activation was 14.7 months, and oral narrative skills were examined at 63 months. It was found that early implanted children developed narrative skills close to those of normal hearing children.

Unit 42.1 Primer on congenital sensorineural hearing loss

(1) Which of the following is *not* a pathological finding in infants with SNHL related to an *in utero* infection?
   (a) atrophy of the organ of Corti
   (b) ossification of the stapes footplate
   (c) cochleosaccular dysplasia
   (d) atresia of the ear canal
   (e) damage to spiral ganglion neurones

(2) A range of factors can lead to SNHL in neonates. Name *one* metabolic cause and *one* pharmacological cause of congenital SNHL.

(3) Not all children with SNHL are good candidates for cochlear implantation. Which of the following are contra-indications for cochlear implantation?
   (a) active middle ear disease
   (b) presence of a cleft palate
   (c) severe intellectual disability
   (d) cochlear aplasia
   (e) presence of a speech disorder

(4) The children with cochlear implants in Nittrouer et al.'s (2014b) study displayed problems in the use of bound morphemes. Give *three* examples of these morphemes.

(5) It was stated above that age at cochlear implantation is a significant factor in language outcome. Describe *two* other factors that influence language outcome in children with cochlear implants.

Client history

Chelsea is a 49-year-old white female. She is the second of seven children who were born and raised in a rural community in northern California. She has severe-to-profound, congenital, sensorineural hearing loss. However, her condition was misdiagnosed in childhood as mental retardation or intellectual disability. Chelsea's mother was advised by professionals to have her institutionalised. However, her mother firmly believed her daughter to be deaf and ignored this advice, raising her instead at home with her siblings. At home, she learned to cook and do housework, and helped her mother raise the younger siblings. Admission to local schools and a school for the deaf was denied. At 32 years of age, Chelsea was referred to a neurologist and speech-language pathologist by a social worker who became aware of her situation. To that point, she had not received any formal education and had not acquired any language. She was subsequently fitted with bilateral hearing aids, and started an intensive programme of oral and signed language instruction. She also received instruction in mathematics and other academic subjects. At the time of the current study, Chelsea was living at home with her parents and was working on a part-time basis as an assistant in a veterinarian's office.

Unit 42.2 Client history

(1) Chelsea's situation is similar to that of so-called feral children in that she has not received exposure to language during the developmental period. However, her situation also differs in a significant respect from these children. What is that respect?

(2) Explain how the respect you have identified in your response to (1) may have had a protective effect on certain of Chelsea's language and communication skills.

(3) Based on your knowledge of first language acquisition, which of the following aspects of language are most likely to be irretrievably compromised in Chelsea as a result of the absence of auditory stimulation in the developmental period?
   (a) phonology
   (b) pragmatics
   (c) vocabulary
   (d) syntax
   (e) morphology

(4) Chelsea received amplification in the form of bilateral hearing aids for the first time at 32 years of age. What factor is likely to limit the effectiveness of these aids at this stage of her life?

(5) Chelsea's case would be unlikely to arise today because of the use of neonatal hearing screening. What two tests undertaken as part of this screening would have detected Chelsea's sensorineural hearing loss?

Cognitive and language assessment

Between July 1980 and July 1989, several standardised tests were performed to assess Chelsea's cognitive and language skills. The Wechsler Adult Intelligence Scale – Revised (WAIS-R; Wechsler, 1981) was performed on four occasions between 1980 and 1987. Chelsea's performance IQ on the WAIS-R ranged from 77 to 89. Five performance subtests were undertaken on each occasion: picture completion; picture arrangement; block design; object assembly; and digit symbol. Each subtest has specific task demands. For example, during picture arrangement the examinee must arrange pictures from left to right to tell a story, while during block design the examinee must arrange blocks to match the design formed by the examiner or shown on a card. Between 1981 and 1987, the Raven's Coloured Progressive Matrices (Raven, 1984) were also conducted on four occasions. Out of a maximum score of 36, Chelsea achieved scores between 24 and 29. The Peabody Picture Vocabulary Test (PPVT; Dunn, 1959; Dunn and Dunn, 1981) was conducted on nine occasions between 1980 and 1983. On five of these occasions, the test was administered with the use of signing. Chelsea's vocabulary age on each administration of the test, and whether or not signing was used, are displayed below.

Date	Vocabulary age	With or without signing
July 1980	2–3	without
December 1980	3–2	without
April 1981	3–11	without
August 1981	4–3	without
August 1981	5–5	with
October 1981	5–3	with
March 1982	6–10	with
June 1982	5–11	with
January 1983	5–8	with

Finally, the Token Test was conducted on four occasions between 1982 and 1989. Chelsea's performance was best on Parts A to E, with scores ranging from 52 to 65 out of a maximum of 67 achieved. However, on Part F, where there was a maximum score of 96, Chelsea's best score across the four occasions of testing was only 57.

Unit 42.3 Cognitive and language assessment

(1) Which of the following cognitive skills is assessed by means of the *block design* subtest of the WAIS-R?
   (a) sequencing skills
   (b) spatial problem-solving
   (c) whole-to-part discrimination
   (d) non-verbal reasoning
   (e) part-to-whole organisation

(2) Studies suggest that the WAIS-R performance scale IQs of deaf adolescents are higher than those of hearing adolescents, with mean performance IQ of 107 to 109 (Rush et al., 1991). Is this true of Chelsea's performance IQ? How might Chelsea's lower performance IQ be explained?

(3) The Raven's Coloured Progressive Matrices (CPM) was also used to assess Chelsea's cognitive skills. Which of the following are *true* statements about this assessment?
   (a) The CPM requires subjects to select one of six patterns to complete a drawing (matrix) of a pattern.
   (b) The CPM assesses verbal abilities in children.
   (c) The CPM assesses non-verbal abilities in children and adults.
   (d) The CPM is a widely used test of intelligence.
   (e) The CPM examines cognitive development up to the point when an individual can reason by analogy.

(4) Which aspect of language is tested by the PPVT? Is there any evidence that Chelsea's performance on this test is facilitated by the use of signing?

(5) Chelsea's comprehension of commands on the Token Test was particularly impaired in Part F. Several commands from this section of the test are shown below. Identify the linguistic feature that is assessed by means of these commands:
  (a) Put the red circle on the green square.
  (b) Pick up the blue circle or the red square.
  (c) If there is a black circle, pick up the red square.
  (d) Touch the squares slowly and the circles quickly.
  (e) Together with the yellow circle, pick up the blue circle.

Pragmatic assessment

Chelsea's pragmatic language skills were assessed by means of the Pragmatic Protocol (Prutting and Kirchner, 1987). The data for this assessment was a videotaped sample of conversation between Chelsea and her teachers. This conversation took place one and a half years into training when Chelsea still had considerably limited language. Chelsea's performance on the protocol was for the most part appropriate. She was able to respond to directives and initiate queries and comments. She displayed appropriate use and diversity of speech acts. In terms of topic management, there was no opportunity to observe her selection of topics. However, she was able to introduce topics, attempted to maintain them and was able to undertake some topic changes. Chelsea was able to initiate questions and respond to the questions of others. She rarely asked for clarification. Her use of pauses was appropriate. When signing, there was some overlap with the turns of others. She nodded and gestured appropriately and waited for her turn. She often repeated information and was not always informative. The specificity and accuracy of her lexical selection was limited but appropriate. There was no opportunity to examine her use of cohesion. Chelsea was able to adjust her speech style. In terms of intelligibility, her signs were intelligible, but her verbal responses were not always so. Her vocal intensity, vocal quality and fluency were normal and she exhibited almost normal prosody. In terms of her non-verbal behaviours, she maintained normal distance to other communicators and her contacts with them were appropriate. Her body posture and movements were normal, as were her facial expressions and eye gaze.

Unit 42.4 Pragmatic assessment

(1) The Pragmatic Protocol was used to assess Chelsea's pragmatic skills. Which of the following are *true* statements about this protocol?
  (a) The Pragmatic Protocol is a standardised test of pragmatics.
  (b) The Pragmatic Protocol examines verbal and non-verbal pragmatics.
  (c) The Pragmatic Protocol examines understanding of figurative language.
  (d) The Pragmatic Protocol examines conversational repair.
  (e) The Pragmatic Protocol was designed for use with clients who have cognitive-communication disorders.

(2) Given her limited language skills, Chelsea's pragmatic skills are remarkably intact. What does this suggest about the relationship between pragmatic competence and linguistic competence?

(3) For the most part, Chelsea makes appropriate contributions to conversation. However, there is one Gricean maxim which she appears to have difficulty observing. What is that maxim?

(4) Chelsea exhibits almost normal prosody. Give *two* examples (one expressive and one receptive) of how prosody may be used during utterance interpretation in conversation.

(5) From what is known of Chelsea's pragmatic skills, is there any evidence to suggest that she has difficulties in the area of theory of mind? Use *three* findings from the Pragmatic Protocol to provide support for your answer.

Focus on conversational speech

Chelsea's conversational speech was recorded and orthographically transcribed. In this short exchange, Chelsea (C) and the interviewer (I) are signing at the same time as they are speaking:

I: (*addressing second interviewer*) I've told Chelsea for the last two days that I had a gift for her.
C: Gift.
I: From Colorado.
C: Colorado.
I: I remembered! (*presents gift*) Do you want to open it?
C: (*accepts wrapped gift, begins to untie ribbon*)
I: Ribbon.
C: Ribbon.
I: What do you think it is?
C: Think? (*shakes head*)
I: A book. Think it's a book?
C: Book? Don't think.
I: Is it a blouse?
C: Blouse? No. You . . . collar.
I: Collar? Of, a scarf. Yes, for my birthday . . .
C: (*continues unwrapping, still unfolding paper*)
I: There's nothing . . . I tricked you!
C: (*laughs; takes out small box*) Oh! Thank you! (*hugs interviewer*) Jewelry!
I: That is named 'turquoise'. (*finger spells 'turquoise'*)
C: Turquoise.

Unit 42.5 Focus on conversational speech

(1) How would you characterise Chelsea's expressive language? What does her expressive language say about her acquisition of syntax?

(2) How would you characterise Chelsea's articulation of speech?

(3) Chelsea performs a number of non-verbal behaviours during this exchange. Are these behaviours communicative in nature?

(4) Pragmatic language skills are an area of relative strength for Chelsea. Describe *three* instances where Chelsea makes appropriate use of these skills.

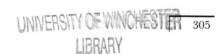

(5) Chelsea's verbal contribution to the exchange consists largely in her repetition of words from the interviewer's utterances and her response to the interviewer's yes–no interrogatives. On one occasion, she deviates from this pattern. Where does this occur, and what is Chelsea attempting to do on this occasion?

Case study 43

Boy aged 4 months with cochlear implants

Introduction

The following exercise is a case study of a boy ('PB') who was studied by May-Mederake and Shehata-Dieler (2013). PB had heredofamilial hearing loss. At 3 months of age, he was fitted with hearing aids with no evident benefit. He received implants at 4;21 months (right ear) and 16 months (left ear). PB's post-implantation speech, language and hearing were examined in detail. The case study is presented in five sections: primer on cochlear implantation; client history; focus on auditory development; focus on speech perception; and focus on language development.

Primer on cochlear implantation

In the United States, cochlear implant devices are approved for use by the Food and Drug Administration (FDA). In 1984, the FDA approved the first cochlear implant for use in adults aged 18 years or older. The first cochlear implant for use in children aged 2 years or older was approved five years later. In 2000, the FDA approved the use of one type of cochlear implant in children as young as 12 months of age. The FDA estimates that as of December 2012, 58,000 adults and 38,000 children in the US have received a cochlear implant (National Institute on Deafness and Other Communication Disorders, 2014). The technology is associated with significant improvements in the quality of life of people who might otherwise derive little benefit from the amplification that hearing aids can provide. Cochlear implantation is also a cost-effective technology. Cheng et al. (2000) estimated that each cochlear implant costs $60,228. In the same year, Mohr et al. (2000) calculated that the lifetime costs of prelingual onset, severe-to-profound hearing impairment exceed $1 million. These costs are accounted for by reduced work productivity and the provision of specialist services. The demonstrable benefits of cochlear implantation combined with its cost-effectiveness have guaranteed this technology a central role in the management of clients with hearing loss.

A cochlear implant consists of two parts. There is an external portion (a sound processor) and an implanted portion (an internal receiver-stimulator). The sound processor contains a microphone and a magnet. The magnet has an associated radiofrequency coil which connects to the implanted portion. The coil stimulates an active electrode that is placed into the scala tympani of the cochlea through a cochleostomy (Grisel and Samy, 2010: 55). These different components are shown in Figure 43.1.

Not every child or adult with hearing loss is a suitable candidate for cochlear implantation. Audiometric threshold, speech recognition performance, age and auditory progress

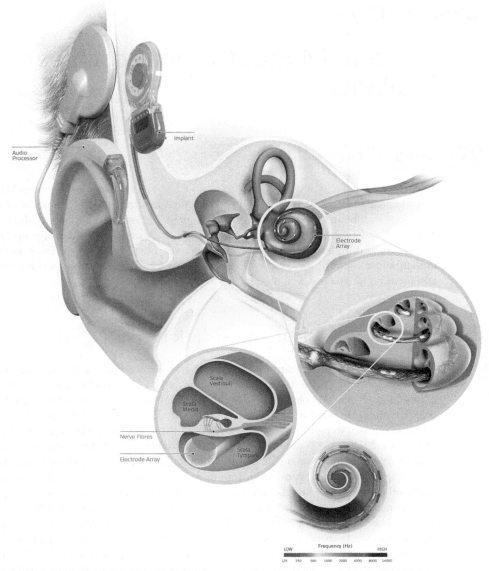

Figure 43.1 Diagram showing the components of a cochlear implant. Image provided courtesy of MED-EL.

with hearing aids are just some of the many criteria that are used to determine candidacy (René, 2011). Paediatric candidacy includes the following criteria: the presence of bilateral, profound hearing loss in children 12 months or older; lack of development of auditory skills; minimal hearing aid benefit; no medical contra-indications; and enrolment in an education programme which emphasises auditory development. Word recognition scores should generally be less than 30% in children over 25 months. Implantation can occur earlier than 12 months if a child experiences trauma or meningitis and is at risk of labyrinthitis ossificans (Grisel and Samy, 2010). Adult candidacy is based on the following criteria: the presence of bilateral, severe-to-profound hearing loss in adults aged 18 years or older; minimal benefit from hearing aids (as indicated by sentence recognition scores less than 60% in the best-aided condition); and no medical contra-indications (Grisel and Samy, 2010).

Cochlear implantation is associated with gains in speech perception, language development, academic achievement and quality of life, although exceptions do exist (e.g. Sarant et al., 2015; Wu et al., 2015). Sparreboom et al. (2015) examined 24 children who underwent sequential bilateral cochlear implantation. These children obtained age-appropriate language scores notwithstanding a period of unilateral deafness. O'Donoghue et al. (2000) examined 40 children whose mean age at implantation was 52 months. The mean number of words per minute perceived increased from 0 before implantation to 44.8 five years after implantation. This represented a significant increase in speech perception over time. King et al. (2014) reported improved quality of life which is independent of speech perception scores in 98 English-speaking adults who received a second cochlear implant between 2000 and 2011. The extent of post-implantation gains is influenced by a range of factors including socioeconomic background, ethnicity, parental input and educational environment (DesJardin and Eisenberg, 2007; Langereis and Vermeulen, 2015; Wu et al., 2015).

Unit 43.1 Primer on cochlear implantation

(1) Cochlear implants are used to treat clients who have severe-to-profound sensorineural hearing loss (SNHL). Which of the following are *true* statements about this type of hearing loss?
   (a) SNHL can be caused by atresia of the ear canal.
   (b) SNHL can be managed in some cases with the use of hearing aids.
   (c) SNHL may be caused by congenital malformation of the inner ear.
   (d) SNHL is the most significant type of hearing loss in clients with palatal clefts.
   (e) SNHL is found in elderly clients with presbycusis.

(2) During cochlear implantation a mastoidectomy and a cochleostomy are performed. Explain what these procedures are designed to achieve.

(3) Paediatric candidacy for cochlear implantation includes an age restriction of 12 months or older. However, implantation can occur earlier than 12 months if a child is at risk of labyrinthitis ossificans. Explain what this condition is and why it necessitates earlier implantation.

(4) Improvements in academic achievement post-implantation are likely to be mediated by gains in language. Which aspects of language in particular contribute to academic achievement? Is there any evidence that these aspects display improvements following cochlear implantation?

(5) It was described above how several factors including socioeconomic background, ethnicity, parental input and educational environment influence the extent of gains after cochlear implantation. Is there any evidence that a client's cognitive ability also plays a role in post-implantation gains?

Client history

PB is a male subject with prelingual hearing loss which is heredofamilial in nature. He was recruited from the Department of Otolaryngology and Cochlea Implantat Centrum, Süd, Würzburg, Germany. PB was raised in a monolingual, German-speaking environment. At 3 months of age, he was fitted with hearing aids with no apparent benefit. His first implant was performed at 4;21 months in the right ear. At 16 months of age, he was implanted in the left ear. The implants were MED-EL COMBI 40+ and a behind the ear TEMPO+ speech processor. The first fitting for both implants took place within 1.5 months after implantation. No surgical complications were reported. PB has no additional needs. He is neurologically and intellectually age appropriate as determined by the German version of the non-verbal intelligence test SON-R 2.5-7 (Tellegen et al., 2007).

Unit 43.2 Client history

(1) PB has hereditary hearing loss. Which of the following are *true* statements about this type of hearing loss?
  (a) Hereditary hearing loss is always sensorineural in nature.
  (b) Hereditary hearing loss only occurs in the presence of a syndrome.
  (c) Hereditary hearing loss may be prelingual or postlingual in nature.
  (d) Hereditary hearing loss only displays autosomal dominant inheritance.
  (e) Hereditary hearing loss can be conductive and sensorineural in nature.

(2) Which of the paediatric candidacy criteria for cochlear implantation does PB clearly satisfy?

(3) How can we tell that PB does not have hearing loss in the presence of a syndrome?

(4) PB underwent sequential bilateral cochlear implantation. Is there any evidence in the clinical literature that (i) *bilateral* implantation has advantages over *unilateral* implantation, and that (ii) *sequential* implantation has advantages over *simultaneous* implantation?

(5) PB had no complications as a result of implantation. However, complications can arise from this procedure. Describe *three* such complications.

Focus on auditory development

A range of assessments was used to assess PB's auditory behaviour. The LittlEARS Auditory Questionnaire (Coninx et al., 2003) was administered at three-monthly intervals up to 24 months of age. At the first interval, a score of 0 was achieved. This steadily increased up to 34 at 24 months of age, which was commensurate with German normative values. PB showed minimal response with a hearing aid prior to implantation. His reactions in free field with both hearing aids were inconsistent at 0.5, 1 and 2 kHz at 100–120 dB. PB's aided responses three months after fitting the first implant were at 0.5 to 4 kHz 65–80 dB. There was continual improvement in his aided responses in free field. He reacted at 45–55 dB six months after the first fitting of the first implant. He reacted at 35–40 dB 18 months after the first fitting of his first implant and six months after the fitting of his second implant. Throughout the follow-up period, PB's aided thresholds remained stable. After the fitting of the second implant, PB's sound localisation abilities showed continuous improvement. PB was able to localise 100% of signals from four loudspeakers six months after fitting. This response was consistent after nine and 18 months of binaural hearing experience.

Unit 43.3 Focus on auditory development

(1) An understanding of terms in audiology is essential for speech-language pathologists. Three such terms are 'free field', 'aided hearing' and 'binaural hearing'. Give a definition of each of these terms.

(2) Which class of speech sounds – consonants or vowels – would PB be able to perceive best prior to implantation? Give a reason for your answer.

(3) Prior to implantation, PB's reactions in free field with both hearing aids did not exceed 2 kHz or 2000 Hz. After receiving his first implant, PB's aided responses extended to 4 kHz or 4000 Hz. Using your knowledge of the frequency of speech sounds, which sounds is PB able to perceive for the first time after implantation?

(4) PB's sound localisation abilities improved after the fitting of the second implant. Explain why this improvement occurred.

(5) The LittlEARS Auditory Questionnaire was used to assess PB's auditory development. Which of the following are *true* statements about this questionnaire?
(a) The questionnaire is completed by hearing professionals.
(b) The questionnaire examines hearing in a child's natural environment.
(c) The questionnaire records preverbal auditory development.
(d) The questionnaire is completed by parents and caregivers.
(e) The questionnaire examines hearing in implanted children prior to 24 months.

Focus on speech perception

A range of assessments was also used to examine PB's speech perception before and after implantation. These were the Mainzer Kindersprachtest (Grimm et al., 2000), the Listening in Progress (LiP) Profile and the Monosyllabic-Trochee-Polysyllabic (MTP) test. The Mainzer is a closed- or open-set German speech discrimination test. Words are presented to subjects who must repeat them or identify them by means of picture cards. The LiP and the MTP are part of the Evaluation of Auditory Responses to Speech (EARS) test battery (Coninx et al., 2003). The LiP assesses auditory detection, discrimination, and early identification abilities in relation to both environmental sounds and speech. Both single words and phonemes are tested. The MTP is a closed-set test that assesses the recognition of words with different syllabic patterns. The LiP and the MTP were conducted in a quiet room under normal ambient noise conditions.

On the Mainzer Test 28 months after the fitting of the first implant, PB reached 80% monosyllabic and bisyllabic word discrimination scores at 70 dB. PB's LiP Profile scores were 0% preoperatively, 4% at 1 month, 6% at 3 months, 28% at 6 months, 52% at 12 months and 62% at 18 months. At 12 and 18 months, PB scored 100% on the 3-word and 6-word tests of the MTP test. At 24 months, he scored 100% on the 12-word test of the MTP. Also at 24 months, PB scored 80% on the open-set monosyllable test. A score of 100% was reached on both the closed- and open-set monosyllable tests at 28 months.

Unit 43.4 Focus on speech perception

(1) Respond with *true* or *false* to each of the following statements about PB's speech perception evaluation:
   (a) PB's evaluation examined speech sounds only.
   (b) PB's evaluation required verbal and non-verbal responses.
   (c) PB's evaluation examined only monosyllabic words.
   (d) PB's evaluation was conducted under free-field conditions.
   (e) PB's evaluation examined perception at phoneme, syllable and word level.

(2) Both open-set and closed-set tests were used to evaluate PB. What is the difference between these tests? Which of these tests is more difficult for hearing impaired clients?

(3) Describe *one* factor which an audiologist must consider when using a word recognition test in children.

(4) At 12 and 18 months, PB scored 52% and 62%, respectively, on the LiP Profile. However, at the same ages he scored 100% on the 3-word and 6-word tests of the MTP test. How do you explain this difference in performance in these two closed-set tests?

(5) Sainz et al. (2003) also used the LiP Profile and the MTP test to examine the auditory performance of 140 children who received cochlear implants. These investigators were particularly interested in the 'initial drop' phenomenon, a decrease of auditory performance that can occur immediately after first fitting. Is there any evidence of this phenomenon in PB's case?

Focus on language development

PB's receptive and expressive language skills were assessed by means of the Sprachen-twicklungtest (SETK; Grimm, 2001) and the German adaptation of the Test of the Reception of Grammar (TROG-D). The SETK is an age-specific test for children aged 2 to 5 years. Among the subtests included in the SETK are word and sentence comprehension and production, memory span for words, morphological syntax and encoding semantic relations. The TROG-D assesses the reception of grammar in children aged 3 to 10;11 years. The understanding of 18 sentence constructions is examined, with each construction assessed four times using different test stimuli. The Aktiver Wortschatztest (AWST-R; Kiese-Himmel, 2005) is a test of expressive vocabulary for German-speaking children between 3 and 5.5 years of age. Subjects are shown pictures, depicting nouns and verbs, to which they produce a one-word response.

At 2;10 years, PB was assessed on the SETK-2. No result was obtained for the Sentence Production subtest, as PB refused to cooperate. On the three other subtests – Word Comprehension; Sentence Comprehension; and Word Production – PB was either within or greater than the normative range of hearing children. The Sentence Comprehension and Encoding of Semantic Relations subtests of the SETK 3–5 were conducted at 3;4

and 3;6 years, respectively. Once again, PB's performance was within the normative range of hearing children. At 4;0 years, PB scored within the normative range of the following subtests of the SETK 4–5: Morphological Syntax; Sentence Comprehension; and Sentence Memory. PB achieved a score of 4 for word order on the Memory Span subtest, which was also within the normative range. At 4;3 years, the TROG-D was performed, with PB's performance in the normative range. At 3;8 years, PB achieved a score on the AWST-R which was higher than the average of the normative group of hearing children.

Unit 43.5 Focus on language development

(1) PB's language assessment examined several aspects of expressive and receptive language. Some of these aspects are presented below. Give at least *one* example of an assessment or subtest within an assessment that was used to assess each of these aspects:
  (a) expressive vocabulary
  (b) receptive syntax
  (c) expressive semantics
  (d) receptive vocabulary
  (e) expressive morphology

(2) PB clearly has normal linguistic competence as measured by formal language tests. What aspect of language is not assessed by these tests? Is there any evidence that this aspect may be impaired in children with cochlear implants who nevertheless perform well on language tests?

(3) Which test result(s) indicate(s) that PB has intact phonological short-term memory?

(4) PB's strong language performance does not occur in all children after cochlear implantation. Describe *one* factor which reduces the probability that a good language outcome will be achieved after implantation.

(5) PB did not cooperate during the Sentence Production subtest of the SETK-2. There is no suggestion that this lack of cooperation was part of a wider behavioural problem on PB's part. But is there any evidence that hearing impaired children with or without implants experience increased behavioural problems?

Case study 44

Girl aged 11 years with central auditory processing disorder

Introduction

The following exercise is a case study of a girl ('Sally') who was studied by Sharma and Purdy (2007). Sally's auditory processing was first assessed at 7;9 years. This was on account of her learning difficulties despite having normal intelligence. The case study is presented in five sections: primer on central auditory processing disorder; developmental and medical history; cognitive and language profile; audiological assessment and amplification; focus on auditory processing assessment and habilitation.

Primer on central auditory processing disorder

In 2005, a technical report was published by the American Speech-Language-Hearing (ASHA) Working Group on Auditory Processing Disorders. The report defined (central) auditory processing or (C)AP as 'the efficiency and effectiveness by which the central nervous system (CNS) utilises auditory information' (American Speech-Language-Hearing, 2005c). The definition continued:

(C)AP includes the auditory mechanisms that underlie the following abilities or skills: sound localisation and lateralisation; auditory discrimination; auditory pattern recognition; temporal aspects of audition, including temporal integration, temporal discrimination (e.g., temporal gap detection), temporal ordering, and temporal masking; auditory performance in competing acoustic signals (including dichotic listening); and auditory performance with degraded acoustic signals.

(Central) auditory processing disorder or (C)APD was subsequently defined in the report as 'difficulties in the perceptual processing of auditory information in the CNS as demonstrated by poor performance in one or more of the above skills'.

Few studies have examined the epidemiology of (C)APD. Chermak and Musiek (1997) estimated that (C)APD occurs in 2 to 3% of children, with a boy:girl ratio of 2:1. The prevalence is greater in specific clinical populations. Iliadou et al. (2009) reported APD in 43.3% of a population of 127 children with learning difficulties. Keller et al. (2006) found APD in 61% of 18 children with non-verbal learning disability. Bergemalm and Lyxell (2005) found (C)APDs in 58% of 19 subjects who had sustained a closed head injury 7 to 11 years earlier. This high prevalence is all the more noteworthy on account of the fact that most participants did not report any signs of auditory impairment. Quaranta et al. (2014) reported (C)APD in 14.3% of 488 subjects older than 65 years. Alzheimer's disease was significantly associated with (C)APD in these subjects. Hariri et al. (1994) found central auditory dysfunction, as indicated by failure on dichotic competing sentence testing, in 17

(68%) of 25 stroke patients. The failure rate on this testing was similar for left and right stroke, and for temporal and non-temporal lobe involvement.

There is considerable controversy surrounding the aetiology of (C)APD. Although definite causal factors have not been identified, certain factors appear to place children at an increased risk of (C)APD. Among these factors are premature birth, otitis media with effusion and the presence of a craniofacial anomaly. Amin et al. (2015) examined 60 children with (C)APD. Fifteen of these children were premature and 45 were full-term. The premature children in this study had a higher total number of failed (C)APD tests compared with the term children. Children who experience otitis media in the first year of life have been found to have auditory processing problems (Maruthy and Mannarukrishnaiah, 2008). Ma et al. (2016) examined 147 school-aged children with non-syndromic cleft lip and/or palate and 60 craniofacially normal children. Children with isolated cleft palate achieved the lowest scores on a parental questionnaire of auditory problems. This was consistent with a higher index of suspicion for (C)APD. Not all studies have linked these factors to the aetiology of (C)APD. Dawes et al. (2008) examined 32 children diagnosed with APD. These investigators found that none of the aetiological factors investigated, including history of otitis media, adverse obstetric history or familial history of listening problems, predicted APD group membership.

Finally, children with (C)APD often exhibit other neurodevelopmental disorders including dyslexia, ADHD and language disorder. APD coexisted with developmental dyslexia in 25% of the 127 children who were examined by Iliadou et al. (2009). Sharma et al. (2009) examined 68 children with suspected APD. Problems in all three areas of APD, language impairment and reading disorder were present in 47% of these children. Similar patterns of deficit across these disorders have also been reported to occur. Dawes and Bishop (2010) found similarly high levels of attentional, reading and language problems in children with an APD diagnosis and children with dyslexia. Ferguson et al. (2011) examined normally hearing children who were diagnosed with APD or specific language impairment. In general, there was no difference between these children on a range of test measures and parental report. This finding led Ferguson et al. to conclude that the children had been 'differentially diagnosed based on their referral route rather than on actual differences' (211).

Unit 44.1 Primer on central auditory processing disorder

(1) Respond with *true* or *false* to each of the following statements about (C)APD:
   (a) (C)APD is a type of peripheral hearing impairment in children and adults.
   (b) (C)APD may arise as a result of meningitis.
   (c) (C)APD is more common in certain ethnic groups.
   (d) (C)APD may be found in individuals with neurodegenerative disorders.
   (e) (C)APD has few implications for academic attainment in children.

(2) There are *two* ways in which children with craniofacial anomalies are at an increased risk of (C)APD. Explain each of these ways.

(3) Bergemalm and Lyxell (2005) reported a high prevalence of (C)APDs in individuals who sustained a closed head injury. However, these individuals did not report any signs of auditory impairment. Explain this finding based on your knowledge of traumatic brain injury (TBI).

(4) In terms of the aetiology of APD, there seems to be a distinction between those cases where there is a clear neurological aetiology and cases where aetiology and risk factors

are not clear and APD is more akin to a neurodevelopmental disorder. Give *one* example of each type of APD.

(5) An issue which has not been addressed by investigators is if (C)APD deteriorates over time. Yet, it cannot simply be assumed that (C)APD remains static in individuals with the disorder. In which of the conditions examined above is (C)APD likely to worsen over time?

Developmental and medical history

Sally's mother had a normal pregnancy. However, Sally was born small for gestational age (SGA, 2470 g). At the time of her birth, Sally had hypothermia and low blood sugar. She was kept in the special care nursery for 48 hours. She had jaundice for which no treatment was recommended. Sally also did not suck or swallow for 12 hours. For the first four months, Sally's mother reported that she gained less weight than expected and also slept a lot. Her muscle tone was low. Motor milestones were somewhat delayed. At 10 months, Sally started sitting. At 14 months, she was walking. At 7;9 years, when Sally was first assessed for APD, she was wearing special shoes to improve her feet posture. Sally was reported by her mother to still stumble into things and fall over.

Sally received her first set of grommets at 18 months. A further two sets of grommets were inserted between 28 months and 4 years. At 24 months, a CT scan was performed. It showed normal left and right internal auditory meatus. At 7;4 years, Sally received a diagnosis of frontal lobe epilepsy following an EEG that showed spikes in the frontal area. Anti-epileptic medication was started.

Unit 44.2 Developmental and medical history

(1) Sally was born small for her gestational age. What evidence is there that low birth weight is a risk factor for (C)APD?

(2) Sally has not achieved two motor milestones at the expected chronological ages. Describe the extent of her delay in each case.

(3) Does Sally exhibit any other risk factor for (C)APD apart from low birth weight? Provide evidence to support your answer.

(4) What *two* factors suggest that Sally's auditory processing problems may have a neurological aetiology?

(5) A CT scan performed at 24 months excluded any abnormality of the left and right internal auditory meatus (IAM). What is the IAM? What abnormality of the IAM can be detected by the use of a CT scan?

Cognitive and language profile

At the request of her paediatrician, Sally's intelligence was assessed at 7;2 years. The Wechsler Intelligence Scale for Children–III (WISC–III; Wechsler, 1992) was used for this purpose. It revealed that Sally was functioning in the average range. Sally obtained average scores on the Vocabulary and Comprehension subtests. However, her score for verbalising the relationship between concepts was more than one standard deviation below the mean. Also, Sally achieved a score of 6 on the short-term memory task when 7 to 13 is considered to be the average range. Sally achieved significantly better scores on performance tasks such as picture arrangement, reflecting her superior performance on non-verbal tasks.

As part of an assessment of her auditory processing skills at 7;9 years, Sally's vocabulary and reading were assessed. On the Peabody Picture Vocabulary Test-III (PPVT-III; Dunn and Dunn, 1997), Sally obtained a score of 109. This is an average score which is consistent with her WISC-III results. To assess reading fluency and accuracy, the Wheldall Assessment of Reading Passages (WARP; Madeline and Wheldall, 2002) was used. Sally was only able to read 16 words per minute. Children of Sally's chronological age can normally read between 51 and 109 words per minute. Reading accuracy for regular and irregular words, and non-words was assessed by means of the Castles' Word/Nonword Test (Castles and Coltheart, 1993). Sally had difficulty reading all of these word types.

Unit 44.3 Cognitive and language profile

(1) Which of the following are *true* statements about Sally's performance on the WISC-III?
   (a) Sally's verbal IQ is superior to her performance IQ.
   (b) Sally's intellectual functioning is in the normal range.
   (c) Sally has difficulty with abstract relationships.
   (d) Sally has a deficit of episodic memory.
   (e) Sally can recognise cause and effect relationships between depicted events.

(2) Sally exhibits significant difficulties in reading. Which of her WISC-III results might explain these difficulties?

(3) Which of the following aspects of language is assessed by means of the PPVT-III?
   (a) receptive syntax
   (b) expressive vocabulary
   (c) expressive semantics
   (d) receptive vocabulary
   (e) expressive syntax

(4) Sally's ability to read regular words, irregular words and non-words was assessed. Why is it important to include each of these word types in an assessment of reading?

(5) Sally's score on the PPVT-III was consistent with her WISC-III results. How would you explain this?

Audiological assessment and amplification

At 6 months, Sally's hearing was assessed using visual reinforcement orientation audiometry (VROA). At 4 kHz, reliable responses were observed down to 25 dB HL. At 500 Hz and 1 kHz, responses were unreliable but were possibly present at 60 dB HL to 70 dB HL. Sally had significant negative pressure in both ears on the day of VROA testing.

Given the inconclusive nature of her results, Sally was referred for auditory brainstem response (ABR) audiometry. Sally received her first set of grommets around 12 months later. Electrocochleography (ECoG) and ABR were conducted around the same time. At the time of ECoG and ABR, no infection or effusion was evident. Sally's ECoG thresholds to click stimuli were 20 and 30 dB nHL for left and right ears, respectively. ECoG action potentials were reported to be 'normal shaped'. At 500 Hz and 1 kHz, precise threshold estimation was difficult. Thresholds were estimated to be 40 dB HL and 50 dB HL in the left and right ears, respectively. Sally's mild hearing loss was presumed to be conductive based on the ECoG input–output characteristics. The ABR revealed a delay in the wave I–V interwave interval in the right ear compared to the left ear. The wave V inter-aural latency difference was 0.36 ms. The I–V delay in the right ear and the inter-aural wave V asymmetry were of concern and a CT scan was conducted. This revealed normal middle and inner ear structures.

At 22 months, Sally was fitted with bilateral low gain programmable behind-the-ear hearing aids. Soon afterwards, Sally started to babble and use repetitive vocalisations. At 2;6 years, transient click-evoked otoacoustic emission testing was first performed. This showed very robust emissions for both right and left ears. It was recommended that Sally discontinue use of her hearing aids. However, this recommendation was disregarded by Sally's mother who believed her daughter's listening was noticeably worse when she did not wear her aids. By 5 years of age, Sally's pure-tone hearing thresholds were within normal limits and had been so for a period of time. Given the normalisation of peripheral hearing thresholds, the audiologist withdrew the hearing aids.

Unit 44.4 Audiological assessment and amplification

(1) Several investigations of Sally's hearing were conducted. Five of the investigative techniques that were employed are listed below. Give a short description of each technique:
  (a) visual reinforcement orientation audiometry
  (b) auditory brainstem response audiometry
  (c) electrocochleography
  (d) otoacoustic emission testing
  (e) CT scan

(2) On the day of VROA testing, Sally had significant negative pressure in both ears. What technique is used to measure middle ear pressure? What does negative middle ear pressure indicate?

(3) VROA testing at 6 months revealed that Sally had superior hearing at 4 kHz, while her hearing at 500 Hz and 1 kHz was altogether poorer. The perception of which class of speech sounds – vowels or consonants – is most compromised by this pattern of hearing?

(4) ABR audiometry revealed that Sally had I–V delay in her right ear and inter-aural wave V asymmetry. This was a cause of concern and a CT scan was recommended. What conditions, consistent with these ABR results, might a CT scan serve to eliminate?

(5) Why do you think the audiologist recommended the withdrawal of Sally's hearing aids?

Focus on auditory processing assessment and habilitation

At 7;9 years, Sally's auditory processing abilities were extensively evaluated. The evaluation included behavioural observations, reading and vocabulary tests, behavioural auditory processing assessments, and electrophysiology. The results of the reading and vocabulary tests were examined (at pp. 316–17) and will not be considered further below.

Behavioural observations: During testing, Sally was cooperative. She appeared to have low self-esteem, and spoke deliberately and softly when asked questions. The mother reported that with the exception of responses to questions, Sally was difficult to understand if you were not familiar with her. This was consistent with the observation during testing that Sally's casual conversation with her mother was unclear. When spoken to directly, however, Sally was intelligible. Sally's mother completed the Children's Auditory Processing Performance Scale (CHAPPS). This is a questionnaire which serves as a screening tool for APD. It is used to assess how the child's listening ability compares to that of classroom peers (Smoski et al., 1992). Parents and teachers rate listening under a range of conditions on a 6-point scale. Sally's mother indicated that she had difficulty with auditory memory/sequencing and when listening in noise.

Behavioural Auditory Processing Assessments: The following three standardised behavioural tests were used to assess auditory processes: Dichotic Digit Test Version 2 (DDT; Musiek, 1983); Frequency Pattern Test (FPT; Musiek, 1994); and the Random Gap Detection Test (RGDT; Keith, 2000). Sally's FPT scores were 26.6% (right ear) and 13.3% (left ear). Scores for the age range 7 years to 8;9 years should be better than 35%. At 70% (right ear) and 75% (left ear), Sally's DDT scores were within the normal range for 7-year-olds. Sally was unable to detect gaps in the RGDT tonal stimuli.

Electrophysiology: Obligatory and discriminative (mismatch negativity) cortical evoked responses were recorded in response to speech, tonal and complex tonal stimuli. To elicit mismatch negativity and obligatory cortical responses, six deviant (i.e. infrequent) stimuli were delivered monaurally to the right ear. Sally exhibited robust obligatory cortical auditory evoked responses to all the sounds and her MMN was absent for all sounds. However, the diagnostic significance of this latter finding is somewhat uncertain. Sally's cortical response latencies for speech stimuli were typical for a child of her age.

On the basis of the above findings, it was decided that Sally should be fitted with an FM device (Phonic Ear™ Easy Listener) for a three-month period. Her mother reported six months later that Sally enjoyed wearing the device. Her speech was noted to be clearer and she was communicating more at home and at school. Three years later during a telephone conversation, Sally's mother said that she wore the device for one year in total and then rejected it for aesthetic reasons. Since ceasing use of the FM unit, Sally's mother reported deterioration in her speech clarity. Her academic progress was also reported to be very slow.

Unit 44.5 Focus on auditory processing assessment and habilitation

(1) One of the behavioural observations was that Sally had difficulty listening in noise. Is this a common observation of the parents of children with APD?

(2) A further behavioural observation was that Sally has difficulty with auditory memory. Which cognitive finding in 44.3 is this observation consistent with?

(3) The results of which *two* of Sally's behavioural auditory processing assessments fell outside the normal range? What auditory processes are examined by means of these assessments? Do these auditory processes hold diagnostic significance for APD?

(4) Sally's mismatch negativity was absent for all sounds. However, the diagnostic significance of this finding was described as being 'uncertain'. Using evidence from the literature, expand on why this is the case.

(5) To address her auditory processing difficulties, Sally was fitted with an FM device, the Phonic Ear™ Easy Listener. What is this device designed to achieve? What benefits are derived from the use of an FM device for individuals with auditory processing problems?

Section F

Psychiatric disorders

Case study 45

Girl aged 8 years with selective mutism

Introduction

The following exercise is a case study of a girl ('Mimi') who was studied by Giddan et al. (1997). At 8 years of age, Mimi was referred to a school programme for the treatment of selective mutism. Selective mutism is a complex condition in which a child can be completely mute in one or more settings (typically, school), despite communicating effortlessly in other settings. The case study is presented in five sections: primer on selective mutism; client history; communication status; psychological intervention; and speech and language intervention.

Primer on selective mutism

Despite being known to the psychiatric community for over a century, selective mutism is still a poorly understood condition which has not been extensively investigated. The disorder is rare, with prevalence rates oscillating between 0.47% and 0.76% in research studies (Viana et al., 2009). The disorder is more commonly found in females than in males, with the female:male sex ratio reported to be in the region of 1.6–3:1 (Busse and Downey, 2011). The cause of the disorder is unknown. However, a number of factors appear to put children at increased risk of developing selective mutism. These factors include a background of migration, complications during pregnancy and delivery, delayed motor development and toilet training, premorbid speech and language disorders, behavioural abnormalities, comorbid diagnoses (such as enuresis and sleeping and eating disorders), a family history of selective mutism, and a pattern of interaction characterised by withdrawal, anxiety, depression and schizoid type behaviours (Unruh and Lowe, 2007). Reflecting a consistent finding of elevated anxiety in children with selective mutism, the Diagnostic and Statistical Manual of Mental Disorders classified selective mutism as an anxiety disorder for the first time in its fifth edition (DSM-5; American Psychiatric Association, 2013).

Although diagnostic criteria in DSM-5 state that selective mutism must not be better accounted for by a communication disorder, the presence of communication problems does not preclude a diagnosis of selective mutism in a particular case. Indeed, it is now widely acknowledged that children with the disorder exhibit a range of structural language deficits and pragmatic and discourse impairments. Cohan et al. (2008) studied 130 children aged 5 to 12 years with selective mutism. The children in this study scored in the clinically significant range for syntax problems on the syntax subscale of the Children's Communication Checklist-2 (Bishop, 2003). Manassis et al. (2007) examined the language skills of 6- to 11-year-old children with selective mutism. These children scored significantly lower on standardised language measures than children with anxiety and normal controls.

Klein et al. (2013) reported an expressive narrative language deficit in 42% of a sample of 33 children aged 5 to 12 years with selective mutism. McInnes et al. (2004) found that children with selective mutism used fewer story elements (i.e. settings, initiating events, internal responses) during their production of narratives than children with social phobia.

Unit 45.1 Primer on selective mutism

(1) The epidemiology of selective mutism exhibits a feature which is not in most communication disorders or conditions that give rise to communication disorders (e.g. ADHD, ASD). What is that feature?

(2) Explain how a background of migration might increase a child's risk of developing selective mutism.

(3) Explain why it is too simplistic to attribute a direct, causal role to anxiety within the aetiology of selective mutism.

(4) The speech and language skills of children with selective mutism are rarely investigated in research studies. Why do you think this is the case?

(5) Respond with *true* or *false* to each of the following statements about language in selective mutism:
  (a) Receptive language skills are superior to expressive language skills.
  (b) Language disorder is related to intellectual disability.
  (c) Syntax and semantics are the most impaired aspects of language.
  (d) Language disorder is related to a theory of mind deficit.
  (e) Children with selective mutism have impaired social communication.

Client history

Mimi was 8 years old when she was referred to the school programme for the treatment of selective mutism. She was repeating her second grade and had displayed three years of silence in regular public school classes by that stage. Since the age of 3, she had not spoken to anyone outside her home. When communication became necessary, Mimi used handwritten notes in class and limited gestures. There was no spoken language used in school either during speech therapy or in individual sessions. However, Mimi did communicate without difficulty with certain family members at home.

Mimi's family situation and relationships were significant in several respects. Mimi's father, who spoke Spanish, left the family home when she was young. When she was 2 years old, Mimi fell and cut the inside of her mouth on the metal leg of a chair. This injury necessitated stitches. Mimi was hospitalised for over a week with a high fever when she was 3 years old. She had many needle sticks during her hospitalisation, and was frightened and did not speak. It was at this stage that Mimi stopped speaking entirely to people outside her immediate family. At 4 years of age, Mimi and her family moved to another state. Mimi's mother remarried. At the time of treatment, Mimi had four older siblings, but was the only child living at home. The relationship between Mimi and her mother was highly enmeshed. They participated jointly in most social activities. Outside the home, Mimi's mother often spoke for her and related her experiences to other people. Mimi's mother encouraged her dependence on her by continuing to bathe her and managing many aspects of her life. Mimi was not required to undertake any chores.

Unit 45.2 Client history

(1) The average age of referral of children with selective mutism is between 6 and 8 years, but the onset of the disorder is usually earlier at preschool (Sluckin, 2000). Mimi's profile is consistent with this typical pattern. What factors may explain the late referral of these children to speech-language pathology?

(2) Notwithstanding her lack of spoken language, certain behaviours suggest that Mimi is still positively inclined towards communication with others. What are those behaviours?

(3) Which feature of Mimi's family background suggests that she exhibits at least one risk factor for selective mutism?

(4) Which features of Mimi's history may have contributed to her anxiety in speaking?

(5) Were there any aspects of Mimi's familial relationships that may have served to perpetuate her mutism once it had developed?

Communication status

At the point of entry to the school programme, Mimi would not talk in public places and on the telephone. She also would not talk to some relatives and even to her best friend, who would sometimes stay overnight at her home. Mimi's reason for not speaking was communicated in a written note: 'When I was little my mother told me don't talk to strangers'. However, a home video-recording of Mimi which was made by her mother revealed that she would speak with animation in that setting.

Like other children with selective mutism, Mimi had speech and language problems. Her communication milestones were reportedly normal. A home video when Mimi was 9 years of age revealed that she had significant phonological and syntactic problems. Mimi distorted the /l/ and /r/ phonemes. She omitted /s/ in plurals, possessives and present tense verbs. Her utterances displayed immature syntax: 'This a boy'; 'This one name Andy'; 'I'm gonna talk about what family do'. These problems had not been addressed in therapy because of her mutism. Mimi had significant pragmatic deficits. Other people had to assume the role of questioner, with Mimi providing only head nods and shakes for 'yes' and 'no', respectively. Mimi's language problems and lack of participation in school placed her at academic risk. At 9 years of age, Mimi should have been in the fourth grade. However, she was only in the third grade and even then was performing at second-grade level in reading, spelling and mathematics.

Unit 45.3 Communication status

(1) The written note that Mimi wrote to explain why she didn't speak is as revealing of her use of language as it is of the reasons for her silence. What aspect of language use does this note indicate is intact in Mimi?

(2) Mimi's communication milestones were reported to be normal. Give *three* examples of such milestones.

(3) Mimi has difficulty with the production of the /l/ and /r/ phonemes. What is this difficulty likely to be? Is its presence in a child of 9 years of age a cause for concern?

(4) In the home video Mimi produces a number of spoken utterances. On the basis of these utterances, identify *three* aspects of immature syntax in Mimi's expressive language.

(5) Mimi has significant pragmatic deficits. Why do you think children with selective mutism are at risk of pragmatic deficits?

Psychological intervention

Mimi was initially seen by a child psychiatry fellow. A total of 10 therapy sessions resulted in improvements in her non-verbal communication skills. As a result of this therapy, Mimi was able to participate in pantomime activities in the classroom, attend with eye contact when spoken to, raise her hand more frequently in class and use more appropriate gesture. However, there was no improvement in vocalisation. Mimi's therapy was eventually taken over by a psychologist. Stimulus fading was used, with Mimi calling the therapist from home and reporting on voice mail. Early treatment sessions focused on establishing rapport and communication by means of written notes and writing on the chalk board. A response initiation approach was adopted within a month. In this approach, children with selective mutism receive the message that they are required to speak. The therapist then arranges a day when the child will spend the majority of it with the therapist. The child must say one word to the therapist before leaving his or her office. After the child speaks, he or she is reunited with his or her family. This session lasted four hours in Mimi's case. During that time, Mimi became very sad, sat curled up in a ball near the door, cried and hid under a chair. She attempted to bargain with her therapist through the use of written notes: 'I promise I will talk Friday'. At nearly five o'clock, she whispered 'I want to go home'. At that point, she was allowed to call her mother from the office phone and ask her to drive her home. Once whispering was established, Mimi's verbalisations were expanded by having her choose what to say. These messages were printed on cards. Mimi agreed to extend her whispering to her speech-language pathologist, her classroom teacher, an aide, and eventually others in the school environment. Other students also became involved in therapy, and Mimi whispered to them. Mimi along with her therapist wrote a puppet show which was performed to the class. Mimi's classroom participation increased – she took part in group discussions, for example – but this was still in a whispered voice.

After a few months, Mimi's therapy began to use shaping. Other vocalisations were encouraged – coughing, making sounds with a kazoo, producing animal sounds for the puppets. Rather than undertake another long day to elicit voice, Mimi agreed to use voice in speech therapy and the classroom to receive rewards. Although Mimi largely continued to whisper, she did begin to use voice on more occasions in response to a reward system. Each half hour, Mimi produced in a 'normal' voice a list of responses that had been compiled by her and her therapist. Some responses were short (e.g. 'please'), while others involved the recitation of the spelling list. If Mimi did not use normal voice, she lost rewards. To generalise her use of full voice, homework assignments were employed. Further rewards were given if Mimi's mother reported that she had used full voice in community settings.

Eventually, Mimi was encouraged to speak each day to one more person beyond school and home.

Unit 45.4 Psychological intervention

(1) Mimi made a number of early gains in non-verbal communication as a result of therapy. Give *three* reasons why gains in Mimi's non-verbal communication skills are to be encouraged.

(2) As part of Mimi's therapy, stimulus fading was used. What is stimulus fading?

(3) The classroom teacher was involved in Mimi's treatment. The teacher made a number of observations about Mimi in the classroom. Several of these observations are presented below. Which of these statements describe behaviours which might inadvertently reinforce Mimi's mutism?
   (a) Mimi earned class points for following classroom rules about not talking.
   (b) Mimi was a willing helper in class.
   (c) Mimi's classmates tended to speak for her and explain to people that she was 'just shy'.
   (d) Other students tried to be like Mimi by not talking.
   (e) Other students occasionally became frustrated by Mimi's silence.

(4) In the transition from whispering to vocalisation, a technique called shaping was used. What is shaping?

(5) A reward system called 'dyno-bucks' was used in Mimi's treatment. This system is a type of contingency management which allowed Mimi to win prizes in a weekly classroom auction. Explain what is meant by 'contingency management'.

Speech and language intervention

Mimi was seen by the speech-language pathologist twice a week for individual treatment. At first, Mimi was encouraged to use gestures in therapy. Pantomime activities and guessing games on themes such as sports and emotions were used. Mimi readily participated in these activities and appeared to enjoy acting things out. She nodded for 'yes' and 'no'. A game called 'Guess Who?' which involved other students was used. It served to initiate non-verbal communication, regulate other's attention and take turns. However, Mimi still did not attempt to initiate communication and used paper and pencil to communicate. The speech-language pathologist encouraged Mimi to record messages and read stories into a tape recorder. Mimi would only make these recordings when the therapist was outside the room. However, she and the therapist jointly listened to the recordings. At the point when Mimi started to use an audible whisper, her articulation, morphology and syntactic errors became the focus of therapy. A consistent reward system was used if Mimi participated by whispering. Along with another student, Mimi participated in question and answer games and activities that used a visual barrier to encourage verbal description. As whispering continued, Mimi became more animated in conversational exchanges and participated more in the classroom and other school settings. Mimi even went as far as whispering loudly into the intercom to announce the arrival of the school buses to the office. Mimi's daily speaking goals were consistently rewarded when they were achieved. Mimi assisted in setting up tasks to achieve the wider use of speech, greater volume, and more substantial verbal interactions. Full voice in school and in the community was achieved by the spring of Mimi's second school year. This was maintained throughout the summer months and when Mimi returned to her regular education setting in the autumn.

Unit 45.5 Speech and language intervention

(1) Respond with *true* or *false* to each of the following statements:
   (a) Mimi's speech and language intervention followed different steps towards vocalisation from those of her psychological intervention.
   (b) Language goals dominated speech and language intervention.
   (c) Generalisation of vocalisation was successfully achieved.
   (d) Mimi's speech and language intervention included contingency management.
   (e) Articulation dominated speech and language intervention.

(2) Mimi enjoyed guessing games on the theme of emotions. Which key cognitive skill must be intact in order for her to participate successfully in these games?
   (a) the ability to inhibit prepotent responses
   (b) the ability to infer the cognitive mental states of others
   (c) the ability to attribute communicative intentions to a speaker
   (d) the ability to infer the affective mental states of others
   (e) the ability to update information in working memory

(3) How would you characterise Mimi's social communication skills?

(4) To what extent do you think Mimi's speech and language problems are contributing to her mutism? Provide evidence to support your answer.

(5) Give *three* reasons why speech-language pathologists should assess and treat children with selective mutism as part of a multidisciplinary team.

Case study 46

Two boys with attention deficit hyperactivity disorder

Introduction

The following exercise is a case study of two boys ('Adam' and 'Abraham') with attention deficit hyperactivity disorder who were studied by Peets (2009). The boys attended primary school special education classes in a large, urban, publicly funded school system in Toronto. These classes were designed to support children with language impairment. The case study is presented in five sections: primer on attention deficit hyperactivity disorder; language in attention deficit hyperactivity disorder; client language status; focus on narrative production – Adam; and focus on narrative production – Abraham.

Primer on attention deficit hyperactivity disorder

Attention deficit hyperactivity disorder (ADHD) is a neurodevelopmental disorder that has its onset in childhood and can persist into adulthood. The disorder is diagnosed on the basis of symptoms of inattention and hyperactivity and impulsivity which are described in the fifth edition of the Diagnostic and Statistical Manual of Mental Disorders (DSM-5; American Psychiatric Association, 2013). Among the behaviours which are used to identify these symptoms are a failure to pay close attention to details, an inability to remain seated in appropriate situations, and difficulty organising tasks and activities. To receive a diagnosis of ADHD, children must have at least six symptoms from either (or both) the inattention criteria or the hyperactivity and impulsivity criteria in DSM-5. Older adolescents and adults must present with at least five symptoms for a diagnosis to be made. ADHD symptoms must not occur exclusively during the course of schizophrenia or another psychotic disorder, and must not be better explained by another mental disorder or by substance intoxication or withdrawal. Unlike earlier editions of DSM, DSM-5 does not contain exclusion criteria for individuals with autism spectrum disorder.

The prevalence of ADHD has been examined in several epidemiological studies. A recent study by Pastor et al. (2015) in the US estimated that in 2011 to 2013, 9.5% of children aged 4–17 years were diagnosed with ADHD. Within this figure, the prevalence of ADHD in children aged 4–5 years, 6–11 years and 12–17 years was 2.7%. 9.5% and 11.8%, respectively. Among all age groups, the prevalence of diagnosed ADHD was more than twice as high in boys as in girls. There is a complex interplay of genetic and non-genetic factors in the aetiology of ADHD. That there is a genetic susceptibility for ADHD is supported by findings of higher rates of ADHD in parents and siblings of affected probands compared to relatives of unaffected controls, and by higher concordance rates for ADHD in monozygotic than in dizygotic twin pairs (Thapar et al., 2012). Lichtenstein et al. (2010) reported concordance rates for ADHD in monozygotic and dizygotic twin boys of 44% and 10%, respectively. Among environmental factors that have been associated with ADHD are maternally related prenatal risks (e.g. alcohol consumption, smoking and drug use in pregnancy), pregnancy and birth complications (e.g. prematurity and low birth weight) and external agents (e.g. infections, exposure to lead and other toxins) (Thapar et al., 2012).

Comorbid conditions are commonly found in ADHD. These conditions can affect the assessment and treatment of ADHD. In the United States, Larson et al. (2011) examined the comorbidities of 5,028 children with ADHD aged 6–17 years. Learning disability was reported in 46% of these children. Other significant comorbidities were conduct disorder (27%), anxiety (18%), depression (14%) and speech problems (12%). Among these children, 33% had one comorbid disorder, while 16% had two comorbid disorders and 18% had three or more comorbid disorders. Giacobini et al. (2016) reported significant psychiatric comorbidity in Swedish children, adolescents and adults with ADHD. Autism spectrum disorders were the most common comorbidities for younger patients, while substance abuse, anxiety and personality disorder were the most common comorbidities in older patients. There are poor academic, vocational and psychosocial outcomes in children with ADHD. Sayal et al. (2015) reported a 27- to 32-point reduction in GCSE scores in children with ADHD, while in boys with the disorder there was more than a twofold increased likelihood of not achieving five good GCSEs. Tervo et al. (2016) reported less education, more involuntary job dismissals and more alcohol abuse at 30 years of age in a group of 122 subjects with ADHD.

Unit 46.1 Primer on attention deficit hyperactivity disorder

(1) Respond with *true* or *false* to each of the following statements about ADHD:
  (a) ADHD has a higher prevalence in boys than in girls.
  (b) ADHD has a higher prevalence in the first-born offspring of parents.
  (c) ADHD has a higher prevalence in bilingual children.
  (d) There is evidence of familial aggregation in ADHD.
  (e) There is evidence that teratogens can increase the risk of ADHD.

(2) Which of the above findings suggests that the aetiology of ADHD cannot be entirely genetic in nature?

(3) Which of the following comorbid conditions in ADHD is an affective disorder?
  (a) autism spectrum disorder
  (b) conduct disorder
  (c) anxiety
  (d) substance use disorder
  (e) depression

(4) Why is it important for speech-language pathologists to have knowledge of comorbidities in ADHD?

(5) Which of the following is *not* an outcome of ADHD?
  (a) alcohol dependence
  (b) poor academic qualifications
  (c) offending behaviour
  (d) psychotic disorder
  (e) non-professional employment

Language in attention deficit hyperactivity disorder

Children with ADHD often have receptive and expressive language impairments. DaParma et al. (2011) examined the scores of 100 children with ADHD aged 6–16 years on the Clinical Evaluation of Language Fundamentals – 4th edn (CELF-4; Semel et al., 2003). Compared to the typical population on whom the CELF-4 is standardised, a greater proportion of children with ADHD obtained scaled scores ≤ 4 (−2 SDs) on a number of receptive and expressive language measures. These children had problems understanding spoken language, following directions and understanding concepts, and understanding grammatical relationships. Children with ADHD also had trouble formulating sentences, recalling words rapidly and performing word association tasks. Reading and written expression are also impaired in ADHD. In a study of 179 children with ADHD aged 6 to 8 years, Sciberras et al. (2014) reported a higher prevalence of language problems than in controls after adjustment for sociodemographic factors and comorbidities. ADHD children with language problems had poorer word reading than children who had ADHD alone. Martinussen and Mackenzie (2015) reported that young people with ADHD scored significantly lower than a comparison group on a standardised measure of reading comprehension. Poor comprehenders with ADHD exhibited weakness in expressive vocabulary and written expression relative to good comprehenders with ADHD.

Pragmatic and discourse skills are also impaired in children with ADHD. Bruce et al. (2006) used a parental questionnaire to examine language and communication skills in 76 children with ADHD. The majority of these children had pragmatic problems. These problems were associated with some of the core aspects of ADHD symptoms, particularly inattention and impulsiveness. Redmond (2004) examined the conversational profiles of children with ADHD and SLI. Children with ADHD were found to produce significantly more mazes and longer mazes than children with SLI or typically developing children. Mazes included false starts, fillers, revisions and repetitions. Discourse production and comprehension problems are also found in children with ADHD. Rumpf et al. (2012) examined the organisation of narratives in children with ADHD. Only one of 9 children with ADHD (11%) was able to verbalise the core aspects of the story adequately. This contrasted with 27% of children with Asperger's syndrome and 82% of healthy controls. This difference in frequencies was significant and pointed to limited coherence in the narratives of children with ADHD (and Asperger's syndrome also). Berthiaume et al. (2010) found that boys with ADHD were less able than comparison peers to draw inferences, particularly explanatory inferences, which link events in a story. They were also less able than peers to monitor their ongoing comprehension of texts.

Unit 46.2 Language in attention deficit hyperactivity disorder

(1) Respond with *true* or *false* to each of the following statements about language in ADHD:
    (a) Expressive language and receptive language are impaired in ADHD.
    (b) The language impairment in ADHD is limited to syntax and semantics.
    (c) Spoken language and written language are impaired in ADHD.
    (d) Conversational deficits are related to the core symptoms of ADHD.
    (e) Story grammar is disrupted in ADHD.

(2) Children with ADHD are at risk of academic underachievement. Which aspect of their language performance might account for reduced achievement?

(3) The following conversational behaviours are found in children with ADHD. Relate each behaviour to inattention or hyperactivity-impulsivity in ADHD:
   (a) The child with ADHD frequently interrupts others in conversation.
   (b) The child with ADHD has difficulty remaining focused during conversations.
   (c) The child with ADHD often talks excessively during conversation.
   (d) The child with ADHD often does not seem to listen when addressed in conversation.
   (e) The child with ADHD often blurts out answers before questions have been completed.

(4) A child with ADHD tells his teacher a story about his trip to school that morning. He describes how he got up, left the house, climbed into the car and then got dressed and had his breakfast. He also introduces characters into his story with expressions such as 'the woman' and 'the small boy'. Which two aspects of narrative production is this child struggling to observe?

(5) Which of the following cognitive skills is likely to be impaired in the child with ADHD who is unable to establish the motivations of characters in a story?
   (a) planning
   (b) theory of mind
   (c) working memory
   (d) organisation
   (e) inhibition

Client language status

The two children with ADHD in this study – Adam and Abraham – are both monolingual English speakers who live in English-speaking families. Both children met criteria for language impairment which were set by the school board. The parents of these children reported that they were late talkers. The listening comprehension and oral expression subtests of the Oral and Written Language Scale (OWLS; Carrow-Woolfolk, 1995) were used to assess expressive and receptive language. Adam and Abraham scored more than 1.5 standard deviations below the mean on the composite language score of the OWLS and had percentile scores of 4 and 3, respectively. The expressive and receptive scores of these children did not differ significantly.

Unit 46.3 Client language status

(1) Adam and Abraham both live in monolingual English-speaking families. Why is it important for the speech-language pathologist to know the language(s) spoken in these children's home environments?

(2) Adam and Abraham both underwent formal language testing. Describe *three* difficulties that the behaviour of children with ADHD might pose during language testing.

(3) Adam and Abraham were assessed using the Oral and Written Language Scale (OWLS). Which of the following are *true* statements about this assessment?

(a) The OWLS is a standardised language assessment.

(b) The OWLS assesses spoken and written language.

(c) The OWLS assesses motor speech production in children.

(d) The OWLS assesses receptive and expressive language.

(e) The OWLS is a parent-completed language checklist.

(4) Adam and Abraham had percentile scores of 4 and 3, respectively, on the OWLS. What do these scores indicate?

(5) Is the OWLS able to provide a comprehensive assessment of Adam's and Abraham's communication skills? Provide support for your answer.

Focus on narrative production – Adam

Adam and Abraham were identified as having pragmatic difficulties. To examine these difficulties, Peets (2009) also analysed the narrative discourse skills of both children. In the extract below, Adam (A) is talking to his teacher (T) about snow tubing. This extract is part of a longer exchange in which Adam successfully engages the other children present, some of whom ask him questions. Adam is very popular among both teachers and his peer group on account of his vivacious and enthusiastic personality.

A: I went to my cousin's house and when I went to my cousin's house that was later when I when I we went back home for um from snow tubing.

T: Can you tell us about snow tubing?

A: Snow tubing is is freaky.

T: Freaky. Tell us what it's like. What do you do?

A: They uh they have a machine that will they have a hooks that will pull you back up and then you have eight tickets you give one of them to (th)em then you got hold onto a rope they have like a little round thing and then you go they put the put the hook inside and then and then it pulls you back up and then you slide down they put they maybe the if you want to stay straight you tell my parents from up there if you want a spin they he spins you.

Unit 46.4 Focus on narrative production – Adam

(1) It was described in 46.2 how children with ADHD produce mazes – language that contains false starts, fillers, revisions and repetitions. Give *one* example of this linguistic behaviour in the above extract.

(2) Is there any evidence in this extract that Adam understands indirect speech acts? Provide support for your answer.

(3) There are a number of structural language deficits in Adam's verbal output. Give *three* examples of such deficits.

(4) Adam's final turn in the above extract is particularly difficult to follow. One reason why this is the case is that he uses pronouns and other expressions which lack a clear referent. Give *three* examples of this behaviour in the above extract.

(5) Autism spectrum disorder is a common comorbidity in children with ADHD. What feature of Adam's behavioural phenotype indicates that a diagnosis of ASD is not appropriate in his case?

Focus on narrative production – Abraham

Abraham is an equally engaging story teller. In the extract below, he relates to his teacher in the presence of other students (S) an interaction he had with his baby brother.

A: Then I throw the ball at my baby brother.
T: Oh why did you do that?
A: So so he can play with it.
T: Did he like you throwing the ball at him?
A: Yeah because I because when I sometimes throw the ball at him he laughs.
T: So you you just threw it gently.
A: Then then he took the pillow.
S: (unspecified turn)
A: Then I said "look out" then I then he throw the pillow in my face!
   (Students laugh)

Unit 46.5 Focus on narrative production – Abraham

(1) Like Adam, Abraham also displays some structural language deficits. One of these deficits involves the use of verbs. Identify *one* instance where Abraham does not use verbs correctly. Is this a consistent feature of Abraham's expressive output?

(2) Respond with *true* or *false* to each of the following statements:
    (a) Abraham can respond to yes–no interrogatives.
    (b) Abraham uses direct reported speech.
    (c) Abraham cannot respond to wh-interrogatives.
    (d) Abraham interjects on the teacher's turns.
    (e) Abraham produces irrelevant utterances.

(3) Abraham uses a number of conjunctions to link events in his story. Give *two* such conjunctions. Indicate the meaning that is expressed by these conjunctions. Which conjunction is used most by Abraham?

(4) What evidence is there in this extract that Abraham displays quite a sophisticated appreciation of the mental states of others?

(5) Abraham appears to confuse some pronouns in this extract. Give *one* example of where this occurs.

Case study 47

Man aged 26 years with schizophrenia

Introduction

The following exercise is a case study of a man of 26 years of age with schizophrenia who was studied by Hella et al. (2013). Schizophrenia is a serious mental illness which has a lifetime prevalence of approximately 0.3% to 0.7% (American Psychiatric Association, 2013). It is diagnosed when two or more of the following symptoms are present: (1) delusions, (2) hallucinations, (3) disorganised speech, (4) grossly abnormal psychomotor behaviour (including catatonia) and (5) negative symptoms (e.g. diminished emotional expression or avolition) (American Psychiatric Association, 2013). The case study is presented in five sections: personal and medical history; clinical discourse analysis; focus on topic management; focus on reference; and discourse deficits in schizophrenia.

Personal and medical history

The client had a long-term doctor–patient relationship with the first author of the study, and was selected for investigation for this reason. His medication regime had previously included clozapine, which had been discontinued because of side effects. During the study, the client was taking a combination of olanzapine and perphenazine. The client had been hospitalised for treatment several times, most recently just one month prior to the interview that formed the basis of this study. He had previously lived in a rehabilitation unit, but a few months prior to interview had moved into his own apartment. He experienced problems with daily activities. The client's diagnosis was confirmed by the first author of the study following a SCID 1 interview (Structured Clinical Interview for DSM-IV Axis 1 Disorders; First et al., 1995). This same transcribed interview was also used to undertake a PANSS assessment (Positive and Negative Syndrome Scale for Schizophrenics; Kay et al., 1988). From the latter assessment, the following scores were obtained: positive symptoms: 25/49; negative symptoms: 26/49; general psychopathology: 46/112; total: 97/210. The client experienced a relapse of psychosis at the time of the study, and a decision on whether or not to send him to in-patient care was being considered.

Unit 47.1 Personal and medical history

(1) Clozapine is an atypical antipsychotic drug that is used when traditional antipsychotics fail to treat schizophrenia. The client in this case study was treated with clozapine but had to discontinue his use of the drug on account of side effects. Some of these side effects must be considered by the speech-language pathologist. State what these side effects are.

(2) The client exhibited positive symptoms during an assessment with PANSS. Which of the following symptoms in schizophrenia are *positive* symptoms?
(a) delusions
(b) avolition
(c) hallucinations
(d) alogia
(e) thought disorder

(3) Which of the following symptoms in schizophrenia is associated with the contribution of unembellished turns in conversation? By what other term is this symptom known?
(a) delusions
(b) avolition
(c) hallucinations
(d) alogia
(e) thought disorder

(4) Which of the following language impairments are typically associated with thought disorder in schizophrenia?
(a) syntactic deficits
(b) word-finding difficulties
(c) phonological deficits
(d) disorganised discourse
(e) morphological deficits

(5) Like many other individuals with schizophrenia, this client has had difficulties with functioning and independent living. It is increasingly recognised that speech-language pathology has an important role to play in improving the functioning and independence of adults with schizophrenia. Which of the following communication skills are targeted during a SLP intervention that is aimed at achieving these outcomes?
(a) word-retrieval skills
(b) expressive syntax skills
(c) social communication skills
(d) semantic categorisation skills
(e) receptive syntax skills

Clinical discourse analysis

The client's communication skills were assessed using a discourse analytic approach. Two conversation analytic concepts – turn and adjacency pair – were also used in the analysis. A rating scale was developed to detect sequences that were difficult for the addressee in the conversational exchange to follow. Called the Overall Comprehensibility of Turn (OCT), it takes into consideration the Gricean maxims of manner, quantity and relevance. Scoring was conducted by post-interview raters who assumed the viewpoint of the addressee. Scores of 0, 1, 2 and 3 represented transparent, slightly opaque, deviant and infelicitous turns, respectively. A slightly opaque turn was somewhat problematic to understand or contained unexpected elements to some extent. A deviant turn posed notable difficulties for comprehension on account of structural deficiencies, missing or vague propositional content, and unexpected associations of topics and/or referents. An infelicitous turn was completely obscure, contained elements which were totally unrelated or which violated the expectations of the interlocutor. Out of a total of 103 client turns which could be scored, 54 were transparent, 32 were slightly opaque, 9 were deviant and 8 were infelicitous. Three sequences with an accumulation of deviant and infelicitous turns will be examined in units 47.3 and 47.4.

Unit 47.2 Clinical discourse analysis

(1) Why is the use of a discourse analytic approach advisable when examining the language and communication skills of clients with schizophrenia?

(2) The authors of this study state that '[t]wo consecutive and semantically linked addressor-addressee turns make up an adjacency pair' (Hella et al., 2013: 3). Is it the case that the two parts of an adjacency pair must be consecutive? Provide evidence to support your answer.

(3) Classify each of the following conversational behaviours as a violation of relevance, quantity and/or manner. Where the violation is one of quantity, further indicate if the behaviour in question is over-informative or under-informative:

    (a) An interlocutor talks at length about his holiday plans in response to a question about his job as a teacher.

    (b) A pedestrian fails to tell a motorist that the road ahead is closed when he is asked for directions to a church.

    (c) An interlocutor is relating a story to a friend but mixes up the order in which he describes the main events.

    (d) A guest at a dinner party talks incessantly about his new Porsche when the topic of conversation is the company's plans to expand into South America.

    (e) A patient does not tell an emergency doctor he is diabetic when he is asked if he has any health problems.

(4) Missing or vague propositional content is part of the definition of a *deviant* turn. Which of the following utterances contain such content? For the utterances that you select, justify your responses.

    (a) A speaker utters 'I would' in response to the question 'Would you like turkey or chicken?'

    (b) Mary tries to dissuade Bill from going to the pub by saying 'Big Jim will be there'.

    (c) Fran has been talking about her close friends Sue and June. Out of the blue she says 'She has such a gorgeous house'.

    (d) When asked if she is going to the prom, Jackie says 'I will be there'.

    (e) Sally asks her mother 'Can I take the car to the shops?'.

(5) According to the definition of turns used in this investigation, is the turn of B in the exchange below transparent, slightly opaque, deviant or infelicitous? Justify your response.

A: Do you like coming to the day centre?
B: Do you like being married?

Focus on topic management

Certain topics dominated the exchange between the client (C) and the first author (a doctor (D)) of the study. These topics were telepathy and harassment, thinking about words and particularly the names of people and places, and music and lyrics. These topics are evident in the two conversational extracts presented in this unit. In these extracts, irrelevant hesitation markers and signs of overlapped speech have been deleted. Authors' clarifying comments are shown in brackets.

Extract 1

D: Your mother has told me that you feel that they [referring to client's paranoid experiences] don't leave you alone.

C: No, they don't. Well, as J. Karjalainen [a Finnish pop musician] sings in his song: 'Do you remember when we played around with telepathy'. I don't know exactly what telepathy means. But maybe I believe in it a little. But, also my mother has to behave herself, but . . . she is sometimes discourteous in her words and she can be a bit rude. It may be the case that I'm the kind of person that speaks aloud a lot and thinks a lot what to say and so . . .

Extract 2

D: Has anybody else ever tried to harm you or tried to lead you to any kind of trouble?

C: Well, I have not thought about that . . . but not [they have not led me] . . . I have seen harm done and stuff, but people, those guys, let me be physically and mentally on my own . . .

D: Have you ever felt you would be especially important or that you would have abilities that no one else has?

C: Well, it's only that my name is John [altered], which happens to be the kind that others are laughing at. They are laughing right to my face, and then . . .

D: Why would they laugh at the name John?

C: Well, in some way that John that you har-har

D: What does John mean?

C: Well I don't know John [aborted utterance] probably . . . it refers to me and that a bit har-har and so on.

D: I can't quite understand. Can you tell what it is . . .

C: Then on the other hand . . .

D: Uh-huh.

C: . . . there are those X-ers [X-er refers to people from area X and is also client's family name] from Y [province capital] but yeah. As a joke, I kind of imagine that it is a kind of sacred relic that I should not be teased for that [laughs].

D: Do you mean that . . .

C: Yeah.

D: . . . that your name is a relic.

C: Or my family name X-er is one, since I am one [i.e. an inhabitant of province X bearing the province name].

D: Yeah, what does it mean . . .

C: Well . . .

D: . . . that it is a relic.

C: Well, it occurs to me all the time that X is the town [literally: municipality] [erroneous statement, confusion of province and hometown names]. It's definitely the town that is called X [erroneous statement repeated with emphasis] which is always seen on the [television] news . . . rolling [makes rolling gestures with arms]

D: Yeah.

C: X, yes. [Yawning] Well, I also do have other names.

D: What names?

C: I'd rather be some Marko, damn it, if I could myself decide upon taking a name.

D: Why would you change your name?

C: Well I don't know. It only occurred to me that it could be cool to be Marko, if not anything else, damn it.

Unit 47.3 Focus on topic management

(1) In extract 1, the client's turn received an OCT score of 2, i.e. it was judged to be deviant. Explain why this is the case.

(2) Although an unexpected topic intrudes into extract 1, the client also exhibits a number of discourse strengths in this extract. These include (a) the use of ellipsis, and (b) the use of anaphoric reference. Give *one* example of each of these discourse features in extract 1.

(3) How would you characterise the client's management of topic in extract 2?

(4) In extract 2, there are two utterances where the propositional content is particularly vague. Identify the utterances in question, and explain why their propositional content is vague.

(5) The OCT is based on three Gricean maxims: relevance, quantity and manner. However, it is clear that a fourth Gricean maxim – quality – is also problematic for the client in extract 2. Where in this extract is there an anomaly related to the quality maxim?

Focus on reference

A number of referential anomalies (as well as strengths) were identified on the part of the client. Further referential anomalies are evident in extract 3 below.

Extract 3

C: I've been thinking about those that . . . going to work I'm always thinking about. Then some people, well they are stars and the like, they play soccer and we then watch, or they watch it and such like that.

D: Yes, who are watching?

C: Trades/professions I kind of think about.

D: Uh-huh.

C: They are a bit like a group of their own and such. They are jobless.

D: Uh-uh, who are you talking about now?

C: Well, I'm thinking about these kind of things. My father works at the city water works. Workers come to my mind sometimes.

D: Yeah.

C: That's it. Well, that I would want to be a bit better educated, but I am not. Then I am not extremely clever, perhaps. In a way that sometimes, well yes, I do watch something. A group of people can come up with wise things but . . . things are not like that now.

D: Yes. What . . .

C: [yawning] Well, I do have a trade school diploma.

Unit 47.4 Focus on reference

(1) This exchange with the client is difficult to follow on account of referential anomalies. Give *three* examples where the client uses terms which lack a clear referent.

(2) Referential anomalies are not the only reason why this exchange with the client is difficult to follow. There is also an abundance of vague and non-specific vocabulary in use. Give *five* examples of such vocabulary.

(3) Referential anomalies exist alongside a number of intact discourse skills. Such skills include: (a) topicalisation; (b) ellipsis; and (c) anaphoric reference. Give *one* example of each of these discourse skills in extract 3.

(4) Is the client aware that the doctor is having difficulty following him? What evidence are you basing your answer on?

(5) Problems with topic management are also evident in this extract. How would you characterise the client's development of topic in this extract?

Discourse deficits in schizophrenia

The investigators in this study made a number of important observations about the discourse behaviours of this client. The first observation is that this client exhibits language and discourse deficits that are typical of positive-state schizophrenia. A second, and probably more critical, observation is that what appears to be highly disordered discourse on the part of this client is more a reflection of limitations in the addressee's discourse model. Specifically, when an off-line analysis of the client's discourse is performed, it is not as disorganised as an on-line interpretation of his discourse suggests. In this way, although extract 1 contained what appeared to be an unexpected topic intrusion, 'an analysis of background knowledge and contextual links revealed that the intrusive utterance was not as irrelevant as it seemed to be in the on-line situation' (2013: 7). It was merely that these links were not active in the addressee's discourse model. Similarly, in extract 2, the gradual, radial extension of topics in this exchange may be seen to arise from an overreliance on semantic associations which are like those seen in normal language. It is simply that the client is developing lexical–conceptual links that are 'too implicit, extensive or complicated from the viewpoint of a co-speaker' (2013: 7). Finally, in extract 3, the abundance of instances of obscure reference is also explicable in terms of the addressee's discourse model. Quite simply, it would be possible to recover the referents of the expressions in this extract with the addition of further information and structure to the discourse. The point, Hella et al. (2013: 8) argue, is the same throughout: 'disorganized discourse is not merely a consequence of thought disorder of a schizophrenia patient. Rather, it should be regarded as a phenomenon of mutual interaction with possible divergent discourse models.'

Unit 47.5 Discourse deficits in schizophrenia

(1) The investigators concluded that this client exhibits discourse behaviours which are typical of positive-state schizophrenia. Identify these behaviours in the following list:
  (a) referential anomalies
  (b) topic intrusions
  (c) echolalic utterances
  (d) circumlocutions
  (e) lack of linear ordering of propositions

(2) In extract 1, the topic of music intrudes into the client's discourse after having been an earlier topic of conversation. Why might this occur?

(3) The investigators in this study believed that the client's overreliance on semantic associations was responsible for the gradual, radial extension of topics in extract 2. Which of the following terms describes the linguistic behaviour in schizophrenia where sound and/or meaning associations between words are developed?
  (a) circumlocution
  (b) verbal perseveration
  (c) glossomania
  (d) echolalia
  (e) phonemic paraphasia

(4) The presence of multiple instances of obscure reference in extract 3 might have a cognitive explanation in addition to the explanation advanced by the study's investigators. Which of the following cognitive factors might account for this linguistic behaviour?
  (a) working memory deficits
  (b) theory of mind deficits
  (c) difficulty inhibiting a prepotent response
  (d) planning deficits
  (e) impaired self-regulation

(5) The conclusion of this study is that schizophrenic discourse would not appear so disorganised if there were greater alignment between the discourse models of the client and the doctor. This conclusion has an important implication for the management of clients with schizophrenia, including the SLP management of these clients. What do you think this implication is?

Case study 48

Woman aged 24 years with bipolar disorder

Introduction

The following exercise is a case study of a woman ('WM') who was studied by Manning (1999). WM was diagnosed with DSM-IV bipolar disorder not otherwise specified. This diagnosis is used for individuals who experience hypomania without a history of major depressive disorder or a manic episode. WM's condition responded well to valproate therapy. The case study is presented in five sections: primer on bipolar disorder; communication and cognition in bipolar disorder; client history and family background; clinical presentation, diagnosis and treatment; focus on discourse in bipolar disorder.

Primer on bipolar disorder

Bipolar disorder (formerly known as 'manic depression') is a psychiatric disorder in which the patient's mood alters between manic episodes (characterised by euphoria, restlessness, poor judgement and risk-taking behaviour), depressive episodes (characterised by depression, anxiety and hopelessness) and episodes of normal mood (known as euthymia). The disorder is diagnosed on the basis of criteria contained in the Diagnostic and Statistical Manual of Mental Disorders (DSM), which is now in its fifth edition (American Psychiatric Association, 2013). When WM received her diagnosis, it was on the basis of criteria contained in the fourth edition of DSM. According to Angst (2013), one of the shortcomings of this edition was the large proportion of treated patients who had to be allocated to the vague 'not otherwise specified' group. WM is one such patient. In DSM-5, several new subthreshold groups of depression, bipolar disorders and mixed states are now operationally defined (Angst, 2013).

The prevalence of bipolar disorder in the population varies between studies. In a New Zealand study, Wells et al. (2010) reported that the lifetime prevalence of bipolar disorder (types I + II) is 1.7%. Kozloff et al. (2010) recorded a lifetime prevalence of 3.0% in 15–24-year-olds in a Canadian sample. A similar lifetime prevalence of 3.0% was reported by Calvó-Perxas et al. (2015) in a population-based sample in Catalonia, Spain. Reviewing data from the Cross-National Collaboration on major depression and bipolar disorder, Grant and Weissman (2007) found that there were no consistent sex differences in bipolar disorder. In a study of 1,665 subjects with type-I bipolar disorder, Baldessarini et al. (2012) reported that the median age at onset was 23.0 years while the average age was 25.7 ± 11.3 years. Thesing et al. (2015) found that increased family history of psychiatric disorders is associated with earlier age at onset, while negative stressors are associated with later age at onset of the first (hypo)manic episode.

Genetic and environmental risk factors for bipolar disorder have been identified. A history of bipolar affective disorder and other psychiatric disorders, including schizophrenia and schizoaffective disorder, in parents or siblings, is a risk factor for bipolar disorder. Päären et al. (2014) found that a family history of bipolar disorder was the strongest predictor of developing bipolar disorder in adulthood among adolescents with mood disorders. Mortensen et al. (2003) reported that people with a first-degree relative with bipolar affective disorder had a 13.63-fold increased risk of bipolar affective disorder. These investigators also found that children who experienced maternal loss before their fifth birthday had a 4.05 increased risk of bipolar affective disorder. Paksarian et al. (2015) found that the number of years of paternal separation is positively associated with bipolar disorder. Comorbid conditions are common in bipolar disorder. Significant comorbid conditions in community studies are anxiety, substance use and conduct disorders, while eating disorders, ADHD, ASD and Tourette's disorder are comorbid conditions in clinical samples (McElroy, 2004). Migraine, thyroid illness, obesity, diabetes and cardiovascular disease are the most common medical comorbidities (McElroy, 2004).

Unit 48.1 Primer on bipolar disorder

(1) Which of the following statements describes a reason why speech-language pathologists should have a sound working knowledge of bipolar disorder?
   (a) Bipolar disorder has direct implications for language and communication.
   (b) Clients with bipolar disorder often have swallowing problems.
   (c) Clients with bipolar disorder often have motor speech disorders.
   (d) Bipolar disorder is a significant comorbidity in many conditions assessed and treated by speech-language pathologists.
   (e) Bipolar disorder has comorbid conditions of relevance to speech-language pathologists.

(2) Faced with growing budgetary pressures, healthcare systems are increasingly demanding that the provision of services to clients be justified in economic and other terms. How might the provision of speech-language pathology services to clients with bipolar disorder be justified in these terms?

(3) Respond with *true* or *false* to each of the following statements about bipolar disorder:
   (a) Bipolar disorder is only found in adults.
   (b) Bipolar disorder affects men and women in roughly equal numbers.
   (c) Bipolar disorder is diagnosed on the basis of criteria in DSM-5.
   (d) Bipolar disorder has the same lifetime prevalence as schizophrenia.
   (e) Bipolar disorder has an exclusively genetic aetiology.

(4) Name *two* comorbid conditions in bipolar disorder in which there are significant language and communication problems that are assessed and treated by speech-language pathologists.

(5) Clients with bipolar disorder can be treated with lithium carbonate. Which of the following is a potential side effect of this drug?
   (a) dysfluency
   (b) aphonia
   (c) dysarthria

    (d) aphasia

    (e) dysphagia

Communication and cognition in bipolar disorder

Increasingly, studies are documenting a range of communication problems in clients with bipolar disorder. These problems include difficulties with the reception and expression of language. In a study of the prevalence of speech and language problems among patients receiving care from a mental health unit, Emerson and Enderby (1996) recorded language comprehension problems in 33% of their patients with bipolar disorder. Difficulties with spontaneous speech, picture description, naming and fluency were observed in 25%, 25%, 16% and 8% of bipolar patients, respectively. Radanovic et al. (2008) examined the performance in language tests of 33 euthymic elderly patients with bipolar disorder but no dementia. When compared with healthy controls, these patients exhibited a mild but significant impairment in language-related ability scores. In a study that analysed the speech output of schizophrenic, bipolar and depressive patients, Lott et al. (2002) found illogicality in 62.1% of bipolar patients, the highest figure of all three psychiatric diagnoses. Poverty of speech was present in 6.9% of bipolar patients. Poulin et al. (2007) reported the unusual case of a patient with bipolar disorder who presented with agrammatism and foreign accent syndrome.

Language impairments are not just a feature of adult-onset bipolar disorder but are also found in children. McClure et al. (2005) found that paediatric outpatients with bipolar disorder performed more poorly than healthy comparison subjects on the pragmatic judgement subtest of the Comprehensive Assessment of Spoken Language. Sigurdsson et al. (1999) found that adolescents who developed early-onset bipolar disorder were significantly more likely to have experienced delayed language than a group of control subjects with depression but without psychotic features. As well as language problems, motor speech disorders such as dysarthria have also been documented in clients with bipolar disorder. In some cases at least, these disorders appear to be related to the client's drug regimen. Bond et al. (1982) reported the case of a 19-year-old patient who developed persistent dysarthria with coexisting apraxia while taking high dose haloperidol and lithium carbonate. Swallowing disorders are also common in clients with bipolar disorder. Regan et al. (2006) reported that 27% of individuals with bipolar disorder in their study exhibited overt signs of oropharyngeal dysphagia.

There is growing evidence that clients with bipolar disorders exhibit certain cognitive deficits. Some of these deficits involve impairments of executive functions. Peters et al. (2014) examined 68 subjects who met DSM-IV criteria for bipolar I disorder in a depressed or euthymic state. Significant impairment in every domain of executive functioning was found in these subjects. Peters et al. concluded that executive functioning problems are not entirely mood-state dependent. Other cognitive deficits take the form of theory of mind (ToM) impairments. Paediatric patients with type I bipolar disorder have been shown to exhibit deficits in the ability to understand another's mental state, with impaired ToM performance associated with poorer interpersonal functioning (Schenkel et al., 2014). Deficits in emotion recognition and theory of mind have been found in manic, depressed and euthymic bipolar subjects (Samamé, 2013). What relationship, if any, these cognitive deficits have to language impairments in bipolar disorder is uncertain at this time.

Unit 48.2 Communication and cognition in bipolar disorder

(1) Respond with *true* or *false* to each of the following statements about language in bipolar disorder:
  (a) Impairments affect only the expression of language.
  (b) Pragmatic aspects of language may be impaired.
  (c) Language is only impaired during manic and depressive episodes.
  (d) Structural levels of language are unimpaired.
  (e) Language may be impaired during periods of euthymia.

(2) Some of the subjects studied by Lott et al. displayed poverty of speech. What is poverty of speech?

(3) Clients with bipolar disorder can sometimes have iatrogenic dysarthria. Define the term 'iatrogenic dysarthria'.

(4) Explain why Peters et al. concluded that executive functioning problems in bipolar disorder are not entirely mood-state dependent.

(5) Little is known about the relationship between cognitive deficits in bipolar disorder and language impairments. Explain how a theory of mind (ToM) impairment might contribute to pragmatic deficits in bipolar disorder.

Client history and family background

WM is a 24-year-old woman. She has been married for one year to a law enforcement officer. The marriage is her first but her husband's third marriage. Her husband's second wife and child from that marriage live nearby. WM has a difficult relationship with her husband's ex-wife. WM and her husband have a 9-month-old child together. The pregnancy and delivery were uncomplicated. WM reported that her problems with mood began after the birth of her child. WM's general state of health is good. She takes birth control pills and has migraine headaches without aura. These have increased in frequency and duration since giving birth. WM is generally successful in treating her headaches with ibuprofen and rest. She smokes two or three packs of cigarettes per day but does not drink alcohol. She has never used marijuana, cocaine or other illicit substances. She drinks four caffeinated soft drinks per day.

Many of WM's relatives have experienced mood or anxiety problems. Her paternal grandfather was hospitalised on one occasion in a state mental health facility. He was diagnosed with manic depression. WM's father was an alcoholic. WM described him as being mercurial and impulsive, and prone to outbursts and violent behaviour even during extended periods of sobriety. Several other male relatives abused alcohol or cocaine.

Unit 48.3 Client history and family background

(1) Name *one* respect in which WM complies with the demographic profile of individuals who are most likely to develop bipolar disorder.

(2) WM exhibits a common medical comorbidity in bipolar disorder. What is that comorbidity?

(3) Name a significant comorbidity in bipolar disorder which WM does not exhibit.

(4) Which risk factor for bipolar disorder is evident in WM's case?

(5) WM's mood problems had their onset after the birth of her child. What evidence is there that childbirth can serve as a trigger for bipolar disorder?

Clinical presentation, diagnosis and treatment

WM presented with nervousness, headache and insomnia. She reported having difficulty dealing with stressful situations and controlling her temper. She also experienced periods of sadness which were often unexplained. These periods could last a week and could be intense, occurring all day every day. WM reported that she normally 'bounced back' from them. On occasion, her sadness was accompanied by a restless energy and irritability which could result in arguments with her husband's ex-wife. These periods of increased energy could rapidly switch back to an intense, depressed mood. When WM was depressed, she slept excessively and would overeat. She also isolated herself, was unable to get things done and would let the housework go. When depressed, WM was also excessively sensitive to feelings of rejection by others. However, her mood could be lifted temporarily if she engaged in activities she enjoyed. These periods of depressed mood had started since the birth of her child. WM reported that she was cheerful and outgoing prior to this time. There was no prior treatment for mood or anxiety problems.

At the initial interview, WM was dramatic and animated. She spoke for seven minutes uninterrupted in response to the question "What brings you here to see us today?". Her speech was moderately pressured and she changed topics several times. WM was affectively labile and would alternately laugh and cry. There were elements of depression and hypomania in her mood. WM reported frenzied activity into the early hours of the morning. She would talk to friends on the phone and plan social outings. After a period of rest for three or four hours, she would wake up with a pressured desire to 'get things done'. WM was often tearful and irritable during the day. Her judgement was not seriously impaired and she was not involved in self-damaging activities. Reality testing revealed no impairments.

WM was diagnosed with DSM-IV bipolar disorder not otherwise specified. She was prescribed divalproex sodium. After seven days, her headaches stopped and a normal sleep pattern was restored. WM reported greater emotional resilience and felt much less irritable. Over the next four weeks, improvement continued and her depressed moods disappeared. With stabilisation of her mood, WM was able to focus on her psychosocial difficulties with a clinical social worker. After two months of treatment, WM briefly discontinued valproate because of weight gain. Because her mood was normal, she felt that medication might no longer be necessary. The option of discontinuing medication altogether or changing to lithium or carbamazepine was considered. Rather than discontinue valproate therapy and risk a reoccurrence of symptoms with all their negative implications for her job and impending legal issues (WM had decided to get a divorce), WM decided to keep taking her medication and made lifestyle changes (diet and exercise) instead.

Unit 48.4 Clinical presentation, diagnosis and treatment

(1) Describe *three* of WM's non-verbal behaviours which are indicative of a depressed state.

(2) During the initial interview WM displayed pressured speech. What is pressured speech?

(3) Was WM's verbal behaviour during the initial interview indicative of depression or hypomania in her mood?

(4) Respond with *true* or *false* to each of the following statements about WM's communicative skills:
  (a) WM makes appropriate use of turn-taking in conversation.
  (b) WM displays problems with topic management.
  (c) WM exhibits marked deficits in expressive syntax.
  (d) WM displays poverty of speech during the initial interview.
  (e) WM displays clanging during the initial interview.

(5) Did WM struggle to adhere to Gricean maxims during the initial interview? Provide support for you answer.

Focus on discourse in bipolar disorder

Like many other communication disorders, disordered language in clients with bipolar disorder is most usefully examined at the level of discourse. It is during conversation, narratives and other forms of discourse that features such as poverty of speech, pressured speech and referential anomalies are most evident. The following extracts are taken from an interview between a clinical psychology researcher (S) and a 33-year-old woman (B) with mania who was studied by Swartz and Swartz (1987). S is university educated, English-speaking and divorced. The interview was conducted three days after S's admission to a locked women's ward in a large psychiatric hospital. Although S was treated with phenothiazines and lithium, her state had not altered since her admission.

Transcription notation

/	a single slash marks tone–unit boundaries
(. . .)	single brackets indicate taped discourse not included in the transcript
((. . .))	inaudible discourse
hesit-	A dash marks an interruption of a word or phrase not accompanied by a pause
(LAUGHS)	capital letters in brackets indicate paralinguistic phenomena or non-verbal events

Extract 1

S: where have you worked here /
  (. . .)
B: I've last worked last Monday / Nadine Gordimer / signed the admission / ((. . .)) if it's Monday / it must be March / surely it must be March / surely it must be March / surely it must be March / how would you spell Jimmy / my father's name Jimmy /

S: J-i-m-m-y / is that right /

B: or i-e /

S: or i-e / e-y

B: you're right / (REPEATS HER OWN NAME) /

S: sure / (OFFERS S A CIGARETTE) no / I won't have another one / thanks /

B: I bet you will light my cigarette for me / the right way /

S: do you want me to light it for you /

B: a woman would do it that way / a woman would do it that way /

S: light /

B: yes thank you / you watched the same programme on television / as I did / didn't you /

S: which one

B: ((. . .))

S: I don't / I don't have a television /

B: not yet /

S: what were you thinking of / which programme /

B: ((. . .)) you recognise those / who recognise you first / don't you /

S: yes /

B: have you ever been in a locked up ward /

Extract 2

B: are my eyes green or blue /

S: they look - /

B: grey /

S: in between to me / grey /

B: I was born with blue eyes /

S: were you /

B: with my daddy's blue eyes / and my mummy's green eyes / my mummy never let me wear green / she never let me wear green / she never let me wear green / did she / she never let me wear green / did she / ((. . .)) is my mother still alive / is my mother still alive / is my mother still alive /

S: is she /

B: she should be / because she phoned this morning / didn't he phone this morning / she phoned this morning / my daddy ((. . .)) /

S: well / you father brought you those / (CIGARETTES)

B: yesterday he did / yesterday must have been Sunday / if it's Sunday / it must have been the 2nd of March / it's March /

Unit 48.5 Focus on discourse in bipolar disorder

(1) Is there any evidence in these extracts that B does not understand the researcher's questions? Provide support for your answer.

(2) Give *one* example in these extracts where B introduces a topic only to quickly abandon it.

(3) Use data from the above extracts to support each of the following statements:
   (a) B makes appropriate use of linguistic politeness.
   (b) B displays some problems with orientation for time.

    (c) B uses grammatical ellipsis.

    (d) B engages in self-initiated repair of his utterances.

    (e) B makes infelicitous use of questions.

(4) Some of B's verbal output is difficult to follow on account of referential anomalies. Where is this particularly evident in the above extracts?

(5) At what point in the above extracts does B appear to be led from one topic or idea to another on the basis of semantic associations between words?

Appendix A

Answers to questions

Unit 1.1 Primer on cleft lip and palate

(1) (a) true; (b) true; (c) false; (d) false; (e) true
(2) A submucous cleft palate typically involves three deformities: a bifid uvula, a notched posterior hard palate and muscular diastasis of the velum. The majority of individuals with this type of cleft are asymptomatic, although approximately 15% can have velopharyngeal insufficiency (Hopper et al., 2007).
(3) Intellectual disability is often a feature of the syndromes in which cleft palate occurs, e.g. velocardiofacial syndrome (De Smedt et al., 2007). The presence of intellectual disability poses a further compromise to speech acquisition and language development in children who have syndromic clefts of the palate, and is thus of concern to speech-language pathologists.
(4) The two factors which are central to this debate are (1) the benefit of achieving normal velopharyngeal function to optimise speech development against (2) the potential disadvantage of impaired facial growth secondary to early surgical trauma (Hopper et al., 2007).
(5) parts (a), (d) and (e)

Unit 1.2 Speech, language and hearing in cleft lip and palate

(1) parts (a), (c) and (e)
(2) To achieve the articulation of oral plosives, an active articulator (e.g. the tongue) rises and seals firmly against a passive articulator (e.g. the alveolar ridge), completely obstructing the oral airflow. Air pressure then builds up behind this obstruction. However, this build-up of air pressure is only possible when there is complete closure of the velopharyngeal port and air cannot escape through any other means. This situation does not obtain in children with cleft palate. The presence of a short, immobile velum permits intra-oral air to escape through the velopharyngeal port. Also, fistulae can develop in the palate following surgery, and these may also permit the loss of air into the nasal cavities. To avoid this loss of air pressure, children with cleft palate often shift the articulation of oral plosives to the glottis. The glottis is often the only place of articulation in the vocal tract where complete closure of the airstream and build-up of air pressure can be achieved.
(3) The toddlers with cleft palate in this study are selecting to produce words which begin with sonorants as these consonant sounds are easier for them to produce than obstruents.
(4) Three reasons why children with cleft palate are at risk of language delay:

    (i) lengthy periods of hospitalisation – children with cleft palate may have many other medical complications that require hospital treatment. This is particularly the case in children with syndromic cleft palate. If children are hospitalised for weeks or even months after birth, they are not receiving normal language stimulation and are thus at risk of language delay.

    (ii) intellectual disability – intellectual disability is present in many of the syndromes in which cleft palate is a feature. Language acquisition is compromised in children with intellectual disability.

    (iii) speech disorder and hearing loss – impaired speech and hearing have an adverse effect on language acquisition.

(5) (a) false; (b) true; (c) true; (d) false; (e) true

Unit 1.3 Client history

(1) Rachel was born 11 weeks prematurely. Low gestational age is more frequent among newborns with oral clefts than in newborns with no cleft (Wyszynski and Wu, 2002).

(2) Rachel has an isolated cleft of the palate. This type of cleft is more commonly found in girls. So Rachel's cleft type is consistent with the findings of studies of sex differences in clefting.

(3) (a) true; (b) false; (c) false; (d) true; (e) true

(4) Children with cleft palate are at an increased risk of hyperfunctional voice disorders. This is because they misuse their vocal folds in an effort to close the velopharyngeal port or to compensate for poor velopharyngeal closure.

(5) A pharyngoplasty achieves reduction in the velopharyngeal port with no disruption of the velum. It is a surgical procedure for the correction of velopharyngeal incompetence. It is most suitable for patients who have poor medial excursion of the lateral pharyngeal walls and a short anteroposterior component of velar competency (Hopper et al., 2007).

Unit 1.4 Focus on phonological analysis – part 1

(1) Phonotactic structures: 'glasses' CCVCVC; 'string' CCCVC; 'matches' CVCVC. Rachel is able to replicate these phonotactic structures in her spoken productions. Rachel clearly has sufficient phonological knowledge to ensure that each segment in the adult target form is marked in some way, even if that way involves the use of segments that are phonetically distant from those of the target form.

(2) Rachel signals a contrast between the alveolar nasal /n/ and the alveolar plosives /t/ and /d/ through the use of a uvular nasal /ɴ/ and glottal plosive /ʔ/, respectively. This can be seen in the word-initial segments of the following examples:

    'nose' [ɴəʊʐ̊]

    'teaspoon' [ˈʔiʐ̊bʉɴ]

    'dog' [ʔɒʔʰ]

(3) The contrast between the velar nasal /ŋ/ and the velar plosives /k/ and /g/ is also signalled by the use of a uvular nasal /ɴ/ and glottal plosive /ʔ/, respectively. This can be seen in the word-final segments in 'ring' and 'dog' and the word-initial segment in 'cat':

'ring' [ʊɪɴ]
'dog' [ʔɒʔ]
'cat' [ʔæʔ]

(4) In the same way that Rachel uses the glottal plosive /ʔ/ to realise alveolar and velar plosives, she also uses the glottal plosive to realise the voiceless bilabial plosive /p/. This can be seen in the word-initial segment in 'pen' [ʔeɴ]. On occasion, Rachel provides her listeners with an additional visual clue as to the target bilabial segment that she is attempting to produce. She achieves this through the coarticulation of a bilabial closure as can be seen in word-initial and word-medial positions in 'paper' [ˈp͡ʔeɪp͡ʔə].

(5) Apart from glottal stops, bilabial segments are realised as follows in Rachel's speech: [m, ɓ, ʘ, p̃ʰ]. With the exception of [ʘ], what these sounds have in common is that they all involve some degree of nasal airflow. The realisation which is particularly unusual is [ʘ] (and [ʔ͡ʘ]) for /p/. Here, Rachel is using a velaric airstream mechanism to mimic the voiceless bilabial plosive. Because this is a late-appearing feature of Rachel's speech, it is thought that this has arisen as a result of speech therapy which is directed at replacing the glottal stop with /p/.

Unit 1.5 Focus on phonological analysis – part 2

(1) The approximants /j/ and /w/ are correctly realised in Rachel's speech, e.g. 'yes' [jɛʔ] and 'why' [waɪ]. It has already been stated that stops are realised word initially by the glottal plosive [ʔ]. Alveolar fricatives /s/ and /z/ and the postalveolar fricative /ʃ/ are consistently realised in word-initial position as [ɕ̟], e.g. 'shop' [ɕ̟jɒp̃ʰ]. So Rachel does have an effective articulatory strategy for signalling a contrast between stop, fricative and approximant sounds.

(2) The stop–affricate contrast is realised in word-initial position by [ʔ] and [ʔj], respectively. Rachel separately marks the stop and fricative elements in an affricate, e.g. 'chair' [ʔjɛə] and 'jam' [ʔjæm]. Moreover, she displays remarkable consistency in that the stop element in affricates is replaced by the glottal stop in the same way that individual stops are glottalised. Once again, although Rachel's productions are phonetically distant from the target in each case, she is nevertheless able to signal a contrast between stops and affricates.

(3) Rachel's alveolar and postalveolar fricatives are consistently realised as [ɕ̟], e.g. 'Sue' [ɕ̟u] and 'shoe' [ɕ̟u]. So Rachel has not succeeded in consistently signalling an alveolar–postalveolar contrast in her production of fricatives following therapy. However, her post-therapy production is still an improvement on her pre-therapy production in two ways. First, she has succeeded in bringing forward the place of fricative articulation from earlier pharyngeal realisations. Second, Rachel sometimes labialises postalveolar fricatives to signal a contrast between them and alveolar fricatives.

(4) The voicing contrast is marked for the bilabial plosives /p/ and /b/. However, there is no voicing contrast observed for the alveolar plosives /t/ and /d/ or the velar plosives /k/ and /g/. The word-initial phoneme in the productions of 'tea', 'dig', 'key' and 'go' is the glottal stop [ʔ]. Rachel variously signals a voicing contrast between /f/ and /v/. On some occasions, she uses the approximant [ʋ] for /v/ (e.g. 'cover' [ˈʔʊʋə]). On other occasions, a voicing distinction is marked by differing forces

of articulation, with /v/ realised as the strong articulation [f] (e.g. 'a van' [ə ˈfæɴ]) in contrast with the weakly articulated [f] (e.g. 'laughing' [ˈæfɪɴ]).

(5) part (d)

<h2>Case study 2 Girl aged 3;8 years with Kabuki make-up syndrome</h2>

Unit 2.1 History and clinical presentation

(1) (a) The fact that Louise had to have transtympanic drains fitted at 11 and 18 months and then again at 2 years suggests the presence of an otological abnormality; (b) conductive hearing loss; (c) The placement of transtympanic drains serves to ventilate the middle ear. This prevents the build-up of mucus in the middle ear, which can impede the vibration of the ear ossicles, known as the malleus, incus and stapes.

(2) The measurement of otoacoustic emissions can be used to test for the presence of sensorineural hearing loss. The presence of these emissions in Louise's case suggests that the outer hair cells of the cochlea are intact and functioning normally.

(3) Yes, Louise's middle ear defect is related to her palatal abnormality. The presence of a submucous cleft palate suggests a defect of the palatal muscles. It is the contraction of the tensor veli palatini muscles which causes the Eustachian tube to open, permitting ventilation of the middle ear.

(4) Yes, Louise has a generalised hypotonia which could cause a speech disorder of neurogenic aetiology.

(5) Kabuki make-up syndrome is caused by mutations of the MLL2 gene. This gene codifies for an enzyme that regulates embryogenesis and tissue development. This explains the multiple congenital anomalies in the syndrome: abnormal facial features; skeletal anomalies; dermatoglyphic abnormalities; intellectual disability; and postnatal growth deficiency.

Unit 2.2 Clinical assessment

(1) (a) Reynell Developmental Language Scales; (b) GRBAS scale; (c) McCarthy Developmental Scales

(2) During this procedure, a flexible nasolaryngoscope is passed along the nasal passages. It allows the otorhinolaryngologist to directly observe the anatomy of the nasal passages, pharynx and larynx as well as visualise aspects of laryngeal function.

(3) The perceptual attribute is pitch.

(4) It is important for the depicted objects and actions to be part of Louise's vocabulary. If these depicted items are not within her vocabulary, Louise's failure to name them may be related more to vocabulary limitations than to any failure of speech production.

(5) part (b)

Unit 2.3 Communication and cognition profile

(1) *kiss the doll*: comprehension of action–object semantic relation; *beside*: comprehension of spatial preposition; *smallest*: comprehension of terms relating to the size of objects

(2) This particular passive sentence poses difficulty for Louise because it describes an implausible event in the world. Louise can clearly comprehend passive sentences when they describe plausible world events.

(3) part (c)

(4) *will come* (not produced: future tense); *cups* (produced: regular plural noun); *mice* (not produced: irregular plural noun); *dog* (produced: singular noun); *gone* (not produced: past participle); *she* (produced: personal pronoun); *run* (produced: infinitive form); *walks* (not produced: third-person singular verb); *John likes oranges and Mary likes apples* (not produced: compound sentence involving coordination)

(5) parts (d) and (e)

Unit 2.4 Focus on speech production

(1) The hypernasality and nasal emission in Louise's speech is most likely to be related to the presence of a submucous cleft palate. However, given that Louise also exhibits some hypotonia, the involvement of neurological factors cannot be discounted in this articulatory deviance.

(2) (a) Frication; (b) Stopping; (c) Fronting; (d) Backing
   'kruis': frication; 'kop': fronting

(3) Progressive assimilation: /siᵛɑʀɛt/ → /sizɑʀɛt/
   Regressive assimilation: /fits/ → /sis/
   Metathesis: /ᵛitər/ → /ʀitə/
   Syllable deletion: /wɔlkən/ → /wɔk/
   Final consonant deletion: /jɔŋən/ → /ɔŋə/

(4) Word initial /kr/ in 'tap' and 'cross': /kr/ undergoes cluster reduction in 'tap' and frication in 'cross'
   Word medial /rst/ in 'sausages' and 'brush': /rst/ is reduced to /s/ in 'sausages' and to /t/ in 'brush'
   Final syllable /ən/ in 'clouds' and 'boy': /ən/ is deleted in 'clouds' and reduced to /ə/ in 'boy'
   Word initial /k/ in 'head' and 'clock': /k/ undergoes fronting in 'head' and frication in 'clock'
   In short, there is considerable variability in Louise's speech production with one and the same target being differently realised on separate occasions.

(5) 'worsten' /wəs/ – cluster reduction and syllable deletion
   'wolken' /wɔk/ – cluster reduction and syllable deletion
   'jongen' /ɔŋə/ – initial and final consonant deletion

Unit 2.5 Clinical intervention

(1) parts (b) and (c)

(2) There is some basis for the inclusion of a treatment based on principles of motor learning of the type used to treat apraxia of speech. Louise displays high variability in the production of sound distortions which is a feature of apraxia of speech. Also, the presence of a slight general hypotonia suggests that there may be a neurogenic aetiology to Louise's speech production difficulties. A neurogenic aetiology is posited to exist in apraxia of speech.

(3) A phonological treatment that could be used with Louise is the Cycles Phonological Remediation Approach (Hodson, 2010). This is a prominent intervention for the treatment of severe speech sound disorders in preschool and school-age children. Evidence of its efficacy is provided in a study by Rudolph and Wendt (2014). In an investigation of three children with moderate–severe to severe speech sound disorders, Rudolph and Wendt found that two of these children exhibited statistically and clinically significant gains by the end of the intervention phase and at follow-up. There were significant gains at follow-up in the third child. Across all phases of the study, phonologically known targets showed greater generalisation than unknown target patterns.

(4) Kummer (2008) states that blowing and sucking exercises should never be used in the treatment of VPD as they are not effective.

(5) The diagnosis of general developmental delay is not appropriate in Louise's case as she displays normal cognitive functioning. The diagnosis of specific language impairment (SLI) is not appropriate either as Louise exhibits features which preclude a diagnosis of SLI. These features include episodes of otitis media, neurological dysfunction in the form of slight general hypotonia and craniofacial anomalies in the form of a submucous cleft palate.

Case study 3 Girl aged 13 years with developmental dysarthria

Unit 3.1 Primer on developmental dysarthria

(1) (a) infectious; (b) traumatic; (c) genetic; (d) genetic; (e) infectious
(2) (a) articulation; (b) prosody; (c) phonation; (d) articulation and resonation; (e) respiration
(3) language disorder; dysphagia; oral apraxia
(4) (a) true; (b) false; (c) true; (d) false; (e) true
(5) (a) improves or remains static; (b) deteriorates; (c) remains static; (d) remains static; (e) improves

Unit 3.2 Client history and communication status

(1) High-tech communication board: a computerised device that offers speech generation and eye-tracking as well as memory storage of commonly used phrases; Low-tech communication board: a book that allows a user to point to letters and words

  Four factors: (i) presence of sensory impairment (e.g. vision); (ii) presence of cognitive impairment; (iii) user's literacy level; and (iv) presence of physical disability (e.g. hemiplegia)

(2) There is evidence that CB's attitude is similar to that of most AAC users with cerebral palsy. In a study of the perspectives of five AAC users with cerebral palsy, Chung et al. (2012) reported that all of the participants preferred to use their natural speech if possible, and thought that their AAC device was not a replacement for speech.

(3) CB's neurological damage occurs in the upper motor neurones.

(4) One of the effects of spasticity on the larynx is hyperadduction of the vocal folds. A strained–strangled voice occurs when subglottic air is forced through a narrow, tightly constricted larynx in which the vocal folds are excessively adducted.

(5) Because CB is unintelligible in conversation, her communication partner is forced to make repeated requests for clarification. Clarification sequences typically proceed by means of a series of yes–no questions (e.g. 'Do you mean X?'), which puts CB in the role of always responding to the utterances of others. This role is a passive one, from which CB expects only to respond to others and not to initiate communication herself.

Unit 3.3 Focus on spastic dysarthria

(1) parts (a), (c) and (e)

(2) The range and timing of palatal elevation are aberrant in spastic dysarthria, with the result that the velum is unable to make contact with the pharyngeal wall. Hypernasal speech results from the escape of air into the nasal cavities.

(3) birth anoxia

(4) Wit et al. found that the fundamental frequency range of children with perinatal-onset spastic dysarthria was lower than that of children with normal speech. This accounts for the reduced pitch of children with spastic dysarthria.

(5) (a) true; (b) true; (c) false; (d) false; (e) true

Unit 3.4 Intervention

(1) The target sounds are all voiceless consonants. Voiceless consonants have been chosen in order to address the tendency of children with cerebral palsy to voice voiceless consonants. Four of the five target consonants are fricative sounds. Fricatives and affricates pose the greatest articulatory difficulty for children with dysarthria and are a significant source of unintelligibility in their speech production.

(2) In a traditional articulation hierarchy, the production of a target sound progresses through a number of stages. The production of the target sound is first attempted in isolation or in simple syllables, followed by single words, phrases, sentences and finally conversational speech. Progression from one level to the next level in the hierarchy is dependent on the client achieving a certain level of accuracy in sound production which, in the case of CB's treatment, is an accuracy level of 80%.

(3) The assumption which underlies this aim is that improvements in oromotor functions such as tongue elevation and lip pursing will lead to improvements in speech sound production. Evidence in support of this assumption is somewhat tenuous. In a review of theoretical and experimental work in motor speech disorders, Weismer (2006) concluded that support for the view that oromotor, non-verbal tasks could be used to improve speech production processes was 'weak at best', and that frequent appeal to oromotor, non-verbal tasks is 'misguided'.

(4) parts (b) and (c)

(5) Two principles of motor learning: (i) there should be multiple opportunities for the practice of the desired motor movement; (ii) appropriate feedback should be provided regarding the nature of the movement. The implementation of principle (i) in CB's treatment took the form of speech drills in phonetic placement therapy. The implementation of principle (ii) in CB's treatment took the form of visual feedback,

the use of an animated character during sEMG-facilitated biofeedback relaxation therapy.

Unit 3.5 Speech outcome

(1) The finding that both treatments failed to bring about improvement in sentence- or paragraph-level intelligibility is consistent with the evidence base on the efficacy of SLT interventions available to individuals with developmental dysarthria. In a wide-ranging review of research published up to April 2009, Pennington et al. (2009) found no firm evidence of the effectiveness of SLT interventions which aimed to improve the speech of children with dysarthria acquired before 3 years of age.

(2) There is no evidence that CB's functioning or psychological well-being were enhanced by the treatments she received in this study. CB's self-perception of her speech impairment remained unchanged following intervention. She still had moderate concern about her speech disorder following treatment.

(3) Tongue protrusion and lip pursing are both non-speech postures. The fact that these non-speech postures improved in CB when her overall intelligibility did not increase supports the view taken by Weismer (2006) that oromotor, non-verbal tasks do not enhance speech production processes.

(4) Alternate motion rates can be assessed by means of DDK tasks. It is not entirely unexpected that these rates did not decrease significantly following PPT, as phonetic placement therapy aims for accuracy in labial and lingual placement and is not concerned to target the rate of articulatory movements.

(5) During PPT, CB progressed as far as the single-word level in the articulation hierarchy. It was also at the single-word level that there was a significant increase in CB's intelligibility at the end of the study. If PPT had been extended and CB had been able to progress to more advanced levels in the articulation hierarchy, then improvements in her intelligibility beyond the single-word level might have been possible.

Case study 4 Boy with developmental apraxia of speech

Unit 4.1 Primer on developmental apraxia of speech

(1) The absence of neuromuscular deficits sets CAS apart from developmental dysarthria.

(2) To establish the prevalence and incidence of a disorder, it is necessary first to be able to identify the disorder. There has not been widespread clinical consensus on the features of DAS. In the absence of this consensus, it has not been possible to identify all cases of the disorder, with the result that investigators cannot study the epidemiology of DAS.

(3) part (c)

(4) If a speaker with DAS is unable to coordinate the onset of voicing with the positioning of the articulators for the production of a certain speech sound (e.g. /b/), the result may be the devoicing of the sound in question (i.e. /p/).

(5) By reducing their rate of speech, speakers with DAS are able to increase their intelligibility. Speech rate reduction is a compensatory strategy on the part of these speakers.

Unit 4.2 Client history

(1) Both influenza and chickenpox can have neural complications such as encephalitis. Encephalitis could have adverse implications for Zachary's postnatal neurodevelopment.

(2) Zachary developed middle ear infections when he was 3 years old. These infections could put him at risk of conductive hearing loss.

(3) parts (b) and (e)

(4) The following non-speech, oral movements suggest the presence of oral dyspraxia: (i) inability to purse or spread lips on command; (ii) inability to protrude tongue and perform lateral tongue movements; and (iii) inability to use tongue tip to lick upper and lower lips.

(5) A comprehensive multidisciplinary evaluation should examine the following three areas: (i) Zachary's cognitive or intellectual skills; (ii) Zachary's motor skills including oral motor skills; and (iii) Zachary's hearing and other sensory organs.

Unit 4.3 Neurological, adaptive and cognitive evaluation

(1) Zachary displayed some incoordination in running and in placing blocks in a wooden frame. This behaviour suggests that he may have a generalised dyspraxia in addition to an apraxia of speech.

(2) Hypotonia is a reduction of the skeletal muscle tone which is marked by a diminished resistance to passive stretching. Hypotonia can be a feature of developmental dysarthria.

(3) The *Vineland Adaptive Behavior Scales* may be used to diagnose autism spectrum disorder (ASD) and attention deficit hyperactivity disorder (ADHD). There is no evidence to suggest that Zachary has either ASD or ADHD.

(4) perceptual and motor skills

(5) Zachary had to use analysis and synthesis skills in order to work out what blocks needed to be brought together to fit into the wooden frame.

Unit 4.4 Speech, language, hearing and oral mechanism evaluation

(1) The 8th percentile means that 92% of Zachary's peers would score above him on the same test, with only 8% scoring below him. The 14th percentile means that 86% of Zachary's peers would score above him on the same test, with only 14% scoring below him.

(2) Normally developing children can produce 10 words at a mean age of 15.1 months (Nelson, 1973). Zachary has fewer than 10 words at 4 years of age (48 months). He thus has a very severe developmental delay in terms of this language milestone.

(3) To say that Zachary's speech displays frequent homonymous forms means that he repeatedly uses the same spoken form of a number of different lexical items. For example, the child who says [tu] for the words 'shoe', 'two', 'chew', 'stew' and 'Sue' is using homonymous forms.

(4) Zachary was unable to perform non-speech, oral movements such as (i) puffing his cheeks; (ii) lateralising and elevating his tongue inside his mouth; and (iii) pushing the examiner's finger when it was placed against his cheek.

(5) With such poor expressive speech skills, Zachary is a suitable candidate for an intervention based on augmentative and alternative communication.

Unit 4.5 Intervention and outcome

(1) Therapies for sound production disorders in children typically emphasise working on sounds that are stimulable, i.e. children must be capable of imitating target sounds in isolation and in nonsense syllables before they are addressed in therapy. However, the new intervention that Powell (1996) undertook emphasises working on unknown aspects of phonology. So this new treatment approach incorporates stimulability, rather than demanding that it be present before certain sounds are addressed in therapy.

(2) Zachary's earlier treatment involved just two, 30-minute sessions per week. This is a low-intensity therapy which is likely to have contributed to the limited success of this intervention. In support of this view, Campbell (1999: 394) states that 'children with apraxia of speech [require] 81% more individual treatment sessions than children with severe phonologic disorders in order to achieve a similar functional outcome'. Campbell claims that while phonologically disordered children need an average of 29 individual, 45-minute treatment sessions for parents to increase their ratings of their children's speech from having less than half of their speech understood by an unfamiliar listener to having about three-quarters understood, children with apraxia of speech require an average of 151 individual sessions to achieve a similar level of parental estimated speech intelligibility.

(3) Feedback in new intervention: successful imitations of sounds and/or syllables are acknowledged by the clinician. Although we cannot say for sure, it seems likely that this acknowledgement takes the form of verbal feedback. Visual feedback is also effective in interventions for DAS. For example, electropalatography (EPG) may be used to deliver visual feedback on tongue–palate contacts during articulation.

(4) The stimulus items that are used for the stabilisation of inconsistently used sounds in goal 2 are selected with a view to facilitating Zachary's vocabulary development. In goal 3, the design of activities addresses language goals. In goal 4, the maintenance of previously taught sounds is achieved by means of a language stimulation activity. It is in this goal that we see language stimulation assuming priority over speech targets.

(5) (a) true; (b) false; (c) true; (d) false; (e) false

Case study 5 Total glossectomy in a man aged 69 years

Unit 5.1 Primer on oral cancer and glossectomy

(1) (a) false; (b) true; (c) false; (d) false; (e) true
(2) Swallowing and speech are the two factors consistently reported by clients who undergo glossectomy to be most significant to their quality of life (e.g. Fang et al., 2013).
(3) parts (b) and (c)
(4) Following total glossectomy, a bulky flap can achieve propulsion of a bolus into the pharynx during swallowing. However, a large, bulky flap may lack the range and speed of movement that is needed for speech production.

(5) Incidence rates of oral cavity cancer are highest in countries where there is widespread use of tobacco, and are in decline in countries where tobacco use has peaked (Simard et al., 2014).

Unit 5.2 Speech and swallowing following glossectomy

(1) (a) otolaryngologist; (b) speech-language pathologist; (c) radiation oncologist; (d) prosthodontist; (e) oral surgeon
(2) A gastrostomy tube, or G-tube, provides access for long-term enteral nutrition in patients who are unable to eat. The tube is inserted through the skin into the stomach. Different types of tube exist for this purpose (Juern and Verhaalen, 2014). Patients who have a glossectomy are candidates for a gastrostomy tube. This is because their nutritional needs cannot be safely met by means of oral feeding for a period of time after surgery.
(3) These substitutions have a compensatory quality. In the absence of the ability to achieve full closure of the pulmonary airstream at the alveolar ridge, these speakers with glossectomy achieve closure at the glottis and lips instead. Hence, the use of the glottal stop [ʔ] and bilabial stop [p], respectively, for /t/.
(4) On account of their tongue defect, these speakers with glossectomy are not able to achieve the full closure that is needed to produce the alveolar and velar plosives /d/, /k/ and /g/. Instead, they approximate these places of articulation by producing alveolar and velar fricatives, respectively. The voicing of the target velar plosives /k/ and /g/ is strictly observed in the use of the voiceless and voiced velar fricatives [x] and [ɣ], respectively. However, this is not the case in the production of /d/ where the voiceless alveolar fricative [s] is used in place of the voiced alveolar plosive.
(5) According to Barry and Timmermann (1985), post-operative lingual *mobility* is more related to speech acceptability than the *amount* of tongue mass remaining after surgery.

Unit 5.3 Client history

(1) GS is a white male who was diagnosed with oral squamous cell carcinoma (OSCC) when he was 61 years old. The age, ethnicity and sex of this subject are typical of clients who receive a diagnosis of OSCC. In a study of incidence trends of OSCC in the United States, Chaturvedi et al. (2008) reported that the mean age at diagnosis was 61.0 years in HPV-related OSCC and 63.8 years in HPV-unrelated OSCC. Weatherspoon et al. (2015) reported that white males displayed the highest incidence rate of all race/ethnicity–gender groups in a study of oral cancer cases diagnosed in the United States between 2000 and 2010.
(2) (a) false; (b) false; (c) true; (d) false;
(e) false; of 1,113 cases of tongue cancer examined by Krishnatreya et al. (2015), 846 (76.1%) occurred at the base of the tongue and 267 (23.9%) occurred on oral tongue.
(3) There is a high probability that GS resumed oral feeding after total glossectomy. In the absence of additional surgical procedures such as laryngectomy, there is a high probability that oral feeding can be resumed. Rigby and Hayden (2014) reported that after total glossectomy with laryngeal preservation, gastric tube dependency ranges from 30% to 44%.

(4) A local flap is a tissue flap that is lifted close to the defect but retains its original blood supply.

(5) The fact that GS had already complied with two years of speech therapy by the time of this study shows that he has a high level of personal motivation. This will have contributed to his good speech outcome.

Unit 5.4 Focus on articulation and intelligibility

(1) It is uncertain for two reasons that listeners would rate GS's speech to be more unintelligible if they had seen a video-recording as well as heard an audio-recording: (i) the articulatory adjustments that GS makes to signal differences between bilabial and alveolar plosives may be detectable on a close-up video analysis but fail to be detected under natural conditions; and (ii) even if listeners did detect these adjustments, they may not be able to attribute any significance to them in terms of their perception of plosive sounds. On account of (i) and (ii), there may be no significant gain in terms of GS's intelligibility by listeners having access to visual information from a video-recording of GS's speech.

(2) GS is using bilabial protrusion, jaw protrusion and jaw lowering as compensatory articulations. Within his anatomical and physiological limitations, GS is using his spared oral structures, specifically his lips and jaw, to alter the configuration of his vocal tract during the articulation of plosive sounds.

(3) Like GS, some of Barry and Timmermann's subjects used the bilabial plosive /p/ in place of /t/. However, these subjects performed other substitutions which were not used by GS. The glottal stop also took the place of /t/. Furthermore, these subjects used alveolar and velar fricatives on account of their attempts to approximate the contact needed to produce alveolar and velar plosives. This pattern was not observed in GS.

(4) GS underwent a total glossectomy while Barry and Timmermann's subjects had a partial glossectomy. The preservation of tongue tissue in a partial glossectomy means that there is greater lingual mobility for articulation. Accordingly, Barry and Timmermann's subjects were able to approximate alveolar and velar plosive articulations even if they were unable to achieve full closure. This approximation was not possible for GS who had a total glossectomy and a flap repair. Because the latter had limited mobility, GS had little option but to substitute alveolar and velar plosives with bilabial stops.

(5) Not all compensatory articulations that are naturally developed by clients who have a glossectomy are effective in terms of improving intelligibility. Some may even be counterproductive to this aim. To the extent that clients can develop maladaptive patterns of articulation following surgery, the supervision of a speech-language pathologist is required to ensure maximally effective use of post-surgical anatomy.

Unit 5.5 Focus on instrumental and acoustic analyses

(1) Electromyography was performed to confirm the results of video analysis, and specifically the finding that GS protruded his lips more during the articulation of /t, d/ than the articulation of /p, b/. By selecting vowels for use in CV monosyllables that are neutral for lip position, the investigator was ensuring that any lip activity

detected during EMG could be attributed to the consonant sound alone in these syllables.

(2) parts (a), (c) and (e)

(3) The epiglottis is active during the production of vowels. It serves to constrict the pharynx during the production of low vowels.

(4) The finding that listeners could not discriminate between GS's production of bilabial and alveolar plosives – all were perceived as bilabial plosives – is unsurprising given that there is no acoustic distinction between these plosives.

(5) The movement of GS's grafted flap, jaw, pharynx and epiglottis altered the configuration of the vocal tract sufficiently that GS was able to discriminate acoustically between high and low vowels, even if not alveolar and bilabial plosives.

Case study 6 Man aged 39 years with stroke-induced dysarthria

Unit 6.1 Primer on acquired dysarthria

(1) parts (b) and (d)

(2) (a) neoplastic and iatrogenic; (b) infectious; (c) traumatic; (d) iatrogenic; (e) neoplastic and iatrogenic

(3) multiple sclerosis: mixed ataxic-spastic dysarthria
Parkinson's disease: hypokinetic dysarthria
motor neurone disease: mixed flaccid-spastic dysarthria

(4) (a) resonation; (b) articulation; (c) respiration; (d) phonation; (e) prosody

(5) When assessing the suitability of an alternative communication system for a client, speech-language pathologists need to consider: (i) the presence of any physical disability; (ii) the presence of any cognitive deficits; and (iii) the presence of any sensory impairments.

Unit 6.2 Client history and clinical presentation

(1) AB had a type of CVA called an intracerebral haemorrhage. AB's high blood pressure (hypertension) caused one or more arteries within his brain to rupture. This released blood into the brain tissue. This blood forms a clot or haematoma which compresses the surrounding brain tissue, leading to raised intracranial pressure.

(2) spastic weakness: damage to the upper motor neurones
flaccid weakness: damage to the lower motor neurones

(3) parts (a), (c) and (d)

(4) AB's palate was atrophied and foreshortened following his CVA. This would have compromised velopharyngeal closure. AB's wife reported that he had nasal speech prior to his CVA. VPI may thus also have been a feature of AB's premorbid communication.

(5) Most of the motor nuclei of the cranial nerves in the brainstem receive bilateral upper motor neurone innervation. Accordingly, in the presence of unilateral cortico-bulbar lesions, there will still be some innervation to the cranial nerve nuclei and the speech musculature will continue to function adequately. Bilateral cortico-bulbar lesions are

required to eliminate innervation to the cranial nerve nuclei altogether, resulting in a significant dysarthria.

Unit 6.3 Speech evaluation

(1) parts (a), (c) and (e)

(2) AB's uneconomical use of air is evident in (i) inadequate vocal fold adduction, resulting in loss of air through the glottis and a breathy voice, and (ii) inadequate velopharyngeal closure, resulting in loss of air through the velopharyngeal port and hypernasal speech.

(3) (a) perceptual assessment; (b) physiological assessment; (c) acoustic assessment; (d) physiological assessment; (e) perceptual assessment

(4) AB's articulation of plosive sounds is compromised in two ways: (i) AB's velopharyngeal incompetence makes it difficult for him to achieve the build-up of intra-oral air pressure that is needed to produce plosives; and (ii) the limited range of AB's articulatory movements means that the full closure which is needed to produce plosives is replaced by a fricative stricture.

(5) AB is unable to vary the pitch (fundamental frequency) and loudness (intensity) of his voice. These phonatory disturbances create prosodic anomalies, as control of pitch and loudness is essential for the use of stress and intonation in speech.

Unit 6.4 Focus on mixed dysarthria

(1) part (a)

(2) Spasticity compromises the range, speed and force of articulatory movements.

(3) The articulator in which there is combined flaccid and spastic involvement is the soft palate (velum). The effect of spasticity on the palate is a tendency towards downward movement. The effect of flaccidity on the palate is to render it too weak to achieve elevation. An appropriate prosthetic intervention in this case is the use of a palatal lift device.

(4) The same lower motor neurones, namely, the vagus nerves (CN X), innervate both the laryngeal muscles and the levator veli palatini. The lower motor neurone involvement of the palate bilaterally is thus a strong basis for the suggestion that AB's phonatory abnormalities are related to a flaccid condition of the vocal folds.

(5) Indirect laryngoscopy is a technique used to examine the larynx. In mirror laryngoscopy, the examining physician uses gauze to hold the end of the client's tongue while a laryngeal mirror is positioned just below the back of the soft palate as the patient says 'ee'. In patients where this procedure elicits a strong gag reflex, fibreoptic laryngoscopy may be a more appropriate technique. A flexible endoscope is passed transnasally into a position above the larynx. Insertion of the scope may be made more tolerable by the use of a local anaesthetic spray.

Unit 6.5 Assessment issues

(1) parts (a), (b) and (d)

(2) Speakers with dysarthria are usually assessed by familiar listeners such as spouses and carers to have a greater level of speech intelligibility than that determined by unfamiliar listeners. Accordingly, both familiar and unfamiliar listeners should be

involved in an assessment of the intelligibility of the speaker with dysarthria. Scripted tasks (e.g. reading passages) and unscripted tasks (e.g. conversation) should both be used in an assessment of intelligibility. Target words are known by the listener in the former tasks but not in the latter tasks, with the result that speech production during scripted tasks is likely to be judged to be more intelligible than during unscripted tasks. If only scripted tasks are used in an assessment of intelligibility, it is likely that the client's intelligibility level could be overestimated.

(3) Under the reflex section of the FDA-2, one might expect to record the presence of pathological reflexes (e.g. sucking reflex). Under the jaw section, one might expect to record any deviation of the jaw to one side or problems with tongue–jaw coordination.

(4) AB's social and occupational functioning will be adversely affected by his dysarthria. His level of unintelligibility is likely to restrict his communication to such a degree that he withdraws from a range of social interactions. Also, AB suffered his CVA at 39 years of age, an age when most adults are still economically active. Although we are not told what AB's employment was prior to his stroke, his level of unintelligibility is likely to preclude a return to the workplace. The combination of social withdrawal and unemployment is likely to put AB at risk of depression and other psychological problems, thus reducing yet further AB's quality of life.

(5) body structure and function

Case study 7 Man aged 35 years with Wilson's disease

Unit 7.1 Primer on Wilson's disease

(1) In an autosomal recessive disorder, the gene which gives rise to a disorder is found on the autosomes, i.e. the chromosomes which are not the sex chromosomes. In a recessive disorder, both alleles of the gene must be disease alleles in order for the disorder to be expressed or manifested in an individual.

(2) part (b)

(3) In the well-managed client with Wilson's disease, dysarthria is likely to improve over time.

(4) part (b)

(5) (a) prosody; (b) resonation; (c) prosody; (d) articulation; (e) prosody

Unit 7.2 Client history and presentation

(1) Three features of R's history:
   (a) presence of neurological signs
   (b) presence of psychiatric disturbance
   (c) presence of Wilson's disease in a biological relative

(2) R's psychiatric problems directly contributed to his poor compliance with his drug and dietary regimen. These same psychiatric problems are likely to have an adverse impact on R's ability to comply with assessment and intervention in speech-language pathology.

(3) There are two indications that R is at risk of aspiration pneumonia. He displays drooling and dysphagia which suggest that his swallowing mechanism is

compromised to at least some degree. There is likely to be inhalation of oropharyngeal secretions in this case.

(4) Written messages and sign language were of limited effectiveness for R because he would also experience poor manual motor control as a result of Wilson's disease.

(5) social functioning

Unit 7.3 Speech intervention: part 1

(1) part (e)

(2) R's speech skills and impairments will vary with changes in his underlying pathology (Wilson's disease). It is, therefore, important that therapy is sensitive to these changes, and is adjusted to reflect them and their impact on speech production.

(3) parts (a), (c), (d) and (e)

(4) R's psychiatric problems may have contributed to (i) his refusal to consider augmentative and alternative communication in therapy, and (ii) his difficulties in monitoring and evaluating his productions.

(5) The behaviour in question is R's use of gestural communication. This behaviour is described as 'maladaptive' because R's gestures were unsuccessful and confusing and, thus, had little communicative value.

Unit 7.4 Speech intervention: part 2

(1) part (e)

(2) By slowing his speech rate, R has more time in which to make the transitions between speech sounds and to assume the articulatory positions that are needed to produce target sounds.

(3) Blowing exercises are one traditional therapy technique which is used to improve hypernasal speech. It is the conclusion of a Cochrane systematic review that there is currently no good-quality evidence to support or refute the use of such techniques in the management of dysarthria (Sellars et al., 2005).

(4) A palatal lift is a rigid, acrylic appliance which is created by a prosthodontist. It consists of a retainer that covers the hard palate and fastens to the maxillary teeth. There is a lift portion that extends along the oral surface of the soft palate. This portion raises the soft palate posteriorly and superiorly so that it does not have as far as normal to travel in order to close the velopharyngeal port.

(5) The two approaches that were used to ensure generalisation of speech skills beyond the clinic were (i) emphasis on R's monitoring and evaluation of his intelligibility in a range of non-clinical settings, and (ii) the provision of feedback from R's wife and his other communicative partners.

Unit 7.5 Speech outcome

(1) By the end of therapy, R's articulation of individual speech sounds made a relatively minor contribution to his overall intelligibility. This is demonstrated by the fact that even as R's intelligibility was judged to have improved significantly by 1985, his production of consonants and phonemes was still judged to be deviant (imprecise consonants and prolonged phonemes were first- and second-ranked, respectively, in an assessment of deviant speech features in 1985).

(2) Reductions in R's intelligibility during the 10-year period of his intervention could be accounted for by (i) R's failure to alter his daily schedule in order to avoid the speech-aggravating effects of fatigue, and (ii) R's failure to comply with the medical regimen that was needed to manage his underlying neurological disorder.

(3) On account of its extended duration, R's intervention raises pressing questions about its cost-effectiveness. The considerable expenditure that is incurred in this case can be supported by the gains that have been achieved in R's occupational functioning, societal participation and psychological well-being. In terms of occupational functioning, R is in full-time employment by the end of therapy. Not only has this resulted in him no longer requiring disability compensation under social security, but he now has the economic means to support his wife and son. In terms of societal participation, R has been able to assume social roles which were previously denied to him by his severe speech disorder. He is now a husband and father. R's range of communicative partners will also have increased with improvements in communication. With these partners comes an expansion of R's social relationships to others. In terms of psychological well-being, R has been vulnerable to psychiatric disturbance on account of his neurological disorder. The psychological benefits that accrue from his improvements in communication might mitigate the effects of conditions such as depression.

(4) The duration of therapy in R's case posed challenges in terms of monitoring speech progress. One challenge is that several different clinicians assessed R's speech production over the course of 10 years. Unless efforts are made to ensure each clinician is working to the same discriminatory standard, the measurement of speech performance will not be reliable. A second challenge is that speech progress can only be properly documented if exactly the same speaking tasks are used at each point of assessment. If different tasks are used to assess a client's speech, what appears to be an improvement in speech function may simply be a reflection of the different levels of difficulty that attend tasks.

(5) This decision reveals that therapy must be tailored to the needs of individual clients. The use of augmentative or alternative communication, even if effective in R's case, would not have been judged by him to be a satisfactory outcome of therapy. However, in another client with R's same level of speech unintelligibility, the use of AAC may be judged to be acceptable. A speech intervention would not be pursued in this case.

Case study 8 Man aged 71 years with apraxia of speech

Unit 8.1 Primer on apraxia of speech

(1) parts (b) and (d)

(2) Three causes of AOS: traumatic brain injury; cerebral infections (e.g. encephalitis); brain tumours.

(3) parts (c) and (e)

(4) Botha et al. (2014) found that bilateral atrophy of the prefrontal cortex anterior to the premotor area and supplementary motor area was associated with non-verbal oral apraxia. This neuroanatomical area is in close proximity to the premotor area which has been implicated in AOS. This proximity explains why oral apraxia is very common in clients with progressive AOS.

(5) static AOS: cerebrovascular accident

progressive AOS: neurodegenerative disease (e.g. frontotemporal dementia)

Unit 8.2 Medical history

(1) part (d)

(2) A right hemiplegia has the following implications for SLT assessment and intervention: (i) a client will be unable to produce written responses on assessments like the Boston Diagnostic Aphasia Examination (at least not with the preferred hand); (ii) a client will find it difficult to manipulate objects during an assessment like the Token Test; (iii) if a client needs to use an augmentative or alternative form of communication, a right hemiplegia will limit the type of communication system that can be used, e.g. signing and the use of natural gesture will be compromised.

(3) parts (b), (d) and (e)

(4) The lower part of the primary motor cortex does have implications for motor speech production. It contains the part of the motor strip that controls movements of the organs of speech production (e.g. articulators, larynx). If this neuroanatomical area is damaged, a motor speech disorder such as dysarthria may result.

(5) part (c)

Unit 8.3 Early post-stroke period

(1) This client does appear to have apraxia of phonation. The evidence in support of this is: (i) the client exhibited minimal vocalisation in the two-week period following the start of speech-language intervention; (ii) when he started producing automatic verbal responses to tasks, his speech remained aphonic; (iii) at five weeks post-stroke, he had substantial difficulty initiating speech. Problems with the initiation of phonation may account for this difficulty.

(2) (a) true; (b) true; (c) false; (d) false; (e) true

(3) The client's naming is influenced by the frequency (high/low) of the target, the class (open/closed) of the target, and the concreteness or abstractness of the target. We are not given specific information about how these variables influenced the client's naming. He may, for example, find it easier to name a word of high frequency ('dog') over a word of low frequency ('albatross'), a word from an open class like noun ('house') over a word from a closed class like preposition ('with'), and a concrete word ('table') over an abstract word ('trust').

(4) By the end of the fourth week post-stroke the client was able to produce *automatic* verbal responses. This is significant in terms of AOS symptomatology, as automatic speech production is known to be easier than volitional speech production in clients with AOS.

(5) The presence of verbal paraphasias indicates that the client exhibits semantic deficits during naming. In a verbal paraphasia, a client produces a word that is semantically related to the target word.

Unit 8.4 Language assessment

(1) (a) 'hurt hisself' (uses [s] in place of /m/)

(b) 'it's cookie jar' (omits 'a')

(c) 'fo fo folling' (unsuccessfully attempts to correct first vowel in 'falling')

(d) 'She's overflowing the sink' (rather than 'The sink is overflowing')

(e) 'With her?' (replicates intonation of examiner's question)

(2) The client's expressive grammatical difficulties and numerous attempts to correct speech conspire to limit the fluency of his verbal output. This lack of fluency disrupts the intonation pattern and other prosodic features of the client's verbal output.

(3) (a) Wernicke's aphasia – There is a severe impairment of auditory comprehension in this syndrome. However, the client's auditory comprehension of language is relatively good.

(b) conduction aphasia – There is a severe impairment of repetition in this syndrome. However, the client's repetition of words and phrases is relatively good.

(c) Broca's aphasia – There is a severe impairment of syntax (agrammatism) in this syndrome. However, the client does not exhibit agrammatic verbal output.

(d) anomic aphasia – There is a severe word-finding difficulty in this syndrome. However, the client's word-finding skills, as indicated by his naming performance, are relatively intact.

(e) global aphasia – There is severe impairment of expressive and receptive skills in this syndrome. However, the client's language difficulties are mild to moderate in severity.

(4) (a) limb/hand praxis

(b) bucco-facial/respiratory praxis

(c) limb/hand praxis

(d) bucco-facial/respiratory praxis

(e) limb/hand praxis

(5) Written confrontation naming is doubly compromised by a right hemiplegia and limb apraxia. The client's right hemiplegia will cause him to use his non-preferred hand to produce a written response, while his limb apraxia will make it difficult to programme the motor movements that are needed to control his hand.

Unit 8.5 Focus on speech

(1) Speech errors in AOS tend to increase in number as the length of words increases. Accordingly, there are likely to be more speech errors in multisyllabic words than in monosyllabic words.

(2) word-initial position

(3) Because the client engages in aphonic speech production, it is inevitable that he will produce a voiceless phoneme in place of a voiced cognate phoneme. Such an error is not a true substitution as such.

(4) Schwa insertion is a common compensatory tactic among speakers with AOS who appear to use it to modify intra- and inter-syllabic consonant sequences (Miller et al., 2006). It has been argued that by inserting a schwa, speakers with AOS can prolong transition times between consonants, thus enabling these speakers to attain articulatory targets (Miller, 2000).

(5) Speakers with AOS related to cortical lesions display more errors on affricates and fricatives than other manners of articulation, and produce more errors on consonant clusters than on singleton consonants (Ogar et al., 2005). However, the client in this study displayed similar percentages of errors across different phoneme groupings, e.g. consonant clusters, fricatives, nasals, etc.

Case study 9 Woman aged 32 years with foreign accent syndrome

Unit 9.1 Primer on foreign accent syndrome

(1) (a) true; (b) false; (c) true; (d) true; (e) true

(2) The client with FAS, who was studied by Tomasino et al. (2013), is not typical of FAS in general. This client did not display signs of dysarthria, apraxia of speech, or aphasia. However, Aronson (1990) reported that 68% of patients with FAS had their accent embedded in, or following, dysarthria, aphasia, or apraxia of speech. Among Aronson's 13 Mayo Clinic patients, 62% had apraxia of speech as an antecedent to the perception of an accent.

(3) Two examples of articulatory overshoot: (i) the production of velar fricatives as velar stops; (ii) the realisation of the glottal fricative as a glottal stop.

(4) These errors are examples of articulatory undershoot, in which the speaker with FAS does not reach the plosive articulatory targets and produces fricatives in their place.

(5) It is a general aim of communicators to give prominence to new information. This is achieved by placing pitch accents on new information. When speakers with FAS place pitch accents on given information, they are giving prominence to information that is already part of the shared or mutual knowledge of speaker and hearer.

Unit 9.2 Client history and medical investigations

(1) Hearing loss with 'sloping configuration' means that TDF had greater difficulty hearing high frequency tones (on the right of an audiogram) than low frequency tones (on the left of an audiogram). It takes the form of a downward or sloping line on an audiogram.

(2) TDF's first head injury occurred nine years before the onset of her speech problems. It is thus too distant in time to be a cause of TDF's speech problems. The second head trauma was minor in nature, and there was no evidence of it causing a lesion or other neurological damage. It, too, is unlikely to be a cause of TDF's speech problems.

(3) A diagnosis of psychogenic dysphonia is only warranted when there is a perceptible vocal anomaly which arises on account of non-organic or psychological factors. However, in TDF's case, there was no perceptible vocal anomaly, according to the otorhinolaryngologist.

(4) dysarthria

(5) part (d)

Unit 9.3 Language and oral motor evaluation

(1) part (b)

(2) (a) production of automatised sequences such as days of the week
   (b) word and sentence repetition

(3) The telegraphic quality of TDF's expressive language – some articles, prepositions and auxiliaries are omitted – is similar to the symptom of agrammatism in aphasia. However, these omissions are not pervasive enough for TDF's expressive language to be described as agrammatic.

(4) The absence of oral apraxia in TDF's case does not necessarily exclude apraxia of speech. It is possible for a client to have apraxia of speech in the absence of oral apraxia.

(5) aphasia; dysarthria

Unit 9.4 Focus on articulation and prosody

(1) stuttering

(2) apraxia of speech

(3) Monday – devoicing of voiced consonant; always – final consonant deletion; three – consonant cluster reduction; Hawaii – initial consonant deletion; talk – final consonant deletion

(4) Scanning speech is the use of excessive and equal stress on all syllables. It is a term which has been used to describe a prominent characteristic of dysarthria in multiple sclerosis as well as of ataxic dysarthria in general.

(5) Incorrect use of stress in sentences may disrupt TDF's ability to signal information status. In this way, instead of giving prominence to new information in utterances through the use of lexical stress, TDF may place stress on words which convey given information.

Unit 9.5 Focus on accent

(1) grammar

(2) The variability in perceived accents in the listener experiments provides support for the view that FAS is a listener-bound epiphenomenon.

(3) Prosody is largely mediated by neural networks in the right hemisphere (Bryan, 1989). Accordingly, one might expect the prosodic anomalies of FAS to be associated with right-hemisphere damage rather than left-hemisphere damage.

(4) The listener experiments in this study used both scripted data (e.g. reading aloud) and unscripted data (e.g. conversation).

(5) The fact that TDF's foreign accent resolved spontaneously within five months of onset suggests that her speech disorder was psychogenic in origin.

Case study 10 Boy aged 7 years with developmental phonological disorder

Unit 10.1 Primer on developmental phonological disorder

(1) idiopathic origin: part (e)
structural anomaly: part (a)
neurological impairment: part (c)

(2) The prevalence of speech sound disorders varies between studies because there is a lack of clinical consensus on how to classify these disorders (Waring and Knight, 2013). Because some prevalence studies examine all speech sound disorders, while other studies investigate one subgroup of speech sound disorders, the prevalence rates of these disorders can vary markedly between different investigations.

(3) The comorbidity of these disorders tells us that there are commonalities in the genetic, neurobiological or other aetiology of these disorders. The reader is referred to Pennington and Bishop (2009) for further discussion.

(4) The late eight phonemes are /ʃ, ʒ, l, r, s, z, θ, ð/ (Shriberg, 1993).

(5) cluster reduction: part (a)
palatal fronting: part (e)
gliding: part (c)

Unit 10.2 Client background

(1) Jarrod's father had a speech disorder, for which he received speech therapy. Jarrod's maternal grandfather has a history of dyslexia. The aggregation of speech sound disorders and reading disability in Jarrod's family is not unique to his family. Lewis et al. (2006) state that '[s]tudies of the familial aggregation of speech sound disorder have reported a higher percentage of family members affected by speech and language disorders in families of children with speech sound disorder than in control families' (1295).

(2) Jarrod is able to forge friendships with other children. He also has a range of interests. Hence, he does not exhibit the restricted interests and impairments of socialisation that are central to the behavioural phenotype of autism spectrum disorder.

(3) The social difficulties reported by Jarrod's teacher are *secondary* to his communication problems. The social difficulties in autism spectrum disorder are a *primary* feature of the condition.

(4) The fact that familiar listeners (i.e. Jarrod's mother and teacher) do not understand him outside of a known conversational context indicates that his phonological disorder is particularly severe.

(5) non-verbal strategies: Jarrod uses gestures and drawing
metalinguistic device: Jarrod engages in message reformulation. This is a *metalinguistic* device, as Jarrod needs to make judgements *about* language in order to convey the same meaning using words that he can produce.

Unit 10.3 Medical, developmental and educational history

(1) Jarrod did not exhibit feeding difficulties in the developmental period. This suggests that he has normal oromotor control.

(2) These studies have revealed that speech sound disorder is most predictive of ADHD when combined with language impairment. McGrath et al. (2008) found that children aged 4–7 years with speech sound disorder and specific language impairment had higher rates of inattentive ADHD symptoms than those with speech sound disorder only. Lewis et al. (2012) reported that children with moderate-to-severe speech sound disorder had higher ratings of inattention and hyperactivity/impulsivity than children with no speech sound disorder. However, language impairment was more predictive of ADHD symptoms than the severity of speech sound disorder.

(3) An allergy or upper respiratory tract infection can cause congestion and swelling of the Eustachian tube, nasopharynx and nasal mucosa. If the Eustachian tube isthmus (the narrowest portion) becomes obstructed, middle ear secretions can build up behind the obstruction. Bacterial and viral infection of these secretions can cause

suppurative otitis media. To prevent this sequence of events, otorhinolaryngologists (ENT consultants in the UK) make a small incision in the tympanic membrane during a procedure known as a myringotomy. The middle ear is cleared of debris and a pressure equalising tube (grommet) is inserted in the membrane to create a temporary aperture. This tube keeps the middle ear ventilated and normally prevents a recurrence of otitis media. The ear drum naturally expels the tube after a period of time with the result that the procedure may need to be repeated (as happened in Jarrod's case).

(4) (i) Jarrod's mother reported that he enjoys a number of activities. She also said that he has been willing to address the school at assembly even though he is not understood. Jarrod's teacher reported that he participates in classroom activities and group discussions.

(ii) Jarrod has been teased by other children about his speech difficulties.

(iii) Jarrod's teacher reported that he is sensitive about his communication problems and he has had reduced self-esteem which has improved as a result of his attendance at an Intensive Language Class.

(5) Children with speech sound disorder have an increased risk of reading disability. Peterson et al. (2009) examined the literacy outcome of 86 children with histories of speech sound disorder. The study also included 37 control children with no histories of speech sound disorder. Reading disability was significantly more prevalent in the group of children with speech sound disorder (22.1%) than in the group of control children (5.4%).

Unit 10.4 Speech, language and cognitive evaluation

(1) (a) gliding; final consonant deletion
   (b) initial consonant deletion; final consonant deletion
   (c) cluster reduction; substitution of alveolar nasal by bilabial nasal; glottal stop replacement
   (d) cluster reduction; glottal stop replacement
   (e) substitution of bilabial nasal by velar nasal

(2) part (d)

(3) Poor non-word repetition suggests that Jarrod's phonological working memory is impaired.

(4) Phonological awareness is impaired in children with reading difficulties. That phonological awareness is impaired in Jarrod is indicated by his performance on the Sutherland Phonological Awareness Test. Jarrod scored 18 on this assessment when the average score range for his age is 33–45.

(5) (a) false; (b) true; (c) true; (d) false; (e) true

Unit 10.5 Focus on articulation and phonology

(1) (a) 'pig' [beɪ]
   (b) 'television' [tstʌʔæbbedn̩]
   (c) 'legs' [jeɡ̊]
   (d) 'goldfish' [doʊbɡ̊]
   (e) 'house' [hæʊ]

Final consonant deletion affects syllable structure.

The age at which these phonological processes are suppressed is indicated in brackets: prevocalic voicing (3;0 years); stopping of /v/ (3;6 years); gliding (5;0 years); fronting (3;6 years) and final consonant deletion (3;3 years). In other words, all these processes are normally suppressed by 7 years of age.

(2) (a) 'jam' [dʒæm]
  (b) 'legs' [jeɡ̊]
  (c) 'sock' [j:ɒk]
  (d) 'foot' [b̥ʊʔ]
  (e) 'zebra' [jebwʌ:]

(3) reduction of consonant cluster: 'zebra' [jegbʌ:]
  deletion of consonant cluster: 'legs' [jeɡ̊]

(4) (a) false; (b) true; (c) true; (d) false; (e) false

(5) final consonant deletion: 'pig' [dɕ:]
  gliding: 'around' [gʌwæ̃ʊ̃]
  Jarrod displays inconsistency in his production of 'pig' in the context of single words and connected speech.

Case study 11 Girl aged 7 years with phonological disorder

Unit 11.1 Primer on phonological disorder in languages other than English

(1) The universal pattern of phonological acquisition (at least in terms of manner of articulation) can be represented as follows: stops > nasals > fricatives > affricates > liquids. The Turkish order of acquisition conforms to this pattern in that stops are acquired before nasals. However, the Turkish order of acquisition differs from this pattern in that affricates are acquired before fricatives.

(2) (a) stopping; (b) affricate stopping; (c) consonant assimilation; (d) syllable-final consonant /ŋ/ deletion; (e) affrication

(3) parts (b), (c) and (e)

(4) The chronological ages at which suppression of these phonological processes occurs in Turkish are largely similar to the ages at which their suppression occurs in English. In English, reduplication (before 3 years), prevocalic voicing (3;0 years) and fronting (3;6 years) are suppressed early. The suppression of cluster reduction (4;0 years) and liquid deviation (5;0 years) occurs later.

(5) Brosseau-Lapré and Rvachew (2014)

Unit 11.2 Client history

(1) It is important for a speech-language pathologist to know if D is monolingual or bilingual because there is some limited evidence that bilingual children are at an increased risk of speech sound disorder. In a systematic review of studies over a 50-year period, Hambly et al. (2013) found limited evidence to suggest that bilingual children develop speech at a slower rate than their monolingual peers. As well as differences in the rate of speech sound acquisition, this review also identified

differences between monolingual and bilingual children in the patterns of their sound errors.

(2) Three motor milestones: begins to sit without support (6 months); crawls (9 months); walks alone (18 months).

(3) This description may be taken to exclude a condition like cleft lip and palate. More generally, it excludes any craniofacial disorder that compromises the structure of the oral cavity and articulators.

(4) developmental dysarthria; developmental verbal dyspraxia (childhood apraxia of speech)

(5) parts (a) and (c)

Unit 11.3 Speech evaluation

(1) (a) fronting; (b) stopping, affrication, devoicing; (c) stopping; (d) fronting, stopping; (e) affrication

(2) (a) [fugãw] → [tudãw] 'oven'
    (b) [igréʒa] → [idédʒa] 'church'
    (c) [aʒúda] → [atúda] 'help'
    (d) [azúleʒu] → [atúledʒu] 'tile'
    (e) [guardaʃúva] → [dadatúta] 'umbrella'

(3) cluster reduction: [igréʒa] → [idédʒa] 'church'

(4) [guardaʃúva] → [dadatúta] 'umbrella'

(5) (a) true; (b) false; (c) true; (d) false; (e) false

Unit 11.4 Focus on systematic sound preference

(1) /ʃ/ and /ʒ/ are realised as [ʧ] and [ʤ], respectively. These realisations occur before the vowels [a] and [u] in syllable initial within word position.

(2) /ʃ/ and /ʒ/ are differently realised in (8) to (10). These sounds are both realised as [t]. It is clear from these productions that /ʃ/ and /ʒ/ are realised as [t] in syllable initial word initial position.

(3) This pattern of realisation is not maintained in (11) to (15). In these productions, /ʃ/ and /ʒ/ are both realised as [t].

(4) In (11) to (15), /ʃ/ and /ʒ/ are realised as [t] because they occur in a stressed syllable. The general rule that captures the pattern of realisation of /ʃ/ and /ʒ/ across (1) to (15) can be stated as follows: /ʃ/ and /ʒ/ are realised as [ʧ] and [ʤ] *unless* they occur in syllable initial word initial position (in which case they are realised as [t]), and *unless* they occur in a stressed syllable (in which case they are realised as [t]). In other words, the [ʧ] and [ʤ] realisations are only found when /ʃ/ and /ʒ/ occur in syllable initial within word position and in an unstressed syllable.

(5) In (16) to (21), there is velar fronting of /k/ and /g/ to [t] and [d], respectively. The fact that [t] and [d] in the single-word productions in (19) to (21) are not replaced by [ʧ] and [ʤ], as we would expect them to be based on the pattern identified in question 4, is an indication that velar fronting is a completely separate process in D's phonological system. So we end up with [atí] and not [aʧí] as we would expect, given that [t] is occurring in syllable initial within word position and in a stressed syllable.

Unit 11.5 Assessment issues

(1) An informal assessment procedure was used to assess D's phonology. D produced spontaneous descriptions of thematic pictures from which a sample of 210 words was obtained for analysis. The selection of an informal assessment procedure was almost certainly motivated by the lack of availability of formal phonological assessments in Brazilian Portuguese.

(2) A *reliable* phonological assessment consistently gives the same results about a child's phonology when the test is administered under identical circumstances. A *valid* phonological assessment measures the specific phonological skills that it is designed to measure. A *norm-referenced* phonological assessment compares the phonological skills of a client to those of a representative sample of individuals of the same age and possibly same sex as the client. This representative sample is known as the normative group.

(3) Two disadvantages in using informal procedures to assess phonology in multilingual children with speech sound disorder: (i) informal procedures are unlikely to test all sounds in a language in all word positions; (ii) informal procedures are not strictly replicable. Because these procedures do not employ the same set of stimuli on each occasion of use, informal procedures cannot be used to chart a child's progress in phonological therapy over time.

(4) A phonological assessment developed for English might contain stimulus items which lie outside the cultural experience of children who are native speakers of other languages.

(5) Puerto Rican Spanish and Mexican Spanish are two different dialects. In terms of assessment development, it is important to understand if there are different phonological norms and other processes at work in children who speak these dialects of Spanish.

Case study 12 Boy aged 4;8 years with specific language impairment

Unit 12.1 Primer on specific language impairment

(1) The expression 'diagnosis by exclusion' means that SLI is a type of negative diagnosis that obtains when all causes of language disorder (e.g. hearing loss, intellectual disability) have been excluded in a particular case. Bishop (2001: 369) states that '[w]here delayed or deviant language learning has no obvious cause, and where development is proceeding normally in other respects, the term 'specific language impairment' (SLI) is used. This is in part a *diagnosis by exclusion* (i.e. the child has language difficulties that are not associated with hearing loss, physical handicap, acquired brain damage, autistic disorder or more general learning difficulties), (italics added).

(2) The variation in SLI prevalence across studies may be explained by the use of different diagnostic criteria. Where less restrictive criteria are used, the prevalence of SLI can be expected to increase.

(3) (i) Child B uses a subject pronoun (albeit an incorrect one), while Child A is unable to use a subject pronoun at all ('her' is used instead of 'she').

   (ii) Child B uses an auxiliary verb, which is omitted in Child A's utterance.

(4) (a) object pronoun 'her' used in place of subject pronoun 'she'
    (b) omission of auxiliary verb 'is'
    (c) Two possibilities:
        (i) 'She is building a block': omission of auxiliary verb 'is' and indefinite article 'a'
        (ii) 'She has a building block': omission of lexical verb 'has' and indefinite article 'a'
    (d) omission of auxiliary verb 'did'
    (e) omission of auxiliary verb 'is'
       grammatical morpheme: progressive *-ing*
(5) (a) false; (b) false; (c) true; (d) true; (e) false

Unit 12.2 Client history and cognitive-linguistic profile

(1) Two conditions which can be excluded as a cause of DF's language problems:
(i) hearing loss (DF passed hearing screenings); and (ii) intellectual disability (DF scored within normal limits on the Leiter-R).

(2) It is important to understand socioeconomic status and maternal education in this case as studies have found a relationship between these factors and a child's language ability. In a longitudinal study of 1,910 infants recruited at 8 months in Melbourne, Australia, Reilly et al. (2010) found that low maternal education levels and socioeconomic status predicted adverse language outcomes at 4 years.

(3) (a) morphology; (b) syntax; (c) syntax; (d) morphology; (e) syntax
The SPELT-3 is particularly suited to an assessment of children with SLI, because it is a sensitive measure of expressive morphosyntax which is impaired in these children.

(4) This finding can be explained by the fact that children with expressive SLI have intact receptive vocabulary: 'Findings from studies employing status assessment measures indicate that children with expressive SLI demonstrate good receptive vocabulary' (Evans and MacWhinney, 1999: 118).

(5) Children with SLI have limitations in cognitive skills known as executive functions (Im-Bolter et al., 2006; Roello et al., 2015).

Unit 12.3 Focus on narrative production

(1) Three morphosyntactic deficits:
    narrative 1: 'I get to hold' (use of present tense 'get' instead of past tense 'got')
    narrative 2: 'He going to jump' (omission of auxiliary 'is')
    narrative 2: 'I know the frog going to jump' (omission of auxiliary 'is')

(2) To produce an autobiographical memory narrative, a narrator must have a mental representation of a past event. Such a representation is not needed when producing a storybook narrative, as the events in the story are visually represented for the narrator. The former type of narrative is thus more cognitively challenging for the narrator than the latter type of narrative. This explains why DF produces an uninformative narrative about his camping holiday, and a more informative narrative based on the wordless picture book.

(3) In the storybook narrative, DF's mother utters 'look at that'. DF reveals his understanding of the deictic function of this demonstrative pronoun by producing an utterance which identifies the referent of 'that' (the frog). Then DF utters 'He going to

jump into that'. His use of the demonstrative pronoun to refer to a feature of the picture confirms that he also has mastery of the deictic function of this expression.

(4) mental state language: *remember* (mother); *think* (mother); *know* (DF)
In order to comprehend and produce mental state language, DF must have theory of mind skills (i.e. the ability to attribute mental states both to his own mind and to the minds of others).

(5) Four question types:
(i) yes–no questions (e.g. 'Do you think the frog is going to jump on his face?')
(ii) wh-questions (e.g. 'what's he looking for?')
(iii) tag questions (e.g. 'that's not going to be good, is it?')
(iv) prosodic questions (e.g. 'He's looking for a frog?')

Unit 12.4 Focus on maternal language in SLI

(1) DF's mother produces the following utterance at the end of the autobiographical memory narrative: 'And you got to hold the black walkie talkie'. This response serves to reinforce DF's utterance, while simultaneously correcting his incorrect use of the present tense verb 'get'.

(2) Two strategies: (i) affirmation of DF's utterance followed by a question (e.g. 'Yeah, what's he looking for?'); (ii) expansion of DF's single-phrase response ('A frog') into a grammatical sentence ('He's looking for a frog?').

(3) For the strategies identified in response to question (2), strategy (i) is intended to encourage DF to expand his narrative, while strategy (ii) is used to provide DF with a linguistic model that will facilitate his development of expressive syntax.

(4) (a) false; (b) false; (c) true; (d) true; (e) true

(5) There are no examples of phonological recasts in the narratives between DF and his mother. However, DF's mother does use a lexical recast when she produces the utterance 'And you got to hold the black walkie talkie' at the end of narrative 1.

Unit 12.5 Impact and outcomes in SLI

(1) If DF's poor expressive language skills mean that he cannot make himself understood to his peers, it is likely that he will attempt to initiate interaction through a range of non-verbal means. Some of these means might include taking a toy from a child or forcefully intruding into the play of others. These clumsy attempts at initiating interaction with others may lead to conflict between DF and his peers, conflict which DF will be unable to negotiate on account of his poor expressive language skills. These poor social encounters with others, which are set in motion by DF's impaired expressive language skills, are likely to result in a reduced ability on DF's part to forge social relationships with others.

(2) Strong expressive and receptive language skills are vital to successful classroom participation. Children like DF who have impaired expressive language may feel inhibited in responding to a teacher's questions in class or may fail to ask for assistance with tasks. This behaviour may be misinterpreted as social withdrawal or a lack of interest on the part of the child. If receptive language is impaired, a child may be unable to follow a teacher's instructions in class. This behaviour may be misinterpreted as defiant behaviour which might incur penalties and sanctions. In each case, poor classroom participation is a consequence of impaired language skills.

(3) Reduced academic attainment is likely to mediate the relationship between specific language impairment and poor vocational outcomes.

(4) parts (b) and (d)

(5) The clinical value of findings from impact and outcome studies is the role that these findings can play in improving language services to individuals with SLI. Specifically, clinicians can use findings of adverse, long-term impacts of SLI to support the case for early language interventions to preschool children with SLI. If these interventions are delivered at an intensity which can produce significant language gains, it may be possible to mitigate many of the serious, lifelong consequences of SLI.

Case study 13 Boy with pragmatic language impairment

Unit 13.1 History and initial assessment

(1) Tony has been exposed to a bilingual language environment during his development. Although Tony's parents have always spoken English to him, this does not preclude their use of Twi when talking to each other.

(2) parts (b) and (d)

(3) part (b)

(4) Five behaviours which are consistent with a diagnosis of autism spectrum disorder are: poor social skills (Tony had poor eye contact and did not relate to children or adults); use of echolalia; recitation of pop songs and nursery rhymes; inability to initiate conversation and respond in conversation; and a lack of imaginative play.

(5) Motor development – Tony has the motor skills to dress and toilet himself.

Unit 13.2 Language profile at 3;10 to 4;4 years

(1) The lack of pointing to indicate or request things, and the failure to bring objects to show to another person suggest that Tony may have impaired theory of mind.

(2) Tony's verbal comprehension score on the Reynell places him below the 1-year level. His receptive vocabulary exceeds 80 words, which is the level expected of typically developing children by 12 months of age (Fenson et al., 1994). So, there is no discrepancy between Tony's receptive language level on the Reynell and as measured by his receptive vocabulary.

(3) Given a lack of positive results from an electroencephalogram (EEG), a diagnosis of Landau–Kleffner syndrome (LKS) now appears increasingly unlikely. This is because there is a close relationship between aphasia and abnormal EEG activity in LKS.

(4) parts (a), (c) and (e)

(5) part (b)

Unit 13.3 Language profile at 5;2 to 5;7 years

(1) part (b)

(2) Mechanical reading ability is the ability to read written language without processing it for meaning. Tony's excellent articulatory (phonological) memory supports this ability.

(3) In order to use ellipsis appropriately, Tony must be aware that he can elide certain phrases and constructions which his hearer will be able to fill in. In order to do this, Tony must be sure that his hearer has these phrases and constructions as part of his discourse representation. That is, Tony must have an understanding of his hearer's discourse knowledge.

(4) use of pronoun reversal (e.g. 'you' for 'I')

(5) We are told in unit 13.2 that Tony has good visual memory – he could recall 4/5 objects. And we are told in unit 13.3 that he has excellent auditory (phonological) memory. So it appears unlikely that reduced auditory–visual memory capacities explain Tony's difficulties in dealing with the multiple conceptual demands of the RDLS. Of course, this still leaves open the possibility that reduced semantic memory may play a role.

Unit 13.4 Language profile at 6;5 to 7;0 years

(1) part (d)

(2) Tony's inability to cope with situation change is consistent with ASD symptoms.

(3) Humour, banter and teasing all involve the use of non-literal language. If Tony does not understand this language, he is at risk of being upset by the playful teasing of his peers.

(4) Tony's inability to spontaneously change or add anything to a set of acting instructions suggests a lack of cognitive flexibility on his part.

(5) Pragmatists and theorists draw upon a script or schema. This is a body of knowledge of the actors, entities and events that we associate with certain scenarios. For example, a restaurant script leads us to expect to find waiters, menus and tables and different food courses within this particular scenario.

Unit 13.5 Focus on pragmatics

(1) (a) Extract 1: 'Hi Ken'
    (b) Extract 2: 'Daddy cut your hair'
    (c) Extract 6: 'Tony is sick'
    (d) Extract 2: 'Daddy cut your hair'
    (e) Extract 6: 'Judy talk mummy'

(2) Ellipsis: Extract 5: '[Alex is] playing with a bus'
    Pronoun for self-reference: Extract 6: 'Can I talk to mummy?'

(3) (a) Extract 2: 'Daddy cut your hair'
    (b) Extract 4: 'Flowers'
    (c) Extract 4: 'Wind it up . . . jump inside'
    (d) Extract 6: 'Judy talk mummy'
    (e) Extract 6: 'Can I talk to mummy?'

(4) In extract 7, Tony is able to identify that Carl is frightened. This suggests he has a reasonably intact affective ToM capacity.

(5) Tony does not appear to understand questions that interrogate the *consequences* of actions (e.g. What would happen to your teeth if you were always eating lots of sweets?) and the *cause* of events and actions (e.g. Why [is Carl crying]?).

Case study 14 Girl with pragmatic language impairment

Unit 14.1 History, hearing and cognitive evaluation

(1) parts (a), (c) and (d)
(2) conductive hearing loss
(3) The achievement of motor milestones (e.g. crawling, walking) was normal.
(4) The fact that both of Lena's brothers have severe developmental language disorders suggests that genetic factors may play a significant role in the aetiology of her own language disorder.
(5) part (a) phonology

Unit 14.2 Language profile at 5;6 years

(1) part (d) semantic paraphasia. Where Lena fails to repeat a target word, she uses a word that has a semantic relationship to one of the target words (e.g. *chair* is related to 'lamp'; *water* is related to 'swimming').
(2) Lena can produce the following consonant clusters:
    /kl/ word initial ('clothes')
    /br/ word initial ('braids')
    /bl/ word initial ('black')
    /ŋk/ word final ('pink')
(3) Lena has greater expressive than receptive lexical semantic deficits. This is evidenced by the fact that she struggles to produce words belonging to certain semantic categories (e.g. food, clothes), but can classify pictures of objects correctly.
(4) Phonology: Lena uses visual feedback to help her discriminate phonemes. Syntax: Lena's participation in tasks that required the comprehension of grammatical constructions was poor in the absence of visual support.
(5) Sentence connectors confer coherence on narratives by linking their constituent sentences in time, space, causality, consequence and a number of other relations. Examples include 'Paul went to the show. <u>Afterwards</u>, he briefly visited his parents' (time) and 'The performance was terrible. <u>So</u> we left the theatre early' (consequence).

Unit 14.3 Language profile at 6;6 years

(1) Exchange 1: (d) consequence
    Exchange 2: (a) causation
(2) The script which appears to dominate Lena's responses is that of a set of directives or instructions issued by a parent or teacher, e.g. 'you may go out'; 'you may not run'.
(3) The three respects in which Lena's response in exchange 2 is problematic are (1) omission of the inflectional suffix in 'she go[es]'; (2) omission of the inflectional suffix in 'ask[s]'; and (3) incorrect use of the preposition 'with'.
(4) It is less likely that a lack of sentence connectors accounts for Lena's narrative production difficulties at 6;6 years than at 5;6 years. This is because sentence connectors are beginning to emerge at 6;6 years. Also, Lena's specific narrative difficulties include the omission of story events and their narration in an illogical order, neither of which is related to the use (or otherwise) of sentence connectors.

(5) Visual (and possibly tactile) cues appear to facilitate naming for Lena, in that she is able to produce the names of clothes that she is wearing, but is unable to produce the names of clothes which are not present in the situation.

Unit 14.4 Language profile at 8;0 years

(1) circumlocution; Lena produces *old wagon bike* for 'wheelchair'.
(2) Lena's own experience serves as a familiar script. She superimposes this script on narratives because she does not understand the events and relationships between actors in those narratives.
(3) (a) *locked* for 'hasp'
    (b) *strainer* for 'funnel'
    (c) *heather* for 'fern'
    (d) *the kings* for 'pyramid'
(4) Lena can make appropriate use of cohesion during the production of narratives. For example, in the following utterance she uses a personal pronoun and a possessive determiner to refer to her cats: 'My <u>Misse and Murre</u> <u>they</u> could climb up the tree in <u>their</u> sharp claws'.
(5) Lena's comprehension of language is good on the Token Test but poor during connected discourse (e.g. narrative, conversation). This is typical of the child with a diagnosis of semantic-pragmatic disorder or pragmatic language impairment.

Unit 14.5 Focus on pragmatics

(1) (a) true; (b) false; (c) false; (d) true; (e) false
(2) Topicalisation occurs in 'Flowers . . . on the apple trees I think are beautiful to see'. Lena's language problems mean she needs extra time to produce and comprehend utterances. The topic–comment structure of this utterance might assist Lena by giving her the extra time she needs to plan what she wants to say about the topic of the utterance.
(3) Lena displays problems with world knowledge during this exchange when (1) she thinks that autumn follows spring and (2) she appears not to know that there are leaves on the ground in autumn.
(4) There are two referential anomalies in the utterance 'everybody went out and played and <u>she</u> throw snowballs on the wall and <u>it</u> was red'. There are no clearly identified referents for either pronoun.
(5) (a) 'Winter and then spring then autumn and then spring . . . usually many days are passing': In this utterance, Lena responds correctly to the question 'What season comes after autumn?' but then proceeds to convey information that has not been requested by the examiner.
    (b) 'At day nursery when was winter then everybody went out and played and she throw snowballs on the wall and it was red': In this utterance, Lena has returned to the topic of winter, even though the examiner has indicated a termination of this topic by asking what it is like in spring.
    (c) 'What sort of pen is this?': When Lena poses this question, it marks an abrupt change of topic.
    (d) 'What is it like in the winter?' and 'what season is it when it is like this outside?': When these wh-interrogatives are posed to Lena, there is a pause before she is

able to produce a response. In each case, the pause suggests Lena needs time to decode the question and plan its response.

(e) 'she throw snowballs on the wall and it was red': Lena uses pronouns such as 'she' and 'it' when it is clear the examiner does not have the requisite knowledge to establish their referents. This suggests that Lena has limited awareness of the examiner's knowledge state.

Case study 15 Man aged 47 years with developmental dyslexia

Unit 15.1 Primer on developmental dyslexia

(1) parts (a), (b) and (e)
(2) (a) Reading problems occur in the presence of intellectual disability.
  (b) Reading and spelling problems are caused by a neurological injury.
  (c) Reading and spelling problems occur in the presence of a sensory deficit (hearing loss).
  (d) Reading problems are related to the onset of epilepsy.
  (e) Reading problems occur in the presence of intellectual disability.
(3) Occupational, social and psychological functioning are all adversely affected in adulthood in individuals with developmental dyslexia (de Beer et al., 2014).
(4) parts (a), (c) and (e)
(5) Comorbid conditions in developmental dyslexia can reveal common underlying aetiologies between dyslexia and disorders such as ADHD at the cognitive and genetic levels.

Unit 15.2 Client history

(1) On the assumption that JR's business involves carpentry and joinery, he has pursued skilled, manual work. Adults with developmental dyslexia tend to pursue non-professional careers where the literacy demands are low.
(2) JR's intellectual functioning is in the normal range.
(3) Although there is little specific information given, it is clear from JR's pursuit of a non-academic route – carpentry and joinery at a technical college – that he experienced limited academic success at school.
(4) absence of a head injury and a neurological disorder
(5) There is familial aggregation of reading and spelling problems. Such aggregation supports a genetic aetiology of dyslexia.

Unit 15.3 Cognitive and language assessment

(1) JR's performance on the Raven's Progressive Matrices indicates that he has average non-verbal intelligence.
(2) JR was able to name 33 of 36 objects correctly on a naming test. This performance does not indicate the presence of anomia.

(3) (a) JR is able to use the facts that the woman is wearing a sleeveless dress and that the window is open to infer that it must be a sunny day.

(b) JR uses the word 'mishap' to describe the children's behaviour. While 'mishap' conveys the sense of them having an unfortunate accident, it does not convey the fact that they are misbehaving when their mother is not watching them. 'Mischief' conveys the latter behaviour more appropriately.

(c) The picture displays the words 'cookie jar'. However, JR uses the word 'cake'.

(d) JR is able to use the mother's eye gaze to infer that she does not *know* that the sink is overflowing.

(e) JR is able to use his script knowledge of kitchens to draw the inference that a cooker should be present.

(4) JR's semantic memory is intact as evidenced by his ability to generate the names of a considerable number of animals and things in one minute. JR's phonological memory is not intact as evidenced by his difficulty in producing words which begin with the letters 'f' and 's' in one minute.

(5) In normal subjects, forward digit span is traditionally considered to be 7 with an approximate standard deviation of 2. In other words, correctly repeating 5–9 digits forward is considered to be normal (Scott, 2011). JR's forward digit span of 5 thus falls within the normal range for verbal working memory.

Unit 15.4 Focus on reading

(1) pivot – visual paralexia
grotesque – neologism
fascinate – morphological paralexia
systematic – visual paralexia
metamorphosis – neologism

(2) There are three forms of evidence that JR is unable to use a phonological reading route:

(i) JR was only able to read four unfamiliar, low-frequency words on a regular word test, in which words can only be read by applying grapheme-to-sound rules.

(ii) JR has considerable difficulty reading non-words, which are not in the semantic system and must be read by applying grapheme-to-sound rules.

(iii) JR was unable to read words when they were presented in typewritten letters in lower case and in the reverse order. A sequential analytic method, in which individual graphemes are identified along with their corresponding phonemes, is needed to read these words. The fact that JR was unable to employ this method is further evidence that he has problems with the phonological reading route.

(3) Irregular words like *ache* and *psalm* cannot be read correctly via the application of grapheme-to-sound rules, and must be read via the semantic system. JR was able to read seven such words correctly. This shows that his semantic reading route is relatively intact.

(4) JR is using whole-word recognition to read high-frequency regular words, thus avoiding use of the impaired phonological reading route (grapheme-to-sound rules). Owing to their lack of familiarity for JR, low-frequency regular words cannot be read by whole-word recognition. Instead, these words must be read via the impaired phonological route.

(5) part (b)

Unit 15.5 Focus on spelling

(1) JR's reading age on the Schonell is 12 years 6 months. However, his spelling age is 10 years 2 months. His spelling performance is therefore worse than his reading performance.

(2) cuisine: phonologically valid
leopard: phonologically valid
ritual: phonologically valid
health: omission of letter

menace: vowel error

(3) JR's relatively strong performance on the spelling of regular words suggests that his phonological route for spelling is intact to a large extent. This is not consistent with what we know about JR's reading skills, where the phonological route was impaired.

(4) JR's spelling of regular words suggested that the phonological spelling route was relatively intact. However, if this were the case, then JR would have been expected to achieve a better performance on the spelling of non-words – JR spelled only 52% of these correctly. The wider conclusion that we can draw from these findings is that the phonological spelling route is working to some degree even if it is not completely intact.

(5) Like the phonological spelling route, the graphemic spelling route is functioning with reduced efficiency in JR. This is suggested by the fact that JR achieved 47% accuracy on the spelling of irregular words, the spelling of which takes place by means of the graphemic spelling route.

Case study 16 Boy aged 5;6 years with FG syndrome

Unit 16.1 History and medical assessment

(1) JB sat at 15 months, walked at 26 months and used phrases at 3 years. However, normally developing children are able to sit without support for long periods of time between 6 to 9 months, are able to walk while holding an adult's hand between 6 to 9 months, and are able to produce two-word utterances between 18 to 24 months. So JB's motor and language development is markedly delayed.

(2) Aspiration pneumonia suggests that JB may have a swallowing disorder (dysphagia). This should be a concern for the speech-language pathologist who assesses JB.

(3) conductive hearing loss; JB has small, underdeveloped, low-set ears which suggests that his otological development may not be normal.

(4) part (c)

(5) part (d)

Unit 16.2 Cognitive and developmental assessment

(1) One of the functions of the corpus callosum is to integrate visual inputs to one cerebral hemisphere with the motor outputs of the other cerebral hemisphere (Berlucchi et al., 1995). This permits fast visuomotor integration to occur. However, in individuals like JB who have a congenital defect of the corpus callosum, this integration proceeds more slowly along extracallosal pathways.

(2) Walking and moving one's arms are gross motor skills. Writing and drawing are fine motor skills.

(3) It is stated in unit 16.1 that JB is ambidextrous. This suggests that he may have bilateral representation of language.

(4) The pragmatic interpretation of utterances draws heavily on visual and other non-linguistic information. For example, to establish the referent of the deictic expression *you* in the utterance 'Do you want more coffee?', a hearer has to know who is present in the physical context. Similarly, a hearer might use a speaker's facial expression to establish that the utterance 'What a delightful child!' is produced with sarcastic intent. In a client with agenesis of the corpus callosum, this visual information may not be successfully integrated with linguistic information, leading to impairments of pragmatic interpretation.

(5) JB's excellent personal-social skills indicate that a diagnosis of autism spectrum disorder would not be appropriate in his case. In fact, his personal-social skills exceed his chronological age on the Denver Developmental Screening.

Unit 16.3 Language assessment at 25 to 34 months

(1) At 34 months, JB's receptive language skills exhibit a delay of 14 months. In other words, JB at 34 months has the receptive language skills of a child of 20 months of age. Sentences with an *agent–action–object* structure are understood by normally developing children for the first time between 24 and 36 months of age. So it is highly unlikely that JB will be able to comprehend a sentence like 'The mummy feeds the baby' at 34 months.

(2) At 34 months, JB's expressive language skills exhibit a delay of 14 months. In other words, JB at 34 months has the expressive language skills of a child of 20 months of age. The relational terms *more* and *no* appear in the two-word utterances of normally developing children for the first time between 18 and 24 months of age. So JB may well be able to produce utterances such as 'more juice' at 34 months.

(3) parts (b), (d) and (e)

(4) parts (a) and (d)

(5) JB's language problems place him at risk of social devalue when he does not have the requisite language skills to forge social relationships with his peers. If JB's language problems at 34 months are still present when he enters formal education, he will also experience a lack of academic achievement, as he will not have the language skills he needs to access the curriculum.

Unit 16.4 Language assessment at 44 to 54 months

(1) JB is producing distorted speech sounds and his speech displays mild hypernasality. These difficulties point to the presence of a mild dysarthria.

(2) JB compensates for his poor language skills by (a) touching his listeners to gain their attention, and (b) using gesture to augment his limited verbal output.

(3) When making a request to push the equipment cart around the room one more time, JB uses 'please'. This indicates a relatively well-developed sense of politeness constraints in conversation.

(4) Three linguistic immaturities:

JB omits the preposition in 'I sleep [in] uncle bed'

JB omits the possessive determiner in 'I sleep [my] uncle bed'

JB omits the genitive ('s) in 'uncle bed' and 'uncle room'

(5) JB omits function words like prepositions (*in*), possessive determiners (*my*) and conjunctions (*and*). Alongside the retention of content words such as nouns (*uncle*) and verbs (*go*), this confers a telegraphic quality on JB's expressive language.

Unit 16.5 Language assessment at 67 months

(1) semantic memory

(2) JB's expressive language contains many pauses and fillers. Also, during his naming of objects such as watch and match, JB produces circumlocutions. Both features suggest that JB has a word-finding difficulty.

(3) Immature linguistic forms:

JB omits the inflectional suffix *–es* ('Puppy dog <u>go</u> bite')

JB uses an onomatopoeic form ('It go <u>woof woof</u>')

JB uses an incorrect subject pronoun ('<u>They</u> go pee-pee')

(4) JB tells the examiner in his first turn that he has a doggie. Yet, it is a presupposition of the examiner's utterance in her first turn that she already knows that JB has a dog. JB appears to be unaware of this presupposition of the examiner's utterance.

(5) JB is able to produce the names of six animals during a verbal fluency task. Additionally, even as he fails to name a chicken and a shovel correctly, he produces words that are semantically related to these targets ('duck' and 'rake', respectively). Both features suggest that JB has relatively intact knowledge of the semantic categories of words.

Case study 17 Boy with Floating-Harbor syndrome

Unit 17.1 Medical history and evaluation

(1) Apgar scores are based on five functions in the neonate: breathing effort; heart rate; muscle tone; reflexes; and skin colour. Each of these functions is scored 0, 1 or 2. The 1-minute score determines how well the baby tolerated the birthing process. The score at 5 minutes indicates how well the baby is doing outside the womb. The total Apgar score ranges from 1 to 10, with scores of 7, 8 or 9 considered to be normal.

(2) The boy's height and weight at 3 years of age are such that less than 3% of children of the same age will have a height and weight below him, while 97% will have a height and weight above him.

(3) The philtrum is the groove that runs from the top of the upper lip to the nose. The columella connects the apex of the nose to the philtrum of the upper lip.

(4) part (b)

(5) A ToRCH assay was undertaken and was normal. This result excludes a number of neonatal infections including the following: toxoplasmosis, rubella, cytomegalovirus, herpes simplex and HIV.

Unit 17.2 Cognitive and language profile

(1) The boy is able to use his stronger non-verbal cognitive capacities to facilitate communication. He does this by using mimicry and gestures to compensate for his poor expressive language skills.

(2) (b) The car is <u>in</u> the garage (spatial preposition)
   (d) The book is <u>on</u> the table (spatial preposition)
   (e) The girl sleeps <u>during</u> the day (temporal preposition)

(3) The boy does not understand colour words like *red* and *yellow*.

(4) As the boy attempts to repeat longer sentences – that is, sentences which are grammatically complex – his production of speech sounds deteriorates. This reveals a trade-off between grammar or syntax on the one hand and phonology on the other hand.

(5) The boy is likely to omit the Italian equivalents of the inflectional suffixes –*s* (in 'boys') and –*ing* (in 'running').

Unit 17.3 Speech evaluation

(1) The GRBAS scale was used to undertake a perceptual assessment of the boy's voice quality.

(2) parts (a), (b) and (e)

(3) The function of the boy's velopharyngeal port is somewhat compromised. The palate displays hypomobility and is poorly coordinated with other articulatory movements, resulting in moderate nasal emission on pressure sounds such as plosives.

(4) The boy is able to produce all seven Italian vowels correctly. The production of vowels is invariably distorted in childhood apraxia of speech.

(5) As pressure sounds, fricatives may be compromised by the palatal abnormality which results in moderate nasal emission on all pressure sounds. Also, the boy's production of fricatives may be further compromised by his open bite malocclusion.

Unit 17.4 Speech and language intervention

(1) Three advantages of a multidisciplinary approach to intervention:
   (a) Speech and language skills are often affected by other aspects of function and development (e.g. hearing, motor development). An intervention that neglects these aspects is likely to have to have an adverse impact on the gains in speech and language that are possible.
   (b) The input of other medical and health professionals can explain a client's regression in treatment or failure to make progress when such progress should be possible. Factors like depression can impact negatively on a client's progress in treatment and are most successfully identified and managed by the team's clinical psychologist.
   (c) It may not be possible to remediate speech and language skills in the absence of prior work on a client's cognitive problems or behavioural issues. Only a multidisciplinary team can decide what problems and issues are a barrier to progress in speech and language and, as such, must be prioritised within intervention.

(2) executive functions

(3) part (e)
(4) parts (c) and (e)
(5) Consonant harmony is a process whereby consonants which are not string adjacent assimilate to one another, usually in place features. There are different types of consonant harmony including velar harmony (e.g. [gɔg] for 'dog') and labial harmony (e.g. [bɛːp] for 'bed'). By around 3 years 9 months, consonant harmony is usually eliminated from the speech of typically developing children.

Unit 17.5 Outcome of intervention

(1) The boy's improved speech and language skills may also be attributed to maturation in areas such as neurodevelopment.
(2) Work on this boy's oromotor skills may have contributed to the disappearance of nasal emission in his speech. However, his developing phonological knowledge may also have contributed to its disappearance.
(3) drawing and writing
(4) A short attention span and receptive language difficulties compromised an early assessment of the boy's intellectual functioning. By the end of intervention, attention span and receptive language had improved, and were unlikely to compromise an assessment of intellectual functioning in consequence.
(5) Literacy skills, namely reading and writing, are particularly important in terms of achieving access to the school curriculum.

Case study 18 Woman aged 28 years with autism

Unit 18.1 Primer on autism spectrum disorder

(1) The prevalence of an illness or condition is the number of individuals who have the condition at any moment. The incidence of a condition is the number of new cases in a period of time, usually one year.
(2) The incidence of ASD is increasing because of better case ascertainment. That is, clinicians are becoming more skilled in recognising the symptoms of ASD and diagnosing the disorder.
(3) Comorbid conditions in ASD are of relevance to speech-language pathologists because many of them (e.g. ADHD, intellectual disability) have implications for communication apart from ASD.
(4) (a) subject relative clause (complex syntax)
    (b) idiom (figurative utterance)
    (c) object relative clause (complex syntax)
    (d) metaphor (figurative utterance)
    (e) idiom (figurative utterance)
(5) Normally developing children follow the gaze of adults because they believe them to be intentional agents who entertain mental states about people and things in the world. Moreover, children can only learn words when they are presented as part of an intentional act of naming by adults – simply hearing a word in the presence of an object is not sufficient for word learning to occur. Children with ASD do not attribute

intentional significance to the gaze of others, with the result that their word learning is compromised.

Unit 18.2 Client history and cognitive-communication status

(1) Mary did not engage in spontaneous play, preferring instead to perseveratively waggle objects.
(2) Mary displayed a lack of interest in her peers and elder sibling.
(3) part (d)
(4) parts (a) and (e)
(5) Mary has a mild intellectual disability.

Unit 18.3 Focus on topic management

(1) The topic of the mini-olympics is clearly familiar to Mary who is able to discuss it with ease (lines 3 to 6). Moreover, she is given the opportunity to do so by two open-ended questions from the researcher (lines 1 and 2). Mary's extended response to that question mentions badminton with Amy which the researcher then attempts to topicalise through the use of a question in line 7. Mary takes this topic in a different direction in line 11 when she begins to talk about the advocacy group where a card was signed for Amy's birthday. Amy provides thematic continuity with the prior topic of badminton. In line 17, the researcher introduces an ancillary topic by asking about Amy's age. It is only in line 29 that the researcher returns to the topic of Amy's birthday. The reintroduction of this topic is indicated by the researcher's use of the discourse marker 'so' at the beginning of line 29.
(2) (a) personal reference – line 18: 'she was twenty nine' ('she' refers to Amy)
   (b) demonstrative reference – line 1: 'what happens at those then' ('those' refers to mini-olympics)
   (c) ellipsis – line 8: 'yes she does [. . .]' ('play badminton' is elided)
   (d) conjunctions – lines 13–14: 'Amy was cutting her cake . . . and we sang' ('and' is a conjunction)
   (e) lexical reiteration – lines 12–15: 'we signed a birthday card for Amy . . . Amy was cutting her cake cutting her birthday cake . . . and we all sang happy birthday to Amy' (repetition of 'birthday', 'cake' and 'cutting')
(3) In extract 2, Mary's ability to contribute to the topic of discussion between lines 17 and 32 sharply declines. This is manifested in her use of a series of brief, low component turns such as 'just a joke' (line 18) and 'she was just saying it' (line 24). While Mary has difficulty maintaining the topic at this point, the researcher manages to maintain it through the use of four question turns such as 'why did she say that' (line 17) and 'why did she make a joke like that' (line 22).
(4) Between lines 11 and 15 in extract 2, Mary uses direct reported speech on two occasions:
   'she (Gloria) says to me "what's that?"'
   'she (Gloria) says to Amy "what's that? Is that a cake or is that a piece of . . . or is it a rabbit?"'
   Of course, Mary's use of 'rabbit' in the second instance of direct reported speech is the source of the researcher's misunderstanding from line 17 onwards. However, this

does not detract in any way from Mary's effort to use direct reported speech as a means of animating her account of Amy's birthday cake for the researcher.

(5) In extract 3, Mary makes extensive use of repetition to maintain the topic of housework. This includes repetition of lexemes such as 'lounge room' and 'downstairs' (and their variants 'dining room' and 'stairs'), as well as repetition of syntactic structures such as 'I hoovered' with a range of direct objects. Repetition is also a feature of the other extracts. For example, in extract 2 there is extensive repetition of relative clauses introduced by 'that' between lines 33 and 38: 'that we bought with Kirsty' (lines 33 to 34); 'that we bought with Kirsty Barker' (line 35); 'that we had it after tea last night' (line 38).

Unit 18.4 Focus on conversational overlaps

(1) After a pause of 1.37 seconds, the researcher legitimately feels entitled to develop the topic of conversation by asking Mary a question ('what colour?'). However, it seems that Mary is still processing her earlier utterance at line 1, which she appears to view as being incomplete. Mary's overlap in line 4 is designed to achieve the completion of that utterance.

(2) The overlap in extract 2 arises because Mary appears to view her response ('I just do sometimes') to the researcher's question in line 3 as informationally inadequate, and wants to convey more information to the researcher about her reasons for not wanting to go swimming. In extract 1, the overlap occurs because Mary is simply continuing an earlier turn, while in extract 2 Mary is dissatisfied with an earlier response and wishes to expand upon it.

(3) That slowed cognitive processing may explain the overlaps in extracts 1 and 2 is supported by two features of these exchanges. First, both overlaps relate to Mary's prior utterances which she still seems to be processing at the point at which processing should be complete. Second, both overlaps are preceded by lengthy pauses which the researcher legitimately interprets to mean that she can ask Mary questions. Even after these pauses have elapsed, Mary can still be seen to be processing her earlier utterances, suggesting that her cognitive processing is slowed.

(4) In extract 3, Mary's overlap appears to pre-empt what the researcher is about to utter. If anything, this suggests a degree of cognitive anticipation on Mary's part. In this case, an explanation of Mary's overlaps based on slowed cognitive processing does not appear valid.

(5) In extract 4, the researcher uses overlapped talk to indicate a revised understanding of Mary's message based on further information which Mary has provided. The purpose of the researcher's overlapped talk is thus quite different from the purposes that are served by Mary's overlapped talk.

Unit 18.5 Focus on conversational pauses

(1) In extract 1, the first of Mary's long pauses appears to be on account of lexical retrieval problems. That Mary is having difficulty retrieving the word 'event' is suggested by her prolongation of the vowel on 'the' and her use of the filler 'errr'. In conjunction with the pause of 3.66 seconds, these features buy Mary additional processing time in which to retrieve the word 'event'. Having retrieved the word

'event', Mary's second long pause in this extract appears to be related to the further planning of her utterance. Mary appears to need time to plan what it is she wants to say about the event.

(2) The first pause of 3.28 seconds is a grammatical pause as it occurs at a grammatical boundary between two clauses: 'they went to the speak up advocacy group' and 'we signed a birthday card for Amy'. The second pause of 2.9 seconds is a non-grammatical pause as it occurs in the middle of a verb phrase: 'Amy was (2.9) cutting her cake'.

(3) Three features which suggest that pauses are related to a word search:

Prolongation of sound in 'ss-'

Use of filler 'errrr'

Use of word ('apple') that is semantically related to the target word ('fruit')

Mary's sound prolongation and use of the filler 'errrr' give her additional processing time in which to conduct a word search. The retrieval of a word that is semantically related to the target word suggests that Mary is conducting a lexical search during which other activated words are produced.

(4) The first of the researcher's questions in extract 4 concerns the name of a British prime minister. Politics is an area of particular interest for Mary, so we can assume she has an extensive store of knowledge in this area. The long pause of seven seconds reflects the time that is needed by Mary to search this extensive store of knowledge before she is able to produce an answer. The second of the researcher's questions concerns an aspect of English literature, about which Mary appears to have little knowledge. Because her knowledge store is small or even non-existent, Mary does not need to conduct an extensive search in order to produce the response 'I don't know'. The pause that precedes this response is shorter as a result.

(5) The pause of 2.15 seconds in extract 5 appears to be used for dramatic effect by Mary and is not related to cognitive processing constraints. This pause serves to foreground the name 'Elly Grey'. Mary builds the suspense further by telling the researcher 'guess what'. She then goes on to repeat the name and narrate what Elly Grey did.

Case study 19 Girl with Sturge–Weber syndrome

Unit 19.1 Primer on epilepsy in Sturge–Weber syndrome

(1) parts (b) and (d)

(2) parts (a), (d) and (e)

(3) Three neurological deficits:

Hemiparesis – a child with weakness or paralysis in one side of the body will be unable to use a manual signing system or manipulate symbols on a computer keyboard.

Visual field deficit – a child with a visual field deficit may not be able to scan pictures on a communication board or computer screen.

Intellectual or cognitive disability – a child with low IQ or cognitive deficits may be unable to learn how to use certain AAC systems. Such a child may fail to understand what symbols may be taken to represent or how to use computer technology or a communication board.

(4) part (e)

(5) Mariotti et al.'s client only had mildly impaired language skills even though the language-dominant left hemisphere was removed. The boy studied by Vargha-Khadem et al. displayed considerable language gains by the non-dominant right hemisphere following left hemidecortication.

Unit 19.2 Medical history

(1) The trigeminal nerve is cranial nerve (CN) V. It provides motor innervation to the muscles that control the mandible, the tensor veli palatini muscle of the velum and the tensor tympani muscle of the middle ear. CN V also mediates sensation from the head, jaw, face, some of the sinuses and tactile sensation from the anterior two thirds of the tongue.

(2) The plum-coloured cortex and the dense purple arachnoid are significant in that they reveal the presence of vascular anomalies in both these structures.

(3) parts (a), (c) and (e)

(4) If a hemispherectomy is performed early, cerebral specialisation will not have taken place. It is likely that the right hemisphere will be able to assume many of the functions of the excised left hemisphere.

(5) part (c)

Unit 19.3 Language and cognitive assessment

(1) CA's spastic hemiplegia might limit her ability to undertake the manual expression subtest of the ITPA, as she will struggle to produce certain gestures. Visual field deficits in children with SWS might compromise picture identification in a vocabulary comprehension test such as the PPVT.

(2) use of the inflectional suffix –s (dogs)

(3) part (d)

(4) (a) passive negative
    (b) active affirmative
    (c) active negative
    (d) passive affirmative
    (e) passive negative

(5) (a) parts 2 and 4
    (b) parts 3 and 5

Unit 19.4 Language and cognitive profile

(1) There is no evidence of a dissociation of auditory and visual modalities in CA's comprehension of language. This is because auditory reception and visual reception are developed to similar, albeit delayed levels.

(2) (a) false; (b) true; (c) true; (d) false; (e) false

(3) CA can comprehend sentences when normal subject–verb–object (SVO) word order occurs. SVO word order occurs in active sentences. However, in passive sentences SVO word order is reversed, explaining CA's poorer comprehension performance on these sentences.

(4) The fact that CA's performance on the Token Test deteriorates markedly in part 5, when the syntactic complexity of the test items is increased, suggests that syntactic complexity plays a more decisive role than informational load for CA on this test.

(5) part (d)

Unit 19.5 Focus on narrative discourse production

(1) (a) 'she knocked on the door' (pronoun should be 'he')
    (b) 'she said, "um- hello-" No- he said, "who's there?"'
    (c) CA states that the grandmother answered the door *before* she asked 'Who's there?'
    (d) 'she put on all her clothes and everything like that'
    (e) 'And then the wolf said, "who is it?"'

(2) CA fails to relate that Little Red Riding Hood thought her grandmother sounded funny and she wondered if she had a cold. This story element involves an exercise in mind-reading on CA's part – CA must be able to attribute mental states to Little Red Riding Hood in order to understand what she was *thinking* and *wondering* about her grandmother. The omission of this story element might suggest that CA has some difficulties in theory of mind.

(3) In her narration, CA states that the bears went to Baby Bear's room *after* Goldilocks has already been discovered in Baby Bear's bed. This misrepresentation suggests that CA does not fully comprehend the temporal meaning of 'and then' – that one event (the visit to Baby Bear's bed) must *precede* another event (the discovery of Goldilocks in the bed).

(4) Upon discovery by the bears, Goldilocks' affective mental state is one of *fear*. However, CA does not succeed in representing this particular mental state. Instead, she characterises Goldilocks' mental state as one of *surprise* and *astonishment*.

(5) CA makes excessive use of 'and then' to link clauses and events in her stories. This type of conjunction expresses a temporal meaning and is more typical of the language of a child much younger than CA.

Case study 20 Man aged 47 years with temporal lobe epilepsy

Unit 20.1 Primer on post-encephalitic epilepsy

(1) parts (b) and (d)
(2) true
(3) false
(4) true
(5) part (c)

Unit 20.2 Medical history

(1) viral encephalitis
(2) DL's receptive aphasia may have compromised an assessment of his orientation. In order to assess orientation, an individual must be able to answer questions such as

'What year is it?' (orientation to time) and 'Where are you?' (orientation to place). These questions may not be understood by the client with receptive aphasia.

(3) (a) Bacterial meningitis is not likely to be a cause of DL's neurological problems because his cerebrospinal fluid examination was normal.

(b) A metabolic disorder is not likely to be a cause of DL's neurological problems because his thyroid function tests and organ function tests were normal.

(c) Cerebrovascular disease is not likely to be a cause of DL's neurological problems because his vasculitis screen was normal.

(4) Wernicke's area

(5) DL's receptive aphasia appears to be mild. This is suggested by the fact that he was able to continue reading – he was able to understand written language – and by the family report that he was able to follow all but the most difficult discussions.

Unit 20.3 Cognitive assessment

(1) (a) attention
    (b) language
    (c) orientation
    (d) recall
    (e) language
(2) Written language is superior to spoken language in DL's case.
(3) parts (a) and (b)
(4) parts (a), (c) and (e)
(5) This behaviour is characterised as DL displaying inconsistent insight into his situation.

Unit 20.4 Language assessment

(1) parts (a), (d) and (e)
(2) Five features of fluent, jargon aphasia: fluent spontaneous speech; poor sentence repetition; impaired comprehension; lack of awareness of communication difficulties; impaired confrontation naming
(3) Three types of paraphasic error:
     Verbal (semantic) paraphasia in which there is a semantic relationship between the uttered and target words (e.g. 'wife' for *husband*)
     Literal (phonemic) paraphasia in which sounds are substituted, added or rearranged so that there is a sound resemblance between the uttered and target words (e.g. 'stowcan' for *snowman*)
     Neologistic paraphasia in which there is a preponderance of neologisms ('new words') in spoken output (e.g. 'pargoney' for *park*)
(4) Three changes in DL's communication skills with the onset of seizure activity:
     DL begins to use gesture to communicate
     DL starts to produce neologistic jargon
     DL's verbal comprehension markedly diminishes
(5) Copying a drawing is a test of constructional praxis. Constructional praxis is a function of the right hemisphere. This skill remains intact as it is unaffected by DL's seizure activity in the left temporal lobe.

Unit 20.5 Focus on expressive language

(1) The dominant theme of DL's spontaneous language production is the loss of his language and cognitive skills.

(2) DL makes repeated use of 'I lost my concentration' and 'I'm just now concentrating', which may be instances of verbal perseveration.

(3) During picture description DL is able to monitor and repair his verbal output when he says 'I don't know if I can figure out if he's a girl <u>I mean a boy</u>'.

(4) Pronoun anomalies during picture description:
   '<u>she</u>'s claiming' (does 'she' refer to the woman or the girl?)
   'he's asking <u>him</u>' (there is only one male person in the picture, so 'him' lacks a referent)
   '<u>he</u>'s a girl' ('he' is the incorrect subject pronoun)

(5) DL is unlikely to have theory of mind deficits. That DL's theory of mind is intact is suggested by his extensive use of mental state language such as:
   'I don't <u>understand</u> them'
   'To <u>interpret</u> what he's doing'
   'I don't <u>know</u>'
   'I can <u>figure</u> out'
   'I <u>mean</u> a boy'

Case study 21 Girl aged 10 years with traumatic brain injury

Unit 21.1 Primer on paediatric traumatic brain injury

(1) parts (c) and (d)

(2) (a) swallowing
   (b) communication
   (c) motor
   (d) communication
   (e) sensory

(3) Lip and tongue pressure transduction systems can be used to measure lip and tongue function in dysarthria.

(4) (a) phonation
   (b) resonation
   (c) prosody
   (d) articulation
   (e) respiration

(5) There is evidence that discourse deficits in children with TBI are related to cognitive deficits in executive function. For example, working memory has been shown to correlate with the ability of children with TBI to summarise the gist of a story and recall discourse content (Chapman et al., 2006).

Unit 21.2 Client history

(1) The brain, blood and cerebrospinal fluid inside the skull constitute a fixed space. In some cases of TBI, oedema and/or haemorrhage into this fixed space cause elevated

intracranial pressure. Hemicraniectomy can reduce this pressure by allowing oedematous tissue to expand outside the neurocranium, thereby preventing fatal internal displacement of brain tissue and subsequent herniation. The procedure involves temporary removal of a large part of the skull which exposes the underlying cerebral hemisphere.

(2) A subdural haematoma is a blood clot that develops between the surface of the brain and the dura mater, the tough, outermost membrane of the meninges. A clot of this type is usually caused by stretching and tearing of veins on the surface of the brain. An epidural (or extradural) haematoma occurs when a blood clot forms underneath the skull but on top of the dura mater. A clot of this type usually results from a tear in an artery that runs just under the skull called the middle meningeal artery. An epidural haematoma is typically associated with a skull fracture.

(3) A right hemiplegia will compromise DG's communication skills in the following respects: (i) it will limit her ability to produce written language (assuming, of course, that DG uses her right hand for writing); and (ii) it will limit her ability to use natural gesture to communicate.

(4) A right hemiplegia must be considered in the SLT management of DG in the following respects: (i) a language assessment that requires written responses must be performed using the non-preferred hand; and (ii) should an augmentative and alternative communication system be necessary, a system must be chosen that does not require the use of the paralysed arm.

(5) parts (a), (c) and (e)

Unit 21.3 Speech, language and hearing assessment

(1) DG's language difficulties do not appear to be related to hearing loss. Even though DG was unable to comply with the requirements of pure-tone audiometry, there is evidence that she has adequate hearing for language comprehension. DG displayed adequate orienting responses to free-field pure tones. Also, she displayed normal responses to environmental sounds.

(2) part (e)

(3) parts (a) and (c)

(4) DG does not have an oral apraxia. She was able to protrude, lateralise and elevate her tongue in imitation of the examiner.

(5) DG's ability to visually match geometric objects, numbers, and pictures indicates that she has intact visual perceptual skills. These skills are mediated by the right cerebral hemisphere which is not damaged in DG.

Unit 21.4 Therapeutic programme

(1) The use of all language modalities might be advantageous as a principle of language intervention in general because: (i) clients can have impairments of auditory, written and signed language, with each requiring direct remediation; (ii) the combined use of auditory, written and signed language may facilitate clients in accessing the semantic system, where a single language modality may not suffice; and (iii) a period of therapy that involves all language modalities may reveal one to make a greater contribution to a client's overall communicative effectiveness than others.

(2) fields

(3) It is likely that DG will perform these activities well. This will provide the therapist with an opportunity to reinforce her correct responding with a view to maintaining this response rate in later activities.

(4) regular words

(5) DG needs to access her semantic system in order to match auditory stimuli to pictures and objects.

Unit 21.5 Post-intervention language skills

(1) By the end of therapy, DG was able to match words with pictures or objects and match pictures or objects with words with 90% and 95% accuracy, respectively. DG could not perform these same tasks at the beginning of therapy. This indicates an improvement in word semantics.

(2) DG's receptive language skills are superior to her expressive language skills. This same receptive–expressive gap is seen in normally developing children who display comprehension of aspects of language before they can produce them.

(3) DG was able to write both regular words (e.g. 'brush') and irregular words (e.g. 'comb').

(4) phonemic cuing

(5) DG's case tends to disconfirm this statement. By 10 years of age, DG had clearly not reached the upper limit in her language recovery. Indeed, DG displayed evidence of considerable language gains at 10 years of age.

Case study 22 Girl aged 9;11 years with right cerebellar tumour

Unit 22.1 Diagnosis and medical intervention

(1) parts (a) and (b)

(2) poor balance

(3) parts (a), (b), (d) and (e)

(4) parts (a), (b) and (d)

(5) The cerebellum may also be compromised by trauma and infection.

Unit 22.2 Assessment battery

(1) (a) proverb; (b) idiom; (c) metaphor; (d) idiom; (e) metaphor

(2) part (c)

(3) (a) semantic; (b) pragmatic; (c) elaborative; (d) semantic; (e) elaborative

(4) (a) lexical ambiguity:
  'They sat down for a rest beside the bank'
  (bank = side of river; financial building)

   (b) structural ambiguity:
  'Put the milk in the jug in the fridge'
  (on one reading the jug is outside the fridge; on the other reading the jug is inside the fridge)

    (c) lexical and structural ambiguity:
       'I said I would file it last week'
       (file = place document in filing cabinet; smooth surface of wood, etc.)
       (on one reading the saying was done last week; on the other reading the filing was
          done last week)
(5) promise ('I will be at the party tonight')
    warning ('The bull is in the field')
    request ('Can you tell me the time?')

Unit 22.3 Language evaluation at 10;9 years

(1) (a) CELF-3; (b) PPVT-III; (c) CELF-3; (d) TOWK; (e) CELF-3
(2) This characterisation is too simplistic because the results of the Test of Language
    Competence reveal that aspects of both receptive and expressive pragmatics are
    intact in this girl.
(3) (a) hot–cold; (b) employer–employee; (c) ascend–descend; (d) absent–present
(4) A routine language evaluation tends to examine structural language skills, which are
    intact in this girl. If such an evaluation does not include an assessment of language
    in more challenging contexts, then it is likely that this girl's language difficulties
    would go undetected. Such contexts might include an assessment of conversation and
    other forms of discourse (e.g. narrative production). These assessments are certainly
    more time-consuming to perform than structural language tests. However, they are
    also more revealing of the type of cognitive-language problems that this girl is
    displaying.
(5) (a) false; (b) false; (c) false; (d) true; (e) false

Unit 22.4 Language evaluation at 11;9 years

(1) The structural and functional brain changes that are associated with the
    administration of radiotherapy are likely to have made the single, biggest contribution
    to the decline in this girl's high-level language skills.
(2) This case illustrates that it cannot be assumed that the language skills of children with
    cerebellar tumours remain static following surgery and radiotherapy. Accordingly,
    speech-language pathologists must commit to the long-term assessment of these skills,
    with consequent adjustment or resumption of therapy depending on the results of
    such assessment.
(3) A girl of 11;9 years is approaching adolescence. This is a stage in life when social
    communication skills come under increasing demands as young people attempt to
    forge significant peer relationships and to negotiate conflict with their peers. The type
    of high-level language skills that are compromised in this girl will make a particularly
    important contribution to the development of strong social communication
    skills.
(4) affective theory of mind
(5) There is now considerable evidence that there are adverse, long-term psychosocial
    implications for children who develop brain tumours in areas such as suicide ideation,
    employment, independent living and dating/marital status (Brinkman et al., 2013;
    Frange et al., 2009; Maddrey et al., 2005).

Unit 22.5 Cognitive functions of the cerebellum

(1) agrammatism and anomia

(2) One of the CELF-3 subtests requires children to list as many words as possible within a given category in one minute (a test of category or verbal fluency). The girl in this case study displayed intact performance across all areas of the CELF-3. So it can be concluded that her verbal fluency is not impaired.

(3) Differences in the linguistic performance of the girl in the case study and the other subjects reported in unit 22.5 may be accounted for by tumour type (e.g. ependymoma versus astrocytoma), tumour location (e.g. right or left cerebellar hemispheres) and language assessments (e.g. the Hundred Pictures Naming Test may not be as challenging as the tests used to assess naming in the subjects in unit 22.5).

(4) Affective functioning was assessed through an examination of empathy in the Test of Problem Solving.

(5) Children with cerebellar tumours must be treated as part of a multidisciplinary team. Speech-language pathologists must work closely with other professionals, particularly neuropsychologists, if the wide array of language and cognitive problems in these clients are to be addressed successfully.

Case study 23 Woman with post-irradiation speech and language disorder

Unit 23.1 History and referral

(1) parts (a), (c) and (e)

(2) parts (a), (b) and (d)

(3) Three structural changes: necrosis; atrophy; and calcification

(4) The velopharyngeal port is malfunctioning to cause the client's hypernasal speech. A neurogenic aetiology is the basis of the client's velopharyngeal incompetence.

(5) A palatal lift device has a posterior bulb structure which serves to elevate a weakened or paralysed soft palate (velum). The elevation achieved by the bulb structure reduces the degree of movement that the velum must perform in order to make contact with the nasopharyngeal wall, a movement which closes off the velopharyngeal port to pulmonary air. A palatal lift device was probably unsuccessful in this case because the client's velum was completely immobile as a result of her underlying neurological impairment.

Unit 23.2 Neurological and neuroradiological evaluation

(1) vagus nerve; three branches: pharyngeal branch; exterior superior laryngeal nerve branch; recurrent nerve branch. The pharyngeal branch is compromised in this client so producing hypernasal speech.

(2) part (c)

(3) The Babinski reflex occurs in children up to 2 years old. When the sole of the foot is firmly stroked, the big toe moves upwards or towards the top surface of the foot and the other toes fan out. As children mature, the reflex disappears. Its presence in an adult is a sign of neurological damage, specifically within the pyramidal system.

(4) The lenticular nucleus is a lens-shaped mass that consists of the putamen and globus pallidus. Along with the caudate nucleus, the putamen and globus pallidus form the basal ganglia, a set of nuclei which is located deep in the cerebral hemispheres. The basal ganglia is involved in the regulation of cortically initiated motor activity, cognition and emotion. The ventrolateral nucleus is a nucleus in the thalamus which is important in the regulation of volitional movements.

(5) The cerebral ventricles are a series of interconnected, fluid-filled spaces that lie at the core of the forebrain and brainstem. The ventricles are filled with cerebrospinal fluid which percolates through the ventricular system and flows into the subarachnoid space (space between the meninges known as the arachnoid mater and pia mater) through perforations in the thin covering of the fourth ventricle.

Unit 23.3 Neuropsychological evaluation

(1) parts (b), (d) and (e)
(2) (d) pragmatics: the client is likely to have difficulty understanding figurative language such as metaphors and idioms
    (e) discourse: the client is likely to have difficulty expressing causal relations between events during narrative production
(3) The client has problems abstracting 'general' from 'specific' information. This cognitive skill is required in order to establish the gist of a story.
(4) A score below the 10th percentile means that over 90% of adults would achieve a higher score than the client on the Rey Figure test.
(5) parietal lobes

Unit 23.4 Speech evaluation

(1) parts (b), (c) and (d)
(2) Speech-language pathologists calculate diadochokinetic rates as a means of assessing an individual's ability to perform alternating articulatory movements. Typically, a client is timed as they produce rapid syllable repetitions such as /pə, tə, kə/.
(3) (a) true; (b) false; (c) true; (d) false; (e) false
(4) The client was observed to speak quickly, with noticeable breaks in fluency and short phrase length. All three features indicate that there is reduced respiratory support for speech.
(5) The client displayed a marked reduction in the length of phonation. This is likely to be related to reduced respiratory support for speech production.

Unit 23.5 Language evaluation

(1) The client's repetition abilities were relatively well preserved. Combined with the lack of phonemic paraphasias during naming, this suggests that the phonological level of language is intact.
(2) The naming errors are semantic paraphasias. The presence of these errors suggests that there is disruption to the lexical/semantic level of language. The severe impairment in word (category) fluency (<20th percentile) further suggests that the lexical/semantic level of language is disrupted.

(3) These errors appear to be related to a visual–perceptual disorder in that the client has produced words that have a visual similarity to the target.

(4) Semantic cues are unlikely to facilitate this client's naming given her evident difficulties at the lexical/semantic level of language.

(5) The client is unlikely to be an informative communicator. Compared to normal subjects, she displays a reduction in both the efficiency of information transfer and the amount of information transferred.

Case study 24 Woman aged 66 years with Wernicke's aphasia

Unit 24.1 Primer on Wernicke's aphasia

(1) part (b)

(2) parts (b), (c) and (d)

(3) The left superior temporal gyrus is the neuroanatomical location of Wernicke's area. A lesion of this area is not always associated with Wernicke's aphasia.

(4) neologism (pargoney)

(5) verbal paraphasia ('run' for *ride*)

Unit 24.2 Client history and presentation

(1) There is an increased likelihood that RC may have right-hemisphere language dominance because she is left-handed. In healthy individuals, the incidence of right-hemisphere language dominance has been found to increase linearly with the degree of left-handedness, from 4% in strong right-handers to 15% in ambidextrous individuals and 27% in strong left-handers (Knecht et al., 2000). However, brain imaging showed that RC has left-hemisphere language dominance. Two CT scans confirmed the presence of lesions in the left cerebral hemisphere as the cause of RC's language problems.

(2) RC's lesions are found in the posterior portion of the first temporal gyrus and the anterior portion of the supramarginal gyrus. Neither of these lesions compromises the anterior temporal lobes, which we can assume to be intact in RC.

(3) Four linguistic impairments:
> use of neologistic jargon
> poor auditory comprehension
> poor repetition of language
> poor awareness and monitoring of communication problems

(4) RC is unlikely to register verbal and non-verbal cues which indicate that she is not being understood by her conversational partner. These cues include requests for clarification (verbal cue) and puzzled facial expressions (non-verbal cue). In the absence of detection of these cues, RC is unable to correct her incomprehensible output.

(5) RC may use rising pitch when making statements, with the result that they are understood by a listener to be questions.

Unit 24.3 Pre-intervention language assessment

(1) (a) oral commands; (b) automatised sequences; (c) responsive naming; (d) complex ideational material; (e) reading comprehension of sentences

(2) melodic line within the rating scale profile

(3) The slightly better performance of RC on the picture-word match subtest than on other subtests suggests that the visual modality may be beneficially used during intervention. During this test, the examiner points to a picture without naming it, and asks the patient to find its name among four printed words.

(4) phonological short-term memory

(5) Three distinctions:
> animate – inanimate (e.g. camel – comb; octopus – bed)
> high frequency – low frequency (e.g. house – sphinx; toothbrush – pelican)
> natural entity – artefact (e.g. volcano – dart; cactus – wheelchair)

Unit 24.4 New language intervention

(1) In a picture categorisation task, a subject is given a number of pictures and is asked to group them according to categories like fruit, clothes and transport. This task is aimed at developing a subject's knowledge of semantic fields.

(2) parts (a), (b) and (e)

(3) The anterior temporal lobes can support comprehension of visually presented material (written words and pictures) in individuals with Wernicke's aphasia (Robson et al., 2014). This neuroanatomical area is intact in RC, who has lesions of the posterior portion of the first temporal gyrus and the anterior portion of the supramarginal gyrus.

(4) Three aspects of word knowledge:
> orthography, e.g. Are the words 'boy' and 'boy' the same or different?
> semantic field, e.g. Do 'pants' and 'dress' belong to the same category?
> grammatical class, e.g. Do 'pen' and 'write' belong to the same word class?

(5) Increasing contextual and linguistic redundancy should improve RC's comprehension as there is additional linguistic and non-linguistic information that RC can use to establish the meaning of sentences.

Unit 24.5 Post-intervention language assessment

(1) RC was able to avail herself of contextual cues in natural conversation to aid her comprehension of language. These same cues are not available during language testing on the BDAE. The facilitation of these cues in natural conversation accounts for her improved comprehension in that situation even though RC's test scores did not reveal an improvement in auditory comprehension.

(2)
> 'scissors' /kʌtmæn/ (contains 'cut')
> 'flower' /blumpat/ (contains 'bloom')
> 'pencil' /pɛnres/ (contains 'pen')
> 'drinking' /kʌpʌp/ (contains 'cup')
> 'cactus' /prɪkəl/ (contains 'prickle')

(3) In an active sentence like *The man kicked the dog* there is simple subject–verb–object word order. However, this word order is reversed (i.e. object–verb–subject) in a

passive sentence like *The dog was kicked by the man.* The reversal of the SVO word order explains RC's greater difficulty in understanding passive voice sentences. A non-reversible passive sentence like *The mouse was chased by the cat* is usually more easily understood by an aphasic client than a reversible passive sentence like *The lorry was followed by the van.* This is because the misinterpretation of the roles of 'cat' and 'mouse' in the non-reversible passive sentence is rendered unlikely by real-world knowledge (i.e. it is usually cats who chase mice, and not the other way round). This is not the case for 'lorry' and 'van' in the reversible passive sentence.

(4) Informational load and syntactic complexity are the two factors that explain RC's performance in the comprehension of instructions. As informational load (the number of words) and the syntactic complexity of instructions increase, RC's comprehension of instructions decreases. Of these two factors, syntactic complexity is the most influential one in terms of RC's comprehension. This is indicated by the fact that RC displayed better comprehension of a seven-word instruction that contains the coordinating conjunction 'and' than a six-word instruction that contains the preposition 'with'.

(5) Wh-interrogatives are more conceptually demanding than yes–no interrogatives. This is because they require the understanding of concepts such as a thing (*What . . . ?*), a person (*Who . . . ?*), a time (*When . . . ?*) and a place (*Where . . . ?*). The more conceptually demanding nature of wh-interrogatives probably explains RC's greater difficulty in understanding these questions over yes–no interrogatives.

Case study 25 Woman aged 41 years with Broca's aphasia

Unit 25.1 History and initial assessment

(1) parts (a), (b) and (d)
(2) Visual information is analysed in the dominant parietal lobe, which is usually in the left hemisphere. The CT scan revealed that HW's ischaemic infarct extended to the left parietal lobe.
(3) parts (a), (c) and (e)
(4) poor sentence repetition
(5) There is evidence that clients with aphasia experience elevated levels of psychological distress including depression and anxiety (Shehata et al., 2014) and a reduction in their social relationships (Fotiadou et al., 2014). These psychosocial aspects are now addressed as part of the management of clients with aphasia.

Unit 25.2 Assessment at 15 months post-onset: part 1

(1) HW's single-word and sentence-level comprehension is intact. Her comprehension of nouns and verbs is unproblematic. HW's performance on the TROG and the Token Test suggests that her comprehension of sentences is also effectively intact.
(2) HW's inability to name items like *pagoda* and *centaur* on the Graded Naming Test is more likely to reflect a limitation in her premorbid vocabulary than any deficit in word-finding. This is because HW achieved 100% naming accuracy on the Boston Naming Test and her performance on the Graded Naming Test was comparable to that of normal controls.

(3) part (c)

(4) HW engages in circumlocution when she is unable to produce the names of these actions.

(5) There is a possible visual basis to HW's error in that the face veil may have caused HW to recall an image of a soldier with his face covered for reasons of camouflage and protection. The left parietal lobe damage that was identified in unit 25.1 may contribute to this visual error.

Unit 25.3 Assessment 15 months post-onset: part 2

(1) At 15 months post-onset, HW achieved a percentile score of 100 on a verbal memory test (see unit 25.2). When first assessed, HW had a weak verbal memory. An improvement in verbal memory most likely accounts for HW's stronger word and sentence repetition skills at 15 months.

(2) During sentence repetition, closed-class words are most compromised for HW. This can be seen in the sentence 'In the classroom all children were talking aloud', where the auxiliary verb (*were*) and the inflectional suffix (*-ing*) were omitted during HW's repetition. Additionally, HW replaces an adverb (*aloud*) with an adjective (*loud*).

(3) Subject noun phrases are vulnerable to repetition (e.g. The old man the old man is begging for money). On one occasion, repetition finds HW correcting her verbal output. The correction takes the form of the inclusion of a definite article (Policeman the policeman fastens handcuffs).

(4) (a) The teacher writes [a] word on the blackboard.
　　(b) Use of *teapot* for *coffeepot*
　　(c) The boy the boy drops a vase [and] cries.
　　(d) Ellipsis should be used in: The man is lying on the couch to [he is] smoking a pipe [he is] reading the newspaper.
　　(e) Use of *vase* for *glass*

(5) Circumlocutions occur in the following:
　　　　use of *fasten handcuffs* for *arrest*
　　　　use of *has a boot on the hook* for *fishes a boot*

Unit 25.4 Focus on spontaneous speech: part 1

(1) HW can comprehend:
　　(a) Prosodic questions: You also encounter problems when making a sentence?
　　(b) Requests for clarification: What do you mean, too fast?
　　(c) Yes–no interrogatives: Do you do that on purpose?
　　(d) Wh-interrogatives: Why don't you do that?
　　(e) Indirect speech acts: Can you tell me what are your problems? (a request)

(2) HW is able to establish the referents of the demonstrative pronouns in the following utterances:
　　　　Why don't you do that? *That* refers to *speak in correct sentences.*
　　　　And looking for words, is that difficult? *That* refers to *looking for words.*
　　　　Do you do that on purpose? *That* refers to *leave words out.*
　　　　That's why you talk in short sentences? *That* refers to *difficulty looking for words.*
　　　　You do hear that? *That* refers to *what you say wrongly.*

(3) Mental state language in HW's expressive output:

'difficult words er to <u>think</u> yes doesn't soon occur to me'

'before the time I did <u>know</u> writing down'

'I write down nothing <u>remembers</u> me'

The use of mental state language suggests that HW has an intact theory of mind capacity.

(4) HW makes extensive use of filled pauses. This indicates that she is searching for words and wants to retain her turn while doing so.

(5) (a) 'I <u>says</u> wrongly'

   (b) 'Er I [am] too fast to talk'

   (c) 'I leave [the words/them] out'

   (d) 'to think yes [it] doesn't soon occur to me'

   (e) 'Er [I am] too fast to talk'

Unit 25.5 Focus on spontaneous speech: part 2

(1) HW first tells the interviewer that she will not give presents at Christmas. She then goes on to say that she gives presents of 10 guilders to people at Christmas. HW first tells the interviewer that she sold her house in March. Later in the conversation, she tells the interviewer that she moved in March.

(2) When the interviewer says 'That is the oldest <u>one</u>, isn't it?', HW understands that *one* is a substitute for *child*. Also, when HW says 'Ah big <u>one</u> big <u>one</u> behind the house', HW is using *one* as a substitute for *garden*. In other words, HW can understand substitution when it is used by the interviewer, and can use substitution in her own utterances.

(3) HW uses direct reported speech ('I want in the attic') to relate to the interviewer a row between her children, Reinier and Renate, about occupancy of the bedroom in the attic.

(4) HW is able to engage in self-initiated and other-initiated repair of utterances:

   Self-initiated repair:

   'fifteen meters width seventeen <u>no seven meters</u>'

   Other-initiated repair:

   HW: Er room er ninety meters no

   INT: No, that seems very large

   HW: <u>No nine meters</u> all thresholds gone oh nice

   This other-initiated repair also contains an element of self-initiated repair (see 'no' at the end of HW's first turn).

(5) (a) 'we [are] saving pennies'

   (b) 'In the pan tasty <u>things</u> snacks tasty'

   (c) 'Er three ground floor first [floor . . .] bedrooms two shower'

   (d) 'now tiles on [the] roof'

   (e) 'Reinier row about [. . .] I want in the attic'

Case study 26 Man with stroke-induced Broca's aphasia

Unit 26.1 History and communication status

(1) The lesion that causes Broca's aphasia affects the third frontal convolution of the left frontal lobe. This location is called Broca's area. The damage from a CVA often

extends posteriorly to the most inferior part of the motor strip that controls voluntary movements of the right side of the body. Because of the organisation of the motor strip, the face and arm on the right are most likely to be affected by this extended damage.

(2) Roy makes extensive use of filled pauses (. . . uh . . .) which reveal he is struggling to find certain words. Filled pauses help Roy to retain his turn as he searches for words.

(3) Notwithstanding his severe expressive language problems, Roy can still communicate effectively as he retains the use of content words. These words, which include nouns and adverbs, convey most meaning to a listener.

(4) In conversational situations, Roy is able to use a range of contextual cues to facilitate his comprehension of language. These same cues are reduced or absent altogether during language testing.

(5) He uses mime to good effect when he mimes falling over.

Unit 26.2 Assessment battery

(1) parts (b), (c) and (d)

(2) *The boy runs*: one-argument structure
Thematic role: the boy (agent)
The woman cooks the meal: two-argument structure
Thematic roles: the woman (agent); the meal (theme)
The man put the book on the shelf: three-argument structure
Thematic roles: the man (agent); the book (theme); the shelf (goal)

(3)   *teeth*: an object that has a close semantic relation to the target verb
scratching: an action that is related to the target action
nails: an object that is related to the action distractor

(4) The scene that is depicted in the cookie theft picture is intended to elicit a description that captures a specific moment in time. The subject who describes the individual events in the picture, such as the woman drying the plate and the boy climbing onto the stool, is doing so within a static frame. The subject who is describing events in a cartoon strip must capture the development of these events over time. The progressive character of this description sets the cartoon strip description task apart from the cookie theft picture description task.

(5) Adults with aphasia may struggle with turn-taking and repair in conversation. These features may be overlooked if only tasks that elicit monological discourse are included within an assessment of language and communication.

Unit 26.3 Focus on agrammatism

(1) semantic paraphasias

(2) *Jill gave the book to the woman* contains the verb 'give' which has a three-argument structure. Roy was unable to produce any sentences on the TRIP which contained verbs with a three-argument structure.

(3) Three ways in which expressive language is compromised by agrammatism:
omission of determiner 'the'
omission of auxiliary verb 'is'
omission of inflectional suffix '-ing'

(4) This difference can be accounted for by the different test administration of the TRIP and the VAST. The TRIP provides a model of all target responses at the outset of the

test, while the VAST only provides a single practice item at the beginning of each subtest. This is likely to have facilitated Roy's performance on the TRIP.

(5) Roy cannot produce the verbs 'cutting' and 'raking', so he produces the nouns 'scissors' and 'hoe' to capture objects in the pictures instead.

Unit 26.4 Discourse production

(1) Roy produces two consecutive discourse markers 'so' and 'then'. These are followed by a standard storytelling phrase 'all of a sudden' and the noun 'spell'. The use of level intonation between each of these elements indicates that there is more to come, with the falling intonation after 'spell' indicating the completion of Roy's turn. Through a combination of these linguistic units and prosody, Roy succeeds in relating an event in the 'Cinderella' story in the absence of any verb production.

(2) Roy utters the name of an object ('plate') that is related to the verb ('drying') that he cannot produce. He then follows this noun with a complex mime.

(3) Roy succeeds in constructing a relatively fluent unit by combining an adverb ('actually') with a first person pronoun and cognitive verb ('I thought'). He then states the noun 'dog' to communicate his initial belief that it was the dog disappearing under the table, with the comment 'but no' to indicate that he was mistaken. Roy makes extensive use of subject pronouns and cognitive verbs (e.g. 'you know'). Their ease of production for him confers fluency on his otherwise severely agrammatic output.

(4) In extract D, Roy uses reported speech ('quick, I know') to convey the actions of the host in the situation. He follows this with symbolic noise ('oooooh') to convey the hostess's crying and then produces the verb 'crying' itself. He then uses further reported speech ('never mind') to convey the female guest's efforts to console the hostess.

(5) part (b)

Unit 26.5 Conversational data

(1) Roy uses a noun-initial strategy whereby he utters 'racing', 'Newmarket' and 'Epsom' first, followed by 'anywhere', indicating that he has attended racing in a large number of locations. The strategy of incrementally building his message continues when he states that he ('but me') has not attended Ascot ('Ascot, no'). Di's contribution to the exchange can be described as one of facilitating her father's turn through the use of back-channel behaviours ('yeah', 'mm'), then summarising his message, and finally giving him an opportunity to accept or reject her summary ('you've never been have you'). After Roy accepts her summary, Di produces a final comment ('perhaps you can go next year dad').

(2) Roy uses an adjective-initial strategy in this exchange whereby he begins with an adjective 'interesting actually'. This stands as an evaluation of Di's job as a nursery nurse. He then justifies this evaluation by providing a reason through the use of the conjunction 'because'. The reason 'now me I think no, special' is an admission that he (Roy) could not do Di's job as you have to be special to do it. Di's contribution to the exchange remains unchanged from extract A. She supports Roy in his turn through the use of back-channel behaviour. She then summarises what she believes his message to be, and provides him with an opportunity to accept or reject her

summary ('what working with children'). After Roy accepts her summary, Di produces a comment ('not everyone can do it').

(3) (a) Roy states 'two weeks' (a noun phrase)
    (b) Roy establishes that the referent of 'it' in 'it'll be a good night' is Di's birthday party.
    (c) Roy comprehends Di's use of '<u>this</u> weekend' (temporal deixis)
    (d) Roy uses 'I <u>know</u>' (mental state language)
    (e) Roy utters 'two weeks <u>innit</u>' (innit = isn't it?)

(4) (a) false; (b) false; (c) true; (d) false; (e) true

(5) (a) Roy describes past visits to racing at Newmarket and Epsom.
    (b) Roy expresses his opinion that it takes someone special to be a nursery nurse.
    (c) Roy confirms that Di's birthday party will take place in two weeks.
    (d) Roy evaluates Di's job as 'interesting'.
    (e) Roy supports Di's conversational turns through the use of back-channel behaviour (see 'yeah' in extract C).

Case study 27 Man aged 41 years with non-fluent aphasia

Unit 27.1 Medical and communication history

(1) Most brain emboli are distributed in the territory of the MCA, which is the main and most direct branch of the internal carotid artery (Garcia et al., 1998: 46). This is why strokes of the MCA territory are so common. The poorer functional outcomes associated with MCA strokes arise because of the presence of aphasia and apraxia in left-sided MCA lesions, and neglect and agnosia in right-sided MCA lesions (Ng et al., 2007). These conditions make a good recovery from a stroke more difficult to achieve.

(2) The lesion localisation in Broca's aphasia is usually in the left inferior frontal cortex, anterior to the motor strip. The motor strip controls voluntary movements of the articulators and other structures involved in speech production (e.g. larynx). If the damage that causes Broca's aphasia extends to involve the motor strip, a client may have apraxia of speech as well as Broca's aphasia.

(3) Five features which are consistent with a diagnosis of Broca's aphasia: (1) impaired verbal fluency; (2) word-finding deficit; (3) agrammatic verbal output; (4) client is aware of communication difficulties; and (5) auditory comprehension is superior to expressive language.

(4) BB is only able to produce nouns (e.g. boy, window) and set phrases ('don't know'). There is no verb production and words from all other grammatical classes (e.g. determiners, prepositions, conjunctions) are absent.

(5) parts (b) and (d)

Unit 27.2 Assessment battery

(1) The examiner gave BB this instruction as she wanted to see if he could produce verbs in the absence of their arguments.

(2) The pictures depicted only animate actors and inanimate patients in order that BB had to produce sentences like *The man kicked the ball*. The pictures required BB to produce irreversible sentences only.

(3) In order to generate a sentence around a verb, BB must produce the arguments that attend a particular verb. This may be one argument (e.g. <u>Tim</u> smiles), two arguments (e.g. <u>The boy</u> hid <u>the book</u>) or three arguments (e.g. <u>The man</u> gave <u>the comb to the girl</u>).

(4) The man hit the boy.

(5) This task is attempting to assess if BB recognises the integrity of the phrase. So, for example, in the sentence *Paula bought some chocolate in the shop*, 'some chocolate' and 'in the shop' constitute phrases (noun and prepositional phrases, respectively), while 'bought some' and 'chocolate in' do not.

Unit 27.3 Assessment findings

(1) BB's performance in this task shows that his retrieval and production of verbs in the absence of their arguments are relatively intact. 'Running' (a gerund) is an example of the form that BB's 'doing' words took.

(2) (a) push; writing; drink; climb; eat
(b) *kicking* 'push'; *writing* 'read'; *drinking* 'eat'
(c) writing
(d) *The girl is writing a letter:* writing . . . /r/ . . . /r/ . . . read . . . **girl**
The boy is climbing a ladder: me! (indicating boy) no . . . **boy** /k/ . . . climb up . . . yes!
The boy is drinking orange: /b/ . . . **boy** . . . ah! . . . boy is . . . /i/ . . . eat . . . no . . . um
(e) *The boy is riding the bike:* girl . . . no **boy** . . . **bike** . . . well . . . um . . . boy . . . um
The boy is digging the garden: /g/ . . . /g/ . . . don't know . . . (cued 1st syll.)
garden . . . **boy** . . . is . . . no

(3) On SVO picture description, BB was able to produce seven actor arguments. However, no actor arguments were produced when he was provided with the infinitive form of the verb. This difference can be explained as an effect of the task – BB was given a verb and started his sentence construction with the verb in each case. On SVO picture description, BB produced three patient arguments. This increased to seven patient arguments on the infinitive verb task. Three of these arguments were semantic paraphasias (*book* 'letter'; *apple* 'food'; *orange* 'beer'). There is little evidence on either of these tasks of BB being able to consistently access and use verb argument structure.

(4) A simple active reversible sentence: *The man chases the boy*. The reason this type of sentence is difficult for BB to understand is that either noun phrase could be the actor in the sentence, and BB must use his knowledge of argument structure to determine which one is the actor. However, BB's knowledge of argument structure is disrupted. This deficit is confirmed by the results of the Word Order Test. When presented with a sentence and asked to match it to one of three pictures, BB consistently selected the picture in which the arguments were reversed.

(5) BB is able to recognise the constituents of phrases, allowing him to segment sentences according to their different phrases. However, because he does not understand how phrases relate to each other within sentences, he is unable to construct grammatical sentences from individual phrases.

Unit 27.4 Language intervention

(1) Intransitive verbs were used to introduce the concept of actor because the actor is the only obligatory argument in these verbs. The absence of other arguments simplifies the production for the client.

> *The girl cries* (human subject); *The dog barks* (animal subject)

(2) Transitive verbs have an obligatory theme.

> *The woman knocked the door* (the woman = WHO? the door = WHAT?)

(3) Verbs like 'put' are three-argument verbs. The therapist used sentences in which the prepositional phrase appears at the beginning of the sentence (<u>In the garden</u> Robert grew herbs) and at the end of the sentence (Robert grew herbs <u>in the garden</u>) in order to avoid a situation in which the client learns (erroneously) that it is always the final argument in the sentence that answers to the question 'where?'.

(4) <u>At midnight</u> the bomb exploded (when?)
Sally went to Paris <u>for a conference</u> (why?)
He bolted <u>quickly</u> through the door (how?)
The pragmatic constraint on sentence production is that these elements are optional and are introduced depending on the informational needs of the listener.

(5) In an irreversible passive voice sentence (e.g. *The ball was kicked by the boy*), world knowledge alone indicates that the boy is responsible for the action of the verb and that the ball is the recipient of that action. No knowledge of the meaning relations expressed by the arguments in the sentence is required in order to decode the sentence successfully. In reversible passive voice sentences (e.g. *The boy was chased by the man*), knowledge of the meaning relations expressed by the arguments is required for successful decoding to occur. This is why the therapist introduced irreversible passives before reversible passives in therapy.

Unit 27.5 Language performance during therapy

(1) *Cookie theft picture description:*
'woman drying the washing up'
'water falling to the floor'
'the window is open'
'girl wants one'
Narrative production: In all three examples, the actor is missing.
'sold potatoes'
'drive van to Cambridge'
'pack the van'

(2) (a) 'boy is kicking the ball'
  (b) BB utters 'girl' for *boy*
  (c) 'the girl . . . no boy . . . is eating an apple'
  (d) 'the boy is . . . eh . . . um . . . oh . . . a ladder no!'
  (e) 'the girl . . . is writing . . . a letter . . . to . . . eh . . . friend' ('to a friend' is an optional argument)

(3) On the Word Order Test in July 1985, BB is still making argument errors when asked to rearrange sentence elements and when required to match a spoken sentence to one of three pictures. The errors all appear to involve the reversal of arguments.

(4) prepositions (e.g. <u>on</u> concrete floor)
  determiners (e.g. <u>the two</u> cups)
  auxiliary verbs (e.g. the girl <u>is</u> reaching up)
  actor arguments (e.g. <u>the woman</u> is washing up)
  main verbs (e.g. the boy is <u>reaching</u> for cookies)

(5) Three discourse anomalies: (i) A topic shift occurs when BB starts to talk about his stroke during a narrative about his previous employment; (ii) BB uses repetitive language when he talks about driving to Cambridge and selling chips; (iii) BB uses the pronoun 'we' in the absence of a clear referent.

Case study 28 Man aged 60 years with right hemisphere damage

Unit 28.1 Primer on right-hemisphere language disorder

(1) parts (a), (b) and (e)

(2) (a) metaphor; (b) idiom; (c) conventional implicature; (d) sarcasm; (e) indirect speech act

(3) Speakers use intonation and other aspects of prosody to signal different types of speech acts. For example, a speaker can use one and the same utterance (e.g. Bob is in town) as a statement or a question, and it is the use of prosody which signals which speech act the speaker expects to obtain in a particular case. Clients with RHD who make poor use of prosody can expect some of their utterances to be misunderstood by hearers during communication.

(4) Phonology, morphology and syntax are well preserved in RHD. The preservation of these aspects of language sets RHLD apart from classical aphasia.

(5) (a) true; (b) false; (c) true; (d) false; (e) true

Unit 28.2 Right-hemisphere language assessment

(1) Myers states that adults with RHD 'miss the implication of [a] question and respond in a most literal and concrete way'. This statement corresponds to the finding that adults with RHD have difficulty understanding indirect speech acts. For example, such an adult may reply 'yes' to the question 'Can you sit down?', a response which suggests that he has failed to grasp that this is a request to sit down.

(2) Myers remarks that the components of a narrative could not be 'integrated into a whole'. This description suggests a problem with weak central coherence on the part of Myers' subjects.

(3) Humour is often based on non-literal language. To the extent that the understanding of non-literal language is compromised in adults with RHD, one might expect to find a failure to appreciate humour in these subjects.

(4) Emotional prosody conveys information about the affective state with which an utterance is produced. So the single utterance 'John is very late' can express quite different affective states, ranging from anger to sadness and happiness, depending on the emotional prosody with which the utterance is produced in a particular context. The use of linguistic prosody can cause one and the same utterance to be a statement

on one occasion of use and a question on another occasion. Linguistic prosody conveys a speaker's communicative intention, not his or her affective state.

(5) The utterances *This homework is a nightmare* and *The stressed lawyer was a steam kettle* would be assessed in the understanding of metaphors in the MEC.

Unit 28.3 Client history and assessment

(1) After initial investigation, OP went on to develop epilepsy and bilateral brain lesions. Because his neurological damage extended beyond the right cerebral hemisphere, and occurred in the presence of epilepsy, OP was no longer judged to be a suitable participant in an investigation of language disorder in stroke-induced right hemisphere damage.

(2) In indirect speech act 1, Louise is requesting her husband to wash the car. When explicitly asked by the examiner which interpretation applies to this speech act, OP opts for the literal interpretation ('I'd probably go with option A'). However, it is clear from his extended response that he does have some appreciation of the intended, non-literal interpretation of the speech act. This is indicated through utterances such as 'it would be convenient to wash the car' and 'she's [. . .] imposing an assigned chore, regarding the husband'.

(3) In indirect speech act 2, Mr Martinez is requesting his spouse to answer the phone. Throughout the exchange with the examiner, there is evidence that OP is pulled between two different interpretations of this speech act. OP begins by repeating information which is provided by the examiner ('He's busy'). He then appears to veer towards the intended interpretation of the speech act when he says 'it's assumed that he wants his wife'. A little later, the intended interpretation is directly stated: 'what's suggested is that she should answer the phone'. That both interpretations are salient for OP is confirmed by the utterance 'he's says both things'.

(4) In indirect speech act 3, OP draws the inference that Martin needs the glasses in order to watch television. It is this inference which motivates Martin to request his wife to bring him his glasses from the table.

(5) Before he arrives at the intended interpretation of indirect speech act 4, OP dwells on the work relationship between Peter and his secretary. OP reports that within this relationship, the secretary is under a 'work obligation' to comply with her boss's requests.

Unit 28.4 Focus on metaphor

(1) OP's understanding of the metaphor in the utterance 'My friend's mother-in-law is a witch' is concrete and literal in nature. In his attempt to characterise the meaning of this metaphor, OP refers only to conventional attributes of witches which are embodied in the semantic meaning of the word 'witch', e.g. inclusion in religious sects, the practice of black magic.

(2) OP displays some awareness that his interpretation of the metaphor may not be accurate. This occurs when he denies that having many brooms is part of the meaning of the metaphor: 'My friend's mother-in-law has many brooms . . . no!'. However, OP's awareness is limited and inconsistent. For as soon as he denies one of the conventional attributes of a witch as part of the meaning of the metaphor, he goes

on to accept another conventional attribute – the practice of black magic – as part of the metaphor's meaning.

(3) OP makes use of egocentric discourse throughout this exchange. He immediately replaces the neutral term 'friend' with the familial term 'son-in-law'. OP also describes at some length aspects of his personal experience which are of no interest to the examiner, e.g. marital relationships and relationships between a couple and their daughter.

(4) OP does not use humour appropriately in this exchange with the examiner. OP's laughter at the end of his second turn suggests that he finds his own remarks humorous. However, the examiner's response in the next turn suggests that whatever humour OP thinks he has conveyed, it has not been interpreted as such by the examiner.

(5) OP's use of referring expressions makes a significant contribution to his discourse difficulties. In OP's second turn in the exchange, he introduces the terms 'she', 'her marriage', and 'her husband', all of which lack clear referents. OP is aware of this and immediately establishes a referent by saying 'I'm referring to the mother-in-law of my son-in-law'. But this correction arrives late, and only after the examiner has had to establish a suitable referent. Other referential anomalies include the use of a definite noun phrase in the absence of a referent in 'Because the woman is separated' (what woman?), and the unclear referent of the pronoun in 'she's now a poor lady' (the woman or the daughter).

Unit 28.5 Focus on narrative discourse

(1) Prior to the utterance beginning 'And so he went down . . . ', OP's narrative is highly repetitive. OP does little more than continually state that the farmer was digging a hole/well with a shovel and pick.

(2) OP fails to narrate the main events in the story. All the events which follow the collapse of the well are omitted. These include the farmer placing his shirt and cap on the edge of the well and then hiding in the tree, a neighbour coming along and calling out for help, and the efforts of friends to dig the farmer out of the well.

(3) The following remark by OP suggests that he may be experiencing visuo-perceptual deficits: 'objects that don't look like what we call shovel and pick'.

(4) OP's introduction of the farmer into the narrative is skilfully achieved through the use of an indefinite noun phrase: 'There was a farmer who was digging . . . '. The use of an indefinite noun phrase is a standard narrative device for the first mention of story characters.

(5) (a) false; (b) true; (c) false; (d) true; (e) false

Case study 29 Man aged 24 years with closed head injury

Unit 29.1 Primer on traumatic brain injury

(1) Five causes of TBI in children and adults:
    (i) violent assaults, particularly among young males
    (ii) abusive head trauma in violently shaken infants

    (iii) sports injuries in contact sports like boxing and rugby

    (iv) combat-related injuries in military personnel

    (v) parturitional injuries sustained during and secondary to foetal delivery

(2) In an epidural haematoma blood accumulates and forms a clot between the skull and the dura mater (the outer of the three meninges). In a subdural haematoma blood accumulates and forms a clot between the dura mater and the arachnoid mater (the middle membrane of the three meninges).

(3) (a) a blunt head trauma – sensorineural hearing loss

    (b) a blast-related brain injury – sensorineural and conductive hearing loss (the tympanic membrane can be perforated by a blast, causing a conductive hearing loss)

(4) Three reasons why speech-language pathologists do not routinely assess domains like discourse in clients with TBI:

    (i) The analyses that are needed to assess discourse are both labour- and time-intensive to perform.

    (ii) While clinical tests of structural language skills are in abundance, there are few clinical tools available for the assessment of pragmatics and discourse.

    (iii) Speech-language pathologists have limited knowledge of pragmatics and discourse in comparison to phonology, syntax and semantics. SLP curricula do not include pragmatics and discourse as standard, with the result that clinicians do not feel particularly well equipped to assess these aspects of language.

(5) Executive function deficits are so common in individuals who sustain TBI because the frontal lobe regions and their related circuitry are particularly vulnerable to TBI pathophysiology. These regions are widely implicated in a range of executive functions.

Unit 29.2 Client history and cognitive-communication status

(1) (a) true; (b) false; (c) true; (d) true; (e) false

(2) apraxia of speech

(3) parts (c) and (e)

(4) parts (a), (c) and (d)

(5) The subject's intellectual functioning is within the normal range. Intellectual functioning was assessed by means of the Raven's Colored Progressive Matrices.

Unit 29.3 Pragmatic and discourse assessment

(1) part (e)

(2) The subject's word-finding difficulty explains the lack of specificity and accuracy exhibited on the Pragmatic Protocol. In the absence of retrieval of specific words, clients with anomic aphasia (like this subject with CHI) use non-specific vocabulary like 'thing' and 'stuff'.

(3) Prosody plays a vital role in conveying a speaker's intended meaning. For example, a speaker's use of intonation can convey to a listener that he or she intends the utterance 'What a delightful child!' to be a sarcastic comment on the boisterous boy in the room. Similarly, a speaker's use of primary stress on the word 'bull' in the utterance 'There's a bull in the field' conveys to a listener that the speaker intends his or her

utterance to be a warning rather than simply a description of a state of affairs. It is for this reason that prosody is one of the pragmatic parameters assessed in the Pragmatic Protocol.

(4) Clients with TBI are known to have problems with a number of abstract cognitive operations. These operations include abstract reasoning and abstracting meaning from a text to arrive at the gist of a story (Anderson and Catroppa, 2005; Cook et al., 2014).

(5) Findings which support clinical impression of tangential, repetitive, uninformative discourse:

> Tangential: 11.4% and 13.8% of issues introduced by the subject with CHI are unrelated to the monologue topic. The normal control subject does not introduce any issues that are unrelated to the monologue topic.
>
> Repetitive: 11.4% and 12.1% of the issues introduced by the subject with CHI are reintroduced. In effect, the subject is revisiting or repeating issues that have already been dealt with in the monologue. This compares to only 5.4% and 2.4% of reintroduced issues by the normal control subject.
>
> Uninformative: The percentage of ideational units which contain new information is low for the subject with CHI (48.8% and 56.0%) in comparison with the normal control subject (83.9% and 79.4%). The subject with CHI produces a higher percentage of ideational units which contain no new information than the normal control subject (12.7% and 9.7%, respectively, in the concrete condition) and introduces a smaller percentage of new issues than the normal control subject (77.1% and 94.6%, respectively, in the concrete condition).

Unit 29.4 Focus on conversation: part 1

(1) non-specific lexemes: 'people'; 'things'; 'somewhere'
(2) The subject uses grammatical ellipsis in the utterance 'no I haven't [been to a Halloween party]'.
(3) incomplete utterances:
> incomplete prepositional phrase: 'coming through [. . .]'
> incomplete verb phrase: 'who [. . .] things'
> incomplete verb phrase: 'you go [. . .]'

(4) The speech-language pathologist expands her question in her second turn because she appears to treat the subject's response ('uh') as an indication that he has not understood the question. However, this response on the part of the subject may not indicate a lack of comprehension so much as a word-finding difficulty.
(5) The subject with CHI uses personal pronouns ('you go') and demonstrative pronouns ('that's . . . good looking costume') in the absence of clear referents.

Unit 29.5 Focus on conversation: part 2

(1) (a) 'it seemed to ah, (2.0) over'
　　(b) 'you put everything in[to it]'
　　(c) 'it seemed to ah'
　　(d) 'I really get into it'
　　(e) 'that's a big circle'

(2) part (c)
(3) Markers of sympathetic circularity:
       ('well') 'well it's <u>like</u> . . . art'
       ('and') 'and that's what you're doing . . . <u>you know</u>'
       ('kinda') '<u>kinda</u> go over'
(4) The subject only links clauses through the use of 'and': 'you jus' sit down . . . <u>and</u> you really concentrate . . . <u>and</u> you put everything in . . . <u>and</u> it . . . seems . . . like . . . <u>and</u> that's what you're doing'.
(5) The speech-language pathologist uses her final turn in the exchange to summarise the message which she believes the subject with CHI has been attempting to communicate. She marks the beginning of her summarisation through the use of the discourse marker 'so'. She then presents her summary by way of a yes–no question which requires only a simple confirmation or rejection on the part of the subject. This summarisation strategy allows the speech-language pathologist to check her understanding of what the subject is saying in a way which places limited demands on the subject's communication skills – he only needs to express his agreement or disagreement with the therapist's summary.

Case study 30 Woman aged 87 years with early-stage Alzheimer's disease

Unit 30.1 Primer on Alzheimer's disease

(1) parts (a) and (e)
(2) The language impairment in AD is described as a 'cognitive-communication disorder' as it is related to the cognitive deficits that occur in AD: 'Communication is affected because the pathophysiologic processes of AD disrupt information generation and processing. Patients are said to have a "cognitive-communication" problem because progressive deterioration of cognition interferes with communication' (Bayles and Tomoeda, 2013: xiv).
(3) part (c)
(4) false
(5) parts (b), (d) and (e)

Unit 30.2 Language in Alzheimer's disease

(1) (a) true; (b) false; (c) true; (d) false; (e) false
(2) parts (a) and (d)
(3) primary progressive aphasia; cognitive
(4) part (d)
(5) The Boston Diagnostic Aphasia Examination (Goodglass et al., 2001) is a standard aphasia test battery. These batteries should be supplemented by other assessments as the language impairments of clients with AD often go beyond deficits in structural language. Specifically, pragmatic and discourse deficits in AD are not readily revealed by aphasia batteries.

Unit 30.3 Focus on language in Alzheimer's disease

(1) (a) 'yes I did [drive all the way by myself]'
    (b) Nurse: 'Did you stop?' Martha: 'we stopped here and there'
    (c) 'to X-county and <u>further up</u>'
    (d) 'I don't have any mon-'
    (e) 'I was so <u>afraid</u>'

(2) Two linguistic features which suggest that Martha is experiencing word-finding problems: (i) the use of vague language (e.g. 'to X-county and <u>further up</u>') and (ii) the use of filled pauses before content words (e.g. 'that small e:h Volkswagen').

(3) (a) '<u>along</u> the road'
    (b) 'the <u>newest</u> one'
    (c) 'I have taken my driving test <u>so</u> I had my license'
    (d) 'it was the newest one <u>that we took</u>'
    (e) '<u>I have been driving</u> too of course'

(4) In extract 2, Martha is able to produce the names of three different types of berry: strawberries; lingonberries; and bilberries.

(5) Catherine supports Martha in the construction of her narrative by (i) producing backchannel sounds (e.g. 'mm'), and (ii) producing evaluative statements (e.g. 'that wasn't a bad thing'). The former behaviour indicates to Martha that Catherine is listening and that she wants Martha to continue her story. The latter behaviour indicates that Catherine appreciates the content of what Martha is saying.

Unit 30.4 Discourse in Alzheimer's disease

(1) (a) idiom; (b) metaphor; (c) idiom; (d) proverb; (e) metaphor

(2) (a) relation – The client states that her daughter will travel to Spain.
    (b) manner – The client relates events in the wrong order when she begins her response by saying that an ambulance took her home.
    (c) quantity – The client's response is under-informative.

(3) Topic development is compromised in the client with AD who produces uninformative utterances in conversation. This client is unable to contribute to the propositional development of a topic.

(4) (a) The speaker fails to use ellipsis and utters 'I would like a coffee' when 'a coffee' would suffice.
    (b) The speaker uses anaphoric reference incorrectly, as it is not clear if 'it' refers to the blouse or to the cardigan. The speaker also uses substitution incorrectly, as it is not clear if 'one' takes the place of blouse or cardigan.
    (c) The speaker uses cataphoric reference incorrectly, as it is not clear if 'it' refers to the cathedral or to the castle.
    (d) The speaker uses ellipsis incorrectly, as it is not clear which action B is prepared to undertake.
    (e) The speaker uses anaphoric reference incorrectly, as it is not clear if 'it' refers to the blue dress or to the pink hat.

(5) In order to establish that the speaker who utters 'What a delightful child!' in the presence of a disruptive 5-year-old does so with sarcastic intent, a hearer must be able to attribute certain mental states to the mind of the speaker. Two such states are that the speaker believes that the child is anything but delightful and that the speaker who

entertains this *belief* and produces this utterance has a *communicative intention* to be sarcastic. The attribution of these mental states to the mind of the speaker requires an intact theory of mind capacity. Because this capacity is often disrupted in clients with AD, it is difficult for these clients to interpret sarcastic utterances.

Unit 30.5 Focus on discourse in Alzheimer's disease

(1) In lines (1), (2) and (4), Martha utters 'he said'. The referent of the personal pronoun 'he' is unclear as it could be her husband, her driving teacher or her driving examiner in this context. In line (9), Catherine says 'I never dare think about <u>that</u>'. The referent of the demonstrative pronoun 'that' is unclear, as Martha's subsequent request for clarification indicates.

(2) In line (10), Martha makes a request for clarification when she says 'come again?' to Catherine. In order to make requests for clarification, Martha must be able to monitor her comprehension of another speaker's utterances. Monitoring understanding of someone else's utterances demands the possession of metacognitive and metalinguistic skills on Martha's part.

(3) Martha is skilled at using direct reported speech. For example, in line (2) she utters: '"You you took the driving test easily" he said'.

(4) In line 17, Martha utters 'And then we drove up to eh'. Martha uses the conjunction words 'and then' to indicate that she bought the car first *and then* went on a road journey in it.

(5) In line (11), Catherine says 'You're so lucky' while pointing at Martha. This gesture enables Catherine to indicate clearly that Martha is the intended referent of the pronoun 'you'. In line (12), Catherine produces a vague gesture which does not facilitate the communication of her message. This gesture is repeated in line (14).

Case study 31 Man aged 36 years with AIDS dementia complex

Unit 31.1 Personal and medical history

(1) part (a)

(2) parts (a), (d) and (e)

(3) Warren has experienced pneumonia, which may be caused by the aspiration of food and liquids. Also, he has had oral candida which can be a cause of dysphagia.

(4) cytomegalovirus (CMV) infection

(5) Warren is a regular user of marijuana. This may also contribute to his cognitive problems.

Unit 31.2 Cognitive and psychological profile

(1) (a) false; (b) false; (c) true; (d) false; (e) false

(2) parts (a), (d) and (e)

(3) parts (c) and (d)

(4) Depression can be an independent cause of communication problems.

(5) parts (b) and (d)

Unit 31.3 Language and communication profile

(1) parts (b) and (e). Both are metaphorical utterances.
(2) part (b)
(3) parts (b) and (e)
(4) Warren's word-finding problems might explain his use of non-specific vocabulary on CDA. Specifically, when a client struggles to find a specific word, s/he substitutes non-specific vocabulary like 'thing' and 'stuff' in its place.
(5) part (a)

Unit 31.4 Focus on conversation

(1) Referential disturbances do contribute to the researcher's difficulty in following what Warren is saying. For example, there are no clear referents of the adverb 'there' and the pronoun 'it' in the following utterance: 'So I've added there as well and the years come along and I didn't remember doing either of the first two so I did it again [...]'. However, Warren is also able to use reference appropriately, as in this example of anaphoric reference: 'I added a year at my birthday, didn't celebrate it so therefore I forgot about it'.
(2) Warren makes use of several mental state verbs including 'I forgot about it', 'I didn't remember' and 'I thought'. The fact that Warren is able to use these verbs in relation to himself suggests that he is able to attribute mental states to his own mind.
(3) (a) 'Someone pointed out'
     (b) 'In September as a halfway between two ages I start saying what the next one is'
     (c) 'and a new set of batteries that were still in the package so that guaranteed the calculator was working properly'
     (d) 'I went "no, I'm not I'm 34"'
     (e) 'I was 34 last year and 33 last year'
(4) Warren appropriately uses an indefinite noun phrase on the first mention of a new person or object, and a definite noun phrase on a subsequent mention, e.g. 'I'm gonna get me a calculator and a new set of batteries that were still in the package so that guaranteed the calculator was working properly'.
(5) parts (b), (c) and (e)

Unit 31.5 Impact of ADC on communicative competence

(1) The AIDS control tends to use minimal, but nonetheless informative and relevant responses to questions, e.g. 'Foreign service'. Warren does make relevant, informative responses to questions, e.g. 'Oh when I had the business, cleaning the building'. However, after making such a response, he can then engage in a lengthy digression, as is evident at the end of the second conversational extract.
(2) When the researcher states 'that must've been very interesting', this is a comment which requires some further development by the AIDS control. However, it is effectively neglected by this speaker, who proceeds to describe the type of work he did.
(3) (a) True: Warren can respond to grammatical questions (e.g. 'What would be the longest job you had?') and prosodic questions (e.g. 'And that was when you were in your twenties?').

   (b) False: Warren is able to make use of anaphoric reference, e.g. 'My great
         grandmother was born into a family that was indentured to a castle near
         Salisbury, Newcastle. Well she was supposed to be a house servant'.
   (c) True: The AIDS control uses a lexical error when he states 'I'm a public service'.
   (d) False: The AIDS control can make use of anaphoric reference, e.g. ''cause X um
         and Australia are connected now with visas they don't need uh like people to issue
         them'.
   (e) True: Warren engages in play on the meaning of words when he uses 'common
         sense' and 'there's nothing common about this little black duck'. The two senses
         of 'common' are *plain, ordinary good judgement* and *vulgar and coarse*, respectively.
(4) For the AIDS control, 'foreign service' appears to activate 'public service'. For
      Warren, 'common sense' appears to activate 'nothing common about this little black
      duck'.
(5) part (c)

Case study 32 Man aged 76 years with Parkinson's disease

Unit 32.1 Primer on Parkinson's disease

(1) (a) hypophonia; (b) bradykinesia; (c) micrographia; (d) substantia nigra; (e) theory of
      mind
(2) Dopamine is a neurotransmitter. In the central nervous system, it is involved in the
      control of locomotion, cognition, affect and neuroendocrine secretion.
(3) (a) respiration; (b) prosody; (c) phonation; (d) articulation; (e) prosody
(4) (b) sarcasm; (d) metaphor
(5) All utterance interpretation involves establishing the communicative intention that
      motivated a speaker to produce an utterance. A communicative intention is a type of
      mental state. Clients with PD who have ToM deficits will be unable to attribute this
      mental state to the mind of a speaker who produces an utterance, and will experience
      problems with pragmatic understanding in consequence.

Unit 32.2 Client history and communication status

(1) part (c)
(2) Saldert et al. (2014: 712) characterise intelligibility as a measure of speech signal
      effectiveness, and comprehensibility as the listener's understanding of the semantic
      content of an utterance produced in a communicative context.
(3) A listener can use contextual cues to help him understand the speaker during
      an assessment of comprehensibility. These same cues are not available to the
      listener during an assessment of intelligibility. A speaker can thus have greater
      comprehensibility than might be suggested by his intelligibility.
(4) executive function skills
(5) This result reveals that the comprehension of both structural and pragmatic aspects
      of language is impaired in Parkinson's disease.

Unit 32.3 Focus on word-finding difficulties

(1) Three features of Robert's pauses which indicate that they are related to a word search:
  (a) duration – several pauses are particularly prolonged, suggesting that Robert is using them to facilitate a word search
  (b) location – several pauses occur immediately before the production of content words such as verbs ('read') and nouns ('purposes'), which are difficult for Robert to produce (see semantic fluency score)
  (c) filler – one of Robert's pauses is followed by a filler ('eh'), which helps him retain his turn as he searches for a word

(2) Non-specific vocabulary:
  'it was <u>some</u> priest'
  'purposes or influ- or <u>something</u>'
  'elderly persons <u>and such</u>'

(3) Robert uses a circumlocution when he produces 'elderly persons and such who are living on those pension schemes' to refer to *pensioners*.

(4) Robert uses pronouns in the absence of clear referents. This includes possessive pronouns ('part of <u>their</u> work') and personal pronouns ('<u>it</u> was a moment of'). The absence of referents contributes to the listener's difficulty in understanding Robert.

(5) In her final turn in the extract, Sonja attempts to bring the conversation back to her earlier enquiry about singing. This is the last point in the exchange where there was mutual understanding between Robert and Sonja. Sonja's desire to return to this point is indicated by her emphasis on the word 'hymns' and by the preface 'no but', which is used in an effort to re-direct Robert away from his troublesome talk.

Unit 32.4 Focus on conversational repair

(1) Non-specific vocabulary:
  'it is good for <u>such</u>'
  'refer to certain <u>things</u>'
  'may speak quite freely on such <u>things</u>'

(2) Problematic reference assignment:
  'what you feel about <u>that</u>' (no referent for demonstrative pronoun)
  '<u>it</u> is good for such' (no referent for personal pronoun)
  '<u>it</u> is not much' (no referent for personal pronoun)

(3) Sonja's repair strategy assumes the following form. She provides Robert with a suggestion about what he means, based on her understanding of what he has been struggling to communicate up to that point in the exchange. Robert is merely required to accept or reject her suggestion, thus reducing his communicative burden. Sonja's first suggestion is rejected by Robert. She then offers a second suggestion, which Robert accepts. The repair strategy is effective in establishing common ground between Robert and Sonja.

(4) As described in (3), the repair strategy sees Sonja presenting Robert with a series of suggestions about what it is that he is attempting to communicate. For his part, Robert either accepts or rejects each of Sonja's suggestions. However, the word 'or' at the end of each of Sonja's utterances (e.g. 'so you had some discussions after <u>or</u>?') suggest that she may have been attempting to provide Robert with a forced choice (i.e. 'Do you

mean X or Y?'). But in each case Robert moves so swiftly to either accept or reject the X element of the forced choice that the Y component is abandoned by Sonja.

(5) Five instances of mental state language:

> Robert: 'what you <u>feel</u> about that'
> Robert: 'you don't <u>know</u>'
> Robert: 'you shouldn't (1.1) <u>understand</u>'
> Sonja: 'I <u>see</u> so you had'
> Sonja: 'I <u>see</u>'

In Sonja's utterances, the verb 'see' has the meaning of *understand*. Robert's ability to use and comprehend mental state language suggests that he has a relatively intact theory of mind.

Unit 32.5 The role of the conversation partner

(1) Sonja is providing Robert with an alternative ('the organ or the piano?'). This is an example of category 5: *guess / completion / suggestion*.

(2) In unit 32.4, there are two instances of the strategy called *guess / completion / suggestion* when Sonja makes two suggestions to Robert which he then either accepts or rejects.

(3) The strategy called *response token* occurs in unit 32.3 when, after an extended and difficult turn by Robert, Sonja utters 'mm' while subtly nodding.

(4) The strategy called *topic shift* occurs in unit 32.3, when Sonja shifts the topic away from what Robert has been trying unsuccessfully to communicate to her, back to the original topic of the singing that occurred in the church.

(5) response token – not related to initiation of or participation in repair
contribution for flow – not related to initiation of or participation in repair
topic shift – not related to initiation of or participation in repair
open-class initiation of repair – request a clarification or modification of the message by the client
guess / completion / suggestion – provide client with solutions
elaboration / specification – provide client with solutions

Case study 33 Man aged 37 years with Huntington's disease

Unit 33.1 Primer on Huntington's disease

(1) parts (b), (d) and (e)
(2) part (e)
(3) bradykinesia (slowness of movement)
(4) (a) false; (b) true; (c) false; (d) true; (e) true
(5) Clients with HD who have neuropsychiatric disorders may have reduced compliance with SLT interventions relating to dysphagia and communication.

Unit 33.2 Client history

(1) ER's children have a 1 in 2 chance of developing HD. Because HD is an autosomal dominant disorder, half the offspring of parents in which one parent has the defective gene will develop HD.

(2) The presence of chorea affecting ER's arms and face is likely to compromise his ability to use manual gestures and facial expressions during communication.

(3) Apathy and visual gaze difficulties are assessed by the neuropsychiatric and motor components of the UHDRS, respectively.

(4) Dysarthria and executive function deficits in clients with HD may be assessed by the motor and cognitive components of the UHDRS, respectively.

(5) ER's occupational and social functioning have been compromised by HD. ER has had to cease working on account of HD. ER's social functioning has been compromised as he is living in a residential care facility which has isolated him from his family (with the exception of contact with his mother).

Unit 33.3 Communication status

(1) ER's respiratory control for speech is most likely to be compromised by his severe truncal chorea.

(2) Background noise is an environmental challenge to ER's intelligibility. It is difficult for ER to address this challenge because he has difficulty varying loudness. ER will be unable to increase his loudness to counteract the effects of background noise.

(3) (a) true; (b) false; (c) false; (d) false; (e) false

(4) The two aspects of ER's pragmatic skills which might be explained by his apathy are (i) his reliance on his communication partner to initiate topics, and (ii) his production of a reduced quantity of output.

(5) The fact that ER's ratings of his communicative effectiveness were consistent with those of nursing staff and speech-language pathologists suggests that his perception of his communicative strengths and weakness is intact. ER's accurate perception of his communicative skills can be used to encourage self-monitoring of performance during intervention.

Unit 33.4 ICF framework

(1) parts (c) and (d)

(2) The results of ER's communication assessment are recorded under body structures and functions in the ICF framework.

(3) Reduced initiation leads ER not to participate in the talking group unless directly invited to do so. Reduced initiation should be classified as a cognitive deficit under body structures and functions.

(4) Social factors – an estranged family situation – account for ER's current difficulties in his relationship with his children. Speech factors will contribute to difficulties in this relationship in the future.

(5) ER is already familiar with augmentative and alternative communication (AAC) in the form of communication books. He is likely to have a positive response to AAC in his own case.

Unit 33.5 Communication goal setting

(1) The development of a legacy item allows ER to address a participation restriction in the form of not being able to perform the social role of a father to his children.

(2) Goal (2) is intended to address environmental factors that were identified during interviews with ER's mother. Specifically, the use of a mobile phone will allow ER to have conversations with his mother in quieter locations than had hitherto been possible.

(3) The factor which is common to these themes is cognitive deficits in HD and their adverse impact on communication.

(4) Goal (3) is intended to address the adverse impact that ER's apathy and reduced initiation has on communication. Specifically, by extending invitations to ER to attend the weekly talking group, there is less of a requirement for him to initiate this particular activity.

(5) ER's apathy is a personality change which reduced his ability to initiate communication with others.

Case study 34 Boy aged 4 years with developmental stuttering

Unit 34.1 Primer on developmental stuttering

(1) parts (a) and (d)

(2) In order to explain this finding, the process of natural recovery must occur more often in girls than in boys.

(3) Probandwise concordance is defined as the risk of an illness or disorder (in this case, stuttering) in the co-twin of a proband-twin. The fact that concordance rates are consistently higher in monozygotic (genetically identical) twins than in dizygotic (genetically non-identical) twins is evidence that stuttering has a genetic aetiology.

(4) The presence of comorbid conditions in stuttering must be considered by speech-language pathologists during assessment, diagnosis and treatment. For example, the SLP will need to determine during assessment if there is a distinct articulation disorder apart from the speech anomalies associated with stuttering. If such a disorder is present, the SLP will need to decide if articulation should be targeted in treatment before or alongside the speech anomalies of stuttering.

(5) parts (a), (b) and (e)

Unit 34.2 Client history

(1) DL's onset is typical of stuttering. It is stated in unit 34.1 that 95% of the risk for stuttering onset is over by age 4 (Yairi and Ambrose, 2013).

(2) Stuttering is also present in four of DL's biological relatives. This pattern of familial aggregation indicates that DL has an increased genetic risk of stuttering.

(3) The history revealed that DL has immature attention and delayed speech motor processes. There are also behaviour management difficulties in DL's case. The two comorbid conditions suggested by this history are attention deficit disorder (possibly ADHD) and articulation disorder.

(4) The family's recent, stressful move is an environmental factor that may be contributing to DL's stutter.

(5) parts (a), (b) and (e)

Unit 34.3 Speech and language evaluation

(1) DL's percentage of stuttered words is 8.4%. This figure indicates that he is at risk of continuing to stutter. Clinicians also calculate a client's percentage of stuttered syllables as a means of assessing stuttering severity.

(2) The dysfluencies in the utterance 'Its its ha-ha-haaa:vn't got got a window' can be characterised as follows: part-word repetition (ha-ha), whole-word repetition (got got) and sound prolongation (haaa:).

(3) (a) true; (b) false; (c) false; (d) true; (e) true

(4) Three verbal behaviours:
  (i) DL's father uses extended, linguistically complex explanations. Given his receptive language problems, DL is unlikely to comprehend these explanations.
  (ii) DL's mother and father make excessive use of questions. Questions are likely to be challenging for DL's expressive language skills as they require a response. Other speech acts such as comments are less challenging as they do not place DL under an expectation to respond. Also, unless they are carefully chosen, questions may not be understood by DL.
  (iii) DL's mother frequently interrupts him. This suggests a lack of awareness of the difficulties that DL faces in producing spoken language.

(5) Two cognitive skills which are likely to be taxed by parental behaviours are *memory* and *speed of information processing*. DL's father takes lengthy turns and uses lengthy explanations, both of which are likely to exceed DL's memory capacity. His mother and father use a fast speech rate which is likely to exceed DL's speed of information processing.

Unit 34.4 Parent–child interaction therapy

(1) During the first six weeks when no direct therapy was undertaken, measures of the number of dysfluencies per 100 words were regularly taken. This enabled the clinician to establish a no-treatment baseline which could be used to assess the effects of treatment.

(2) DL displayed concomitant non-verbal behaviours such as facial grimacing when he produced stuttered speech. These behaviours, which can only be identified through video-recordings, would have assisted the authors of the study in identifying dysfluencies in DL's speech.

(3) part (c)

(4) Parental use of questions and imperatives was discouraged, and the use of comments was encouraged. Questions were discouraged as they place demands on DL's receptive and expressive language skills, which are known to be significantly delayed. Comments do not demand a response and so they are less challenging for DL in linguistic terms. The father is excessively directive in his interaction with DL. In order to reduce the father's directiveness, the use of imperatives was discouraged and replaced by comments. Comments permit DL to make an active contribution to communication, whereas imperatives consign him to a role in which he is merely complying with the father's commands during play. It should be noted that the use of questions also allowed the parents to direct DL's behaviour. Reduction of the use of questions would have had the effect of decreasing the parents' directiveness with DL.

(5) The purpose of the final five weeks, during which no new information or advice was offered, was to assess the maintenance of treatment effects.

Unit 34.5 Speech outcome

(1) The non-significant result in Phase A indicates that DL's dysfluency was not resolving spontaneously, i.e. without direct intervention.

(2) An intervention which takes as its baseline a single measure of dysfluency at one point in time is likely to overestimate or underestimate the child's actual level of dysfluency. To overcome the inconsistency of early dysfluency in young children, investigators and clinicians must measure the number of dysfluencies produced across several points in time.

(3) Even in the absence of formal language test results, there is some evidence that DL's language skills did improve following parent–child interaction therapy. At the end of 17 weeks, DL was reported to be using more utterances and longer (more complex) utterances.

(4) The demands on DL's speech production system took the form of a pattern of parental interaction which unnecessarily taxed his motor planning and language skills. The aim of parent–child interaction therapy was to reduce these particular environmental demands. At the same time, developmental maturation and the linguistic stimulation provided by PCI therapy jointly bolstered DL's capacities. Intervention thus achieved a reduction in DL's rate of dysfluencies by simultaneously reducing the demands on DL's speech production system and increasing DL's motor speech and language capacities.

(5) DL was producing more utterances and more complex utterances towards the end of the study. As the complexity and amount of DL's linguistic output increase, it is to be expected that his rate of dysfluencies will also increase.

Case study 35 Man aged 29 years with acquired stuttering

Unit 35.1 Primer on acquired stuttering

(1) That there is a significant gender bias among adults with developmental stuttering – a male-to-female ratio of 4:1 – has been recognised for some time. (It should be noted that Yairi and Ambrose (2013) state that this ratio is considerably smaller in very young children near stuttering onset.) However, there is no evidence of a similar gender bias in adults with acquired stuttering.

(2) parts (b) and (d)

(3) part (d)

(4) whole-word repetition; part-word repetition

(5) developmental; choral; auditory

Unit 35.2 Client history and presentation

(1) On the basis of this history and presentation, Mr A appears to have acquired psychogenic stuttering. This is supported by two findings: (i) Mr A reported

considerable work-related stress, and (ii) a comprehensive neurological evaluation was negative.

(2) part (c)

(3) increase in vocal pitch; writing problems

(4) This impairment of writing is suggestive of micrographia in Parkinson's disease. Micrographia is an abnormal reduction in writing size which is specific to Parkinson's disease.

(5) electroencephalography (EEG)

Unit 35.3 Speech pathology evaluation

(1) Mr A's repetitions differ from the iterations of developmental stuttering in the following ways:
   (i) Mr A's repetitions were present on *every* word and syllable, whereas the iterations of developmental stuttering only occur on *some* words and syllables.
   (ii) Mr A's repetitions involve full syllables and words, whereas the repetitions of developmental stuttering involve sound elements that are smaller than full syllables (e.g. phonemes or phonemes and a schwa vowel).

(2) In developmental stuttering sound prolongations or perseverations occur. However, this is not a feature of Mr A's stuttered speech.

(3) Mr A's stuttering behaviour differs from developmental stuttering in the following three respects:
   (i) Choral reading did not alter Mr A's stuttering. Choral reading can induce immediate fluency in the person with developmental stuttering.
   (ii) Mr A did not display secondary characteristics or accessory features. These characteristics are often found in the person with developmental stuttering.
   (iii) Mr A did not display avoidance behaviour or fear of words and/or situations. Both of these behaviours are often found in the person with developmental stuttering.

(4) Fasciculations appear as random, irregular, twitching movements on the surface of the tongue. These movements are caused by involuntary contractions of small bundles of muscle fibres under the surface of the tongue. Fasciculations are indicative of lower motor neurone damage.

(5) There is no comorbid aphasia in Mr A's case. His expressive and receptive language skills are intact.

Unit 35.4 Psychiatric and neurological evaluation

(1) The psychiatric intervention employed pharmacological and behavioural strategies. Neither set of strategies resulted in speech improvement.

(2) The four cardinal signs of Parkinson's disease are resting tremor, bradykinesia, rigidity and postural instability. Mr A displays all four cardinal signs:
   Resting tremor – Mr A exhibited a tremor at rest in both arms and a slight tremor at rest in the right leg.
   Bradykinesia – Mr A displayed slowness of tongue movements and his finger to nose movements were slow.
   Rigidity – Mr A's face was without expression.
   Postural instability – Pushing on Mr A's chest and back produced mild instability with no reflexive compensatory movements of his arms.

(3) The symptoms of Parkinson's disease are typically caused by dopamine deficiency. However, SPECT scanning revealed that Mr A had normal proportions of dopamine in his brain. It must, therefore, be concluded that dopamine receptors in the brain are no longer functioning, or that Mr A's symptoms do not have a biochemical basis.

(4) The palpebral fissures (distance between upper and lower eyelids) are wider than normal and blinking is infrequent. Eyes have a staring appearance on account of these features, and because spontaneous ocular movements are lacking. The patient's facial muscles exhibit an unnatural immobility.

(5) parts (c) and (e)

Unit 35.5 Fluency therapy

(1) parts (c) and (d)

(2) Relaxation techniques were used to address Mr A's vocal pitch anomalies. The fact that Mr A's pitch anomalies improved while other aspects of his stuttered speech did not indicates that these anomalies were likely secondary to his anxiety about his speech disorder rather than a symptom of a parkinsonian-like syndrome.

(3) A soft contact aims to achieve gentle and tension-free contact between the articulators. Sounds which are made with visible articulators such as the lips and teeth are employed to instruct clients in the use of this technique. The clinician can demonstrate the distinction between hard and soft contact by contrasting the tension that occurs during a tense, forceful production of /b/ in 'big' with the altogether less tense and less effortful contact that is used during a soft production of the same sound.

(4) The respiratory–phonatory mechanism is targeted by continuous breath flow which leads to the use of voicing by humming vowels and nasal continuants.

(5) Mr A's fluency intervention aims to increase his rate of speech.

Case study 36 Boy with developmental cluttering

Unit 36.1 Primer on cluttering

(1) parts (a), (d) and (e)

(2) part (c)

(3) In order to study the prevalence and incidence of a disorder, investigators must be able to identify it. However, there has been a lack of clinical consensus on the speech features and other behaviours which constitute cluttering. This lack of consensus has limited the extent to which it has been possible to conduct epidemiological investigations of cluttering.

(4) The person who clutters is collapsing syllables. This behaviour is known as telescoping or the coarticulation of syllables.

(5) true

Unit 36.2 Client history

(1) Three motor milestones: begins to sit without support (6 months); crawls (9 months); walks alone (18 months).

(2) Michael has a reading disorder. Reading problems are often found in people who clutter.

(3) Michael's mother reported that there was a family history of fast talking and stuttering. This indicates that Michael was probably at an elevated genetic risk of having a communication disorder.

(4) unusually fast speech rate

(5) The intervention for speech intervention was probably only minimally effective because there didn't appear to be a proper understanding of the nature of Michael's speech difficulties, namely, that they were related to cluttering.

Unit 36.3 Pre-intervention speech-language evaluation

(1) This description captures the telescoping or coarticulation of syllables and sounds in cluttering.

(2) oral motor coordination skills

(3) This finding is confirmed by the fact that there was an improvement in Michael's speech when a recorder was introduced into the evaluation.

(4) The checklist finding that there is a lack of self-awareness in people who clutter explains why many individuals need to have their communication problems pointed out by others before they seek professional help.

(5) Topic management was judged to be impaired in Michael.

Unit 36.4 Cluttering therapy

(1) The motoric and linguistic components of cluttering are both reflected in the intervention that Michael received. The motoric component of the intervention involved work on Michael's oral motor coordination skills. The linguistic component of the intervention included a focus on language skills such as narrative production and topic maintenance.

(2) Three cognitive components of intervention: (i) focus on concentration and memory; (ii) improving awareness; and (iii) emphasis on thought organisation.

(3) The school speech-language pathologist delivered a motor speech intervention with a focus on articulation and prosody. The hospital speech-language pathologist delivered a cognitive-linguistic intervention.

(4) The American Speech-Language-Hearing Association (2005b) defines central auditory processing disorder as 'difficulties in the processing of auditory information in the central nervous system (CNS) as demonstrated by poor performance in one or more of the following skills: sound localisation and lateralisation; auditory discrimination; auditory pattern recognition; temporal aspects of audition, including temporal integration, temporal discrimination (e.g., temporal gap detection), temporal ordering, and temporal masking; auditory performance in competing acoustic signals (including dichotic listening); and auditory performance with degraded acoustic signals'.

(5) In order to narrate a story, a narrator must be able to plan and organise (or sequence) not just the key events in a story but also the linguistic utterances which will be needed to convey these events. These cognitive-linguistic processes are impaired in people who clutter.

Unit 36.5 Post-intervention speech-language evaluation

(1) A prosodic aspect which had clearly improved following therapy was Michael's speech rate, which was reduced. However, Michael's volume or loudness, which had been minimally aberrant before therapy, was more noticeably aberrant following therapy.

(2) Michael's pragmatic language skills did appear to improve as a result of intervention. His topic maintenance skills improved – he did not deviate from topic as he did at his first evaluation. Also, Michael was able to sequence events where previously his language output had been disorganised.

(3) auditory memory; awareness

(4) Michael engaged in rapid, repetitive eye blinking in association with linguistic revisions and other speech production difficulties. This behaviour is suggestive of the secondary characteristics or accessory features that are found in stuttering.

(5) At re-evaluation Michael frequently kept his hands in front of his mouth and did not always maintain good eye contact. The emergence of these behaviours can be explained as follows. As Michael's awareness of his communication difficulties increases, he is more likely to experience a sense of social unease about them. This sense of unease is likely to be exacerbated by the fact that Michael is approaching adolescence, a life phase where his communication difficulties will set him apart from his peers.

Case study 37 Man aged 51 years with contact granuloma

Unit 37.1 Primer on organic dysphonia

(1) (a) infectious disease
    (b) laryngeal trauma
    (c) neurodegenerative disorder
    (d) infectious disease
    (e) neurodegenerative disorder

(2) (a) endocrine disorder
    (b) pharmacological agent
    (c) auto-immune disease
    (d) endocrine disorder
    (e) pharmacological agent

(3) parts (b) and (d)

(4) vocal fold bowing in presbylarynx

(5) Three occupational groups: teachers; singers; actors
    Laryngeal pathology: vocal nodules

Unit 37.2 Client history

(1) In gastroesophageal reflux, transient relaxation of the lower oesophageal sphincter allows a bolus of refluxate to move from the stomach into the oesophagus. This bolus contains acid and pepsin, which is the primary enzyme of the stomach. If the upper oesophageal sphincter (called the cricopharyngeus) is not functioning normally, this

bolus spills into the larynx and pharynx, causing LPR. The airway epithelium, including the epithelium of the larynx, is fragile and more easily damaged by gastric reflux than the oesophageal epithelium. The corrosive effect of reflux on this epithelium leads to the development of a number of laryngeal pathologies. Laryngeal pathology linked to LPR: laryngeal carcinoma

(2) Vocal hyperfunction: vocal fatigue; hoarseness after teaching a long class
   Laryngopharyngeal reflux: sensation of a lump in the throat in the morning

(3) parts (a), (c) and (e)

(4) (a) false; (b) true; (c) true; (d) true; (e) false

(5) part (e)

Unit 37.3 Voice evaluation

(1) Description 1: open quotient
   Description 2: voice onset time

(2) Stroboscopy is used to examine fine movement of the vocal folds and the mucosal wave. A microphone is placed on the neck of the patient. It allows the frequency of a strobe flashing light to be matched to the frequency of vocal fold vibration. The 'slow-motion' image is captured by a flexible endoscope or a 60° or 70° rigid telescope inserted into the mouth.

(3) part (a)

(4) The presence of a contact granuloma might be expected to increase a speaker's mean expiratory airflow as there will be inadequate adduction of the vocal folds. A successful intervention, which achieves improved glottal contact during adduction, might be expected to result in a decrease in a speaker's mean expiratory airflow.

(5) parts (a), (c) and (e)

Unit 37.4 Voice therapy

(1) The emphasis of physiological voice therapy is on directly exercising and manipulating the different systems involved in voice production: 'The hallmark of physiologic voice therapy is direct physical exercise and manipulations of the laryngeal, respiratory, and the resonance systems in an effort to improve voice quality' (Stemple et al., 2000: 331).

(2) This accommodation is addressed by the VFE which aims to improve the balance among the subsystems for voice production.

(3) 'Vocal function exercises promote a glottal closure pattern (barely adducted/abducted arytenoids) that enhances efficient vocal fold vibration through the use of a semioccluded posturing of the vocal tract' (Patel et al., 2012: 741).

(4) The cricothyroid muscle activates during pitch elevation. It is this laryngeal muscle that is exercised during gliding from a low to a high fundamental frequency.

(5) There is some evidence that vocal function exercises are effective in treating clients with voice disorders. Gorman et al. (2008) reported that vocal function exercises achieved an improvement in vocal aerodynamics in elderly men with voice problems. Roy et al. (2001) found that teachers with voice disorders who received vocal function exercises reported a significant reduction in mean Voice Handicap Index scores. They also reported more overall voice improvement and greater ease and clarity in

their speaking and singing voice following vocal function exercises than teachers with voice disorders who received vocal hygiene only.

Unit 37.5 Post-intervention vocal function

(1) Open quotient is the duration of the cycle during which the vocal folds remain open divided by the duration of the entire cycle. If the folds are open for the entire cycle, as they were in PT's case before treatment, it is not possible to arrive at a calculation of open quotient.

(2) Image B corresponds to the pre-therapy description. Image A corresponds to the post-therapy description.

(3) These findings suggest that acoustic measurements are somewhat insensitive to the impact of a contact granuloma on PT's vocal function.

(4) There was a 4.07% increase in PT's respiratory volume following VFEs. This suggests that these exercises were successful in training PT how to breathe to his maximum capacity for voice production.

(5) A speech-language pathologist might defend the cost-effectiveness of PT's voice therapy in the following terms. He or she could argue that even a mildly deviant voice quality could put PT at risk of psychological distress (e.g. depression) which, in turn, might require him having to take time off work. There are economic consequences for PT and his employer if he is on sick leave. These economic consequences could be averted if PT received timely voice therapy.

Case study 38 Woman aged 50 years with psychogenic dysphonia

Unit 38.1 Primer on psychogenic dysphonia

(1) parts (b) and (d)

(2) Three medical and health professionals:
otorhinolaryngologist
speech-language pathologist
psychotherapist/clinical psychologist/psychiatrist

(3) parts (a), (c) and (e)

(4) Psychogenic dysphonia is frequently misdiagnosed because (i) it is preceded by conditions such as acute laryngitis and allergy/asthma symptoms, and (ii) acute laryngitis and psychogenic dysphonia create similar perceptual aberrations in the voice.

(5) part (b)

Unit 38.2 Client history

(1) parts (c) and (e)

(2) Ms S reports experiencing low mood and feelings of anxiety.

(3) occupational functioning

(4) Ms S is a teaching assistant at a local school. This is an occupation which places high vocal demands on individuals and places them at risk of organic disorders such as vocal nodules. Until a complete laryngological assessment has been conducted, an organic disorder of this type cannot be excluded as a cause of Ms S's voice disorder.

(5) It is known that psychogenic dysphonia is frequently misdiagnosed. This may account for the limited success of Ms S's previous interventions.

Unit 38.3 Voice assessment

(1) part (b)

(2) A good volitional cough indicates that Ms S is able to achieve adequate adduction of the vocal folds.

(3) The fact that Ms S has worse GRBAS scale scores during speaking than during phonation indicates that there is likely to be a psychogenic aetiology to her disorder. If an organic abnormality was the cause of Ms S's voice problems, her GRBAS scale scores would be the same during speaking and phonation.

(4) These values are within the normal range for someone of Ms S's age and sex (Xue et al., 2008).

(5) Ms S's maximum phonation duration of 4 seconds is not within the normal range. The maximum phonation duration of a woman aged 50 years should be 21.34 seconds (standard deviation: 5.66) (Gallena, 2007).

Unit 38.4 Psychological assessment

(1) Ms S has considerable issues around speaking out and having her voice heard. She feels she cannot express her opinions and thoughts to her spouse or to her wider family. Her voice is not heard or is dismissed as having no worth.

(2) Communication is also one of the ways in which conflict is expressed between Ms S and her spouse. They both express anger by not talking to each other for days.

(3) Fluctuations in Ms S's vocal symptoms are reflective of her emotional state. During joint sessions with her spouse, Ms S's voice was hoarse and became aphonic when an argument occurred.

(4) Ms S has received the attention and concern of her children, and particularly her daughters, on account of having a voice disorder. This is a possible secondary gain for Ms S of her dysphonia.

(5) There is evidence that a combined treatment involving psychotherapy and speech therapy is more effective than speech therapy alone. Martins et al. (2014) found that all patients with psychogenic dysphonia in their study showed remission of vocal symptoms after speech therapy and psychological treatment. However, when speech therapy was used alone, only 12.5% of patients reported vocal symptom improvement.

Unit 38.5 Therapeutic programme

(1) parts (b) and (e)

(2) The expression 'soft contact' refers to a type of vocal fold adduction where the vocal folds are gently adducted to achieve the onset of voicing. It is the opposite of a type of vocal fold adduction called hard glottal attack.

(3) During a discussion of vocal hygiene, clients are made aware of environmental and behavioural factors which can have an adverse impact on the voice. This can include the dehydrating effects of caffeine, alcohol, heating and certain drugs (e.g. anti-histamines) on the vocal fold mucosa, the carcinogenic and other effects of tobacco smoke on the laryngeal mechanism, and the vocal fold damage which can be caused by persistent coughing and throat clearing.

(4) Clients with psychogenic dysphonia can make compensatory maladjustments which put the laryngeal mechanism at risk of organic pathologies. For example, they may begin to recruit laryngeal muscles that are not normally involved in vocal fold adduction. To avoid the use of potentially damaging vocal patterns, voice clients must be educated about voice misuse.

(5) GRBAS scale scores of zero across all parameters indicate that Ms S's voice was perceptually normal by the termination of treatment.

Case study 39 Man aged 62 years with laryngeal carcinoma

Unit 39.1 Primer on laryngeal carcinoma

(1) Historically, as male smoking rates have declined, female smoking rates have increased. The Office for National Statistics in the UK reports that in 1974, 51% of men smoked compared with 41% of women. In 2011, 21% of men smoked compared with 19% of women. A 10 percentage point difference in 1974 has narrowed to a 2 percentage point difference in 2011. This gender-related trend in smoking rates is the most likely explanation of the fact that women are representing an increasing proportion of cases of laryngeal cancer over time.

(2) Piselli et al.'s subjects exhibit the following risk factors for laryngeal cancer: (i) as liver transplant recipients, they had immunosuppression, and (ii) these subjects had alcoholic liver disease, indicating excessive alcohol consumption.

(3) In gastroesophageal reflux disease, transient relaxation of the lower oesophageal sphincter allows a bolus of refluxate to move from the stomach into the oesophagus. This bolus contains acid and pepsin, which is the primary enzyme of the stomach. If the upper oesophageal sphincter (called the cricopharyngeus) is not functioning normally, this bolus spills into the larynx and pharynx, causing laryngopharyngeal reflux. The airway epithelium, including the epithelium of the larynx, is fragile and more easily damaged by gastric reflux than the oesophageal epithelium. The corrosive effect of reflux on this epithelium leads to the development of laryngeal carcinomas.

(4) part (c)

(5) (a) false; (b) true; (c) true; (d) false; (e) true

Unit 39.2 Client history

(1) Most new laryngeal cancers are diagnosed in people aged between 55 and 64 years. At 62 years of age, MT falls within this age range. Most laryngeal cancers also develop in men. So in terms of both age and sex, MT conforms to the demographic profile of individuals who are most likely to develop laryngeal cancer.

(2) MT has smoked cigarettes for 40 years and also consumes alcohol, both of which are lifestyle risk factors for laryngeal cancer.

(3) Because of its capacity to disrupt the vibratory pattern of the vocal folds, a glottic carcinoma will cause hoarseness at an early stage in tumour development. Supraglottic and subglottic carcinomas will only cause hoarseness at a later stage of tumour development when the tumour has invaded the glottis.

(4) The term 'odynophagia' refers to the symptom of painful swallowing. It derives from the Greek words *odyno* (pain) and *phagein* (to eat). The term 'otalgia' refers to ear pain. It can be caused by conditions in the ear itself (primary otalgia) or, as in the case of laryngeal cancer, can be referred from other locations in the head and neck (referred otalgia).

(5) Three other symptoms of laryngeal cancer:
  (i) *stridor* is a harsh, vibratory sound of variable pitch which is caused by partial obstruction of the respiratory passages. Inspiratory stridor indicates obstruction of the airway above the glottis and is a symptom of many vocal fold pathologies including laryngeal carcinoma. Expiratory stridor indicates obstruction in the lower trachea.
  (ii) *dyspnoea* is a subjective sensation of difficulty breathing. As well as being a symptom of laryngeal carcinoma, it can also be a sign of cardiac, respiratory and neuromuscular disease.
  (iii) *haemoptysis* is the coughing of blood from a source below the glottis. This can take the form of blood-streaked sputum or a significant haemorrhage. Haemoptysis can be a symptom of a range of pathologies including laryngeal and lung cancer.

Unit 39.3 Medical evaluation and diagnosis

(1)

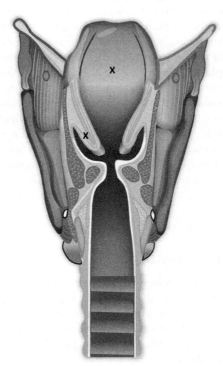

(2) A supraglottic laryngectomy is warranted in MT's case. This is because the tumour involves the epiglottis and left false vocal fold. Additionally, neck dissection will need to be performed to address the cervical lymph node which contains squamous cell carcinoma clusters.

(3) After supraglottic laryngectomy, MT is likely to experience dysphagia. His poor dentition will serve as an aggravating factor at the oral stage of swallowing as it will compromise his ability to form a bolus of safe consistency for swallowing.

(4) Panendoscopy is an examination of the upper part of the aerodigestive tract. It can include any of the following procedures: rhinoscopy, nasopharyngoscopy, inspection of the oral cavity and oropharynx, direct laryngoscopy and hypopharyngoscopy, oesophagoscopy and bronchoscopy. The procedure can be performed in order to biopsy a tumour that is not accessible under local anaesthesia in the clinic. This was not necessary in MT's case as a biopsy was performed during laryngoscopy. The procedure is also performed to rule out an associated malignancy. In MT's case, the presence of a second primary tumour was excluded by means of panendoscopy.

(5) The TNM staging system stands for Tumour (T), Node (N) and Metastasis (M). MT's tumour was classified as T2N1M0. T2 indicates that the tumour has invaded more than one portion of the supraglottis or glottis and there is abnormal vocal cord movement. N1 indicates that there is metastasis in a single ipsilateral lymph node which is less than 3 cm. M0 indicates that there is no distant metastasis.

Unit 39.4 Medical and surgical management

(1) The aspect of MT's post-surgical rehabilitation which will be of most concern to the speech-language pathologist is swallowing. This is because clients who are treated with supraglottic laryngectomy have acceptable voice quality on perceptual and subjective assessment (Topaloğlu et al., 2014). Instead, it is swallowing function that is most compromised by this surgical procedure. Prades et al. (2005) examined 110 patients who had standard and extended supraglottic laryngectomies. Pulmonary complications due to aspiration were observed in 6% of patients with standard supraglottic laryngectomy, 15% of patients with laterally extended supraglottic laryngectomy and 19% of patients with anteriorly extended supraglottic laryngectomy.

(2) The pharyngeal stage of swallowing is most compromised after supraglottic laryngectomy. This is because a standard supraglottic laryngectomy involves the resection of the following structures: the hyoid bone, the epiglottis, the valleculae, the aryepiglottic folds, the upper third of the thyroid cartilage and the false vocal cords (Schweinfurth and Silver, 2000). Some of these structures (e.g. the epiglottis) are involved in the protection of the airway during the pharyngeal stage of swallowing. Also, the removal of these structures results in the loss of supraglottic sensation. This can lead to improper timing of upper oesophageal relaxation. If this occurs, entry of the bolus into the oesophagus may be hindered, resulting in aspiration (Schweinfurth and Silver, 2000).

(3) MT received postoperative radiotherapy. This is likely to contribute to any swallowing problems. Alicandri-Ciufelli et al. (2013) examined the swallowing function of 32 patients who underwent partial laryngectomies between June 2003 and November 2010. Postoperative radiotherapy was the only factor that was found to influence swallowing function. Radiotherapy statistically significantly affected dysphagia score and penetration aspiration in these patients.

(4) Transoral laser supraglottic laryngectomy is an alternative procedure to open (transcervical) supraglottic laryngectomy. A number of studies have compared the voice and swallowing outcomes of these two approaches. Cabanillas et al. (2004) reported no significant difference in swallowing capacity in 26 patients who were treated with a transoral approach and 26 patients who underwent transcervical supraglottic laryngectomy. Peretti et al. (2006) compared functional outcomes in 14 patients who underwent endoscopic supraglottic laryngectomy by carbon dioxide laser for selected T1–T3 supraglottic squamous cell carcinomas and 14 patients who were treated with open-neck supraglottic laryngectomy. There were no statistically significant differences between the two groups in the results of a comprehensive voice analysis, the M.D. Anderson Dysphagia Inventory, complication and aspiration rates. Significant differences between the groups were found for video nasal endoscopic examination of swallowing, videofluoroscopy, hospitalisation, feeding tube duration and tracheotomy duration. Peretti et al. concluded that endoscopic supraglottic laryngectomy had a significantly lower functional impact on swallowing than open-neck supraglottic laryngectomy.

(5) MT's neck specimen revealed extracapsular spread. Extracapsular extension in squamous cell carcinoma nodal metastases usually predicts worse outcome (Lewis et al., 2011).

Unit 39.5 Focus on post-laryngectomy communication

(1) (a) true; (b) true; (c) false; (d) false; (e) true

(2) Role functioning, social functioning and mental health have all been found to contribute to quality of life in clients after laryngectomy (Singer et al., 2014; Perry et al., 2015). As well as making a direct contribution to quality of life, effective alaryngeal communication can also make an indirect contribution by way of improving clients' role functioning, social functioning and mental health.

(3) (a) electronic larynx; (b) voice prosthesis; (c) oesophageal speech; (d) voice prosthesis; (e) voice prosthesis

(4) Because they depend on the vibratory capacity of the PE segment, oesophageal voice and the use of a tracheoesophageal voice prosthesis are the methods of alaryngeal communication that are most compromised by PE stenosis. PE stenosis also compromises swallowing function.

(5) To be considered a candidate for TEVP, a client must have functional manual dexterity and functional visual acuity, or at least have access to a carer who has these skills.

Case study 40 Male-to-female transgender adolescent aged 15 years

Unit 40.1 Primer on gender dysphoria and transsexual voice

(1) Studies which base their estimates of the prevalence of gender dysphoria on the number of individuals who attend gender clinics are likely to be underestimating the

true prevalence of gender dysphoria in the general population. This is because there are individuals who experience gender dysphoria and do not present themselves to specialist clinics for treatment.

(2) (a) true; (b) false; (c) true; (d) true; (e) false

(3) fundamental frequency

(4) parts (b) and (d)

(5) part (b)

Unit 40.2 Client history

(1) (a) true; (b) false; (c) true; (d) false; (e) true

(2) In males, there are abrupt changes in voice characteristics between Tanner stages G3 and G4 (Harries et al., 1997). By the time LA is seen at 15;3 years of age for voice and communication therapy, she has already experienced the changes associated with voice mutation.

(3) LA had poor voice-related quality of life at the point of referral to a university voice clinic. LA reported that her voice caused her embarrassment, made her feel less feminine, and got in the way of her living as a female.

(4) LA was identified as a female speaker in face-to-face interaction 70% of the time. However, when visual stimuli were not available, and listeners had to identify LA's gender from auditory–perceptual characteristics of her voice on the phone, the identification of LA as a female dropped to just 50%.

(5) Abusive vocal behaviours are associated with hyperfunctional dysphonias. Acid reflux and alcohol and tobacco use can place an individual at risk of organic laryngeal pathologies. LA's voice clinicians need to know about these factors in order to establish whether she is at risk of organic and hyperfunctional voice disorders.

Unit 40.3 Voice evaluation

(1) parts (a), (c), (d) and (e)

(2) It is important to include different speech tasks in a voice assessment as there is evidence that vocal parameters vary across tasks. Watts et al. (2015) examined cepstral/spectral acoustic measures in adult males in two speech tasks: production of sustained vowels and reading of a connected speech stimulus. Older men displayed significantly greater Cepstral/Spectral Index of Dysphonia measures than younger men in connected speech but not during sustained vowel production. Abu-Al-makarem and Petrosino (2007) found that mean speaking fundamental frequency of young Arabic men was significantly higher during reading than in spontaneous speech.

(3) Studies have shown that mean speaking fundamental frequency is associated with the perception of the gender of the speaker more than other acoustic measures. In a study of male, female and transgendered subjects, Gelfer and Mikos (2005) found that gender identifications were based on fundamental frequency, even when fundamental frequency and formant frequency information was contradictory. Skuk and Schweinberger (2014) examined the relative importance of four acoustic parameters – fundamental frequency, formant frequencies, aperiodicity and spectrum level – on voice gender perception. The strongest cue related to gender perception was

fundamental frequency followed by formant frequencies and spectrum level. Aperiodicity did not influence gender perception.

(4) part (b) (see Gelfer (1999) for discussion)

(5) There is evidence that speaking rate and loudness are greater in men than in women (Brockmann et al., 2008; Jacewicz et al., 2010). In order for LA to be perceived as female, it is likely that there will need to be some modification of her speaking rate and loudness.

Unit 40.4 Voice and communication therapy

(1) LA's clinician will be aiming to avoid the use of clavicular breathing. This is the least efficient pattern of breathing for voice production. Clavicular breathing relies on the neck accessory muscles. The shoulders elevate during inhalation and breathing can be effortful.

(2) Modifications of oral resonance in male-to-female transsexuals can increase perception of the speaker as female. Carew et al. (2007) examined the effectiveness of an oral resonance therapy that targeted lip spreading and forward tongue carriage in 10 male-to-female transsexuals. Listener ratings of recordings made pre- and post-therapy indicated that the majority of participants were perceived to sound more feminine following treatment.

(3) (a) true; (b) false; (c) false; (d) false; (e) true

(4) Male-to-female transsexuals are at an increased risk of voice disorder because they can develop maladaptive vocal patterns in an effort to achieve pitch elevation. The educational aspect of LA's intervention, and specifically the information that LA received about abusive vocal behaviours, is intended to reduce this risk.

(5) LA's breathy voice quality might be explained by these endoscopic and stroboscopic findings.

Unit 40.5 Communication outcomes

(1) LA's voice therapy was highly effective as it produced a significant improvement in her voice-related quality of life. LA's voice improved from a pre-therapy level where it was negatively affecting her life to a severe degree to a post-therapy level where she reported a positive change in attitude and self-perception.

(2) If LA's suprahyoid and laryngeal tension had been allowed to persist, LA would have been placed at risk of developing a hyperfunctional voice disorder. Palmer et al. (2012) reported that there were indications of vocal hyperfunction in all the male-to-female transsexuals in their study, either by self-report or on laryngeal examination.

(3) High shimmer values confirm the impression of breathiness.

(4) Upon completion of treatment, LA's mean fundamental frequency is just within the low end of the mean fundamental frequency range of natal females (i.e. 197–227 Hz).

(5) LA's speaking rate decreased from 282 wpm at the start of therapy to 200 wpm by the end of therapy. This reduction in rate might have facilitated LA in making the modifications in tongue position that were necessary to bring about a change in resonance.

Case study 41 Boy aged 19 months with Goldenhar syndrome

Unit 41.1 Primer on Goldenhar syndrome

(1) malformation of the ear ossicles; conductive hearing loss
(2) hearing loss; intellectual disability
(3) abnormalities of the semicircular canals
(4) microtia; atresia of the external auditory canal. Atresia can cause a maximum conductive hearing loss of 40–50 dB (Ackley, 2014).
(5) cochlear hypoplasia

Unit 41.2 Client history

(1) George was the second of triplets. Twinning and multiple births are risk factors for Goldenhar syndrome or OAVS.
(2) Aspiration pneumonia is an infectious process caused by the inhalation of oropharyngeal secretions that are colonised by pathogenic bacteria. Its relevance to the speech-language pathologist is that it suggests the presence of dysphagia in clients.
(3) OAVS is related to disturbances in the first and second branchial arches during embryogenesis. The key period for these disturbances to arise is 30–45 days of gestation (Gorlin et al., 2001: 790). This is very early in a pregnancy and long before George's mother was administered ritodrine at seven months in order to inhibit premature labour.
(4) language development; motor development; cognitive development
(5) parts (c) and (d)

Unit 41.3 Clinical presentation

(1) Clefts of the lip and palate are also embryological malformations of the first and second branchial arches. This explains their presence alongside OAVS.
(2) Three cerebral anomalies: (i) interventricular and periventricular haemorrhages; (ii) hydrocephalus; (iii) frontal and temporal cortical atrophy.
(3) cerebrospinal fluid; ventricles
(4) parts (a), (c) and (d)
(5) parts (a) and (d)

Unit 41.4 Speech, language and hearing assessment

(1) George's difficulties with speech production are compromising his expressive language skills. This explains the receptive–expressive gap in his language performance.
(2) George makes use of gestural and physical prompts to facilitate his impaired comprehension of language.
(3) George has right ear atresia. So his responses on audiological testing cannot be on account of his right ear.
(4) George's limited phonetic inventory is likely to be on account of (i) his malformed articulatory anatomy and (ii) his conductive hearing loss.

(5) Velopharyngeal incompetence is the likely articulatory basis of George's hypernasal voice and audible nasal emission.

Unit 41.5 Post-therapy communication status

(1) George did not have intellectual disability which would adversely affect language acquisition and limit progress in therapy.

(2) George has intact pragmatic language skills at his second evaluation. He is able to use language appropriately, and displays a range of speech acts (e.g. requests).

(3) At his first evaluation, George was only able to produce the bilabial and velar nasals (/m/, /ŋ/). At his second evaluation he is able to produce a number of other sounds in addition to these nasal sounds. These sounds include the alveolar nasal /n/, bilabial and velar plosives /b, k, g/ and the glide /w/.

(4) Surgical intervention for velopharyngeal incompetence: palatoplasty
Prosthetic intervention for velopharyngeal incompetence: palatal lift or obturator

(5) George had a behavioural age of 22.4 months on the Wisconsin Behavior Rating Scale. The WBRS uses a 3-point rating scale to assess each of the following areas: gross and fine motor skills; expressive and receptive language; play skills; socialisation; domestic activities; eating; toileting; dressing and grooming. Several of these areas (e.g. socialisation and play skills) are particularly sensitive to the deficits of autism. The fact that George achieved a score on this assessment which exceeded his chronological age of 19 months suggests that he does not have autism.

Case study 42 Woman aged 49 years with congenital sensorineural hearing loss

Unit 42.1 Primer on congenital sensorineural hearing loss

(1) parts (b) and (d)

(2) hyperbilirubinaemia (metabolic cause); neomycin (pharmacological cause)

(3) parts (a), (c) and (d)

(4) bound morphemes: -s (e.g. walks); -ed (e.g. walked); -ing (e.g. walking)

(5) Duration of cochlear implant experience and the amount of hearing available to a child before implantation are significant factors in determining language outcome (Nicholas and Geers, 2007).

Unit 42.2 Client history

(1) Chelsea's lack of exposure to language during the developmental period was on account of her sensory (hearing) impairment. However, she was otherwise brought up in a supportive family environment where she received normal social stimulation from her parents and siblings. The situation of feral children is quite different. They have been exposed to situations of extreme neglect where social as well as linguistic stimulation is lacking.

(2) Chelsea's social communication skills may have been protected on account of the normal social stimulation that she received within her family. As a key contributor to those skills, pragmatic language may also be relatively intact.

(3) parts (a), (d) and (e)

(4) At 32 years of age, there will be reduced plasticity of the auditory cortex. This will limit the capacity of the auditory cortex to process and recognise verbal and non-verbal auditory stimuli.

(5) otoacoustic emission testing; automated auditory brainstem response testing

Unit 42.3 Cognitive and language assessment

(1) parts (b) and (e)

(2) Even Chelsea's highest performance IQ of 89 falls short of the range 107 to 109 which is typical of deaf adolescents. Chelsea's lower performance IQ compared to deaf adolescents probably reflects her lack of formal education and amplification, both of which are normally accessed by deaf individuals.

(3) parts (a), (c), (d) and (e)

(4) The PPVT examines receptive vocabulary. Chelsea's performance on this test is facilitated by the use of signing. In August 1981, the test was conducted with and without signing. The use of signing increased Chelsea's vocabulary age by over one year.

(5) Alongside the comprehension of colours (red, green), shapes (circle, square) and actions (put, touch), these commends are assessing the comprehension of the following aspects of language:
  (a) locative preposition 'on'
  (b) coordinating conjunction 'or'
  (c) conditional 'if'
  (d) adverbs 'slowly' and 'quickly'
  (e) two-word preposition 'together with'

Unit 42.4 Pragmatic assessment

(1) parts (b) and (d)

(2) The fact that Chelsea's pragmatic skills are relatively intact in the presence of her limited language suggests that pragmatic competence is largely independent of linguistic competence.

(3) maxim of quantity

(4) Expressive prosody: The use of a specific intonation pattern may change a statement into a question. For example, when uttered with rising pitch at the end, the utterance 'John is leaving tomorrow' may be used to ask a question.
Receptive prosody: The hearer who can detect the placement of stress and increased vocal intensity on the word *delightful* in the utterance 'What a delightful child!' is able to establish that the speaker of this utterance intends it to stand as a sarcastic remark.

(5) Chelsea exhibits a number of pragmatic skills which suggest that she has no deficits in theory of mind. The ability to introduce and develop topics in conversation, the ability to respond appropriately to speech acts such as directives, and the ability to use facial expressions appropriately all require the ability on Chelsea's part to attribute cognitive and affective mental states both to her own mind and to the minds of

others. The fact that all three of these pragmatic skills are intact in Chelsea suggests that she has no deficits in theory of mind.

Unit 42.5 Focus on conversational speech

(1) Chelsea is producing language at a single-word level. Her inability to link two words together suggests that she has not acquired the syntax of language. The single exception is 'Don't think' which, in its use of both an auxiliary verb and negative 'not', far exceeds the grammatical complexity of her other utterances in the exchange.

(2) After such an extended period of auditory stimuli deprivation, Chelsea's articulation of speech is unlikely to be completely intact. However, on the basis of this short exchange, we can at least say that her speech production is not so poor that she is unintelligible to the interviewer. It is clear that the interviewer understands each of her single-word utterances, and does not have to ask her to repeat unintelligible words.

(3) A number of the non-verbal behaviours that Chelsea uses have no communicative function, e.g. unwrapping the gift. However, other non-verbal behaviours do have a communicative function, such as when she shakes her head to indicate to the interviewer that she doesn't know what the gift is.

(4) Chelsea displays an appreciation of the dyadic structure of conversation in that she exchanges turns appropriately with the interviewer. Chelsea also displays an appreciation of humour in conversation when she laughs at the interviewer's statement that she has tricked her. Chelsea also understands that there are politeness constraints at work in conversation when she thanks the interviewer for her gift.

(5) When Chelsea utters 'You . . . collar', she is attempting to ask the interviewer about the scarf she is wearing (or a scarf she previously wore). This utterance sees Chelsea move beyond her role as a passive respondent in the exchange to one where she takes control, if only momentarily, by asking the interviewer a question.

Case 43 Boy aged 4 months with cochlear implants

Unit 43.1 Primer on cochlear implantation

(1) parts (b), (c) and (e)

(2) To achieve electrode placement during cochlear implantation, a postauricular mastoidectomy (removal of mastoid bone) is performed to gain access to the inner ear. A small opening is made in the cochlea (cochleostomy) anterior/inferior to the round window to permit placement of the electrode into the scala tympani.

(3) Labyrinthitis ossificans is the formation of new bone in the fluid-filled scalae of the cochlea. The scala tympani in the basal turn of the cochlea is the most frequent area of ossification. This condition is a hindrance to cochlear implantation as it makes electrode insertion difficult. Accordingly, earlier implantation is recommended before significant ossification has occurred. Labyrinthitis ossificans related to meningitis is associated with the greatest amount of ossification (Green et al., 1991).

(4) Reading, spelling and writing are the aspects of language that contribute most to academic achievement. Evidence for improvements in these aspects of language following cochlear implantation is mixed. Geers and Hayes (2011) examined reading, spelling and expository writing in 112 high school students who received cochlear

implants as pre-schoolers. Although these adolescents performed within or above the average range for hearing peers on reading tests, they were poorer spellers and expository writers than hearing peers. Venail et al. (2010) reported delayed reading and writing in 19 of 74 (26%) prelingually deaf children who received cochlear implants before 6 years of age.

(5) The contribution of an individual's cognitive ability to post-implantation gains is both supported and refuted by studies. Sarant et al. (2014) reported that higher cognitive ability was associated with significantly better language outcomes in 91 children with unilateral or bilateral cochlear implants. In a study of 114 postlingually deaf adult cochlear implant recipients, Holden et al. (2013) found that cognitive ability was significantly and positively related to outcome, measured in terms of word recognition scores. However, after controlling for age, cognition no longer affected outcome.

Unit 43.2 Client history

(1) parts (c) and (e)

(2) PB satisfies the criterion that he derived no apparent benefit from the use of hearing aids.

(3) We can tell that PB does not have hearing loss in the presence of a syndrome as he has no additional needs and is neurologically and intellectually age appropriate.

(4) In relation to (i), there is evidence that clients who undergo unilateral cochlear implantation perform poorly in binaural hearing tasks such as speech understanding in the presence of background noise and the ability to localise the source of sounds. Bilateral cochlear implants can restore these abilities (Peters et al., 2004). In relation to (ii), evidence is less definitive, as the benefits and disadvantages of sequential and simultaneous implantation have not been well researched: 'there are no developmental studies that have examined the advantages and disadvantages of sequential versus simultaneous implantation in a systematic way' (Sharma et al., 2007: 218). For their part, Sharma et al. (2007) reported no difference between sequential and simultaneous implantation: 'Our results suggest that bilateral implantation, whether simultaneous or sequential, occurring within the sensitive period of 3.5 years, takes place within a central auditory nervous system that shows a high degree of developmental plasticity' (223).

(5) Complications have been reported in 19% of cochlear implant recipients (Theunisse et al., 2014). Three such complications are bacterial meningitis, mastoiditis and facial palsy (Farinetti et al., 2014).

Unit 43.3 Focus on auditory development

(1) The term 'free field' describes a region in space where sound may propagate free from any form of obstruction. It is a homogeneous medium that lacks boundaries or reflecting surfaces. The term 'aided hearing' describes an individual's hearing when using hearing aids or a cochlear implant. The term 'binaural hearing' describes the perception of sound by stimulation in two ears. Binaural hearing allows individuals to understand speech in silence and noisy conditions and is an essential requirement for spatial hearing and sound localisation.

(2) Prior to implantation, PB displayed some aided hearing in the lower frequencies. Vowels are produced at these frequencies. Accordingly, they would have been the class of speech sounds that PB was able to perceive best prior to implantation.

(3) The voiceless alveolar and velar plosives /t, k/ have frequencies between 2000 and 4000 Hz. The fricative sounds /f, s, h, ð/ have frequencies between 4000 and 8000 Hz. It is likely that PB would have been able to perceive all these speech sounds for the first time after implantation.

(4) Sound localisation requires the use of binaural hearing. This hearing became available to PB for the first time following the fitting of his second cochlear implant.

(5) parts (b), (c), (d) and (e)

Unit 43.4 Focus on speech perception

(1) (a) false; (b) true; (c) false; (d) false; (e) true

(2) In closed-set tests, the number of response alternatives is limited to a small set, usually between 4 and 10 depending on the procedure used. By contrast, there is an unlimited number of response alternatives in open-set tests. Accordingly, open-set tests are more difficult for hearing impaired clients.

(3) The audiologist who is using a word recognition test must ensure that the target words are all within the receptive vocabulary of the children assessed by means of the test.

(4) Unlike the MTP test which only examines word recognition, the LiP Profile also examines phoneme recognition. Because of the reduced redundancy of phonemes, phoneme recognition is more difficult than word recognition. This greater difficulty may explain PB's reduced performance on the LiP Profile relative to the MTP test.

(5) PB's LiP Profile scores suggest that he did not experience the 'initial drop' phenomenon. However, this phenomenon cannot be excluded based on these scores alone, as the LiP Profile scores of Sainz et al.'s subjects also did not show a decrease of auditory performance immediately after first fitting. A significant temporary decrease after initial fitting, however, was observed in the scores on the MTP test in Sainz et al.'s subjects. There was no evidence of a decrease in PB's MTP test scores at 12, 18 and 24 months.

Unit 43.5 Focus on language development

(1) (a) AWST-R; Word Production subtest of the SETK-2
    (b) TROG-D; Sentence Comprehension subtest of the SETK-2
    (c) Encoding of Semantic Relations subtest of the SETK 3–5
    (d) Word Comprehension subtest of the SETK-2
    (e) Morphological Syntax subtest of the SETK 4–5

(2) Pragmatics is not assessed by the formal language tests that were used to evaluate PB. Yet, there is evidence that pragmatics can be impaired in implanted children who perform within normal limits on formal language tests. Nicastri et al. (2014) examined discourse inferencing skills and metaphor comprehension in 31 children with unilateral cochlear implants who attained a normal language level. There was no significant difference between these children's discourse inferencing skills and the inferencing skills of 31 normal hearing matched peers. However, children with

cochlear implants performed significantly below their normal hearing peers in verbal metaphor comprehension.

(3) PB has normal memory for sentences and a normal memory span for words. These results indicate that PB has intact phonological short-term memory.

(4) The presence of developmental disabilities (e.g. autism) reduces the likelihood that a good language outcome will be achieved following cochlear implantation. Cruz et al. (2012) examined 188 deaf children. Among these children, 85% had a single diagnosis of severe-to-profound hearing loss and 15% had an additional disability. Although deaf children with and without additional disabilities experienced significant improvement in their oral language skills post-implantation, children with developmental disorders such as autism made slower progress in language.

(5) There is substantial evidence that hearing impaired children without implants experience elevated levels of behavioural problems. Barker et al. (2009) reported more behavioural difficulties in 116 severely and profoundly deaf children than in normally hearing children. The hearing impaired children in this study had all been referred for cochlear implant surgery. Even after cochlear implantation there is evidence of elevated levels of behavioural problems in children. Wu et al. (2015) examined behaviour problems in 60 Mandarin-speaking children with cochlear implants. Significantly more children with implants had problems with aggressive behaviour and overall behaviour than in a normative sample.

Case study 44 Girl aged 11 years with central auditory processing disorder

Unit 44.1 Primer on central auditory processing disorder

(1) (a) false; (b) true; (c) false; (d) true; (e) false

(2) Two ways in which children with craniofacial anomalies are at an increased risk of (C)APD: (i) Many craniofacial anomalies occur in the context of syndromes in which there are CNS defects (e.g. Goldenhar syndrome). These defects can include (C)APD; and (ii) children with craniofacial anomalies are at an increased risk of otitis media with effusion. OME has also been linked to (C)APD.

(3) Awareness of injury-related deficits is limited in children, adolescents and adults with TBI (Lewis and Horn, 2013; Lloyd et al., 2015). This lack of awareness explains the failure of these subjects with closed head injury to report any signs of auditory impairment.

(4) neurological aetiology – APD related to stroke-induced brain damage
neurodevelopmental disorder – APD in children with learning difficulties

(5) (C)APD is likely to worsen over time in those individuals with neurodegenerative disorders such as Alzheimer's disease.

Unit 44.2 Developmental and medical history

(1) There is evidence that low birth weight is a risk factor for (C)APD. Davis et al. (2001) compared the audiological function of children with very low birth weight (< or

= 1500g) to that of children with normal birth weight (> 2499g). Children with very low birth weight had higher rates of some central auditory processing problems than children of normal birth weight. There were no significant differences between these children in rates of hearing impairment, abnormal tympanograms, figure–ground problems or digit recall.

(2) Normally developing infants are able to sit alone without support between 5 and 6 months. Sally started sitting at 10 months. Normally developing infants are able to walk while holding an adult's hand between 6 and 9 months. Sally was walking at 14 months.

(3) Grommet insertion indicates that Sally has otitis media with effusion. OME is another risk factor for (C)APD.

(4) The presence of low muscle tone (hypotonia) and frontal lobe epilepsy suggests that Sally's auditory processing problems may have a neurological aetiology. (C)APDs have been reported in a number of epilepsies including clients with temporal lobe epilepsy and generalised and partial seizures (Han et al., 2011; Ortiz et al., 2009).

(5) The IAM is the opening of the internal auditory canal, a canal in the temporal bone that transmits nerves and blood vessels from within the posterior cranial fossa to the hearing mechanism. An acoustic neuroma (or vestibular schwannoma) can be detected by a CT scan. This is a benign tumour that typically arises from the vestibular portion of the eighth cranial nerve. As an acoustic neuroma expands, it fills the IAM and compresses the cochlear and facial nerves.

Unit 44.3 Cognitive and language profile

(1) parts (b), (c) and (e)

(2) The WISC-III revealed that Sally has impaired short-term memory. This impairment might explain her reading difficulties. In a meta-analysis of studies that examined the academic, cognitive and behavioural performance of children with and without reading disabilities, Kudo et al. (2015) found that short-term memory was one of a number of specific cognitive processes that significantly moderated overall group effect size differences.

(3) part (d)

(4) Regular words (e.g. 'hit') can be read by means of grapheme-to-phoneme rules. The lexicon does not need to be accessed in order to read these words but it can be accessed. Irregular words (e.g. 'yacht') can only be read by accessing the lexicon. If these words are read using grapheme-to-phoneme rules, mispronunciations will result. Non-words (e.g. 'splank') can only be read by using grapheme-to-phoneme rules as they have no entry in the lexicon. Because there are different reading routes for different types of words, each type must be separately examined in an assessment of reading.

(5) As well as measuring receptive vocabulary, the PPVT-III has also been used to provide an estimate of verbal intelligence. This would explain why Sally's PPVT-III score is consistent with her WISC-III results. However, Strauss et al. (2006) remark that '[a]lthough the PPVT-III is still used occasionally as an IQ estimate, its use in this way is not recommended' (951).

Unit **44.4** Audiological assessment and amplification

(1) (a) Visual reinforcement orientation audiometry (VROA) is suitable for infants who are developmentally 7 or 8 months to 3 years of age. The child is taught or conditioned to turn his or her head when a sound is heard. To achieve initial conditioning, stimuli are presented at moderately high levels, with the audiologist waiting until the child looks for the source of sound. As a reward, the child is shown a colourful, moving puppet or toy under illumination. This reinforces the child's turning behaviour or orientation. Once this conditioned response is reliable, stimuli can be presented at steadily decreasing levels until an auditory threshold is reached.

(b) In auditory brainstem response (ABR) audiometry, an evoked potentials measurement of the auditory nervous system is conducted. Through electrodes taped to the skull, signals are delivered to each ear independently. Microvolt sensory responses from the auditory nerve and brainstem are detected through these electrodes. Slight modifications of the auditory brainstem response technique permit measurement of the middle latency response, an evoked response that occurs between the brainstem and auditory cortex.

(c) Electrocochleography (ECoG) measures gross potentials that originate from the vicinity of the cochlea. These potentials include the cochlear microphonic and the summating potential, and the whole nerve action or compound action potential which corresponds to wave I of the ABR. A small needle electrode is placed through the tympanic membrane and on the promontory (the bulge in the medial wall of the middle ear, inferior to the stapes). The electrode may also be placed on the tympanic membrane and in the ear canal. The technique is most often used for intra-operative monitoring of the cochlea and the eighth cranial nerve and in the diagnosis of Ménière's disease.

(d) Otoacoustic emission testing is a technique which can be used to test for the presence of sensorineural hearing loss in newborns. It is based on the observation that the cochlea can actually generate sounds (technically, emissions) either spontaneously (spontaneous otoacoustic emissions) or in response to acoustic stimulation (evoked otoacoustic emissions). These emissions are absent in mild inner ear deafness.

(e) Computerised axial tomography (a CAT or CT scan) is a technique in which an x-ray source produces a narrow, fan-shaped beam of x rays to irradiate a section of the body. On a single rotation of the x-ray source around the body, many different 'snapshots' are taken. These are then reconstructed by a computer into a cross-sectional image of internal organs and tissues for each complete rotation. CT scanning has many uses in the management of otological disorders, including middle ear cholesteatoma, inner ear aplasia and mastoiditis related to chronic middle ear infection.

(2) Tympanometry is a quantitative technique for measuring the mobility or compliance of the tympanic membrane as a function of changing air pressures in the external auditory canal. It can be used to establish middle ear pressure through the measurement of the amount of air pressure in the external auditory canal that is needed to achieve maximum mobility of the eardrum. Negative middle ear pressure is associated with middle ear pathology, specifically acute otitis media, which can cause conductive hearing loss.

(3) Vowels are low frequency sounds (they extend a little above 1000 Hz), while consonants are high frequency sounds (they extend only a little below 1000 Hz). Sally's hearing is poorest at 500 Hz and 1 kHz, so the perception of vowels will be most compromised for her.

(4) A CT scan might serve to eliminate the presence of an acoustic neuroma and perinatal encephalopathy. Both conditions are consistent with the ABR results obtained (Romero et al., 2008; Shih et al., 2009).

(5) Sally's hearing aids provided amplification which was not required. If it continued, this amplification would cause noise-induced hearing loss through the destruction of outer and inner hair cells in the cochlea.

Unit 44.5 Focus on auditory processing assessment and habilitation

(1) Difficulty listening in background noise is frequently reported by the parents of children with APD. In a study of 19 children with APD, Ferguson et al. (2011) reported that the most common difficulty indicated by parents of these children was listening in background noise. This difficulty occurred in 13 (68.4%) of children.

(2) Sally achieved a score of 6 on the short-term memory task of the WISC-III when 7 to 13 is considered to be the average range. The behavioural observation that Sally has difficulty with auditory memory is consistent with this cognitive finding.

(3) Sally's performance on the Frequency Pattern Test (FPT) and the Random Gap Detection Test (RGDT) fell outside the normal range. The FPT and the Duration Pattern Test (DPT) are both used in clinical settings to assess an individual's ability to discriminate temporal order or sequence in stimuli. In these tests, subjects are instructed that they will hear sets of three consecutive tones which vary in pitch or duration. Subjects are required to verbalise the tonal patterns by indicating the frequency patterns (e.g. high–low–high, low–low–high) and the duration patterns (e.g. long–short–long, short–short–long). The RGDT is used to assess temporal resolution in clinical settings: 'Auditory temporal resolution ability enables the detection of changes in the duration of a sound stimulus and/or the detection of gaps inserted in an auditory stimulus' (Dias et al., 2012: 175).

The FPT, DPT and the RGDT hold diagnostic significance for APD. In this way, Iliadou et al. (2008) arrived at a diagnosis of CAPD in a young girl who was preterm at birth on the basis of severe deficits in three non-speech temporal tests – frequency and duration pattern tests and the random gap detection test.

(4) Aaronson and Bernier (2013) define mismatch negativity (MMN) as 'an event-related potential evoked in response to a perceived change in sensory stimuli. It is commonly elicited in an oddball paradigm in which a standard stimulus is paired with a deviant stimulus, the standard being presented the majority of instances' (1878). The reason that the absence of MMN for all sounds has uncertain diagnostic significance is that MMN can be absent in children with disorders other than APD. And even children with APD can display intact MMN. For example, Muniz et al. (2015) reported that all typically developing children in their study exhibited an MMN response. However, so too did 84% of individuals in an APD group and 76% of individuals in a group with specific language impairment.

(5) The Easy Listener personal FM system can be used with hearing aids or as a stand-alone hearing system. The device can help combat background noise, distance to sound source, and/or reverberation, all of which can interfere with speech understanding in individuals with APD. Johnston et al. (2009) examined children with APD who were fitted with FM devices for home and classroom use. Prior to FM use, these children exhibited significantly lower speech perception scores, decreased academic performance and psychosocial problems in comparison to a control group matched for age and gender. Following FM use, these children displayed improved speech perception in noisy classroom environments as well as significant academic and psychosocial gains. Moreover, after prolonged FM use, there was also improvement in the unaided (no FM device) speech perception of these children.

Case study 45 Girl aged 8 years with selective mutism

Unit 45.1 Primer on selective mutism

(1) The higher prevalence of selective mutism in females than in males sets this condition apart from a range of disorders in speech-language pathology which are more commonly found in males. These disorders include communication disorders such as specific language impairment and developmental phonological disorder, and conditions such as ADHD and ASD which have communication deficits as part of their phenotype.

(2) Children with a background of migration encounter a new language and culture in the areas in which they settle. A lack of proficiency in the new language of an area and a lack of familiarity with aspects of its culture may reduce these children to silence rather than be exposed to the negative reactions of members of the settled population.

(3) It is too simplistic to attribute a direct, causal role to anxiety within the aetiology of selective mutism for three reasons. First, children can display anxiety but not develop selective mutism. Second, the co-occurrence of anxiety and selective mutism may be because anxiety is a consequence of a child having selective mutism. Third, the co-occurrence of anxiety and selective mutism may be on account of a third variable (e.g. genetic factors) which is an independent cause of both anxiety and selective mutism.

(4) The mutism of these children makes it difficult for researchers and clinicians to obtain samples of expressive language for analysis. Children with selective mutism are unlikely to produce responses during language testing, participate in conversation with clinicians or generate extended language in the form of narratives. Audio- and video-recordings of children at home are often the only source of expressive language.

(5) (a) true; (b) false; (c) false; (d) false; (e) true

Unit 45.2 Client history

(1) A number of factors may explain the late referral of children with selective mutism. First, family physicians (general practitioners) and health visitors are usually the first professionals that parents turn to with concerns about their children's development

and well-being. However, awareness of selective mutism among these professionals is low. Second, parents may discount their concerns because children with selective mutism continue to communicate normally at home. Third, communication disorders such as speech sound disorders often have significant implications for communication which cannot be easily overlooked (e.g. severe unintelligibility). These implications are not a feature of selective mutism, with the result that parents may be inclined to respond with less urgency to their children's mutism.

(2) Even in the absence of spoken language Mimi displays a willingness to communicate with others through handwritten notes and the use of gestures.

(3) The fact that Mimi's father spoke Spanish suggests that she has a background of immigration.

(4) There are factors in Mimi's history which may have interacted with each other to produce her anxiety in speaking. Her mouth trauma led to a medical intervention (stitches). A later medical intervention for a high fever provoked considerable anxiety on account of the many needle sticks that Mimi received. By association Mimi may have come to link her anxiety around medical procedures to the mouth injury that necessitated some of these procedures and, ultimately, to the act of speaking itself.

(5) Mimi's mother assumed the role of communicator for her daughter, thus removing any need for Mimi to communicate for herself. Mimi's mother also anticipated her every need and managed her life to such an extent that communication for Mimi became unnecessary.

Unit 45.3 Communication status

(1) Mimi's note reveals that she is able to use direct reported speech. She writes: 'my mother told me "don't talk to strangers"'.

(2) Three communication milestones:
Babbling (6–9 months)
Use of first words (12–18 months)
Use of two-word utterances (18–24 months)

(3) It is likely that Mimi is engaging in the gliding of the liquids /l/ and /r/. The gliding of liquids normally resolves around 5 years of age. Its presence in a child of 9 years is a cause for concern.

(4) Three aspects of immature syntax:
Omission of 'is' as a copular verb (e.g. 'This [is] a boy')
Omission of determiner (e.g. 'what [my] family do')
Omission of genitive (e.g. 'This one['s] name Andy')

(5) Because children with selective mutism do not have experience of conversation, they do not get practice in a range of conversational skills. These skills include turn-taking, conversational openings/closings, topic management and the use of a range of speech acts. These skills largely fall within the pragmatic domain.

Unit 45.4 Psychological intervention

(1) Three reasons why gains in Mimi's non-verbal communication skills are to be encouraged:
(i) Improved non-verbal communication can help Mimi to increase her classroom participation.

    (ii) Non-verbal communication is Mimi's only means of expressing her needs and desires until vocalisation is achieved. In the absence of effective non-verbal communication, Mimi will experience frustration at her inability to communicate. Gains in non-verbal communication should be encouraged in order to avoid this scenario.

    (iii) In the absence of speech, Mimi is at risk of becoming passive in communication, with other people assuming the role of communicator on her behalf. Gains in non-verbal communication will enable Mimi to play an active role in communication.

(2) Stimulus fading is a behavioural technique which has been known for some time to be effective in the treatment of children with selective mutism. Wulbert et al. (1973) used stimulus fading to treat a 6-year-old girl with selective mutism. This girl received reinforcement for responding to demands for verbal and motor responses in the presence of someone who already had stimulus control of such behaviour, while a stranger was slowly faded into stimulus control.

(3) parts (a) and (c)

(4) Shaping is another behavioural technique in the treatment of selective mutism. In this technique, the therapist reinforces mouth movements that resemble speech (Mendlowitz and Monga, 2007).

(5) Contingency management is a reinforcement strategy in behaviour therapy. It involves rewarding verbal behaviour and not reinforcing mute behaviour (Krysanski, 2003).

Unit 45.5 Speech and language intervention

(1) (a) false; (b) false; (c) true; (d) true; (e) false

(2) part (d)

(3) Mimi displays good social communication skills. Mimi's classroom teacher reports that she is well-liked by other students, many of whom have attempted to help her with her mutism. As soon as whispering was established in therapy, Mimi used it to good effect by becoming a more active participant in the classroom and more animated in her conversational exchanges. Mimi's case demonstrates that good social communication skills are possible even in the absence of vocalisation.

(4) Mimi's speech and language problems appear to be making, at most, a relatively minor contribution to her mutism. Evidence in support of this claim includes:

    (i) Mimi communicates freely and easily at home in spite of her immature speech and language skills.

    (ii) Although Mimi's speech and language skills are impaired, they are still more than adequate for spoken communication to occur.

    (iii) There is no evidence from either parental or teacher reports that Mimi experienced early communication failures with peers as a result of her immature speech and language skills. If these failures had occurred, they could have prompted an anxiety reaction around speaking, thus leading to mutism.

(5) Three reasons why speech-language pathologists should assess and treat children with selective mutism as part of a multidisciplinary team:

    (i) The expertise of mental health professionals is needed to understand and manage the anxiety disorder of these children.

(ii) The input of other professionals (e.g. classroom teachers) is needed to identify behaviours which may perpetuate mutism in these children.

(iii) Skills acquired during speech-language intervention must be generalised to the classroom and wider community, and this requires the participation of professionals such as teachers.

Case study 46 Two boys with attention deficit hyperactivity disorder

Unit 46.1 Primer on attention deficit hyperactivity disorder

(1) (a) true; (b) false; (c) false; (d) true; (e) true

(2) The fact that the concordance rate for ADHD in the monozygotic twin boys in the study by Lichtenstein et al. (2010) was 44% and not 100% shows that the aetiology of ADHD cannot be entirely genetic in nature.

(3) parts (c) and (e)

(4) It is important for speech-language pathologists to have knowledge of comorbidities in ADHD for two reasons. First, some comorbid conditions (e.g. speech disorder) are assessed and treated by speech-language pathologists. Second, other comorbid conditions (e.g. depression) might adversely affect an individual's communication skills and compliance with intervention.

(5) part (d)

Unit 46.2 Language in attention deficit hyperactivity disorder

(1) (a) true; (b) false; (c) true; (d) true; (e) true

(2) Academic underachievement in ADHD is best accounted for by poor word reading and written expression in children with ADHD.

(3) (a) hyperactivity–impulsivity; (b) inattention; (c) hyperactivity–impulsivity; (d) inattention; (e) hyperactivity–impulsivity

(4) The child with ADHD is struggling with the following aspects of narrative production: (i) he fails to relate events in the correct temporal order (e.g. he describes how he left the house and got into the car *before* he got dressed and had his breakfast); (ii) he fails to use an indefinite noun phrase (e.g. 'a woman') for the first mention of characters. A listener could legitimately ask 'what woman?' and 'what small boy?'.

(5) part (b)

Unit 46.3 Client language status

(1) It is important for the speech-language pathologist to know the language(s) spoken in these children's home environments, as there is clear evidence that bilingual and multilingual home environments serve to exacerbate the extent of any language impairment. Cleave et al. (2010) found that dual language learners with SLI achieved lower scores on standardised tests of morphosyntax than monolingual children with SLI. Cheuk et al. (2005) found that a multilingual home environment is associated with SLI. In a sample of 326 children with SLI, multilingual exposure significantly

reduced the language quotient and language comprehension standard score of children with SLI.

(2) During language testing, children with ADHD might: (i) fail to listen carefully to instructions about how to perform tasks; (ii) initiate a response before a stimulus utterance has been fully issued; and (iii) might become distracted by background stimuli and lose focus on a task.

(3) parts (a), (b) and (d)

(4) Percentile scores indicate the percentage of individuals in the norm group who scored below the level of the cohort member. So a percentile score of 4 indicates that 4% of the norm group achieved a lower score on the OWLS than Adam. Similarly, a percentile score of 3 indicates that 3% of the norm group achieved a lower score on the OWLS than Abraham.

(5) The OWLS assesses structural aspects of language. It does not examine pragmatic aspects of language and discourse.

Unit 46.4 Focus on narrative production – Adam

(1) Adam's first utterance in the extract is an example of a maze: 'I went to my cousin's house and when I went to my cousin's house that was later when I when I we went back home for um from snow tubing.' It contains repetitions (Adam repeats that he went to his cousin's house), fillers ('um'), and revisions (after repeating 'when I', Adam revises his utterance to become 'we went back home').

(2) There is evidence that Adam understands indirect speech acts. When the teacher says 'Can you tell us about snow tubing?', Adam clearly interprets this utterance as a request on the part of the teacher and not as a question about his ability to describe snow tubing.

(3) Structural language deficits: (i) 'a hooks' – Adam uses an indefinite article with a plural noun; (ii) 'you got hold' – Adam uses the past tense verb 'got' instead of the present tense verb 'get'; (iii) 'you got hold onto a rope' – Adam uses the preposition 'onto' instead of the preposition 'of'.

(4) '<u>they</u> have a machine' (the referent of the pronoun 'they' cannot be identified)
'you tell my parents from up <u>there</u>' (the referent of the adverb 'there' cannot be identified)
'<u>he</u> spins you' (the referent of the pronoun 'he' cannot be identified)

(5) Adam is a highly sociable child who is liked by teachers and peers alike. Notwithstanding his language difficulties, he clearly enjoys relating stories to others and wants to communicate. His strong social skills and desire to communicate indicate that a diagnosis of ASD is not appropriate in his case.

Unit 46.5 Focus on narrative production – Abraham

(1) In the utterance 'I throw the ball at my baby brother', Abraham uses the present tense verb 'throw' instead of the past tense 'threw'. Although Abraham is unable to use the correct past tense form of an irregular verb in this instance, on other occasions he is able to make use of irregular past tense verbs, e.g. 'he <u>took</u> the pillow'.

(2) (a) true; (b) true; (c) true; (d) false; (e) false

(3) Two conjunctions:

'<u>so</u> he can play with it' ('so' is short for 'so that' which has the meaning *reason* or *explanation*)

'<u>then</u> he took the pillow' ('then' has a *temporal* meaning)

Abraham makes most use of the conjunction 'then'.

(4) Abraham displays a sophisticated appreciation of the mental states of others in two ways. First, he understands the teacher when she asks him if his baby brother *liked* having the ball thrown at him. Second, Abraham is able to use his brother's laughter to establish that his mental state is one of *enjoyment*.

(5) In Abraham's final turn in the extract, he uses the pronoun 'I' when he should be using 'he' to describe the actions of his brother – he said 'look out' and he threw the pillow.

Case study 47 Man aged 26 years with schizophrenia

Unit 47.1 Personal and medical history

(1) Side effects of clozapine that must be addressed by the speech-language pathologist include sialorrhoea (drooling) and stuttering.

(2) parts (a), (c) and (e)

(3) part (d); poverty of speech

(4) part (d)

(5) part (c)

Unit 47.2 Clinical discourse analysis

(1) A discourse analytic approach is advisable because clients with schizophrenia exhibit anomalies in areas such as topic management and reference. These areas cannot be adequately assessed using sentence-level formats (as in standardised language batteries) or even by examining local sequences in isolated adjacency pairs.

(2) The two parts of an adjacency pair need not be *consecutive* turns. For example, in the following conversational exchange, the response to the question in turn 1 is not forthcoming until turn 4. What intervenes is another question–answer adjacency pair in turns 2 and 3.

1 A: How much is a scotch on the rocks?
2 B: Would you like a small or large?
3 A: A large
4 B: It's £5.99

(3) (a) relevance; quantity (over-informative)
(b) quantity (under-informative)
(c) manner
(d) relevance; quantity (over-informative)
(e) quantity (under-informative)

(4) (a) The speaker does not indicate which type of poultry (turkey or chicken) he would like. There is missing propositional content.
(c) The referent of the pronoun in '<u>She</u> has such a gorgeous house' is unclear – it could be either Sue or June. There is vague propositional content.

(5) B's utterance is an infelicitous turn, in that it completely violates the expectations of A in the exchange.

Unit 47.3 Focus on topic management

(1) The client's turn was judged to be deviant because it involved 'unexpected associations of topics'. The topics in question are the client's paranoid experiences and music.

(2) (a) Ellipsis: 'they don't [leave me alone]'
      (b) Anaphoric reference: '<u>my mother</u> has to behave <u>herself</u>, but . . . <u>she</u> is sometimes discourteous in <u>her</u> words and <u>she</u> can be a bit rude'.

(3) After an appropriate response to the doctor's initial question, the speaker with schizophrenia pursues a sequence of topics which is characterised by linguistic and other associations between key words and ideas. The speaker's introduction of the topic of his name is somewhat irrelevant as a response to the doctor's question about 'special abilities' and is the start of a chain of topics that is increasingly difficult to follow. After stating that people laugh at his name, and then being unable to clarify this remark for the doctor, the speaker abruptly changes topic to begin talking about people from a certain area. The trigger for this topic change appears to be the fact that people from the area in question have the same name as the speaker's family name. There is then a remark that the speaker's name (this is somewhat unclear) is 'a kind of sacred relic'. When asked by the doctor to clarify this remark, the speaker with schizophrenia shifts the topic again to talk about a town called X which is seen on the news. He then returns to the topic of his name by stating that, if he had a choice, he would rather be known as Marko. When pressed by the doctor about the reason for a name change, the speaker indicates that it would be 'cool' to have this new name. The entire sequence is characterised by a gradual, radial extension of topics.

(4) The propositional content of these utterances in extract 2 is vague:

'I kind of imagine that <u>it</u> is a kind of sacred relic that I should not be teased for <u>that</u>'
'Or my family names X-er is <u>one</u>, since I am <u>one</u>'

In the first utterance, it is unclear if the pronoun 'it' refers to the name or location. The intended referent of the subsequent demonstrative pronoun 'that' is similarly unclear. In the second utterance, the client employs substitution on two occasions in his use of 'one'. The first use of 'one' appears to refer to a relic. However, it is unclear if the second use of 'one' refers to a relic or being an inhabitant of a certain area.

(5) In extract 2, the client exhibits difficulty with the quality maxim when he twice makes the erroneous statement that X is the town.

Unit 47.4 Focus on reference

(1) Referential anomalies are evident in the following utterances:
      '<u>they</u> watch <u>it</u> and such like <u>that</u>' – 'they' most likely refers to *some people* and 'it' most likely refers to *soccer*. However, there is no clear referent of 'that'.
      '<u>They</u> are a bit like a group of <u>their</u> own and such. <u>They</u> are jobless' – the first use of 'they' and 'their' appear to refer to *trades/professions*. However, there is no

clear referent of the second use of 'they', although it must refer to *people who practice trades/professions* if it is to make sense in this context.

'Well, I'm thinking about these kind of things' – there is no clear referent of 'these', as is evidenced by the fact that we are left asking 'What kind of things?'

(2) Vague and non-specific vocabulary is evident in the following utterances:
'they are stars and the like'
'I'm thinking about these kind of things'
'I do watch something'
'A group of people can come up with wise things'
'things are not like that now'

(3) (a) Topicalisation: 'Trades/professions I kind of think about'
(b) Ellipsis: 'but I am not [better educated]'
(c) Anaphoric reference: 'some people, well they are stars'

(4) The client appears to be largely unaware that the doctor is not following him. On two occasions, the doctor asks questions in an effort to establish who the client is talking about: 'who are watching?' and 'who are you talking about now?'. Neither question is adequately addressed by the client.

(5) The client develops topic along the following lines: work – soccer stars – trades and professions – workers – education and intelligence – qualifications. These individual areas are all related to the topic of work and education. In this extract, topic development appears to proceed by means of a series of associations.

Unit 47.5 Discourse deficits in schizophrenia

(1) parts (a), (b) and (e)
(2) There are two possible explanations for the intrusion of the topic of music in extract 1. The topic of music may have sustained its semantic activation in the client's discourse model from earlier in the conversation and intrudes at a later point as a result. Alternatively, the topic of music may be part of the client's psychotic experience which he proceeds to narrate at various points.
(3) part (c)
(4) part (b)
(5) Greater alignment of the doctor's discourse model with that of the client is only possible where the doctor has extensive knowledge of a client. Accordingly, there needs to be continuity in the mental health professionals and speech-language pathologists who work with clients with schizophrenia.

Case study 48 Woman aged 24 years with bipolar disorder

Unit 48.1 Primer on bipolar disorder

(1) parts (a), (d) and (e)
(2) According to one large study, the median and mean ages of onset in bipolar disorder are 23.0 years and 25.7 years, respectively (Baldessarini et al., 2012). The case for the provision of speech-language pathology services to clients with bipolar disorder should be based on the lack of economic productivity that ensues when a disorder

which has its onset for the most part in early adulthood is not successfully treated by a range of support services. Aside from a lack of economic productivity, individuals with bipolar disorder have reduced social functioning. Social roles within families and communities often cannot be successfully performed by clients with this disorder. The provision of SLP services can thus help mitigate some of the adverse economic and social consequences of bipolar disorder.

(3) (a) false; (b) true; (c) true; (d) false; (e) false
(4) autism spectrum disorder; attention deficit hyperactivity disorder
(5) parts (c) and (e)

Unit 48.2 Communication and cognition in bipolar disorder

(1) (a) false; (b) true; (c) false; (d) false; (e) true
(2) Poverty of speech describes substantially reduced verbal output of a speaker. It may manifest itself as minimal, one-word turns in conversation. It is also a feature of schizophrenic language.
(3) 'Iatrogenic dysarthria' describes dysarthria which is caused by medical intervention. Clients with bipolar disorder may develop iatrogenic dysarthria as a result of their drug regimen.
(4) Peters et al. concluded that executive functioning problems in bipolar disorder are not entirely mood-state dependent because some of the subjects in their study were in euthymic (normal) state. Executive functioning problems are, therefore, not confined to depressive and manic episodes in bipolar disorder.
(5) Utterance interpretation depends on a set of cognitive processes referred to as theory of mind. For example, in order to grasp the sarcastic intent of the speaker who utters 'This weather is glorious' in the middle of a thunderstorm, a hearer must be able to attribute certain mental states to the speaker. One such mental state is a belief to the effect that the speaker believes the weather is anything but glorious. All pragmatic interpretation involves mental state attribution of this type. When mental state attribution is impaired, as in clients with ToM impairments, it is likely that pragmatic interpretation will be adversely affected.

Unit 48.3 Client history and family background

(1) WM is 24 years old. She is very close to the median age of onset (23 years) for bipolar disorder in one large study (Baldessarini et al., 2012).
(2) WM has migraines, which are a common medical comorbidity in bipolar disorder.
(3) WM does not have a substance use disorder, which is a significant comorbidity in bipolar disorder.
(4) WM has a biological relative (paternal grandfather) who was diagnosed with manic depression. This is a risk factor for bipolar disorder.
(5) There is good evidence that childbirth can serve as a trigger for bipolar disorder. In a sample of 120,378 women, Munk-Olsen et al. (2012) found that a first-time psychiatric episode in the immediate postpartum period (0–14 days after delivery) significantly predicted conversion to bipolar affective disorder during a 15-year follow-up period.

Unit 48.4 Clinical presentation, diagnosis and treatment

(1) The following non-verbal behaviours are indicative of a depressed state: (i) WM slept excessively; (ii) WM isolated herself (social withdrawal); and (iii) WM was unable to get things done (difficulty initiating activity).

(2) Pressured speech (or press of speech) is excessive speech which is produced at a rapid rate and is difficult to interrupt. It is one of the features of speech in hypomania and mania but rarely occurs in schizophrenia.

(3) WM's verbal behaviour during the initial interview, specifically her pressured speech and topic shifts, were indicative of hypomania in her mood.

(4) (a) false; (b) true; (c) false; (d) false; (e) false

(5) During the initial interview WM spoke for seven minutes uninterrupted in response to the question 'What brings you here to see us today?'. It is likely that this extended response contained irrelevant information (relation maxim). It is also likely that this response was over-informative (quantity maxim). At a minimum, it seems likely that WM had difficulty adhering to Gricean maxims of relation and quantity during the initial interview.

Unit 48.5 Focus on discourse in bipolar disorder

(1) There is some evidence that B does not understand the researcher's questions. In extract 1, the researcher asks a question about *place* ('where have you worked here?') to which B replies with an answer about *time* ('I've last worked last Monday').

(2) In extract 1, B introduces the topic of a television programme. However, after three follow-up turns by the researcher, in which she attempts to identify the particular programme that B is talking about, the topic is abandoned by B.

(3) (a) B responds 'thank you' to the offer of a light in extract 1.
   (b) In extracts 1 and 2, B is consciously trying to work out which month it is.
   (c) B uses grammatical ellipsis when he says in extract 2 'yesterday he did [bring me those cigarettes]'.
   (d) B initiates repair of an utterance in 'I was born with blue eyes [. . .] with my daddy's blue eyes'.
   (e) B asks the researcher questions which she does not have the knowledge to address, e.g. 'is my mother still alive?'

(4) In extract 2, B asks 'didn't he phone this morning?' in the absence of any preceding referent for 'he'. In fact, the referent for 'he' – presumably, daddy – is only introduced subsequently.

(5) In extract 2, B appears to be led by her own talk about her mother's *green* eyes into talk about how her mother would never let her wear *green* clothes.

Appendix B
Suggestions for further reading

Section A Speech disorders

CLEFT LIP AND PALATE

Howard, S. and Lohmander, A. (eds.) (2011) *Cleft Palate Speech: Assessment and Intervention*, Chichester, West Sussex: John Wiley & Sons.

Peterson-Falzone, S.J., Hardin-Jones, M.A. and Karnell, M.P. (2010) *Cleft Palate Speech*, 4th edn, St. Louis, MO: Mosby Elsevier.

Riski, J.E. (2014) 'Cleft lip and palate and other craniofacial anomalies', in L. Cummings (ed.), *Cambridge Handbook of Communication Disorders*, Cambridge: Cambridge University Press, 3–25.

DEVELOPMENTAL DYSARTHRIA

Ballard, K.J. and McCabe, P. (2014) 'Developmental motor speech disorders', in L. Cummings (ed.), *Cambridge Handbook of Communication Disorders*, Cambridge: Cambridge University Press, 383–99.

Hodge, M. (2014) 'Developmental dysarthria', in L. Cummings (ed.), *Cambridge Handbook of Communication Disorders*, Cambridge: Cambridge University Press, 26–48.

Murdoch, B.E. and Horton, S.K. (1998) 'Acquired and developmental dysarthria in childhood', in B.E. Murdoch (ed.), *Dysarthria: A Physiological Approach to Assessment and Treatment*, Cheltenham: Stanley Thornes, 373–428.

DEVELOPMENTAL VERBAL DYSPRAXIA

McNeill, B. (2014) 'Developmental verbal dyspraxia', in L. Cummings (ed.), *Cambridge Handbook of Communication Disorders*, Cambridge: Cambridge University Press, 49–60.

Murray, E., McCabe, P., Heard, R. and Ballard, K.J. (2015) 'Differential diagnosis of children with suspected childhood apraxia of speech', *Journal of Speech, Language, and Hearing Research*, **58** (1): 43–60.

Shriberg, L.D. (2010) 'A neurodevelopmental framework for research in childhood apraxia of speech', in B. Maassen and P. van Lieshout (eds.), *Speech Motor Control: New Developments in Basic and Applied Research*, New York: Oxford University Press, 259–70.

GLOSSECTOMY

Blyth, K.M., McCabe, P., Madill, C. and Ballard, K.J. (2015) 'Speech and swallow rehabilitation following partial glossectomy: A systematic review', *International Journal of Speech-Language Pathology*, **17** (4): 401–10.

Bressmann, T. (2014) 'Head and neck cancer and communication', in L. Cummings (ed.), *Cambridge Handbook of Communication Disorders*, Cambridge: Cambridge University Press, 161–84.

Ward, E.C. and van As-Brooks, C.J. (2014) *Head and Neck Cancer: Treatment, Rehabilitation, and Outcomes*, 2nd edn, San Diego, CA: Plural Publishing.

ACQUIRED DYSARTHRIA

Duffy, J.R. (2013) *Motor Speech Disorders: Substrates, Differential Diagnosis, and Management*, 3rd edn, St. Louis, MO: Elsevier Mosby.

Lowit, A. (2014) 'Acquired motor speech disorders', in L. Cummings (ed.), *Cambridge Handbook of Communication Disorders*, Cambridge: Cambridge University Press, 400–18.

Murdoch, B.E. (2014) 'Acquired dysarthria', in L. Cummings (ed.), *Cambridge Handbook of Communication Disorders*, Cambridge: Cambridge University Press, 185–210.

APRAXIA OF SPEECH

Ogar, J., Slama, H., Dronkers, N., Amici, S. and Gorno-Tempini, M.L. (2005) 'Apraxia of speech: an overview', *Neurocase*, **11** (6): 427–32.

Robin, D.A. and Flagmeier, S. (2014) 'Apraxia of speech', in L. Cummings (ed.), *Cambridge Handbook of Communication Disorders*, Cambridge: Cambridge University Press, 211–23.

Ziegler, W., Aichert, I. and Staiger, A. (2012) 'Apraxia of speech: concepts and controversies', *Journal of Speech, Language, and Hearing Research*, **55** (5): S1485–S1501.

FOREIGN ACCENT SYNDROME

Gurder, J. and Coleman, J. (eds.) (2006) 'Special issue: foreign accent syndrome', *Journal of Neurolinguistics*, **19** (5): 341–430.

Moen, I. (2000) 'Foreign accent syndrome: a review of contemporary explanations', *Aphasiology*, **14** (1): 5–15.

Ryalls, J. and Millar, N. (2015) *Foreign Accent Syndromes: The Stories People Have to Tell*, London and New York: Psychology Press.

Section B Language disorders

DEVELOPMENTAL PHONOLOGICAL DISORDER

Dodd, B. (ed.) (2005) *Differential Diagnosis and Treatment of Children with Speech Disorder*, Chichester, West Sussex: Whurr.

Kamhi, A.G. and Pollock, K.E. (eds.) (2005) *Phonological Disorders in Children: Clinical Decision Making in Assessment and Intervention*, Baltimore, MD: Paul H. Brookes Publishing.

Rvachew, S. (2014) 'Developmental phonological disorder', in L. Cummings (ed.), *Cambridge Handbook of Communication Disorders*, Cambridge: Cambridge University Press, 61–72.

SPECIFIC LANGUAGE IMPAIRMENT

Botting, N. and Conti-Ramsden, G. (2004) 'Characteristics of children with specific language impairment', in L. Verhoeven and H. van Balkom (eds.), *Classification of Developmental Language Disorders: Theoretical Issues and Clinical Implications*, Mahwah, NJ: Lawrence Erlbaum Associates, 23–38.

Ellis Weismer, S. (2014) 'Specific language impairment', in L. Cummings (ed.), *Cambridge Handbook of Communication Disorders*, Cambridge: Cambridge University Press, 73–87.

Leonard, L.B. (2014) *Children with Specific Language Impairment*, 2nd edn, Cambridge, MA: MIT Press.

PRAGMATIC LANGUAGE IMPAIRMENT

Adams, C. (2015) 'Assessment and intervention for children with pragmatic language impairment', in D.A. Hwa-Froelich (ed.), *Social Communication Development and Disorders*, New York and London, 141–70.

Swineford, L.B., Thurm, A., Baird, G., Wetherby, A.M. and Swedo, S. (2014) 'Social (pragmatic) communication disorder: A research review of this new DSM-5 diagnostic category', *Journal of Neurodevelopmental Disorders*, **6** (1): 41.

Van Balkom, H. and Verhoeven, L. (2004) 'Pragmatic disability in children with specific language impairments', in L. Verhoeven and H. van Balkom (eds.), *Classification of Developmental Language Disorders: Theoretical Issues and Clinical Implications*, Mahwah, NJ: Lawrence Erlbaum Associates, 283–306.

DEVELOPMENTAL DYSLEXIA

Christo, C. (2014) 'Developmental dyslexia', in L. Cummings (ed.), *Cambridge Handbook of Communication Disorders*, Cambridge: Cambridge University Press, 88–108.

Peterson, R.L. and Pennington, B.F. (2015) 'Developmental dyslexia', *Annual Review of Clinical Psychology*, **11**: 283–307.

Snowling, M.J. and Stackhouse, J. (eds.) (2006) *Dyslexia, Speech and Language: A Practitioner's Handbook*, 2nd edn, Chichester, West Sussex: Whurr.

LANGUAGE IN INTELLECTUAL DISABILITY

Abbeduto, L. (ed.) (2003) *International Review of Research in Mental Retardation: Language and Communication in Mental Retardation*, San Diego, CA: Academic Press.

Martin, G.E., Klusek, J., Estigarribia, B. and Roberts, J.E. (2009) 'Language characteristics of individuals with Down syndrome', *Topics in Language Disorders*, **29** (2): 112–32.

Short-Meyerson, K. and Benson, G. (2014) 'Intellectual disability and communication', in L. Cummings (ed.), *Cambridge Handbook of Communication Disorders*, Cambridge: Cambridge University Press, 109–24.

LANGUAGE IN AUTISM SPECTRUM DISORDER

Charman, T. and Stone, W. (eds.) (2006) *Social and Communication Development in Autism Spectrum Disorders: Early Identification, Diagnosis, and Intervention*, New York: Guilford Press.

Muma, J. and Cloud, S. (2013) 'Autism spectrum disorders: The state of the art', in J.S. Damico, N. Müller and M.J. Ball (eds.), *The Handbook of Speech and Language Disorders*, Chichester, West Sussex: Wiley-Blackwell, 153–77.

Norbury, N.F. (2014) 'Autism spectrum disorders and communication', in L. Cummings (ed.), *Cambridge Handbook of Communication Disorders*, Cambridge: Cambridge University Press, 141–58.

LANGUAGE IN EPILEPSY

Broeders, M., Geurts, H. and Jennekens-Schinkel, A. (2010) 'Pragmatic communication deficits in children with epilepsy', *International Journal of Language & Communication Disorders*, **45** (5): 608–16.

Deonna, T. (2000) 'Acquired epileptic aphasia (AEA) or Landau–Kleffner syndrome: From childhood to adulthood', in D.V.M. Bishop and L.B. Leonard (eds.), *Speech and Language Impairments in Children: Causes, Characteristics, Intervention and Outcome*, Hove: Psychology Press, 261–72.

Pal, D.K. (2011) 'Epilepsy and neurodevelopmental disorders of language', *Current Opinion in Neurology*, **24** (2): 126–31.

LANGUAGE IN PAEDIATRIC TRAUMATIC BRAIN INJURY

Ewing-Cobbs, L. and Barnes, M. (2002) 'Linguistic outcomes following traumatic brain injury in children', *Seminars in Pediatric Neurology*, **9** (3): 209–17.

McDonald, S., Togher, L. and Code, C. (eds.) (2014) *Social and Communication Disorders Following Traumatic Brain Injury*, 2nd edn, Hove and New York: Psychology Press.

Sullivan, J.R. and Riccio, C.A. (2010) 'Language functioning and deficits following pediatric traumatic brain injury', *Applied Neurospsychology*, **17** (2): 93–8.

LANGUAGE IN CHILDHOOD CANCER

Docking, K., Murdoch, B.E. and Suppiah, R. (2007) 'The impact of a cerebellar tumour on language function in childhood', *Folia Phoniatrica et Logopaedica*, **59** (4): 190–200.

Murdoch, B.E. (1999) *Communication Disorders in Childhood Cancer*, London: Whurr.

Taylor, O.D., Ware, R.S. and Weir, K.A. (2012) 'Speech pathology services to children with cancer and nonmalignant hematological disorders', *Journal of Pediatric Oncology Nursing*, **29** (2): 98–108.

FLUENT AND NON-FLUENT APHASIA

Bastiaanse, R. and Prins, R.S. (2014) 'Aphasia', in L. Cummings (ed.), *Cambridge Handbook of Communication Disorders*, Cambridge: Cambridge University Press, 224–46.

Edwards, S. (2005) *Fluent Aphasia*, Cambridge: Cambridge University Press.

Whitworth, A., Webster, J. and Morris, J. (2014) 'Acquired aphasia', in L. Cummings (ed.), *Cambridge Handbook of Communication Disorders*, Cambridge: Cambridge University Press, 436–56.

RIGHT-HEMISPHERE LANGUAGE DISORDER

Joanette, Y., Ferré, P. and Wilson, M.A. (2014) 'Right hemisphere damage and communication', in L. Cummings (ed.), *Cambridge Handbook of Communication Disorders*, Cambridge: Cambridge University Press, 247–65.

Lehman Blake, M. (2013) 'Communication deficits associated with right hemisphere brain damage', in J.S. Damico, N. Müller and M.J. Ball (eds.), *The Handbook of Speech and Language Disorders*, Chichester, West Sussex: Wiley-Blackwell, 556–76.

Tompkins, C.A., Klepousniotou, E. and Scott, A.G. (2013) 'Nature and assessment of right hemisphere disorders', in I. Papathanasiou, P. Coppens and C. Potagas (eds.), *Aphasia and Related Neurogenic Communication Disorders*, Burlington, MA: Jones & Bartlett Learning.

LANGUAGE IN ADULT TRAUMATIC BRAIN INJURY

Coelho, C. and Youse, K.M. (2007) 'Cognitive-communication rehabilitation following traumatic brain injury', in A.F. Johnson and B.H. Jacobson (eds.), *Medical Speech-Language Pathology: A Practitioner's Guide*, 2nd edn, New York and Stuttgart: Thieme, 71–93.

McDonald, S., Togher, L. and Code, C. (eds.) (2014) *Social and Communication Disorders Following Traumatic Brain Injury*, 2nd edn, Hove and New York: Psychology Press.

Togher, L. (2014) 'Traumatic brain injury and communication', in L. Cummings (ed.), *Cambridge Handbook of Communication Disorders*, Cambridge: Cambridge University Press, 284–99.

LANGUAGE IN DEMENTIA

Bayles, K.A. and Tomoeda, C.K. (2013) *Cognitive-Communication Disorders of Dementia: Definition, Diagnosis and Treatment*, 2nd edn, San Diego, CA: Plural Publishing.

Nickels, L. and Croot, K. (eds.) (2015) *Clinical Perspectives on Primary Progressive Aphasia*, Hove: Psychology Press.

Reilly, J. and Hung, J. (2014) 'Dementia and communication', in L. Cummings (ed.), *Cambridge Handbook of Communication Disorders*, Cambridge: Cambridge University Press, 266–83.

LANGUAGE IN OTHER NEURODEGENERATIVE DISORDERS

Hartelius, L., Jonsson, M., Rickeberg, A. and Laakso, K. (2010) 'Communication and Huntington's disease: qualitative interviews and focus groups with persons with Huntington's disease, family members, and carers', *International Journal of Language & Communication Disorders*, **45** (3): 381–93.

Murdoch, B. and Theodoros, D. (eds.) (2000) *Speech and Language Disorders in Multiple Sclerosis*, London and Philadelphia, PA: Whurr.

Theodoros, D. and Ramig, L. (eds.) (2011) *Communication and Swallowing in Parkinson Disease*, San Diego, CA: Plural Publishing.

Section C Fluency disorders

DEVELOPMENTAL STUTTERING

Howell, P. (2011) *Recovery from Stuttering*, Hove and New York: Psychology Press.

Ward, D. (2016) *Stuttering and Cluttering: Frameworks for Understanding and Treatment*, 2nd edn, Hove: Psychology Press.

Yaruss, J.S. (2014) 'Disorders of fluency', in L. Cummings (ed.), *Cambridge Handbook of Communication Disorders*, Cambridge: Cambridge University Press, 484–98.

ACQUIRED STUTTERING

De Nil, L.F., Jokel, R. and Rochon, E. (2007) 'Etiology, symptomatology, and treatment of neurogenic stuttering', in E.G. Conture and R.F. Curlee (eds.), *Stuttering and Related Disorders of Fluency*, 3rd edn, New York: Thieme, 326–43.

Lundgren, K., Helm-Estabrooks, N. and Klein, R. (2010) 'Stuttering following acquired brain damage: A review of the literature', *Journal of Neurolinguistics*, **23** (5): 447–54.

Ward, D. (2010) 'Sudden onset of stuttering in an adult: neurogenic and psychogenic perspectives', *Journal of Neurolinguistics*, **23** (5): 511–17.

CLUTTERING

Scaler Scott, K. (2014) 'Stuttering and cluttering', in L. Cummings (ed.), *Cambridge Handbook of Communication Disorders*, Cambridge: Cambridge University Press, 341–58.

St. Louis, K.O., Myers, F.L., Bakker, K. and Raphael, L.J. (2007) 'Understanding and treating cluttering', in E.G. Conture and R.F. Curlee (eds.), *Stuttering and Related Disorders of Fluency*, 3rd edn, New York: Thieme, 297–325.

Ward, D. and Scaler Scott, K. (eds.) (2011) *Cluttering: A Handbook of Research, Intervention and Education*, Hove: Psychology Press.

Section D Voice disorders

ORGANIC VOICE DISORDER

Connor, N.P. and Bless, D.M. (2014) 'Functional and organic voice disorders', in L. Cummings (ed.), *Cambridge Handbook of Communication Disorders*, Cambridge: Cambridge University Press, 321–40.

Rammage, L. (2014) 'Disorders of voice', in L. Cummings (ed.), *Cambridge Handbook of Communication Disorders*, Cambridge: Cambridge University Press, 457–83.

Sataloff, R.T. (2005) *Clinical Assessment of Voice*, San Diego, CA: Plural Publishing.

FUNCTIONAL VOICE DISORDER

Baker, J. (2002) 'Psychogenic voice disorders – heroes or hysterics? A brief overview with questions and discussion', *Logopedics, Phoniatrics, Vocology*, **27** (2): 84–91.

Connor, N.P. and Bless, D.M. (2014) 'Functional and organic voice disorders', in L. Cummings (ed.), *Cambridge Handbook of Communication Disorders*, Cambridge: Cambridge University Press, 321–40.

Roy, N. (2003) 'Functional dysphonia', *Current Opinion in Otolaryngology and Head & Neck Surgery*, **11** (3): 144–8.

LARYNGECTOMY

Coffey, M. and Tolley, N. (2015) 'Swallowing after laryngectomy', *Current Opinion in Otolaryngology & Head and Neck Surgery*, **23** (3): 202–8.

Tang, C.G. and Sinclair, C.F. (2015) 'Voice restoration after total laryngectomy', *Otolaryngologic Clinics of North America*, **48** (4): 687–702.

Ward, E.C. and van As-Brooks, C.J. (2014) *Head and Neck Cancer: Treatment, Rehabilitation, and Outcomes*, 2nd edn, San Diego, CA: Plural Publishing.

TRANSSEXUAL VOICE

Adler, R.K., Hirsch, S. and Mordaunt, M. (eds.) (2012) *Voice and Communication Therapy for the Transgender/Transsexual Client: A Comprehensive Clinical Guide*, 2nd edn, San Diego, CA: Plural Publishing.

Azul, D. (2015) 'Transmasculine people's vocal situations: a critical review of gender-related discourses and empirical data', *International Journal of Language & Communication Disorders*, **50** (1): 31–47.

Dacakis, G., Oates, J. and Douglas, J. (2012) 'Beyond voice: perceptions of gender in male-to-female transsexuals', *Current Opinion in Otolaryngology & Head and Neck Surgery*, **20** (3): 165–70.

Section E Hearing disorders

CONDUCTIVE HEARING LOSS

Ackley, R.S. (2014) 'Hearing disorders', in L. Cummings (ed.), *Cambridge Handbook of Communication Disorders*, Cambridge: Cambridge University Press, 359–80.

Hellier, W. (2009) 'The aetiology and management of conductive hearing loss in children and adults', in J. Graham and D. Baguley (eds.), *Ballantyne's Deafness*, Chichester, West Sussex: Wiley-Blackwell, 85–100.

Northern, J.L. and Downs, M.P. (2014) *Hearing in Children*, 6th edn, San Diego, CA: Plural Publishing.

SENSORINEURAL HEARING LOSS

Ackley, R.S. (2014) 'Hearing disorders', in L. Cummings (ed.), *Cambridge Handbook of Communication Disorders*, Cambridge: Cambridge University Press, 359–80.

Burton, M. (2009) 'Acquired sensorineural hearing loss', in J. Graham and D. Baguley (eds.), *Ballantyne's Deafness*, Chichester, West Sussex: Wiley-Blackwell, 101–14.

Saeed, S., Booth, R. and Hill, P. (2009) 'The causes, identification and confirmation of sensorineural hearing loss in children', in J. Graham and D. Baguley (eds.), *Ballantyne's Deafness*, Chichester, West Sussex: Wiley-Blackwell, 127–38.

COCHLEAR IMPLANTATION

Ambrose, S.E., Hamnes-Ganguly, D.M. and Lehnert, K.M. (2009) 'The speech-language specialist on the pediatric cochlear implant team', in L.S. Eisenberg (ed.), *Clinical Management of Children with Cochlear Implants*, San Diego, CA: Plural Publishing, 251–324.

Mellon, N.K. (2009) 'Language and speech acquisition', in J.K. Niparko (ed.), *Cochlear Implants: Principles & Practices*, 2nd edn, Philadelphia, PA: Lippincott Williams & Wilkins, 245–62.

O'Donoghue, G.M. and Pisoni, D.B. (2014) 'Auditory and linguistic outcomes in pediatric cochlear implantation', in S.B. Waltzman and J.T. Roland Jr. (eds.), *Cochlear Implants*, 3rd edn, New York: Thieme.

CENTRAL AUDITORY PROCESSING DISORDER

Bellis, T.J. and Bellis, J.D. (2015) 'Central auditory processing disorders in children and adults', *Handbook of Clinical Neurology*, **129**: 537–56.

DeBonis, D.A. and Moncrieff, D. (2008) 'Auditory processing disorders: An update for speech-language pathologists', *American Journal of Speech-Language Pathology*, **17** (1): 4–18.

Ross-Swain, D. (2013) 'The speech-language pathologist's role in the assessment of auditory processing skills', in D. Geffner and D. Ross-Swain (eds.), *Auditory Processing Disorders: Assessment, Management and Treatment*, San Diego, CA: Plural Publishing, 251–82.

Section F Psychiatric disorders

CHILDHOOD EMOTIONAL AND BEHAVIOURAL DISORDERS

Benner, G.J. and Nelson, J.R. (2014) 'Emotional disturbance and communication', in L. Cummings (ed.), *Cambridge Handbook of Communication Disorders*, Cambridge: Cambridge University Press, 125–40.

McInnes, A. and Manassis, K. (2005) 'When silence is not golden: an integrated approach to selective mutism', *Seminars in Speech and Language*, **26** (3): 201–10.

Westby, C. and Watson, S. (2013) 'ADHD and communication disorders', in J.S. Damico, N. Müller and M.J. Ball (eds.), *The Handbook of Speech and Language Disorders*, Chichester, West Sussex: Wiley-Blackwell, 529–55.

SCHIZOPHRENIA

Bryan, K. (2014) 'Psychiatric disorders and communication', in L. Cummings (ed.), *Cambridge Handbook of Communication Disorders*, Cambridge: Cambridge University Press, 300–18.

Covington, M.A., He, C., Brown, C., Naçi, L., McClain, J.T., Fjordbak, B.S., Semple, J. and Brown, J. (2005) 'Schizophrenia and the structure of language: the linguist's view', *Schizophrenia Research*, **77** (1): 85–98.

France, J. and Kramer, S. (eds.) (2001) *Communication and Mental Illness: Theoretical and Practical Approaches*, London and Philadelphia, PA: Jessica Kingsley Publishers.

BIPOLAR DISORDER

Fine, J. (2006) *Language in Psychiatry: A Handbook of Clinical Practice*, London: Equinox Publishing.

France, J. (2001) 'Depression and other mood disorders', in J. France and S. Kramer (eds.), *Communication and Mental Illness: Theoretical and Practical Approaches*, London and Philadelphia, PA: Jessica Kingsley Publishers, 65–80.

Quattlebaum, P.D., Grier, B.C. and Klubnik, C. (2012) 'Bipolar disorder in children: implications for speech-language pathologists', *Communication Disorders Quarterly*, **33** (3): 181–92

References

Aaronson, B. and Bernier, R. 2013. 'Mismatch negativity', in F.R. Volkmar (ed.), *Encyclopedia of Autism Spectrum Disorder*, New York: Springer, 1878–82.

Aarsen, F.K., Paquier, P.F., Arts, W.-F., Van Veelen, M.-L., Michiels, E., Lequin, M. and Catsman-Berrevoets, C.E. 2009. 'Cognitive deficits and predictors 3 years after diagnosis of a pilocytic astrocytoma in childhood', *Journal of Clinical Oncology* **27**:21, 3526–32.

Aarsen, F.K., Paquier, P.F., Reddingius, R.E., Streng, I.C., Arts, W.-F., Evera-Preesman, M. and Catsman-Berrevoets, C.E. 2006. 'Functional outcome after low-grade astrocytoma treatment in childhood', *Cancer* **106**:2, 396–402.

Abu-Al-makarem, A. and Petrosino, L. 2007. 'Reading and spontaneous speaking fundamental frequency of young Arabic men for Arabic and English languages: a comparative study', *Perceptual and Motor Skills* **105**:2, 572–80.

Abusamra, V., Côté, H., Joanette, Y. and Ferreres, A. 2009. 'Communication impairments in patients with right hemisphere damage', *Life Span and Disability* **12**:1, 67–82.

Ackley, R.S. 2014. 'Hearing disorders', in L. Cummings (ed.), *Cambridge Handbook of Communication Disorders*, Cambridge: Cambridge University Press, 359–80.

Adams, S.G. and Dykstra, A. 2009. 'Hypokinetic dysarthria', in M.R. McNeil (ed.), *Clinical Management of Sensorimotor Speech Disorders*, 2nd edn, New York: Thieme Medical Publishers, 166–86.

Aguilar-Mediavilla, E.M., Sanz-Torrent, M. and Serra-Raventos, M. 2002. 'A comparative study of the phonology of pre-school children with specific language impairment (SLI), language delay (LD) and normal acquisition', *Clinical Linguistics and Phonetics* **16**:8, 573–96.

Ahmed, S., Haigh, A.M., de Jager, C.A. and Garrard, P. 2013. 'Connected speech as a marker of disease progression in autopsy-proven Alzheimer's disease', *Brain* **136**:12, 3727–37.

Albustanji, Y.M., Albustanji, M.M., Hegazi, M.M. and Amayreh, M.M. 2014. 'Prevalence and types of articulation errors in Saudi Arabic-speaking children with repaired cleft lip and palate', *International Journal of Pediatric Otorhinolaryngology* **78**:10, 1707–15.

Alcock, K.J., Passingham, R.E., Watkins, K.E. and Vargha-Khadem, F. 2000. 'Oral dyspraxia in inherited speech and language impairment and acquired dysphasia', *Brain and Language* **75**:1, 17–33.

Alicandri-Ciufelli, M., Piccinini, A., Grammatica, A., Chiesi, A., Bergamini, G., Luppi, M.P., Nizzoli, F., Ghidini, A., Tassi, S. and Presutti, L. 2013. 'Voice and swallowing after partial laryngectomy: factors influencing outcome', *Head & Neck* **35**:2, 214–19.

Allan, B.J., Van Haren, R.M., Wang, B. and Thaller, S. 2015. 'Secondary soft tissue reconstruction', in P.J. Taub, P.K. Patel, S.R. Buchman and M.N. Cohen (eds.), *Ferraro's Fundamentals of Maxillofacial Surgery*, New York: Springer, 313–22.

Allen, M.L., Haywood, S., Rajendran, G. and Branigan, H. 2011. 'Evidence for syntactic alignment in children with autism', *Developmental Science* **14**:3, 540–8.

American Psychiatric Association 2013. *Diagnostic and Statistical Manual of Mental Disorders*, 5th edn, Washington, DC: American Psychiatric Association.

American Speech-Language-Hearing Association 2002. *Consensus Auditory–Perceptual Evaluation of Voice (CAPE-V)*, Rockville, MD: ASHA.

2005a. 'What does the speech-language pathologist or audiologist need to know about genetics when conducting assessments?'. Access Academics and Research, August 2005 (accessed June 2015).

2005b. 'Central auditory processing disorders – the role of the audiologist'. Position statement. Online. Available at: www.asha.org/members/deskref-journals/deskref/default (accessed June 2015).

2005c. 'Technical report: (central) auditory processing disorders'. Online. Available at: www .asha.org/policy/TR2005-00043.htm#sec1.3 (accessed June 2015).

2007. 'Childhood apraxia of speech'. Position statement. Online. Available at: www.asha.org/ policy (accessed June 2015).

2015. 'Speech sound disorders – articulation and phonology'. Online. Available at: www.asha .org/Practice-Portal/Clinical-Topics/Articulation-and-Phonology (accessed June 2015).

Amin, S.B., Orlando, M., Monczynski, C. and Tillery, K. 2015. 'Central auditory processing disorder profile in premature and term infants', *American Journal of Perinatology* **32**:4, 399–404.

Anderson, J.A. 2014. 'Pitch elevation in transgendered patients: anterior glottic web formation assisted by temporary injection augmentation', *Journal of Voice* **28**:6, 816–21.

Anderson, V. and Catroppa, C. 2005. 'Recovery of executive skills following paediatric traumatic brain injury (TBI): a 2 year follow-up', *Brain Injury* **19**:6, 459–70.

Andriessen, T.M., Jacobs, B. and Vos, P.E. 2010. 'Clinical characteristics and pathophysiological mechanisms of focal and diffuse traumatic brain injury', *Journal of Cellular and Molecular Medicine* **14**:10, 2381–92.

Angelillo, N., Di Costanzo, B. and Barillari, U. 2010. 'Speech-language evaluation and rehabilitation treatment in Floating-Harbor syndrome: a case study', *Journal of Communication Disorders* **43**:3, 252–60.

Angst, J. 2013. 'Bipolar disorders in DSM-5: Strengths, problems and perspectives', *International Journal of Bipolar Disorders* **1**:12.

Archibald, L.M.D. and Gathercole, S.E. 2006. 'Prevalence of SLI in language resource units', *Journal of Research in Special Educational Needs* **6**:1, 3–10.

Aronson, A.E. 1990. *Clinical Voice Disorders: An Interdisciplinary Approach*, 3rd edn, Stuttgart and New York: Thieme.

Aronson, A.E. and Bless, D.M. 2009. *Clinical Voice Disorders*, 4th edn, New York: Thieme Medical Publishers.

Aziz, A.A., Shohdi, S., Osman, D.M. and Habib, E.I. 2010. 'Childhood apraxia of speech and multiple phonological disorders in Cairo-Egyptian Arabic speaking children: language, speech, and oro-motor differences', *International Journal of Pediatric Otorhinolaryngology* **74**:6, 578–85.

Azul, D. 2015. 'Transmasculine people's vocal situations: a critical review of gender-related discourses and empirical data', *International Journal of Language & Communication Disorders* **50**:1, 31–47.

Bader, S. 2009. 'Speech and language impairments of Arabic-speaking Jordanian children within natural phonology and phonology as human behaviour', *Poznań Studies in Contemporary Linguistics* **45**:2, 191–210.

Bagwell, K., Leder, S.B. and Sasaki, C.T. 2015. 'Is partial laryngectomy safe forever?', *American Journal of Otolaryngology* **36**:3, 437–41.

Baker, J. 2003. 'Psychogenic voice disorders and traumatic stress experience: a discussion paper with two case reports', *Journal of Voice* **17**:3, 308–18.

Baldessarini, R.J., Tondo, L., Vazquez, G.H., Undurraga, J., Bolzani, L., Yildiz, A., Khalsa, H.-M.K., Lai, M., Lepri, B., Lolich, M., Maffei, P.M., Salvatore, P., Faedda, G.L., Vieta, E. and Mauricio, T. 2012. 'Age at onset versus family history and clinical outcomes in 1,665 international bipolar-I disorder patients', *World Psychiatry* **11**:1, 40–6.

Bali, J., Gheinani, A.H., Zurbriggen, S. and Rajendran, L. 2012. 'Role of genes linked to sporadic Alzheimer's disease risk in the production of β-amyloid peptides', *Proceedings of the National Academy of Sciences of the United States of America* **109**:38, 15307–11.

Barachetti, C. and Lavelli, M. 2011. 'Responsiveness of children with specific language impairment and maternal repairs during shared book reading', *International Journal of Language & Communication Disorders* **46**:5, 579–91.

Barisic, I., Odak, L., Loane, M., Garne, E., Wellesley, D., Calzolari, E., Dolk, H., Addor, M.-C., Arriola, L., Bergman, J., Bianca, S., Doray, B., Khoshnood, B., Klungsoyr, K., McDonnell, B., Pierini, A., Rankin, J., Rissmann, A., Rounding, C., Queisser-Luft, A., Scarano, G. and Tucker, D. 2014. 'Prevalence, prenatal diagnosis and clinical features of oculo-auriculo-vertebral spectrum: a registry-based study in Europe', *European Journal of Human Genetics* **22**:8, 1026–33.

Barker, D.H., Quittner, A.L., Fink, N.E., Eisenberg, L.S., Tobey, E.A., Niparko, J.K. and CDaCI Investigative Team 2009. 'Predicting behaviour problems in deaf and hearing children: the influences of language, attention, and parent–child communication', *Development and Psychopathology* **21**:2, 373–92.

Barlow, K.M., Thomson, E., Johnson, D. and Minns, R.A. 2005. 'Late neurologic and cognitive sequelae of inflicted traumatic brain injury in infancy', *Pediatrics* **116**:2, e174–e185.

Barry, W.J. and Timmermann, G. 1985. 'Mispronunciations and compensatory movements of tongue-operated patients', *British Journal of Disorders of Communication* **20**:1, 81–90.

Bastiaanse, R. 1995. 'Broca's aphasia: a syntactic and/or a morphological disorder: a case study', *Brain and Language* **48**:1, 1–32.

Bastiaanse, R. and Prins, R.S. 2014. 'Aphasias', in L. Cummings (ed.), *Cambridge Handbook of Communication Disorders*, Cambridge: Cambridge University Press, 224–46.

Bastiaanse, R., Edwards, S. and Rispens, J. 2002. *Verb and Sentence Test*, Bury St. Edmunds: Thames Valley Test Company.

Bates, G.P., Dorsey, R., Gusella, J.F., Hayden, M.R., Kay, C., Leavitt, B.R., Nance, M., Ross, C.A., Scahill, R.I., Wetzel, R., Wild, E.J. and Tabrizi, S.J. 2015. 'Huntington disease', *Nature Reviews Disease Primers* **1**, 1–21.

Baxter, A.J., Brugha, T.S., Erskine, H.E., Scheurer, R.W., Vos, T. and Scott, J.G. 2014. 'The epidemiology and global burden of autism spectrum disorders', *Psychological Medicine* **45**:3, 601–13.

Bayles, K.A. and Tomoeda, C.K. 2013. *MCI and Alzheimer's Dementia: Clinical Essentials for Assessment and Treatment of Cognitive-Communication Disorders*, San Diego, CA: Plural Publishing.

Bayley, N. 1969. *Manual for the Bayley Scales of Infant Development*, San Antonio, TX: Psychological Corporation.

Beauchamp, M.H. and Anderson, V. 2013. 'Cognitive and psychopathological sequelae of pediatric traumatic brain injury', in O. Dulac, M. Lassonde and H.B. Sarnat (eds.), *Handbook of Clinical Neurology, Pediatric Neurology*, Part II, Amsterdam: the Netherlands, 913–20.

Beck, A.T., Steer, R.A. and Brown, G.K. 1996. *Beck Depression Inventory-II*, San Antonio, TX: Psychological Corporation.

Beck, A.T., Ward, C.H., Mendelson, M., Mock, J. and Erbaugh, J. 1961. 'An inventory for measuring depression', *Archives of General Psychiatry* **4**:6, 561–71.

Becker, K.P. and Grundmann, K. 1970. 'Investigation on incidence and symptomatology of cluttering', *Folia Phoniatrica* **22**:4, 261–71.

Beeke, S., Wilkinson, R. and Maxim, J. 2007. 'Individual variation in agrammatism: a single case study of the influence on interaction', *International Journal of Language & Communication Disorders* **42**:6, 629–47.

Beery, K. 1989. *Manual for the VMI: Developmental Test of Visual-Motor Integration*, 3rd rev., Cleveland, OH: Modern Curriculum Press.

Beinhardt, S., Leiss, W., Stättermayer, A.F., Graziadei, I., Zoller, H., Stauber, R., Maieron, A., Datz, C., Steindl-Munda, P., Hofer, H., Vogel, W., Trauner, M. and Ferenci, P. 2014. 'Long-term outcomes of patients with Wilson disease in a large Austrian cohort', *Clinical Gastroenterology and Hepatology* **12**:4, 683–9.

Belenchia, P. and McCardle, P. 1985. 'Goldenhar's syndrome: a case study', *Journal of Communication Disorders* **18**:5, 383–92.

Beleza-Meireles, A., Clayton-Smith, J., Saraiva, J.M. and Tassabehji, M. 2014. 'Oculo-auriculo-vertebral spectrum: a review of the literature and genetic update', *Journal of Medical Genetics* **51**:10, 635–45.

Ben-David, A., Ezrati, R. and Stulman, N. 2010. 'Acquisition of /s/-clusters in Hebrew-speaking children with phonological disorders', *Clinical Linguistics & Phonetics* **24**:3, 210–23.

Benninger, M.S., Grywalski, C. and Phyland, D. 2007. 'Rehabilitation of the head and neck cancer patients', in A.F. Johnson and B.H. Jacobson (eds.), *Medical Speech-Language Pathology: A Practitioner's Guide*, 2nd edn, New York: Thieme, 182–202.

Bergemalm, P.O. and Lyxell, B. 2005. 'Appearances are deceptive? Long-term cognitive and central auditory sequelae from closed head injury', *International Journal of Audiology* **44**:1, 39–49.

Berlucchi, G., Aglioti, S., Marzi, C.A. and Tassinari, G. 1995. 'Corpus callosum and simple visuomotor integration', *Neuropsychologia* **33**:8, 923–36.

Berry, W.R., Darley, F.L., Aronson, A.E. and Goldstein, N.P. 1974. 'Dysarthria in Wilson's disease', *Journal of Speech, Language, and Hearing Research* **17**:2, 169–83.

Berthiaume, K.S., Lorch, E.P. and Milich, R. 2010. 'Getting clued in: inferential processing and comprehension monitoring in boys with ADHD', *Journal of Attention Disorders* **14**:1, 31–42.

Bezerra, J.F., Oliveira, G.H., Soares, C.D., Cardoso, M.L., Ururahy, M.A., Neto, F.P., Lima-Neto, L.G., Luchessi, A.D., Silbiger, V.N., Fajardo, C.M., Oliveira, S.R., Almeida, M.D., Hirata, R.D., Rezende, A.A. and Hirata, M.H. 2015. 'Genetic and non-genetic factors that increase the risk of non-syndromic cleft lip and/or palate development', *Oral Diseases* **21**:3, 393–9.

Bhattacharyya, N. 2014. 'The prevalence of voice problems among adults in the United States', *Laryngoscope* **124**:10, 2359–62.

Bianchi, M.T., Dworetzky, B.A. and Bromfield, E.B. 2009. 'Auditory auras in patients with postencephalitic epilepsy: case series', *Epilepsy & Behavior* **14**:1, 250–2.

Bien, C.G., Urbach, H., Schramm, J., Soeder, B.M., Becker, A.J., Voltz, R., Vincent, A. and Elger, C.E. 2007. 'Limbic encephalitis as a precipitating event in adult-onset temporal lobe epilepsy', *Neurology* **69**:12, 1236–44.

Bishop, D.V.M. 1983. *Test for Reception of Grammar*, Manchester: Medical Research Council.
2001. 'Genetic and environmental risks for specific language impairment in children', *Philosophical Transactions of the Royal Society of London* **356**:1407, 369–80.
2003. *The Children's Communication Checklist-2*, London: Psychological Corporation.

Blood, G.W., Ridenour Jr, V.J., Qualls, C.D. and Hammer, C.S. 2003. 'Co-occurring disorders in children who stutter', *Journal of Communication Disorders* **36**:6, 427–48.

Bloodstein, O. and Bernstein Ratner, N. 2008. *A Handbook on Stuttering*, 6th edn, Clifton Park, NY: Thomson Delmar.

Bond, W.S., Carvalho, M. and Foulks, E.F. 1982. 'Persistent dysarthria with apraxia associated with a combination of lithium carbonate and haloperidol', *Journal of Clinical Psychiatry*, **43**:6, 256–7.

Botha, H., Duffy, J.R., Strand, E.A., Machulda, M.M., Whitwell, J.L. and Josephs, K.A. 2014. 'Nonverbal oral apraxia in primary progressive aphasia and apraxia of speech', *Neurology* **82**:19, 1729–35.

Bowers, L., Huisingh, R., Barrett, M., Orman, J. and LoGiudice, C. 1994. *Test of Problem-solving – Elementary*, rev., East Moline, IL: PRO-IDEA.

Brandstorp-Boesen, J., Falk, R.S., Boysen, M. and Brøndbo, K. 2014. 'Long-term trends in gender, T-stage, subsite and treatment for laryngeal cancer at a single center', *European Archives of Oto-Rhino-Laryngology* **271**:12, 3233–9.

Bressmann, T., Jacobs, H., Quintero, J. and Irish, J.C. 2009. 'Speech outcomes for partial glossectomy surgery: measures of speech articulation and listener perception', *Canadian Journal of Speech-Language Pathology and Audiology* **33**:4, 204–10.

Brew, B.J. 1999. 'AIDS dementia complex', *Neurologic Clinics* **17**:4, 861–81.

Bridgemann, E. and Snowling, M. 1988. 'The perception of phoneme sequence: a comparison of dyspraxic and normal children', *British Journal of Disorders of Communication* **23**:3, 245–52.

Brinkman, T.M., Liptak, C.C., Delaney, B.L., Chordas, C.A., Muriel, A.C. and Manley, P.E. 2013. 'Suicide ideation in pediatric and adult survivors of childhood brain tumors', *Journal of Neuro-Oncology* **113**:3, 425–32.

Brockmann, M., Storck, C., Carding, P.N. and Drinnan, M.J. 2008. 'Voice loudness and gender effects on jitter and shimmer in healthy adults', *Journal of Speech, Language, and Hearing Research* **51**:5, 1152–60.

Brosseau-Lapré, F. and Rvachew, S. 2014. 'Cross-linguistic comparison of speech errors produced by English- and French-speaking preschool-age children with developmental phonological disorders', *International Journal of Speech-Language Pathology* **16**:2, 98–108.

Bruce, B., Thernlund, G. and Nettelbladt, U. 2006. 'ADHD and language impairment: a study of the parent questionnaire FTF (Five to Fifteen)', *European Child & Adolescent Psychiatry* **15**:1, 52–60.

Bryan, K.L. 1988. 'Assessment of language disorders after right hemisphere damage', *International Journal of Language & Communication Disorders* **23**:2, 111–25.

1989. 'Language prosody and the right hemisphere', *Aphasiology* **3**:4, 285–99.

1995. *The Right Hemisphere Language Battery*, 2nd edn. London: Whurr.

Bryan, K.L. and Hale, J.B. 2001. 'Differential effects of left and right cerebral vascular accidents on language competency', *Journal of the International Neuropsychological Society* **7**:6, 655–64.

Burkart, C.M., Senchenkov, A. and Wilson, K.M. 2010. 'Laryngeal carcinoma', in M.L. Pensak (ed.), *Otolaryngology Cases: The University of Cincinnati Clinical Portfolio*, New York: Thieme, 127–30.

Busse, R.T. and Downey, J. 2011. 'Selective mutism: a three-tiered approach to prevention and intervention', *Contemporary School Psychology* **15**:1, 53–63.

Bzoch, K. and League, R. 1970. *Receptive–Expressive Emergent Language Scale*, Baltimore: University Park Press.

Cabanillas, R., Rodrigo, J.P., Llorente, J.L., Suárez, V., Ortega, P. and Suárez, C. 2004. 'Functional outcomes of transoral laser surgery of supraglottic carcinoma compared with a transcervical approach', *Head & Neck* **26**:8, 653–9.

Cahill, L.M., Murdoch, B.E. and Theodoros, D.G. 2005. 'Articulatory function following traumatic brain injury in childhood: a perceptual and instrumental analysis', *Brain Injury* **19**:1, 41–58.

Calvó-Perxas, L., Garre-Olmo, J. and Vilalta-Franch, J. 2015. 'Prevalence and sociodemographic correlates of depressive and bipolar disorders in Catalonia (Spain) using DSM-5 criteria', *Journal of Affective Disorders* **184**, 97–103.

Campbell, T.F. 1999. 'Functional treatment outcomes in young children with motor speech disorders', in A.J. Caruso and E.A. Strand (eds.), *Clinical Management of Motor Speech Disorders in Children*, New York: Thieme Medical Publishers., 385–96.

Cantor Cutiva, L.C., Vogel, I. and Burdorf, A. 2013. 'Voice disorders in teachers and their associations with work-related factors: a systematic review', *Journal of Communication Disorders* **46**:2, 143–55.

Cardoso, F. 2014. 'Differential diagnosis of Huntington's disease: what the clinician should know', *Neurodegenerative Disease Management* **4**:1, 67–72.

Carew, L., Dacakis, G. and Oates, J. 2007. 'The effectiveness of oral resonance therapy on the perception of femininity of voice in male-to-female transsexuals', *Journal of Voice* **21**:5, 591–603.

Carlsson, E., Hartelius, L. and Saldert, C. 2014. 'Communicative strategies used by spouses of individuals with communication disorders related to stroke-induced aphasia and Parkinson's disease', *International Journal of Language & Communication Disorders* **49**:6, 722–35.

Carroll, T.L., Gartner-Schmidt, J., Statham, M.M. and Rosen, C.A. 2009. 'Vocal process granuloma and glottal insufficiency: an overlooked etiology?', *Laryngoscope* **120**:1, 114–20.

Carrow-Woolfolk, E. 1995. *Oral and Written Language Scales*, Circle Pines, MN: American Guidance Service.

Carta, M.G., Sorbello, O., Moro, M.F., Bhat, K.M., Demelia, E., Serra, A., Mura, G., Sancassiani, F., Piga, M. and Demelia, L. 2012. 'Bipolar disorders and Wilson's disease', *BMC Psychiatry* **12**:52.

Castles, A. and Coltheart, M. 1993. 'Varieties of developmental dyslexia', *Cognition* **47**:2, 149–80.

Cera, M.L., Ortiz, K.Z., Bertolucci, P.H. and Minett, T.S. 2013. 'Speech and orofacial apraxias in Alzheimer's disease', *International Psychogeriatrics* **25**:10, 1679–85.

Chanson, J.B., Kremer, S., Blanc, F., Marescaux, C., Namer, I.J. and de Seze, J. 2009. 'Foreign accent syndrome as a first sign of multiple sclerosis', *Multiple Sclerosis* **15**:9, 1123–5.

Chapman, S.B., Gamino, J.E., Cook, L.G., Hanten, G., Li, X. and Levin, H.S. 2006. 'Impaired discourse gist and working memory in children after brain injury', *Brain and Language* **97**:2, 178–88.

Chaturvedi, A.K., Engels, E.A., Anderson, W.F. and Gillison, M.L. 2008. 'Incidence trends for human papillomavirus-related and -unrelated oral squamous cell carcinomas in the United States', *Journal of Clinical Oncology* **26**:4, 612–19.

Chen, J.L., Messner, A.H. and Curtin, G. 2008. 'Newborn hearing screening in infants with cleft palates', *Otology & Neurotology* **29**:6, 812–15.

Cheng, A.K., Rubin, H.R., Powe, N.R., Mellon, N.K., Francis, H.W. and Niparko, J.K. 2000. 'Cost–utility analysis of the cochlear implant in children', *Journal of the American Medical Association* **284**:7, 850–6.

Chermak, G.D. and Musiek, F.E. 1997. *Central Auditory Processing Disorders: New Perspectives*, San Diego, CA: Singular.

Cheuk, D.K., Wong, V. and Leung, G.M. 2005. 'Multilingual home environment and specific language impairment: a case-control study in Chinese children', *Paediatric and Perinatal Epidemiology* **19**:4, 303–14.

Chevallier, C., Wilson, D., Happé, F. and Noveck, I. 2010. 'Scalar inferences in autism spectrum disorders', *Journal of Autism and Developmental Disorders* **40**:9, 1104–17.

Chiesi, A., Vella, S., Dally, L.G., Pedersen, C., Danner, S., Johnson, A.M., Schwander, S., Goebel, F.D., Glauser, M., Antunes, F. and Lundgren, J.D. for the AIDS in Europe Study Group 1996. 'Epidemiology of AIDS dementia complex in Europe', *Journal of Acquired Immune Deficiency Syndromes & Human Retrovirology* **11**:1, 39–44.

Choi, J.W., Kim, H.J., Park, H.S. and Kwon, T.G. 2013. 'Congenital macroglossia treated by 2-stage partial glossectomy', *Journal of Craniofacial Surgery* **24**:2, 554–6.

Christo, C. 2014. 'Developmental dyslexia', in L. Cummings (ed.), *Cambridge Handbook of Communication Disorders*, Cambridge: Cambridge University Press, 88–108.

Chung, Y., Behrmann, M., Bannan, B. and Thorp, E. 2012. 'Perspectives of high tech augmentative and alternative communication users with cerebral palsy at the post-secondary level', *SIG 12 Perspectives on Augmentative and Alternative Communication* **21**:2, 43–55.

Cleave, P.L., Girolametto, L.E., Chen, X. and Johnson, C.J. 2010. 'Narrative abilities in monolingual and dual language learning children with specific language impairment', *Journal of Communication Disorders* **43**:6, 511–22.

Cleland, J., Gibbon, F., Peppé, S., O'Hare, A. and Rutherford, M. 2010. 'Phonetic and phonological errors in children with high functioning autism and Asperger syndrome', *International Journal of Speech-Language Pathology* **12**:1, 69–76.

Cohan, S.L., Chavira, D.A., Shipon-Blum, E., Hitchcock, C., Roesch, S.C. and Stein, M.B. 2008. 'Refining the classification of children with selective mutism: a latent profile analysis', *Journal of Clinical Child and Adolescent Psychology* **37**:4, 770–84.

Cohen, M.S., Samango-Sprouse, C.A., Stern, H.J., Custer, D.A., Vaught, D.R., Saal, H.M., Tifft, C.J. and Rosenbaum, K.N. 1995. 'Neurodevelopmental profile of infants and toddlers with oculo-auriculo-vertebral spectrum and the correlation of prognosis with physical findings', *American Journal of Medical Genetics* **60**:6, 535–40.

Coltheart, M., Besner, D., Jonasson, J.T. and Davelaar, E. 1979. 'Phonological encoding in the lexical decision task', *Quarterly Journal of Experimental Psychology* **31**:3, 489–507.

Colton, R.H., Casper, J.K. and Leonard, R. 2006. *Understanding Voice Problems: A Physiological Perspective for Diagnosis and Treatment*, Baltimore, MD: Lippincott Williams & Wilkins.

Comi, A.M. 2007. 'Update on Sturge–Weber syndrome: diagnosis, treatment, quantitative measures, and controversies', *Lymphatic Research and Biology* **5**:4, 257–64.

2011. 'Presentation, diagnosis, pathophysiology, and treatment of the neurological features of Sturge–Weber syndrome', *Neurologist* **17**:4, 179–84.

Coninx, F., Weichbold, V. and Tsiakpini, L. 2003. *LittlEARS Auditory Questionnaire*, Innsbruck, Austria: MED-EL.

Connor, N.P. and Bless, D.M. 2014. 'Functional and organic voice disorders', in L. Cummings (ed.), *Cambridge Handbook of Communication Disorders*, Cambridge: Cambridge University Press, 321–40.

Conrad, A.L., McCoy, T.E., De Volder, I., Richman, L.C. and Nopoulos, P. 2014. 'Reading in subjects with an oral cleft: speech, hearing and neuropsychological skills', *Neuropsychology* **28**:3, 415–22.

Conti-Ramsden, C. Durkin, K., Simkin, Z. and Knox, E. 2009. 'Specific language impairment and school outcomes. I: identifying and explaining variability at the end of compulsory education', *International Journal of Language & Communication Disorders* **44**:1, 15–35.

Conti-Ramsden, G. and Durkin, K. 2012. 'Postschool educational and employment experiences of young people with specific language impairment', *Language, Speech, and Hearing Services in Schools* **43**:4, 507–20.

Conti-Ramsden, G. and Gunn, M. 1986. 'The development of conversational disability: a case study', *British Journal of Disorders of Communication* **21**:3, 339–51.

Conture, E.G. 1997. 'Evaluating childhood stuttering', in R.F. Curlee and G.M. Siegal (eds.), *Nature and Treatment of Stuttering: New Directions*, Boston: Allyn and Bacon, 239–56.

Cook, L.G., Chapman, S.B., Elliott, A.C., Evenson, N.N. and Vinton, K. 2014. 'Cognitive gains from gist reasoning training in adolescents with chronic-stage traumatic brain injury', *Frontiers in Neurology* **5**:87.

Coppens-Hofman, M.C., Terband, H.R., Maassen, B.A., van Schrojenstein Lantman-De Valk, H.M.J., van Zaalen-op't Hof, Y. and Snik, A.F.M. 2013. 'Dysfluencies in the speech of adults with intellectual disabilities and reported speech difficulties', *Journal of Communication Disorders* **46**:(5–6), 484–94.

Corrigan, J.D., Selassie, A.W. and Orman, J.A. 2010. 'The epidemiology of traumatic brain injury', *Journal of Head Trauma Rehabilitation* **25**:2, 72–80.

Cosyns, M., Van Borsel, J., Wierckx, K., Dedecker, D., Van de Peer, F., Daelman, T., Laenen, S. and T'Sjoen, G. 2014. 'Voice in female-to-male transsexual persons after long-term androgen therapy', *Laryngoscope* **124**:6, 1409–14.

Cruz, I., Vicaria, I., Wang, N.-Y., Niparko, J., Quittner, A.L. and CDaCI Investigative Team 2012. 'Language and behavioral outcomes in children with developmental disabilities using cochlear implants', *Otology & Neurotology* **33**:5, 751–60.

Crystal, D. 1997. *Profiling Linguistic Disability*, London: Whurr Publishers.

Cummings, J.L., Benson, D.F., Hill, M.A. and Read, S. 1985. 'Aphasia in dementia of the Alzheimer type', *Neurology* **35**:3, 394.

Cummings, L. 2009. *Clinical Pragmatics*, Cambridge: Cambridge University Press.

(ed.) 2014a. 'Pragmatic disorders and theory of mind', in L. Cummings (ed.), *Cambridge Handbook of Communication Disorders*, Cambridge: Cambridge University Press, 559–77.

2014b. *Pragmatic Disorders*, Dordrecht: Springer.

Da Silva, M.K., Ferrante, C., Van Borsel, J. and de Britto Pereira, M.M. 2012. 'Phonological acquisition of Brazilian Portuguese in children from Rio de Janeiro', *Jornal da Sociedade Brasileira de Fonoaudiologia* **24**:3, 248–54.

Dacakis, G. 2006. 'Assessment and goals', in R.K. Adler, S. Hirsch and M. Mordaunt (eds.), *Voice and Communication Therapy for the Transgender Client*, San Diego, CA: Plural Publishing, 101–26.

Dacakis, G., Oates, J. and Douglas, J. 2012. 'Beyond voice: perceptions of gender in male-to-female transsexuals', *Current Opinion in Otolaryngology & Head and Neck Surgery* **20**:3, 165–70.

Daly, D.A. and Burnett, M.L. 1996. 'Cluttering: assessment, treatment planning, and case study illustration', *Journal of Fluency Disorders* **21**:(3–4), 239–48.

Damico, J.S. 1985. 'Clinical discourse analysis: a functional approach to language assessment', in C.S. Simon (ed.), *Communication Skills and Classroom Success: Assessment of Language-Learning Disabled Students*, San Diego, CA: College Hill Press, 165–206.

Danesh-Sani, S.A., Rahimdoost, A., Soltani, M., Ghiyasi, M., Haghdoost, N. and Sabzali-Zanjankhah, S. 2013. 'Clinical assessment of orofacial manifestations in 500 patients with multiple sclerosis', *Journal of Oral and Maxillofacial Surgery* **71**:2, 290–4.

DaParma, A., Geffner, D. and Martin, N. 2011. 'Prevalence and nature of language impairment in children with attention deficit/hyperactivity disorder', *Contemporary Issues in Communication Science and Disorders* **38**:Fall 2011, 119–25.

Davis, B.L., Jacks, A. and Marquardt, T.P. 2005. 'Vowel patterns in developmental apraxia of speech: three longitudinal case studies', *Clinical Linguistics & Phonetics* **19**:4, 249–74.

Davis, G.A. and Wilcox, M.J. 1981. 'Incorporating parameters of natural conversation in aphasia treatment', in R. Chapey (ed.), *Language Intervention Strategies in Adult Aphasia*, Baltimore: Williams & Wilkins, 169–93.

    1985. *Adult Aphasia Rehabilitation: Applied Pragmatics*, San Diego, CA: College-Hill Press.

Davis, N.M., Doyle, L.W., Ford, G.W., Keir, E., Michael, J., Rickards, A.L., Kelly, E.A. and Callanan, C. 2001. 'Auditory function at 14 years of age of very-low-birth weight', *Developmental Medicine and Child Neurology* **43**:3, 191–6.

Dawes, P. and Bishop, D.V. 2010. 'Psychometric profile of children with auditory processing disorder and children with dyslexia', *Archives of Disease in Childhood* **95**:6, 432–6.

Dawes, P., Bishop, D.V., Sirimanna, T. and Bamiou, D.E. 2008. 'Profile and aetiology of children diagnosed with auditory processing disorder (APD)', *International Journal of Pediatric Otorhinolaryngology* **72**:4, 483–9.

Dawson, J., Stout, C. and Eyer, J. 2003. *Structured Photographic Expressive Language Test*, 3rd edn, DeKalb, IL: Janelle Publications.

Day, L.S. and Parnell, M.M. 1987. 'Ten-year study of a Wilson's disease dysarthric', *Journal of Communication Disorders* **20**:3, 207–18.

De Araújo Pernambuco, L., Espelt, A., Balata, P.M. and de Lima, K.C. 2015. 'Prevalence of voice disorders in the elderly: a systematic review of population-based studies', *European Archives of Oto-Rhino-Laryngology* **272**:10, 2601–9.

De Beer, J., Engels, J., Heerkens, Y. and van der Klink, J. 2014. 'Factors influencing work participation of adults with developmental dyslexia: a systematic review', *BMC Public Health* **14**:77.

De Cuypere, G., Van Hemelrijck, M., Michel, A., Carael, B., Heylens, G., Rubens, R., Hoebeke, P. and Monstrey, S. 2007. 'Prevalence and demography of transsexualism in Belgium', *European Psychiatry* **22**:3, 137–41.

De Renzi, E. and Vignolo, L.A. 1962. 'The token test: a sensitive test to detect receptive disturbances in aphasics', *Brain* **85**:4, 665–78.

De Smedt, B., Devriendt, K., Fryns, J.P., Vogels, A., Gewillig, M. and Swillen, A. 2007. 'Intellectual abilities in a large sample of children with velo-cardio-facial syndrome: an update', *Journal of Intellectual Disability Research* **51**:9, 666–70.

De Smet, H.J., Baillieux, H., Wackenier, P., De Praeter, M., Engelborghs, S., Paquier, P.F., De Deyn, P.P. and Mariën, P. 2009. 'Long-term cognitive deficits following posterior fossa tumour resection: a neuropsychological and functional neuroimaging follow-up study', *Neuropsychology* **23**:6, 694–704.

De Smet, H.J., Catsman-Berrevoets, C., Aarsen, F., Verhoeven, J., Mariën, P. and Paquier, P.F. 2012. 'Auditory-perceptual speech analysis in children with cerebellar tumours: a long-term follow-up study', *European Journal of Paediatric Neurology* **16**:5, 434–42.

Deelman, B.G., Koning-Haanstra, M., Liebrand, W.B.G. and Van Den Burg, W. 1981. *SAN Test. Een afasietest voor auditief taalbegrip en mondeling taalgebruik*, Lisse: Swets & Zeitlinger.

Dennis, M. and Kohn, B. 1975. 'Comprehension of syntax in infantile hemiplegics after cerebral hemidecortication: left hemisphere superiority', *Brain and Language* **2**, 472–82.

Dennis, M. and Whitaker, H.A. 1976. 'Language acquisition following hemidecortication: linguistic superiority of the left over the right hemisphere', *Brain and Language* **3**:3, 404–33.

Dennis, M., Lazenby, A.L. and Lockyer, L. 2001. 'Inferential language in high-function children with autism', *Journal of Autism and Developmental Disorders* **31**:1, 47–54.

DesJardin, J.L. and Eisenberg, L.S. 2007. 'Maternal contributions: supporting language development in young children with cochlear implants', *Ear and Hearing* **28**:4, 456–69.

Di Giacomo, D., De Federicis, L.S., Pistelli, M., Fiorenzi, D., Sodani, E., Carbone, G. and Passafiume, D. 2012. 'The loss of conceptual associations in mild Alzheimer's dementia', *Journal of Clinical and Experimental Neuropsychology* **34**:6, 643–53.

Dias, K.Z., Jutras, B., Acrani, I.O. and Pereira, L.D. 2012. 'Random Gap Detection Test (RGDT) performance of individuals with central auditory processing disorders from 5 to 25 years of age', *International Journal of Pediatric Otorhinolaryngology* **76**:2, 174–8.

Dijkstra, K., Bourgeois, M.S., Allen, R.S. and Burgio, L.D. 2004. 'Conversational coherence: discourse analysis of older adults with and without dementia', *Journal of Neurolinguistics* **17**:4, 263–83.

Dobbinson, S., Perkins, M.R. and Boucher, J. 1998. 'Structural patterns in conversations with a woman who has autism', *Journal of Communication Disorders* **31**:2, 113–34.

Docking, K.M., Murdoch, B.E. and Suppiah, R. 2007. 'The impact of a cerebellar tumour on language function in childhood', *Folia Phoniatrica et Logopaedica* **59**:4, 190–200.

Dodd, B., Crosbie, S., McIntosh, B., Teitzel, T. and Ozanne, A. 2000. *PIPA: Preschool and Primary Inventory of Phonological Awareness*, London: Psychological Corporation.

Dodd, B., Holm, A., Oerlemans, M. and McCormick, M. 1996. *QUIL: Queensland University Inventory of Literacy*, Brisbane: Department of Speech Pathology and Audiology, the University of Queensland.

Dodd, B., Hua, Z., Crosbie, S., Holm, A. and Ozanne, A. 2002. *Diagnostic Evaluation of Articulation and Phonology*, London: Psychological Corporation.

2006. *Diagnostic Evaluation of Articulation and Phonology*, Bloomington, MN: Pearson Assessment.

Dronkers, N.F., Ludy, C.A. and Redfern, B.B. 1998. 'Pragmatics in the absence of verbal language: descriptions of a severe aphasic and a language-deprived adult', *Journal of Neurolinguistics* **11**:(1–2), 179–90.

Duffy, J.R. 1995. *Motor Speech Disorders: Substrates, Differential Diagnosis and Management*, St. Louis, MO: Elsevier Mosby.

2005. *Motor Speech Disorders: Substrates, Differential Diagnosis and Management*, 2nd edn, St. Louis, MO: Elsevier Mosby.

Duffy, J.R., Strand, E.A., Clark, H., Machulda, M., Whitwell, J.L. and Josephs, K.A. 2015. 'Primary progressive apraxia of speech: clinical features and acoustic and neurologic correlates', *American Journal of Speech-Language Pathology* **24**:2, 88–100.

Dunn, L.M. 1959. *The Peabody Picture Vocabulary Test*, Circle Pines, MN: American Guidance Service.

1965. *Peabody Picture Vocabulary Test*, Circle Pines, MN: American Guidance Service.

Dunn, L.M. and Dunn, L.M. 1981. *The Peabody Picture Vocabulary Test*, rev., Circle Pines, MN: American Guidance Service.

1997. *Peabody Picture Vocabulary Test*, 3rd edn, Circle Pines, MN: American Guidance Service.

Durrleman, S., Hippolyte, L., Zufferey, S., Iglesias, K. and Hadjikhani, N. 2015. 'Complex syntax in autism spectrum disorders: a study of relative clauses', *International Journal of Language & Communication Disorders* **50**:2, 260–7.

Dworzynski, K., Remington, A., Rijsdijk, F., Howell, P. and Plomin, R. 2007. 'Genetic etiology in cases of recovered and persistent stuttering in an unselected, longitudinal sample of young twins', *American Journal of Speech-Language Pathology* **16**:2, 169–78.

Dziegielewski, P.T., Ho, M.L., Rieger, J., Singh, P., Langille, M., Harris, J.R. and Seikaly, H. 2013. 'Total glossectomy with laryngeal preservation and free flap reconstruction: objective functional outcomes and systematic review of the literature', *Laryngoscope* **123**:1, 140–5.

Eadie, P., Morgan, A., Ukoumunne, O.C., Ttofari, E.K., Wake, M. and Reilly, S. 2015. 'Speech sound disorder at 4 years: prevalence, comorbidities, and predictors in a community cohort of children', *Developmental Medicine and Child Neurology* **57**:6, 578–84.

Eastwood, P. 1981. The Sheffield computerised articulation test. Unpublished paper.

Ellis Weismer, S. 2014. 'Specific language impairment', in L. Cummings (ed.), *Cambridge Handbook of Communication Disorders*, Cambridge: Cambridge University Press, 73–87.

Emanuelson, I., von Wendt, L., Lundälv, E. and Larsson, J. 1996. 'Rehabilitation and follow-up of children with severe traumatic brain injury', *Child's Nervous System* **12**:8, 460–5.

Emerson, J. and Enderby, P. 1996. 'Prevalence of speech and language disorders in a mental illness unit', *European Journal of Disorders of Communication* **31**:3, 221–36.

Emery, V.O. 2000. 'Language impairment in dementia of the Alzheimer type: a hierarchical decline?', *International Journal of Psychiatry in Medicine* **30**:2, 145–64.

Enderby, P. 1983. *Frenchay Dysarthria Assessment*, California: College Hill Press.

Enderby, P. and Palmer, R. 2008. *Frenchay Dysarthria Assessment*, 2nd edn, Austin, TX: Pro-ed.

Engelter, S.T., Gostynski, M., Papa, S., Frei, M., Born, C., Ajdacic-Gross, V., Gutzwiller, F. and Lyrer, P.A. 2006. 'Epidemiology of aphasia attributable to first ischemic stroke: incidence, severity, fluency, etiology, and thrombolysis', *Stroke* **37**:6, 1379–84.

Erickson, S. and Block, S. 2013. 'The social and communication impact of stuttering on adolescents and their families', *Journal of Fluency Disorders* **38**:4, 311–24.

Evans, J.L. and MacWhinney, B. 1999. 'Sentence processing strategies in children with expressive and expressive-receptive specific language impairments', *International Journal of Language & Communication Disorders* **34**:2, 117–34.

Fang, Q.G., Shi, S., Zhang, X., Li, Z.N., Liu, F.Y. and Sun, C.F. 2013. 'Assessment of the quality of life of patients with oral cancer after pectoralis major myocutaneous flap reconstruction with a focus on speech', *Journal of Oral and Maxillofacial Surgery* **71**:11, 2004.e1–2004.e5.

Farinetti, A., Gharbia, D.B., Mancini, J., Roman, S., Nicollas, R. and Triglia, J.-M. 2014. 'Cochlear implant complications in 403 patients: comparative study of adults and children and review of the literature', *European Annals of Otorhinolaryngology, Head and Neck Diseases* **131**:3, 177–82.

Fenson, L., Dale, P.S., Reznick, J.S., Bates, E., Thal, D.J. and Pethick, S.J. 1994. 'Variability in early communicative development', *Monographs of the Society for Research in Child Development* **59**:5, 1–185.

Ferguson, M.A., Hall, R.L., Riley, A. and Moore, D.R. 2011. 'Communication, listening, cognitive and speech perception skills in children with auditory processing disorder (APD) or specific language impairment (SLI)', *Journal of Speech, Language, and Hearing Research* **54**:1, 211–27.

Ferreres, A., Abusamra, V., Cuitiño, M., Côté, H., Ska, B. and Joanette, Y. 2007. *Protocolo MEC. Protocolo para la Evaluación de la Communicación de Montréal*, Buenos Aires, Argentine: Neuropsi Ediciones.

Fey, M. 1986. *Language Intervention with Young Children*, San Diego, CA: College Hill Press.

Feyereisen, P., Berrewaerts, J. and Hupet, M. 2007. 'Pragmatic skills in the early stages of Alzheimer's disease: an analysis by means of a referential communication task', *International Journal of Language & Communication Disorders* **42**:1, 1–17.

First, M.B., Spitzer, R.L., Gibbon, M. and Williams, J.B.W. 1995. *Structured Clinical Interview for DSM-IV Axis 1 Disorders (SCID)*, Washington, DC: American Psychiatric Press.

Fisher, E.R. and Hayden, M.R. 2014. 'Multi source ascertainment of Huntington disease in Canada: prevalence and population at risk', *Movement Disorders* **29**:1, 105–14.

Fisher, J.P. and Glenister, J.M. 1992. *The Hundred Pictures Naming Test*, Melbourne: Australian Council for Educational Research.

Fletcher, M. and Birt, D. 1983. *Storylines: Picture Sequences for Language Practice*, London: Longman.

Flowers, H.L., Silver, F.L., Fang, J., Rochon, E. and Martino, R. 2013. 'The incidence, co-occurrence, and predictors of dysphagia, dysarthria, and aphasia after first-ever acute ischemic stroke', *Journal of Communication Disorders* **46**:3, 238–48.

Folio, M. and Fewell, R. 1983. *Peabody Developmental Motor Scales*, Texas: Pro-Ed.

Folstein, M.F., Folstein, S.E. and McHugh, P.R. 1975. '"Mini-mental state". A practical method for grading the cognitive state of patients for the clinician', *Journal of Psychiatric Research* **12**:3, 189–98.

Fonseca, R.P., Joanette, Y., Côté, H., Ska, B., Giroux, F., Fachel, J.M., Damasceno Ferreira, G. and Parente, M.A. 2008. 'Brazilian version of the Protocole Montréal d'Évaluation de la Communication (Protocole MEC): normative and reliability data', *Spanish Journal of Psychology* **11**:2, 678–88.

Fortes, F.S., Imamura, R., Tsuji, D.H. and Sennes, L.U. 2007. 'Profile of voice professionals seen in a tertiary health center', *Brazilian Journal of Otorhinolaryngology* **73**:1, 27–31.

Fotiadou, D., Northcott, S., Chatzidaki, A. and Hilari, K. 2014. 'Aphasia blog talk: how does stroke and aphasia affect a person's social relationships?', *Aphasiology*, **28**:11, 1281–300.

Fox, A.V. and Dodd, B. 2001. 'Phonologically disordered German-speaking children', *American Journal of Speech-Language Pathology* **10**:3, 291–307.

Frange, P., Alapetite, C., Gaboriaud, G., Bours, D., Zucker, J.M., Zerah, M., Brisse, H., Chevignard, M., Mosseri, V., Bouffet, E. and Doz, F. 2009. 'From childhood to adulthood: long-term outcome of medulloblastoma patients. The Institut Curie experience (1980–2000)', *Journal of Neuro-Oncology* **95**:2, 271–9.

Frankenburg, W.K., Dodds, J.B. and Fandal, A.W. 1968. *The Revised Denver Developmental Screening Test*, Denver, CO: LADOCA.

Frith, M., Togher, L., Ferguson, A., Levick, W. and Docking, K. 2014. 'Assessment practices of speech-language pathologists for cognitive communication disorders following traumatic brain injury in adults: an international survey', *Brain Injury* **28**:(13–14), 1657–66.

Gabel, R.M., Blood, G.W., Tellis, G.M. and Althouse, M.T. 2004. 'Measuring role entrapment of people who stutter', *Journal of Fluency Disorders* **29**:1, 27–49.

Gallena, S.K. 2007. *Voice and Laryngeal Disorders: A Problem-Based Clinical Guide with Voice Samples*, St. Louis, MO: Mosby Elsevier.

Galski, T., Tompkins, C. and Johnston, M.V. 1998. 'Competence in discourse as a measure of social integration and quality of life in persons with traumatic brain injury', *Brain Injury* **12**:9, 769–82.

Gangji, N., Pascoe, M. and Smouse, M. 2015. 'Swahili speech development: preliminary normative data from typically developing pre-school children in Tanzania', *International Journal of Language & Communication Disorders* **50**:2, 151–64.

Garcia, J.H., Ho, K.-L. and Pantoni, L. 1998. 'Pathology', in H.J.M. Barnett, J.P. Mohr, B.M. Stein and F.M. Yatsu (eds.), *Stroke: Pathophysiology, Diagnosis and Management*, 3rd edn, Philadelphia, PA: Churchill Livingstone, 139–57.

Garro, S.J. and Bradshaw, W.T. 2014. 'Sturge–Weber syndrome: a case study', *Advances in Neonatal Care* **14**:2, 96–102.

Gathercole, S. and Baddeley, A. 1996. *CNRep: The Children's Test of Nonword Repetition*, London: Psychological Corporation.

Geers, A.E. and Hayes, H. 2011. 'Reading, writing, and phonological processing skills of adolescents with 10 or more years of cochlear implant experience', *Ear and Hearing* **32**:(suppl. 1), S49–S59.

Gelfer, M.P. 1999. 'Voice treatment for the male-to-female transgendered client', *American Journal of Speech-Language Pathology* **8**:3, 201–8.

Gelfer, M.P. and Mikos, V.A. 2005. 'The relative contributions of speaking fundamental frequency and formant frequencies to gender identification based on isolated vowels', *Journal of Voice* **19**:4, 544–54.

Gerrard-Morris, A., Taylor, H.G., Yeates, K.O., Walz, N.C., Stancin, T., Minich, N. and Wade, S.L. 2010. 'Cognitive development after traumatic brain injury in young children', *Journal of the International Neuropsychological Society* **16**:1, 157–68.

Giacobini, M., Medin, E., Ahnemark, E., Russo, L.J. and Carlqvist, P. 2016. 'Prevalence, patient characteristics, and pharmacological treatment of children, adolescents, and adults diagnosed with ADHD in Sweden', *Journal of Attention Disorders* doi:10.1177/1087054714554617.

Giddan, J.J., Ross, G.J., Sechler, L.L. and Becker, B.R. 1997. 'Selective mutism in elementary school: multidisciplinary interventions', *Language, Speech, and Hearing Services in Schools* **28**:2, 127–33.

Giora, R., Zaidel, E., Soroker, N., Batori, G. and Kasher, A. 2000. 'Differential effects of right- and left-hemisphere damage on understanding sarcasm and metaphor', *Metaphor and Symbol* **15**:(1–2), 63–83.

Godefroy, O., Dubois, C., Debachy, B., Leclerc, M., Kreisler, A. for the Lille Stroke Program 2002. 'Main characteristics of patients hospitalized in acute stroke units', *Stroke* **33**:3, 702–5.

Goldman, R. and Fristoe, M. 1969. *Goldman–Fristoe Test of Articulation*, Circle Pines, MN: American Guidance Service.

    1986. *Goldman–Fristoe Test of Articulation*, Circle Pines, MN: American Guidance Service.

Goldman, R., Fristoe, M. and Woodcock, R.W. 1970. *Goldman–Fristoe–Woodcock Test of Auditory Discrimination*, Circle Pines, MN: American Guidance Service.

Goldstein, B., Fabiano, L. and Iglesias, A. 2004. 'Spontaneous and imitated productions in Spanish-speaking children with phonological disorders', *Language, Speech, and Hearing Services in Schools* **35**:1, 5–15.

Goldstein, B.A. 2007. 'Phonological skills in Puerto Rican and Mexican Spanish-speaking children with phonological disorders', *Clinical Linguistics & Phonetics* **21**:2, 93–109.

Gonçalves, M.I., Radzinsky, T.C., da Silva, N.S., Chiari, B.M. and Consonni, D. 2008. 'Speech-language and hearing complaints of children and adolescents with brain tumors', *Pediatric Blood & Cancer* **50**:3, 706–8.

Goodglass, H. and Kaplan, E. 1972a. *The Assessment of Aphasia and Related Disorders*, Philadelphia, PA: Lea & Febiger.

    1972b. *Boston Diagnostic Aphasia Examination*, Philadelphia, PA: Lea & Febiger.

    1983a. *The Assessment of Aphasia and Related Disorders*, 2nd edn, Philadelphia, PA: Lea & Febiger.

    1983b. *Boston Diagnostic Aphasia Examination*, 2nd edn, Philadelphia, PA: Lea & Febiger.

Goodglass, H., Gleason, J.B., Bernholtz, N.A. and Hyde, M.R. 1972. 'Some linguistic features in the speech of a Broca's aphasic', *Cortex* **8**:2, 191–212.

Goodglass, H., Kaplan, E. and Barresi, B. 2001. *Boston Diagnostic Aphasia Examination*, 3rd edn, Baltimore: Lippincott Williams & Wilkins.

Gorlin, R.J., Cohen, M.M. and Hennekam, R.C.M. 2001. *Syndromes of the Head and Neck*, 4th edn, New York: Oxford University Press.

Gorman, S., Weinrich, B., Lee, L. and Stemple, J.C. 2008. 'Aerodynamic changes as a result of vocal function exercises in elderly men', *Laryngoscope* **118**:10, 1900–3.

Graetz, P., De Bleser, R. and Willmes, K. 1992. *Akense afasie test*, Lisse: Swets & Zeitlinger.

Graham Jr, J.M., Clark, R.D., Moeschler, J.B. and Rogers, R.C. 2010. 'Behavioral features in young adults with FG syndrome (Opitz-Kaveggia syndrome)', *American Journal of Medical Genetics, Part C, Seminars in Medical Genetics* **154C**:4, 477–85.

Grant, B.F. and Weissman, M.M. 2007. 'Gender and the prevalence of psychiatric disorders', in W.E. Narrow, M.B. First, P.J. Sirovatka and D.A. Regier (eds.), *Age and Gender Considerations in Psychiatric Diagnosis: A Research Agenda for DSM-IV*, Arlington, VA: American Psychiatric Association, 31–46.

Grau, C., Johansen, L.V., Hansen, H.S., Andersen, E., Godballe, C., Andersen, L.J., Hald, J., Møller, H., Overgaard, M., Bastholt, L., Greisen, O., Harbo, G., Hansen, O. and Overgaard, J. 2003. 'Salvage laryngectomy and pharyngocutaneous fistulae after primary radiotherapy for head and neck cancer: a national survey from DAHANCA', *Head & Neck* **25**:9, 711–16.

Green Jr, J.D., Marion, M.S. and Hinojosa, R. 1991. 'Labyrinthitis ossificans: histopathologic consideration for cochlear implantation', *Otolaryngology – Head and Neck Surgery* **104**:3, 320–6.

Grigos, M.I. and Kolenda, N. 2010. 'The relationship between articulatory control and improved phonemic accuracy in childhood apraxia of speech: a longitudinal case study', *Clinical Linguistics & Phonetics* **24**:1, 17–40.

Grimm, H. 2001. *SETK 3–5. Sprachentwicklungtest für drei – bis fünfjährige Kinder. Diagnose von Sprachverarbeitungsfähigkeiten und auditiven Gedächtnisleistungen*, Göttingen, Germany: Hogrefe.

Grimm, H., Aktas, M. and Frevert, S. 2000. *Sprachentwicklungstest für zweijährige Kinder*, Göttingen, Germany: Hogrefe.

Grisel, J.J. and Samy, R.N. 2010. 'Cochlear implant', in M.L. Pensak (ed.), *Otolaryngology Cases*, New York: Thieme, 54–6.

Grunwell, P. 1985. *PACS Phonological Assessment of Child Speech*, London: NFER-Nelson.

Grunwell, P. and Huskins, S. 1979. 'Intelligibility in acquired dysarthria – a neuro-phonetic approach: three case studies', *Journal of Communication Disorders* **12**:1, 9–22.

Hall, P.K., Jordan, L.S. and Robin, D.A. 1993. *Developmental Apraxia of Speech: Theory and Clinical Practice*, Austin, TX: Pro-ed.

Hambly, H., Wren, Y., McLeod, S. and Roulstone, S. 2013. 'The influence of bilingualism on speech production: a systematic review', *International Journal of Language & Communication Disorders* **48**:1, 1–24.

Han, M.W., Ahn, J.H., Kang, J.K., Lee, E.M., Lee, J.H., Bae, J.H. and Chung, J.W. 2011. 'Central auditory processing impairment in patients with temporal lobe epilepsy', *Epilepsy & Behavior* **20**:2, 370–4.

Hancock, A. and Helenius, L. 2012. 'Adolescent male-to-female transgender voice and communication therapy', *Journal of Communication Disorders* **45**:5, 313–24.

Hancock, A.B. and Garabedian, L.M. 2013. 'Transgender voice and communication treatment: a retrospective chart review of 25 cases', *International Journal of Language & Communication Disorders* **48**:1, 54–65.

Hannus, S., Kauppila, T. and Launonen, K. 2009. 'Increasing prevalence of specific language impairment (SLI) in primary healthcare of a Finnish town, 1989–99', *International Journal of Language & Communication Disorders* **44**:1, 79–97.

Hanson, D.M., Jackson, A.W. and Hagerman, R.J. 1986. 'Speech disturbances (cluttering) in mildly impaired males with the Martin-Bell/ fragile X syndrome', *American Journal of Medical Genetics* **23**:(1–2), 195–206.

Hardin-Jones, M. and Chapman, K.L. 2014. 'Early lexical characteristics of toddlers with cleft lip and palate', *Cleft Palate-Craniofacial Journal* **51**:6, 622–31.

Hariri, M.A., Lakshmi, M.V., Larner, S. and Connolly, M.J. 1994. 'Auditory problems in elderly patients with stroke', *Age and Ageing* **23**:4, 312–16.

Harries, M.L.L., Walker, J.M., Williams, D.M., Hawkins, S. and Hughes, I.A. 1997. 'Changes in the male voice at puberty', *Archives of Disease in Childhood* **77**:5, 445–7.

Hartelius, L., Jonsson, M., Rickeberg, A. and Laakso, K. 2010. 'Communication and Huntington's disease: qualitative interviews and focus groups with persons with Huntington's disease, family members, and carers', *International Journal of Language & Communication Disorders* **45**:3, 381–93.

Hashimoto, R., Taguchi, T., Kano, M., Hanyu, S., Tanaka, Y., Nishizawa, M. and Nakano, I. 1999. 'A case report of dementia with cluttering-like speech disorder and apraxia of gait', *Rinsho Shinkeigaku* **39**:5, 520–6.

Hatta, T., Hasegawa, J. and Wanner, P.J. 2004. 'Differential processing of implicature in individuals with left and right brain damage', *Journal of Clinical and Experimental Neuropsychology* **26**:5, 667–76.

Hayden, D. and Square, P. 1999. *VMPAC: Verbal Motor Production Assessment for Children*, San Antonio, TX: Psychological Corporation.

Hebert, L.E., Beckett, L.A., Scherr, P.A. and Evans, D.A. 2001. 'Annual incidence of Alzheimer disease in the United States projected to the years 2000 through 2050', *Alzheimer Disease and Associated Disorders* **15**:4, 169–73.

Heck, J.E., Berthiller, J., Vaccarella, S., Winn, D.M., Smith, E.M., Shan'gina, O., Schwartz, S.M., Purdue, M.P., Pilarska, A., Eluf-Neto, J., Menezes, A., McClean, M.D., Matos, E., Koifman, S., Kelsey, K.T., Herrero, R., Hayes, R.B., Franceschi, S., Wünsch-Filho, V., Fernández, L., Daudt, A.W., Curado, M.P., Chen, C., Castellsaqué, X., Ferro, G., Brennan, P., Boffetta, P. and Hashibe, M. 2010. 'Sexual behaviours and the risk of head and neck cancers: a pooled analysis in the International Head and Neck Cancer Epidemiology (INHANCE) consortium', *International Journal of Epidemiology* **39**:1, 166–81.

Heemskerk, A.-W. and Roos, R.A.C. 2012. 'Aspiration pneumonia and death in Huntington's disease', *PloS Currents* **4**.

Hella, P., Niemi, J., Hintikka, J., Otsa, L., Tirkkonen, J.-M. and Koponen, H. 2013. 'Disordered semantic activation in disorganized discourse in schizophrenia: a new pragma-linguistic tool for structure and meaning reconstruction', *International Journal of Language & Communication Disorders* **48**:3, 320–8.

Helm-Estabrooks, N. 1999. 'Stuttering associated with acquired neurological disorders', in R.F. Curlee (ed.), *Stuttering and Related Disorders of Fluency*, New York: Thieme, 255–68.

Hennersdorf, F., Friese, N., Löwenheim, H., Tropitzsch, A., Ernemann, U. and Bisdas, S. 2014. 'Temporal bone changes in patients with Goldenhar syndrome with special emphasis on inner ear abnormalities', *Otology & Neurotology* **35**:5, 826–30.

Henry, J.D., Phillips, L.H., Crawford, J.R., Ietswaart, M. and Summers, F. 2006. 'Theory of mind following traumatic brain injury: the role of emotion recognition and executive dysfunction', *Neuropsychologia* **44**:10, 1623–8.

Hertrich, I. and Ackermann, H. 1994. 'Acoustic analysis of speech timing in Huntington's disease', *Brain and Language* **47**:2, 182–96.

Hinkka-Yli-Salomäki, S., Banerjee, P.N., Gissler, M., Lampi, K.M., Vanhala, R., Brown, A.S. and Sourander, A. 2014. 'The incidence of diagnosed autism spectrum disorders in Finland', *Nordic Journal of Psychiatry* **68**:7, 472–80.

Hirano, M. 1981. *Clinical Examination of Voice*, New York: Springer Verlag.

Hoang, D.H., Pagnier, A., Guichardet, K., Dubois-Teklali, F., Schiff, I., Lyard, G., Cousin, E. and Krainik, A. 2014. 'Cognitive disorders in pediatric medulloblastoma: what neuroimaging has to offer', *Journal of Neurosurgery Pediatrics* **14**:2, 136–44.

Hodge, M. 2014. 'Developmental dysarthria', in L. Cummings (ed.), *Cambridge Handbook of Communication Disorders*, Cambridge: Cambridge University Press, 26–48.

Hodson, B. 2004. *Hodson Assessment of Phonological Patterns*, 3rd edn, Austin, TX: Pro-Ed.
   2010. *Evaluating and Enhancing Children's Phonological Systems: Research and Theory to Practice*, Wichita, KS: Phonocomp Publishers.

Hoehn, M.M. and Yahr, M.D. 1967. 'Parkinsonism: onset, progression and mortality', *Neurology* **17**:5, 427–42.

Hoffmann, M. and Chen, R. 2013. 'The spectrum of aphasia subtypes and etiology in subacute stroke', *Journal of Stroke and Cerebrovascular Diseases* **22**:8, 1385–92.

Holden, L.K., Finley, C.C., Firszt, J.B., Holden, T.A., Brenner, C., Potts, L.G., Gotter, B.D., Vanderhoof, S.S., Mispagel, K., Heydebrand, G. and Skinner, M.W. 2013. 'Factors affecting open-set word recognition in adults with cochlear implants', *Ear and Hearing* **34**:3, 342–60.

Holm, A. and Crosbie, S. 2006. 'Introducing Jarrod: a child with a phonological impairment', *Advances in Speech-Language Pathology* **8**:3, 164–75.

Holtgraves, T. and McNamara, P. 2010. 'Pragmatic comprehension deficit in Parkinson's disease', *Journal of Clinical and Experimental Neuropsychology* **32**:4, 388–97.

Hopper, R.A., Cutting, C. and Grayson, B. 2007. 'Cleft lip and palate', in C.H. Thorne (ed.), *Grabb and Smith's Plastic Surgery*, 6th edn, Philadelphia, PA: Lippincott Williams & Wilkins, 201–25.

Hough, M.S. 1993. 'Treatment of Wernicke's aphasia with jargon: a case study', *Journal of Communication Disorders* **26**:2, 101–11.

Howard, S.J. 1993. 'Articulatory constraints on a phonological system: a case study of cleft palate speech', *Clinical Linguistics & Phonetics* **7**:4, 299–317.

Hua, Z. and Dodd, B. 2000. 'Putonghua (modern standard Chinese)-speaking children with speech disorder', *Clinical Linguistics & Phonetics* **14**:3, 165–91.

Huntington Study Group 1996. 'Unified Huntington's disease rating scale: reliability and consistency', *Movement Disorders* **11**:2, 136–42.

Hydén, L.-C. and Örulv, L. 2009. 'Narrative and identity in Alzheimer's disease: a case study', *Journal of Aging Studies* **23**:4, 205–14.

Iliadou, V., Bamiou, D.E., Kaprinis, S., Kandylis, D. and Kaprinis, G. 2009. 'Auditory processing disorders in children suspected of learning disabilities – a need for screening?', *International Journal of Pediatric Otorhinolaryngology* **73**:7, 1029–34.

Iliadou, V., Bamiou, D.E., Kaprinis, S., Kandylis, D., Vlaikidis, N., Apalla, K., Psifidis, A., Psillas, G. and St Kaprinis, G. 2008. 'Auditory processing disorder and brain pathology in a preterm child with learning disabilities', *Journal of the American Academy of Audiology* **19**:7, 557–63.

Im-Bolter, N., Johnson, J. and Pascual-Leone, J. 2006. 'Processing limitations in children with specific language impairment: the role of executive function', *Child Development* **77**:6, 1822–41.

International Dyslexia Association 2002. 'Definition of dyslexia'. Online. Available: http://eida .org/definition-of-dyslexia (accessed 8 February 2015).

Jacewicz, E., Fox, R.A. and Wei, L. 2010. 'Between-speaker and within-speaker variation in speech tempo of American English', *Journal of the Acoustical Society of America* **128**:2, 839–50.

Jacks, A., Marquardt, T.P. and Davis, B.L. 2006. 'Consonant and syllable structure patterns in childhood apraxia of speech: developmental change in three children', *Journal of Communication Disorders* **39**:6, 424–41.

Jankovic, J. 2008. 'Parkinson's disease: clinical features and diagnosis', *Journal of Neurology, Neurosurgery & Psychiatry* **79**:4, 368–76.

Jerônimo, G.M., Marrone, L.C. and Scherer, L.C. 2011. 'Narrative discourse comprehension in right hemisphere brain damage: a single case study', *Procedia Social and Behavioral Sciences* **23**, 203–4.

Joanette, Y., Ska, B. and Côté, H. 2004. *Protocole Montréal d'évaluation de la communication (MEC)*, Isbergues, France: Ortho-Edition.

Jodzio, K., Gąsecki, D., Drumm, D.A., Lass, P. and Nyka, W. 2003. 'Neuroanatomical correlates of the post-stroke aphasias studied with cerebral blood flow SPECT scanning', *Medical Science Monitor* **9**:3, MT32–MT41.

Jodzio, K., Łojek, E. and Bryan, K. 2005. 'Functional and neuroanatomical analysis of extralinguistic disorders in right hemisphere-damaged patients', *Psychology of Language and Communication* **9**:1, 55–73.

Johnston, K.N., John, A.B., Kreisman, N.V., Hall, J.W. and Crandell, C.C. 2009. 'Multiple benefits of personal FM system use by children with auditory processing disorder (APD)', *International Journal of Audiology* **48**:6, 371–83.

Jones, E.V. 1984. 'Word order processing in aphasia: effect of verb semantics', *Advances in Neurology* **42**, 159–81.

  1986. 'Building the foundations for sentence production in a non-fluent aphasic', *British Journal of Disorders of Communication* **21**:1, 63–82.

Jones, M.W., Catling, S., Evans, E., Green, D.H. and Green, J.R. 1992. 'Hoarseness after tracheal intubation', *Anaesthesia* **47**:3, 213–16.

Jucker, A.H. 1997. 'The discourse marker well in the history of English', *English Language and Linguistics* **1**:1, 91–110.

Judge, C., O'Donovan, C., Callaghan, G., Gaoatswe, G. and O'Shea, D. 2014. 'Gender dysphoria – prevalence and co-morbidities in an Irish adult population', *Frontiers in Endocrinology* **5**:87.

Juern, J. and Verhaalen, A. 2014. 'Gastrostomy-tube exchange', *New England Journal of Medicine* **370**:18, e28.

Kaipa, R., Robb, M.P., O'Beirne, G.A. and Allison, R.S. 2012. 'Recovery of speech following total glossectomy: an acoustic and perceptual appraisal', *International Journal of Speech-Language Pathology* **14**:1, 24–34.

Kanner, L. 1943. 'Autistic disturbances of affective contact', *Nervous Child* **2**, 217–50.

Kapila, M., Deore, N., Palav, R.S., Kazi, R.A., Shah, R.P. and Jagade, M.V. 2011. 'A brief review of voice restoration following total laryngectomy', *Indian Journal of Cancer* **48**:1, 99–104.

Kaplan, E., Goodglass, H. and Weintraub, S. 1983. *Boston Naming Test*, Philadelphia, PA: Lea & Febiger.

Kasher, A., Batori, G., Soroker, N., Graves, D. and Zaidel, E. 1999. 'Effects of right- and left-hemisphere damage on understanding conversational implicatures', *Brain and Language* **68**:3, 566–90.

Katz, W.F., Garst, D.M. and Levitt, J. 2008. 'The role of prosody in a case of foreign accent syndrome (FAS)', *Clinical Linguistics & Phonetics* **22**:7, 537–66.

Kay, J., Lesser, R. and Coltheart, M. 1992. *Psycholinguistic Assessments of language Processing in Aphasia*, PALPA, Hove: Lawrence Erlbaum.

Kay, S.R., Opler, L.A. and Lindenmayer, J.-P. 1988. 'Reliability and validity of the positive and negative syndrome scale for schizophrenics', *Psychiatry Research* **23**:1, 99–110.

Kazi, R., Prasad, V.M.N., Kanagalingam, J., Georgalas, C., Venkitaraman, R., Nutting, C.M., Clarke, P., Rhys-Evans, P. and Harrington, K.J. 2007. 'Analysis of formant frequencies in patients with oral or oropharyngeal cancers treated by glossectomy', *International Journal of Language & Communication Disorders* **42**:5, 521–32.

Keith, R.W. 2000. *Random Gap Detection Test*, San Antonio, TX: Auditec, St. Louis.

Keller, W.D., Tillery, K.L. and McFadden, S.L. 2006. 'Auditory processing disorder in children diagnosed with nonverbal learning disability', *American Journal of Audiology* **15**:2, 108–13.

Kempster, G., Gerratt, B., Verdolini-Abbott, K., Barkmeier-Kraemer, J. and Hillman, R. 2009. 'Consensus auditory-perceptual evaluation of voice: development of a standardized clinical protocol', *American Journal of Speech-Language Pathology* **18**:2, 124–32.

Kernahan, D.A. and Stark, R.B. 1958. 'A new classification for cleft lip and cleft palate', *Plastic and Reconstructive Surgery and the Transplantation Bulletin* **22**:5, 435–41.

Kertesz, A. 1982. *Western Aphasia Battery*, New York: Grune and Stratton.

Kiese-Himmel, C. 2005. *Aktiver Wortschatztest für 3-bis 5-jährige Kinder*, Göttingen, Germany: Hogrefe.

Kim, H.S., Lyoo, C.H., Lee, P.H., Kim, S.J., Park, M.Y., Ma, H.I., Lee, J.H., Song, S.K., Baik, J.S., Kim, J.H. and Lee, M.S. 2015. 'Current status of Huntington's disease in Korea: a nationwide survey and national registry analysis', *Journal of Movement Disorders* **8**:1, 14–20.

King, N., Nahm, E.A., Liberatos, P., Shi, Q. and Kim, A.H. 2014. 'A new comprehensive cochlear implant questionnaire for measuring quality of life after sequential bilateral cochlear implantation', *Otology & Neurotology* **35**:3, 407–13.

Kirk, S.A., McCarthy, J.J. and Kirk, W.D. 1968. *Illinois Test of Psycholinguistic Abilities*, Urbana, IL: University of Illinois Press.

Kishi, M., Sakakibara, R., Ogata, T. and Ogawa, E. 2010. 'Transient phonemic paraphasia by bilateral hippocampus lesion in a case of limbic encephalitis', *Neurology International* **2**:1, e8.

Klein, E.R., Armstrong, S.L. and Shipon-Blum, E. 2013. 'Assessing spoken language competence in children with selective mutism: using parents as test presenters', *Communication Disorders Quarterly* **34**:3, 184–95.

Klintö, K., Salameh, E.K. and Lohmander, A. 2015. 'Verbal competence in narrative retelling in 5-year-olds with unilateral cleft lip and palate', *International Journal of Language & Communication Disorders* **50**:1, 119–28.

Kluin, K.J., Foster, N.L., Berent, S. and Gilman, S. 1993. 'Perceptual analysis of speech disorders in progressive supranuclear palsy', *Neurology* **43**:3 (Pt 1), 563–6.

Knecht, S., Dröger, B., Deppe, M., Bobe, L., Lohmann, H., Flöel, A., Ringelstein, E.-B. and Henningsen, H. 2000. 'Handedness and hemispheric language dominance in healthy humans', *Brain* **123**:12, 2512–18.

Kollbrunner, J., Menet, A.-D. and Seifert, E. 2010. 'Psychogenic aphonia: no fixation even after a lengthy period of aphonia', *Swiss Medical Weekly* **140**:(1–2), 12–17.

Kozloff, N., Cheung, A.H., Schaffer, A., Cairney, J., Dewa, C.S., Veldhuizen, S., Kurdyak, P. and Levitt, A.J. 2010. 'Bipolar disorder among adolescents and young adults: results from an epidemiological sample', *Journal of Affective Disorders* **125**:(1–3), 350–4.

Krishnatreya, M., Nandy, P., Rahman, T., Sharma, J.D., Das, A., Kataki, A.C., Das, A.K. and Das, R. 2015. 'Characteristics of oral tongue and base of the tongue cancer: a hospital cancer registry based analysis', *Asian Pacific Journal of Cancer Prevention* **16**:4, 1371–4.

Krysanski, V.L. 2003. 'A brief review of selective mutism literature', *Journal of Psychology: Interdisciplinary and Applied* **137**:1, 29–40.

Kudo, M.F., Lussier, C.M. and Swanson, H.L. 2015. 'Reading disabilities in children: a selective meta-analysis of the cognitive literature', *Research in Developmental Disabilities* **40**, 51–62.

Kumin, L. 2006. 'Speech intelligibility and childhood verbal apraxia in children with Down syndrome', *Down's Syndrome, Research and Practice* **10**:1, 10–22.

Kummer, A.W. 2008. *Cleft Palate and Craniofacial Anomalies: The Effects on Speech and Resonance*, 2nd edn, New Albany, NY: Delmar Cengage Learning.

Kuo, C.L., Tsao, Y.H., Cheng, H.M., Lien, C.F., Hsu, C.H., Huang, C.Y. and Shiao, A.S. 2014. 'Grommets for otitis media with effusion in children with cleft palate: a systematic review', *Pediatrics* **134**:5, 983–94.

Kuschmann, A. and Lowit, A. 2012. 'Phonological and phonetic marking of information status in foreign accent syndrome', *International Journal of Language & Communication Disorders* **47**:6, 738–49.

2015. 'The role of speaking styles in assessing intonation in foreign accent syndrome', *International Journal of Speech-Language Pathology*, **17**:5, 489–99.

Kuyper, L. and Wijsen, C. 2014. 'Gender identities and gender dysphoria in the Netherlands', *Archives of Sexual Behavior* **43**:2, 377–85.

Lai, C.H. and Tseng, H.F. 2010. 'Population-based epidemiologic study of Wilson's disease in Taiwan', *European Journal of Neurology* **17**:6, 830–3.

Langereis, M. and Vermeulen, A. 2015. 'School performance and wellbeing of children with cochlear implants in different communicative-educational environments', *International Journal of Pediatric Otorhinolaryngology* **79**:6, 834–9.

Larson, K., Russ, S.A., Kahn, R.S. and Halfon, N. 2011. 'Patterns of comorbidity, functioning, and service use for US children with ADHD, 2007', *Pediatrics* **127**:3, 462–70.

Laska, A.C., Hellblom, A., Murray, V., Kahan, T. and Van Arbin, M. 2001. 'Aphasia in acute stroke and relation to outcome', *Journal of Internal Medicine* **249**:5, 413–22.

Laskaris, S., Sengas, I., Maragoudakis, P., Tsimplaki, E., Argyri, E., Manolopoulos, L. and Panotopoulou, E. 2014. 'Prevalence of human papillomavirus infection in Greek patients with squamous cell carcinoma of the larynx', *Anticancer Research*, **34**:10, 5749–53.

Laws, G., Briscoe, J., Ang, S.Y., Brown, H., Hermena, E. and Kapikian, A. 2015. 'Receptive vocabulary and semantic knowledge in children with specific language impairment and children with Down syndrome', *Child Neuropsychology* **21**:4, 490–508.

Leão, S.H., Oates, J.M., Purdy, S.C., Scott, D. and Morton, R.P. 2015. 'Voice problems in New Zealand teachers: a national survey', *Journal of Voice* **29**:5, 645.e1–645.e13.

Lebrun, Y. 1996. 'Cluttering after brain damage', *Journal of Fluency Disorders* **21**:(3–4), 289–95.

Leder, S.B. 1996. 'Adult onset of stuttering as a presenting sign in a Parkinsonian-like syndrome: a case report', *Journal of Communication Disorders* **29**:6, 471–8.

Lehman Blake, M.T. 2006. 'Clinical relevance of discourse characteristics after right hemisphere brain damage', *American Journal of Speech-Language Pathology* **15**:3, 255–67.

Leong, S.C.L., Pinder, E., Sasae, R. and Mortimore, R. 2007. 'Mucoepidermoid carcinoma of the tongue', *Singapore Medical Journal* **48**:10, e272–e274.

Levisohn, L., Cronin-Golomb, A. and Schmahmann, J.D. 2000. 'Neuropsychological consequences of cerebellar tumour resection in children: cerebellar cognitive affective syndrome in a paediatric population', *Brain* **123**:5, 1041–50.

Lewis, B.A., Freebairn, L.A., Hansen, A.J., Iyengar, S.K. and Taylor, H.G. 2004. 'School-age follow-up of children with childhood apraxia of speech', *Language, Speech and Hearing Services in Schools* **35**:2, 122–40.

Lewis, B.A., Short, E.J., Iyengar, S.K., Taylor, H.G., Freebairn, L., Tag, J., Avrich, A.A. and Stein, C.M. 2012. 'Speech-sound disorders and attention-deficit/hyperactivity disorder symptoms', *Topics in Language Disorders* **32**:3, 247–63.

Lewis, B.A., Shriberg, L.D., Freebairn, L.A., Hansen, A.J., Stein, C.M., Taylor, H.G. and Iyengar, S.K. 2006. 'The genetic bases of speech sound disorders: evidence from spoken and written language', *Journal of Speech, Language, and Hearing Research* **49**:6, 1294–1312.

Lewis, F.D. and Horn, G.J. 2013. 'Traumatic brain injury: analysis of functional deficits and posthospital rehabilitation outcomes', *Journal of Special Operations Medicine* **13**:3, 56–61.

Lewis, F.M., Woodyatt, G.C. and Murdoch, B.E. 2008. 'Linguistic and pragmatic language skills in adults with autism spectrum disorder: a pilot study', *Research in Autism Spectrum Disorders* **2**:1, 176–87.

Lewis, J.S., Carpenter, D.H., Thorstad, W.L., Zhang, Q. and Haughey, B.H. 2011. 'Extracapsular extension is a poor predictor of disease recurrence in surgically treated oropharyngeal squamous cell carcinoma', *Modern Pathology* **24**:11, 1413–20.

Leyhe, T., Saur, R., Eschweiler, G.W. and Milian, M. 2011. 'Impairment in proverb interpretation as an executive function deficit in patients with amnestic mild cognitive impairment and early Alzheimer's disease', *Dementia and Geriatric Cognitive Disorders Extra* **1**:1, 51–61.

Lichtenstein, P., Carlström, E., Råstam, M., Gillberg, C. and Anckarsäter, H. 2010. 'The genetics of autism spectrum disorders and related neuropsychiatric disorders in childhood', *American Journal of Psychiatry* **167**:11, 1357–63.

Lippert-Gruener, M., Weinert, U., Greisbach, T. and Wedekind, C. 2005. 'Foreign accent syndrome following traumatic brain injury', *Brain Injury* **19**:11, 955–8.

Little, B.B. 2006. *Drugs and pregnancy: a handbook*, Boca Raton, FL: CRC Press.

Litwin, T., Gromadzka, G. and Członkowska, A. 2012. 'Gender differences in Wilson's disease', *Journal of the Neurological Sciences* **312**:(1–2), 31–5.

Lloyd, O., Ownsworth, T., Fleming, J. and Zimmer-Gembeck, M.J. 2015. 'Awareness deficits in children and adolescents after traumatic brain injury: a systematic review', *Journal of Head Trauma Rehabilitation* **30**:5, 311–23.

Locke, J. 1980. 'The inference of speech perception in the phonologically disordered child. Part II: some clinically novel procedures, their use, some findings', *Journal of Speech and Hearing Disorders* **45**:4, 445–68.

Lomas, J., Pickard, L., Bester, S., Elbard, H., Finlayson, A. and Zoghaib, C. 1989. 'The communicative effectiveness index: development and psychometric evaluation of a functional communication measure for adult aphasia', *Journal of Speech and Hearing Disorders* **54**:1, 113–24.

Lopez, E., Callier, P., Cormier-Daire, V., Lacombe, D., Moncla, A., Bottani, A., Lambert, S., Goldenberg, A., Doray, B., Odent, S., Sanlaville, D., Gueneau, L., Duplomb, L., Huet, F., Aral, B., Thauvin-Robinet, C. and Faivre, L. 2012. 'Search for a gene responsible for

Floating-Harbor syndrome on chromosome 12q15q21.1', *American Journal of Medical Genetics, Part A* **158A**:2, 333–9.

Lorincz, M.T. 2010. 'Neurologic Wilson's disease', *Annals of the New York Academy of Sciences* **1184**, 173–87.

Lott, P.R., Guggenbühl, S., Schneeberger, A., Pulver, A.E. and Stassen, H.H. 2002. 'Linguistic analysis of the speech output of schizophrenic, bipolar, and depressive patients', *Psychopathology* **35**:4, 220–7.

Lousada, M., Mendes, A.P., Valente, A.R. and Hall, A. 2012. 'Standardization of a phonetic–phonological test for European-Portuguese children', *Folia Phoniatrica et Logopaedica* **64**:3, 151–6.

Lovett, M.W., Dennis, M. and Newman, J.E. 1986. 'Making reference: the cohesive use of pronouns in the narrative discourse of hemidecorticate adolescents', *Brain and Language* **29**:2, 224–51.

Lowit, A. 2014. 'Acquired motor speech disorders', in L. Cummings (ed.), *Cambridge Handbook of Communication Disorders*, Cambridge: Cambridge University Press, 400–18.

Luna-Ortiz, K., Carmona-Luna, T., Cano-Valdez, A.M., Mosqueda-Taylor, A., Herrera-Gómez, A. and Villavicencio-Valencia, V. 2009. 'Adenoid cystic carcinoma of the tongue – a clinicopathological study and survival analysis', *Head & Neck Oncology* **1**:15.

Lyons, M.J., Graham Jr, J.M., Neri, G., Hunter, A.G., Clark, R.D., Rogers, R.C., Moscarda, M., Boccuto, L., Simensen, R., Dodd, J., Robertson, S., DuPont, B.R., Friez, M.J., Schwartz, C.E. and Stevenson, R.E. 2009. 'Clinical experience in the evaluation of 30 patients with a prior diagnosis of FG syndrome', *Journal of Medical Genetics* **46**:1, 9–13.

Ma, X., McPherson, B. and Ma, L. 2016. 'Behavioural signs of (central) auditory processing disorder in children with nonsyndromic cleft lip and/or palate: a parental questionnaire approach', *Cleft Palate-Craniofacial Journal* **53**:2, 147–56.

McAllister, J., Collier, J. and Shepstone, L. 2013. 'The impact of adolescent stuttering and other speech problems on psychological well-being in adulthood: evidence from a birth cohort study', *International Journal of Language & Communication Disorders* **48**:4, 458–68.

McCabe, P.J., Sheard, C. and Code, C. 2008. 'Communication impairment in the AIDS dementia complex (ADC): a case report', *Journal of Communication Disorders* **41**:3, 203–22.

McCardle, P. and Wilson, B. 1993. 'Language and development in FG syndrome with callosal agenesis', *Journal of Communication Disorders* **26**:2, 83–100.

McCarthy, D. 1972. *Scales of Children's Abilities*, San Antonio, TX: Psychological Corporation.

McClure, E.B., Treland, J.E., Snow, J., Schmajuk, M., Dickstein, D.P., Towbin, K.E., Charney, D.S., Pine, D.S. and Leibenluft, E. 2005. 'Deficits in social cognition and response flexibility in pediatric bipolar disorder', *American Journal of Psychiatry* **162**:9, 1644–51.

McDonald, S. 2000. 'Exploring the cognitive basis of right-hemisphere pragmatic language disorders', *Brain and Language* **75**:1, 82–107.

McElroy, S.L. 2004. 'Diagnosing and treating comorbid (complicated) bipolar disorder', *Journal of Clinical Psychiatry* **65**:(suppl. 15), 35–44.

McGinty, A.S., Justice, L.M., Zucker, T.A., Gosse, C. and Skibbe, L.E. 2012. 'Shared-reading dynamics: mothers' question use and the verbal participation of children with specific language impairment', *Journal of Speech, Language, and Hearing Research* **55**:4, 1039–52.

McGrath, L.M., Hutaff-Lee, C., Scott, A., Boada, R., Shriberg, L.D. and Pennington, B.F. 2008. 'Children with comorbid speech sound disorder and specific language impairment are at an increased risk for attention-deficit/hyperactivity disorder', *Journal of Abnormal Child Psychology* **36**:2, 151–63.

McGregor, K.K., Newman, R.M., Reilly, R.M. and Capone, N.C. 2002. 'Semantic representation and naming in children with specific language impairment', *Journal of Speech, Language, and Hearing Research* **45**:5, 998–1014.

Machado, A., Chien, H.F., Deguti, M.M., Cançado, E., Azevedo, R.S., Scaff, M. and Barbosa, E.R. 2006. 'Neurological manifestations in Wilson's disease: report of 119 cases', *Movement Disorders* **21**:12, 2192–6.

McInnes, A., Fung, D., Manassis, K., Fiksenbaum, L. and Tannock, R. 2004. 'Narrative skills in children with selective mutism: an exploratory study', *American Journal of Speech-Language Pathology* **13**:4, 304–15.

MacKay, G. and Shaw, A. 2004. 'A comparative study of figurative language in children with autistic spectrum disorders', *Child Language Teaching and Therapy* **20**:1, 13–32.

McKenna, P. and Warrington, E.K. 1983. *Graded Naming Test*, Windsor: NFER-Nelson.

Mackenzie, I.R.A. 2001. 'The pathology of Parkinson's disease', *BC Medical Journal* **43**:3, 142–7.

McKinnon, D.H., McLeod, S. and Reilly, S. 2007. 'The prevalence of stuttering, voice, and speech-sound disorders in primary school students in Australia', *Language, Speech and Hearing Services in Schools* **38**:1, 5–15.

McLeod, S. and Baker, E. 2014. 'Speech-language pathologists' practices regarding assessment, analysis, target selection, intervention, and service delivery for children with speech sound disorders', *Clinical Linguistics & Phonetics* **28**:(7–8), 508–31.

McLeod, S., Harrison, L.J., McAllister, L. and McCormack, J. 2013. 'Speech sound disorders in a community study of preschool children', *American Journal of Speech-Language Pathology* **22**:3, 503–22.

MacNeil, S.D., Liu, K., Shariff, S.Z., Thind, A., Winquist, E., Yoo, J., Nichols, A., Fung, K., Hall, S. and Garg, A.X. 2015. 'Secular trends in the survival of patients with laryngeal carcinoma, 1995–2007', *Current Oncology* **22**:2, e85–e99.

McNeil, M.R., Robin, D.A. and Schmidt, R.A. 2009. 'Apraxia of speech', in M.R. McNeil (ed.), *Clinical Management of Sensorimotor Speech Disorders*, New York: Thieme Publishers, 249–68.

Maddrey, A.M., Bergeron, J.A., Lombardo, E.R., McDonald, N.K., Mulne, A.F., Barenberg, P.D. and Bowers, D.C. 2005. 'Neuropsychological performance and quality of life of 10 year survivors of childhood medulloblastoma', *Journal of Neuro-Oncology* **72**:3, 245–53.

Madeline, A. and Wheldall, K. 2002. 'Further progress towards a standardised curriculum-based measure of reading: calibrating a new passage reading test against the New South Wales Basic Skills Test', *Educational Psychology* **22**:4, 461–71.

Majorano, M. and Lavelli, M. 2015. 'The use of sophisticated words with children with specific language impairment during shared book reading', *Journal of Communication Disorders* **53**, 1–16.

Maki, Y., Yamaguchi, T., Koeda, T. and Yamaguchi, H. 2013. 'Communicative competence in Alzheimer's disease: metaphor and sarcasm comprehension', *American Journal of Alzheimer's Disease and Other Dementias* **28**:1, 69–74.

Manassis, K., Tannock, R., Garland, E.J., Minde, K., McInnes, A. and Clark, S. 2007. 'The sounds of silence: language, cognition, and anxiety in selective mutism', *Journal of the American Academy of Child and Adolescent Psychiatry* **46**:9, 1187–95.

Manning, J.S. 1999. 'Valproate in bipolar disorder: case examples from a family practice', *Primary Care Companion to the Journal of Clinical Psychiatry* **1**:3, 71–3.

Marchant, J., McAuliffe, M.J. and Huckabee, M.-L. 2008. 'Treatment of articulatory impairment in a child with spastic dysarthria associated with cerebral palsy', *Developmental Neurorehabilitation* **11**:1, 81–90.

Margari, L., Buttiglione, M., Craig, F., Cristella, A., de Giambattista, C., Matera, E., Operto, F. and Simone, M. 2013. 'Neuropsychological comorbidities in learning disorders', *BMC Neurology* **13**:198.

Margulis, A.V., Mitchell, A.A., Gilboa, S.M., Werler, M.M., Mittleman, M.A., Glynn, R.J., Hernandez-Diaz, S. and the National Birth Defects Prevention Study 2012. 'Use of topiramate in pregnancy and risk of oral clefts', *Journal of Obstetrics and Gynecology* **207**:5, 405.e1–405.e7.

Mariën, P., Verhoeven, J., Wackenier, P., Engelborghs, S. and De Deyn, P.P. 2009. 'Foreign accent syndrome as a developmental motor speech disorder', *Cortex* **45**:7, 870–8.

Marignier, S., Lesca, G., Marguin, J., Bussy, G., Sanlaville, D. and des Portes, V. 2012. 'Childhood apraxia of speech without intellectual deficit in a patient with cri du chat syndrome', *European Journal of Medical Genetics* **55**:(6–7), 433–6.

Marini, A. 2012. 'Characteristics of narrative discourse processing after damage to the right hemisphere', *Seminars in Speech and Language* **33**:1, 68–78.

Marini, A., Carlomagno, S., Caltagirone, C. and Nocentini, U. 2005. 'The role played by the right hemisphere in the organization of complex textual structures', *Brain and Language* **93**:1, 46–54.

Mariotti, P., Iuvone, L., Torrioli, M.G. and Silveri, M.C. 1998. 'Linguistic and non-linguistic abilities in a patient with early left hemispherectomy', *Neuropsychologia* **36**:12, 1303–12.

Martin, I. and McDonald, S. 2003. 'Weak coherence, no theory of mind, or executive dysfunction? Solving the puzzle of pragmatic language disorders', *Brain and Language* **85**:3, 451–66.

Martins, R.H.G., Tavares, E.L.M., Ranalli, P.F., Branco, A. and Pessin, A.B.B. 2014. 'Psychogenic dysphonia: diversity of clinical and vocal manifestations in a case series', *Brazilian Journal of Otorhinolaryngology* **80**:6, 497–502.

Martinussen, R. and Mackenzie, G. 2015. 'Reading comprehension in adolescents with ADHD: exploring the poor comprehender profile and individual differences in vocabulary and executive functions', *Research in Developmental Disabilities* **38**, 329–37.

Maruthy, S. and Mannarukrishnaiah, J. 2008. 'Effect of early onset otitis media on brainstem and cortical auditory processing', *Behavioral and Brain Functions* **4**:17.

Matsumoto, N. and Niikawa, N. 2003. 'Kabuki make-up syndrome: a review', *American Journal of Medical Genetics, Part C, Seminars in Medical Genetics* **117C**:1, 57–65.

Matthews, J.L., Oddone-Paolucci, E. and Harrop, R.A. 2015. 'The epidemiology of cleft lip and palate in Canada, 1998 to 2007', *Cleft Palate-Craniofacial Journal* **52**:4, 417–24.

Matthews, S., Williams, R. and Pring, T. 1997. 'Parent–child interaction therapy and dysfluency: a single-case study', *European Journal of Disorders of Communication* **32**:3, 346–57.

Mattingly, E.O. 2015. 'Dysfluency in a service member with comorbid diagnoses: a case study', *Military Medicine* **180**:1, e157–e159.

Max, J.E. 2014. 'Neuropsychiatry of pediatric traumatic brain injury', *Psychiatric Clinics of North America* **37**:1, 125–40.

Mayer, M. 1974. *Frog Goes to Dinner*, New York: Dial Press.

May-Mederake, B. and Shehata-Dieler, W. 2013. 'A case study assessing the auditory and speech development of four children implanted with cochlear implants by the chronological age of 12 months', *Case Reports in Otolaryngology* **359218**.

Mei, C. and Morgan, A.T. 2011. 'Incidence of mutism, dysarthria and dysphagia associated with childhood posterior fossa tumour', *Child's Nervous System* **27**:7, 1129–36.

Memari, A., Ziaee, V., Mirfazeli, F. and Kordi, R. 2012. 'Investigation of autism comorbidities and associations in a school-based community sample', *Journal of Child and Adolescent Psychiatric Nursing* **25**:2, 84–90.

Mendlowitz, S.L. and Monga, S. 2007. 'Unlocking speech where there is none: practical approaches to treatment of selective mutism', *Behavior Therapist* **30**:1, 11–15.

Mentis, M. and Prutting, C.A. 1991. 'Analysis of topic as illustrated in a head-injured and a normal adult', *Journal of Speech and Hearing Research* **34**:3, 583–95.

Mentis, M., Briggs-Whittaker, J. and Gramigna, D. 1995. 'Discourse topic management in senile dementia of the Alzheimer's type', *Journal of Speech, Language, and Hearing Research* **38**:5, 1054–66.

Merrill, R.M., Anderson, A.E. and Sloan, A. 2011. 'Quality of life indicators according to voice disorders and voice-related conditions', *Laryngoscope* **121**:9, 2004–10.

Mihaylova, V., Todorov, T., Jelev, H., Kotsev, I., Angelova, L., Kosseva, O., Georgiev, G., Ganeva, R., Cherninkova, S., Tankova, L., Savov, A. and Tournev, I. 2012. 'Neurological symptoms, genotype-phenotype correlations and ethnic-specific differences in Bulgarian patients with Wilson disease', *The Neurologist* **18**:4, 184–9.

Miller, N. 2000. 'Changing ideas in apraxia of speech', in I. Papathanasiou (ed.), *Acquired Neurogenic Communication Disorders: A Clinical Perspective*, London: Whurr, 173–202.

Miller, N., Lowitt, A. and O'Sullivan, H. 2006. 'What makes acquired foreign accent syndrome foreign?', *Journal of Neurolinguistics* **19**:5, 385–409.

Mohr, P.E., Feldman, J.J., Dunbar, J.L., McConkey-Robbins, A., Niparko, J.K., Rittenhouse, R.K. and Skinner, M.W. 2000. 'The societal costs of severe to profound hearing loss in the United States', *International Journal of Technology Assessment in Health Care* **16**:4, 1120–35.

Møller, L.B., Horn, N., Jeppesen, T.D., Vissing, J., Wibrand, F., Jennum, P. and Ott, P. 2011. 'Clinical presentation and mutations in Danish patients with Wilson disease', *European Journal of Human Genetics* **19**:9, 935–41.

Monetta, L. and Pell, M.D. 2007. 'Effects of verbal working memory deficits on metaphor comprehension in patients with Parkinson's disease', *Brain and Language* **101**:1, 80–9.

Monetta, L., Grindrod, C.M. and Pell, M.D. 2009. 'Irony comprehension and theory of mind deficits in patients with Parkinson's disease', *Cortex* **45**:8, 972–81.

Moore, M.E. 2001. 'Third person pronoun errors by children with and without language impairment', *Journal of Communication Disorders* **34**:3, 207–28.

Moore, S.R., Johnson, N.W., Pierce, A.M. and Wilson, D.F. 2000. 'The epidemiology of tongue cancer: a review of global incidence', *Oral Diseases* **6**:2, 75–84.

Moores, A., Fox, S., Lang, A. and Hirschfield, G.M. 2012. 'Wilson disease: Canadian perspectives on presentation and outcomes from an adult ambulatory setting', *Canadian Journal of Gastroenterology* **26**:6, 333–9.

Morgan, A.T., Mageandran, S-D. and Mei, C. 2010. 'Incidence and clinical presentation of dysarthria and dysphagia in the acute setting following paediatric traumatic brain injury', *Child: Care, Health and Development* **36**:1, 44–53.

Moriarty, B.C. and Gillon, G.T. 2006. 'Phonological awareness intervention for children with childhood apraxia of speech', *International Journal of Language & Communication Disorders* **41**:6, 713–34.

Morris, H. and Ozanne, A. 2003. 'Phonetic, phonological, and language skills of children with a cleft palate', *Cleft Palate-Craniofacial Journal* **40**:5, 460–70.

Morrish, E.C.E. 1988. 'Compensatory articulation in a subject with total glossectomy', *British Journal of Disorders of Communication* **23**:1, 13–22.

Mortensen, P.B., Pedersen, C.B., Melbye, M., Mors, O. and Ewald, H. 2003. 'Individual and familial risk factors for bipolar affective disorders in Denmark', *Archives of General Psychiatry* **60**:12, 1209–15.

Mower, D.E. and Younts, J. 2001. 'Sudden onset of excessive repetitions in the speech of a patient with multiple sclerosis: a case report', *Journal of Fluency Disorders* **26**:4, 269–309.

Mumby, K., Bowen, A. and Hesketh, A. 2007. 'Apraxia of speech: how reliable are speech and language therapists' diagnoses?', *Clinical Rehabilitation* **21**:8, 760–7.

Muniz, C.N.R., Lopes, D.M.B. and Schochat, E. 2015. 'Mismatch negativity in children with specific language impairment and auditory processing disorder', *Brazilian Journal of Otorhinolaryngology* **81**:4, 408–15.

Munk-Olsen, T., Laursen, T.M., Meltzer-Brody, S., Mortensen, P.B. and Jones, I. 2012. 'Psychiatric disorders with postpartum onset: possible early manifestations of bipolar affective disorders', *Archives of General Psychiatry* **69**:4, 428–34.

Murakami, N., Morioka, T., Suzuki, S.O., Hashiguchi, K., Amano, T., Sakata, A., Iwaki, T. and Sasaki, T. 2012. 'Focal cortical dysplasia type IIa underlying epileptogenesis in patients with epilepsy associated with Sturge–Weber syndrome', *Epilepsia* **53**:11, e184–e188.

Murdoch, B.E. 2010. *Acquired Speech and Language Disorders: A Neuroanatomical and Functional Neurological Approach*, 2nd edn, West Sussex: Wiley-Blackwell.

Murdoch, B.E. and Chenery, H.J. 1990. 'Latent aphasia and flaccid dysarthria associated with subcortical and brainstem calcification 20 years post-radiotherapy', *Journal of Neurolinguistics* **5**:1, 55–73.

Murdoch, B.E., Chenery, H.J., Wilks, V. and Boyle, R.S. 1987. 'Language disorders in dementia of the Alzheimer type', *Brain and Language* **31**:1, 122–37.

Murray, L.L. and Lenz, L.P. 2001. 'Productive syntax abilities in Huntington's and Parkinson's diseases', *Brain and Cognition* **46**:(1–2), 213–19.

Murri, A., Cuda, D., Guerzoni, L. and Fabrizi, E. 2015. 'Narrative abilities in early implanted children', *Laryngoscope* **125**:7, 1685–90.

Musiek, F.E. 1983. 'Assessment of central auditory dysfunction: the dichotic digit test revisited', *Ear and Hearing* **4**:2, 79–83.

1994. 'Frequency (pitch) and duration pattern tests', *Journal of American Academy of Audiology* **5**:4, 265–8.

Myers, P.S. 1979. 'Profiles of communication deficits in patients with right cerebral hemisphere damage: implications for diagnosis and treatment', *Clinical Aphasiology Conference*, Phoenix, AZ: BRK Publishers, 38–46.

Myers, R.H. 2004. 'Huntington's disease genetics', *NeuroRx* **1**:2, 255–62.

Nabbout, R. and Juhász, C. 2013. 'Sturge–Weber syndrome', *Handbook of Clinical Neurology* **111**, 315–21.

Naigles, L.R., Kelty, E., Jaffery, R. and Fein, D. 2011. 'Abstractness and continuity in the syntactic development of young children with autism', *Autism Research* **4**:6, 422–37.

National Cancer Institute 2015. *SEER statistics on cancer of the larynx*. Online. Available: seer.cancer.gov/statfacts/html/laryn.html (accessed 29 June 2015).

National Institute on Deafness and Other Communication Disorders 2014. *Cochlear implants*. Online. Available: www.nidcd.nih.gov/health/hearing/pages/coch.aspx (accessed 19 June 2015).

Neilson, R. 2003. *Sutherland Phonological Awareness Test*, rev., Jamberoo, NSW: Author.

Nelson, H.E. and O'Connell, A. 1978. 'Dementia: the estimation of premorbid levels using the new adult reading test', *Cortex* **14**:2, 234–44.

Nelson, K. 1973. 'Structure and strategy in learning to talk', *Monographs of the Society for Research in Child Development* **38**:(1–2), 1–135.

Ng, Y.S., Stein, J., Ning, M.M. and Black-Schaffer, R.M. 2007. 'Comparison of clinical characteristics and functional outcomes of ischemic stroke in different vascular territories', *Stroke* **38**:8, 2309–14.

Nicastri, M., Filipo, R., Ruoppolo, G., Viccaro, M., Dincer, H., Guerzoni, L., Cuda, D., Bosco, E., Prosperini, L. and Mancini, P. 2014. 'Inferences and metaphoric comprehension in unilaterally implanted children with adequate formal oral language performance', *International Journal of Pediatric Otorhinolaryngology* **78**:5, 821–7.

Nicholas, J.G. and Geers, A.E. 2007. 'Will they catch up? The role of age at cochlear implantation in the spoken language development of children with severe-profound hearing loss', *Journal of Speech, Language, and Hearing Research* **50**:4, 1048–62.

Nittrouer, S., Caldwell-Tarr, A., Sansom, E., Twersky, J. and Lowenstein, J.H. 2014a. 'Nonword repetition in children with cochlear implants: a potential clinical marker of poor language acquisition', *American Journal of Speech-Language Pathology* **23**:4, 679–95.

Nittrouer, S., Sansom, E., Low, K., Rice, C. and Caldwell-Tarr, A. 2014b. 'Language structures used by kindergartners with cochlear implants: relationship to phonological awareness, lexical knowledge and hearing loss', *Ear and Hearing* **35**:5, 506–18.

Noffsinger, D., Wilson, R.H. and Musiek, F.E. 1994. 'Department of veterans affairs compact disc recording for auditory perceptual assessment: background and introduction', *Journal of American Academy of Audiology* **5**:4, 231–5.

Norbury, C.F., Griffiths, H. and Nation, K. 2010. 'Sound before meaning: word learning in autistic disorders', *Neuropsychologia* **48**:14, 4012–19.

Nordberg, A., Miniscalco, C., Lohmander, A. and Himmelmann, K. 2012. 'Speech problems affect more than one in two children with cerebral palsy: Swedish population-based study', *Acta Paediatrica* **102**:2, 161–6.

Nussbaum, R.L. and Ellis, C.E. 2003. 'Alzheimer's disease and Parkinson's disease', *New England Journal of Medicine* **384**:14, 1356–64.

Nyberg, J., Peterson, P. and Lohmander, A. 2014. 'Speech outcomes at age 5 and 10 years in unilateral cleft lip and palate after one-stage palatal repair with minimal incision technique – a longitudinal perspective', *International Journal of Pediatric Otorhinolaryngology* **78**:10, 1662–70.

O'Brien, G. and Pearson, J. 2004. 'Autism and learning disability', *Autism* **8**:2, 125–40.

O'Donoghue, G.M., Nikolopoulos, T.P. and Archbold, S.M. 2000. 'Determinants of speech perception in children after cochlear implantation', *The Lancet* **356**:9228, 466–8.

Odell, K.H. and Shriberg, L.D. 2001. 'Prosody-voice characteristics of children and adults with apraxia of speech', *Clinical Linguistics & Phonetics* **15**:4, 275–307.

Oelschlaeger, M.L. and Scarborough, J. 1976. 'Traumatic aphasia in children: a case study', *Journal of Communication Disorders* **9**:4, 281–8.

Office for National Statistics 2013. 'Smoking prevalence among adults has declined by half since 1974'. Online. Available: www.ons.gov.uk/ons/rel/ghs/general-lifestyle-survey/2011/sty-smoking-report.html (accessed 30 June 2015).

Ogar, J., Slama, H., Dronkers, N., Amici, S. and Gorno-Tempini, M.L. 2005. 'Apraxia of speech: an overview', *Neurocase*, **11** (6): 427–32.

Ohl, C., Dornier, L., Czajka, C., Chobaut, J.C. and Tavernier, L. 2009. 'Newborn hearing screening on infants at risk', *International Journal of Pediatric Otorhinolaryngology* **73**:12, 1691–5.

Okuda, B., Kawabata, K., Tachibana, H., Sugita, M. and Tanaka, H. 2001. 'Postencephalitic pure anomic aphasia: 2-year follow-up', *Journal of the Neurological Sciences* **187**:(1–2), 99–102.

Oldfield, R.C. and Wingfield, A. 1965. 'Response latencies in naming objects', *Quarterly Journal of Experimental Psychology* **17**:4, 273–81.

Ortiz, K.Z., Pereira, L.D., de Carvalho Borges, A.C.L. and Vilanova, L.C.P. 2009. 'Nonverbal dichotic test in patients with epilepsy', *Dementia & Neuropsycologia* **3**:2, 108–13.

Päären, A., Bohman, H., von Knorring, L., Olsson, G., von Knorring, A.L. and Jonsson, U. 2014. 'Early risk factors for adult bipolar disorder in adolescents with mood disorders: a 15-year follow-up of a community sample', *BMC Psychiatry* **14**:363.

Paksarian, D., Eaton, W.W., Mortensen, P.B., Merikangas, K.R. and Pedersen, C.B. 2015. 'A population-based study of the risk of schizophrenia and bipolar disorder associated with parent–child separation during development', *Psychological Medicine* **45**:13, 2825–37.

Palmer, D., Dietsch, A. and Searl, J. 2012. 'Endoscopic and stroboscopic presentation of the larynx in male-to-female transsexual persons', *Journal of Voice* **26**:1, 117–26.

Papagno, C., Curti, R., Rizzo, S., Crippa, F. and Colombo, M.R. 2006. 'Is the right hemisphere involved in idiom comprehension? A neuropsychological study', *Neuropsychology* **20**:5, 598–606.

Parellada, M., Penzol, M.J., Pina, L., Moreno, C., González-Vioque, E., Zalsman, G. and Arango, C. 2014. 'The neurobiology of autism spectrum disorders', *European Psychiatry* **29**:1, 11–19.

Parisi, D. and Pizzamiglio, L. 1970. 'Syntactic comprehension in aphasia', *Cortex* **6**:2, 204–15.

Pastor, P., Reuben, C., Duran, C. and Hawkins, L. 2015. 'Association between diagnosed ADHD and selected characteristics among children aged 4–17 years: United States, 2011–2013', *NCHS Data Brief* **201**, 1–8.

Patel, R.R., Pickering, J., Stemple, J. and Donohue, K.D. 2012. 'A case report in changes in phonatory physiology following voice therapy: application of high-speed imaging', *Journal of Voice* **26**:6, 734–41.

Peach, R.K. and Tonkovich, J.D. 2004. 'Phonemic characteristics of apraxia of speech resulting from subcortical hemorrhage', *Journal of Communication Disorders* **37**:1, 77–90.

Peavy, G.M., Jacobson, M.W., Goldstein, J.L., Hamilton, J.M., Kane, A., Gamst, A.C., Lessig, S.L., Lee, J.C. and Corey-Bloom, J. 2010. 'Cognitive and functional decline in Huntington's disease: dementia criteria revisited', *Movement Disorders* **25**:9, 1163–9.

Peets, K.F. 2009. 'Profiles of dysfluency and errors in classroom discourse among children with language impairment', *Journal of Communication Disorders* **42**:2, 136–54.

Penn, C., Watermeyer, J. and Schie, K. 2009. 'Auditory disorders in a South African paediatric TBI population: some preliminary data', *International Journal of Audiology* **48**:3, 135–43.

Pennington, B.F. and Bishop, D.V.M. 2009. 'Relations among speech, language, and reading disorders', *Annual Review of Psychology* **60**, 283–306.

Pennington, L., Miller, N. and Robson, S. 2009. 'Speech therapy for children with dysarthria acquired before three years of age', *Cochrane Database of Systematic Reviews* **4**:CD006937.

Peppé, S., McCann, J., Gibbon, F., O'Hare, A. and Rutherford, M. 2007. 'Receptive and expressive prosodic ability in children with high-functioning autism', *Journal of Speech, Language, and Hearing Research* **50**:4, 1015–28.

Peretti, G., Piazza, C., Cattaneo, A., De Benedetto, L., Martin, E. and Nicolai, P. 2006. 'Comparison of functional outcomes after endoscopic versus open-neck supraglottic laryngectomies', *Annals of Otology, Rhinology, and Laryngology* **115**:11, 827–32.

Perez-Lloret, S., Nègre-Pagès, L., Ojero-Senard, A., Damier, P., Destée, A., Tison, F., Merello, M., Rascol, O. and COPARK Study Group 2012. 'Oro-buccal symptoms (dysphagia, dysarthria, and sialorrhea) in patients with Parkinson's disease: preliminary analysis from the French COPARK cohort', *European Journal of Neurology* **19**:1, 28–37.

Perl, D.P. 2010. 'Neuropathology of Alzheimer's disease', *Mount Sinai Journal of Medicine* **77**:1, 32–42.

Pernon, M., Trocello, J.M., Vaissière, J., Cousin, C., Chevaillier, G., Rémy, P., Kidri-Osmani, K., Fougeron, C. and Woimant, F. 2013. ['Could speech rate of Wilson's disease dysarthric patient be improved in dual task condition?'], *Revue Neurologique* **169**:(6–7), 502–9.

Perry, A., Casey, E. and Cotton, S. 2015. 'Quality of life after total laryngectomy: functioning, psychological well-being and self-efficacy', *International Journal of Language & Communication Disorders* **50**:4, 467–75.

Peters, A.T., Peckham, A.D., Stange, J.P., Sylvia, L.G., Hansen, N.S., Salcedo, S., Rauch, S.L., Nierenberg, A.A., Dougherty, D.D. and Deckersbach, T. 2014. 'Correlates of real world executive dysfunction in bipolar I disorder', *Journal of Psychiatric Research* **53**, 87–93.

Peters, B., Litovsky, R., Lake, J. and Parkinson, A.J. 2004. 'Sequential bilateral cochlear implantation in children', *International Congress Series* **1273**, 462–5.

Peterson, R.L., Pennington, B.F., Shriberg, L.D. and Boada, R. 2009. 'What influences literacy outcome in children with speech sound disorder?', *Journal of Speech, Language, and Hearing Research* **52**:5, 1175–88.

Piacentini, V., Mauri, I., Cattaneo, D., Gilardone, M., Montesano, A. and Schindler, A. 2014. 'Relationship between quality of life and dysarthria in patients with multiple sclerosis', *Archives of Physical Medicine and Rehabilitation* **95**:11, 2047–54.

Pijnacker, J., Hagoort, P., Buitelaar, J., Teunisse, J.-P. and Geurts, B. 2009. 'Pragmatic inferences in high-functioning adults with autism and Asperger syndrome', *Journal of Autism and Developmental Disorders* **39**:4, 607–18.

Piselli, P., Burra, P., Lauro, A., Baccarani, U., Ettorre, G.M., Vizzini, G.B., Rendina, M., Rossi, M., Tisone, G., Zamboni, F., Bortoluzzi, I., Pinna, A.D., Risaliti, A., Galatioto, L., Vennarecci, G., Di Leo, A., Nudo, F., Sforza, D., Fantola, G., Cimaglia, C., Verdirosi, D., Virdone, S., Serraino, D. and the Italian Transplant and Cancer Cohort Study 2015. 'Head and neck and esophageal cancers after liver transplant: results from a multi-center cohort study. Italy, 1997–2010', *Transplant International* **28**:7, 841–8.

Platt, L.J., Andrews, G., Young, M. and Quinn, P.T. 1980. 'Dysarthria of adult cerebral palsy. I. Intelligibility and articulatory impairment', *Journal of Speech, Language, and Hearing Research* **23**:1, 28–40.

Poulin, S., Macoir, J., Paquet, N., Fossard, M. and Gagnon, L. 2007. 'Psychogenic or neurogenic origin of agrammatism and foreign accent syndrome in a bipolar patient: a case report', *Annals of General Psychiatry* **6**:1.

Pouliquen, D., Goldenberg, A., Hannequin, D., Lecointre, C., Lechevallier, J., Cormier-Daire, V. and Martinaud, O. 2012. 'Detailed neuropsychological evaluation in a patient with Floating Harbor syndrome', *Journal of Clinical and Experimental Neuropsychology* **34**:5, 445–52.

Powell, T.W. 1996. 'Stimulability considerations in the phonological treatment of a child with a persistent disorder of speech-sound production', *Journal of Communication Disorders* **29**:4, 315–33.

Power, E., Anderson, A. and Togher, L. 2011. 'Applying the WHO ICF framework to communication assessment and goal setting in Huntington's disease: a case discussion', *Journal of Communication Disorders* **44**:3, 261–75.

Prades, J.M., Simon, P.G., Timoshenko, A.P., Dumollard, J.M., Schmitt, T. and Martin, C. 2005. 'Extended and standard supraglottic laryngectomies: a review of 110 patients', *European Archives of Oto-Rhino-Laryngology* **262**:12, 947–52.

Priefer, B.A. and Robbins, J. 1997. 'Eating changes in mild-stage Alzheimer's disease: a pilot study', *Dysphagia* **12**:4, 212–21.

Pringsheim, T., Jette, N., Frolkis, A. and Steeves, T.D. 2014. 'The prevalence of Parkinson's disease: a systematic review and meta-analysis', *Movement Disorders* **29**:13, 1583–90.

Prutting, C.A. and Kirchner, D.M. 1987. 'A clinical appraisal of the pragmatic aspects of language', *Journal of Speech and Hearing Disorders* **52**:2, 105–19.

Qiu, C., Kivipelto, M. and von Strauss, E. 2009. 'Epidemiology of Alzheimer's disease: occurrence, determinants, and strategies toward intervention', *Dialogues in Clinical Neuroscience* **11**:2, 111–28.

Quaranta, N., Coppola, F., Casulli, M., Barulli, M.R., Panza, F., Tortelli, R., Capozzo, R., Leo, A., Tursi, M., Grasso, A., Solfrizzi, V., Sobbà, C. and Logroscino, G. 2014. 'The prevalence of peripheral and central hearing impairment and its relation to cognition in older adults', *Audiology & Neuro-otology* **19**:(suppl. 1), 10–14.

Rabinowitz, A.R. and Levin, H.S. 2014. 'Cognitive sequelae of traumatic brain injury', *Psychiatric Clinics of North America* **37**:1, 1–11.

Raches, D., Hiscock, M. and Chapieski, L. 2012. 'Behavioral and academic problems in children with Sturge–Weber syndrome: differences between children with and without seizures', *Epilepsy & Behavior* **25**:3, 457–63.

Radanovic, M., Villela Nunes, P., Farid Gattaz, W. and Vicente Forlenza, O. 2008. 'Language impairment in euthymic, elderly patients with bipolar disorder but no dementia', *International Psychogeriatrics* **20**:4, 687–96.

Rafii, M.S. and Aisen, P.S. 2015. 'Advances in Alzheimer's disease drug development', *BMC Medicine* **13**:62.

Ramírez-Crescencio, M.A. and Velásquez-Pérez, L. 2013. 'Epidemiology and trend of neurological diseases associated to HIV/AIDS. Experience of Mexican patients 1995–2009', *Clinical Neurology and Neurosurgery* **115**:8, 1322–5.

Raphael, D.B. and Schoenfeld, F.B. 2006. 'Psychogenic stuttering following a gastric bypass operation: case report', *Jefferson Journal of Psychiatry* **20**:1, 13–21.

Rassiga, C., Lucchelli, F., Crippa, F. and Papagno, C. 2009. 'Ambiguous idiom comprehension in Alzheimer's disease', *Journal of Clinical and Experimental Neuropsychology* **31**:4, 402–11.

Raven, J.C. 1962. *Coloured Progressive Matrices*, London: H.K. Lewis.

1984. *Manual for the Coloured Progressive Matrices*, rev., Windsor, UK: NFER-Nelson.

Redmond, S.M. 2004. 'Conversational profiles of children with ADHD, SLI and typical development', *Clinical Linguistics & Phonetics* **18**:2, 107–25.

2011. 'Peer victimization among students with specific language impairment, attention-deficit/hyperactivity disorder, and typical development', *Language, Speech, and Hearing Services in Schools* **42**:4, 520–35.

Regan, J., Sowman, R. and Walsh, I. 2006. 'Prevalence of dysphagia in acute and community mental health settings', *Dysphagia* **21**:2, 95–101.

Reilly, S., Wake, M., Ukoumunne, O.C., Bavin, E., Prior, M., Cini, E., Conway, L., Eadie, P. and Bretherton, L. 2010. 'Predicting language outcomes at 4 years of age: findings from Early Language in Victoria Study', *Pediatrics* **126**:6, e1530–e1537.

René, G. 2011. 'Who is a cochlear implant candidate?', *Hearing Journal* **64**:6, 16, 18–22.

Rey, A. 1941. 'L'Examen psychologique dans les cas d'encephalopathie traumatique', *Archives de Psychologie* **28**, 215–85.

    1964. *L'Éxam clinique en psychologie*, Paris: Presses Universitaires France.

Reynell, J. 1977. *Reynell Developmental Language Scales*, rev., Berkshire: NFER-Nelson.

Rezzonico, S., de Weck, G., Salazar Orvig, A., da Silva, G.C. and Rahmati, S. 2014. 'Maternal recasts and activity variations: a comparison of mother-child dyads involving children with and without SLI', *Clinical Linguistics & Phonetics* **28**:4, 223–40.

Rhys, C.S. and Schmidt-Renfree, N. 2000. 'Facework, social politeness and the Alzheimer's patient', *Clinical Linguistics & Phonetics* **14**:7, 533–43.

Ribi, K., Reilly, C., Landolt, M.A., Alber, F.D., Boltshauser, E. and Grotzer, M.A. 2005. 'Outcome of medulloblastoma in children: long-term complications and quality of life', *Neuropediatrics* **36**:6, 357–65.

Rigby, M.H. and Hayden, R.E. 2014. 'Total glossectomy without laryngectomy – a review of functional outcomes and reconstructive principles', *Current Opinion in Otolaryngology & Head and Neck Surgery* **22**:5, 414–18.

Riley, G. and Riley, J. 1985. *Oral Motor Assessment and Treatment: Improving Syllable Production*, Austin, TX: Pro-Ed.

Rinaldi, M.C., Marangolo, P. and Baldassarri, F. 2004. 'Metaphor comprehension in right brain-damaged patients with visuo-verbal and verbal material: a dissociation (re)considered', *Cortex* **40**:3, 479–90.

Ripich, D.N., Carpenter, B.D. and Ziol, E.W. 2000. 'Conversational cohesion patterns in men and women with Alzheimer's disease: A longitudinal study', *International Journal of Language & Communication Disorders* **35**:1, 49–64.

Robin, D.A. and Flagmeier, S. 2014. 'Apraxia of speech', in L. Cummings (ed.), *Cambridge Handbook of Communication Disorders*, Cambridge: Cambridge University Press, 211–23.

Robson, H., Zahn, R., Keidel, J.L., Binney, R.J., Sage, K. and Lambon, R.M.A. 2014. 'The anterior temporal lobes support residual comprehension in Wernicke's aphasia', *Brain* **137**:3, 931–43.

Roello, M., Ferretti, M.L., Colonnello, V. and Levi, G. 2015. 'When words lead to solutions: executive function deficits in preschool children with specific language impairment', *Research in Developmental Disabilities* **37**, 216–22.

Rohrer, J.D., Rossor, M.N. and Warren, J.D. 2012. 'Alzheimer's pathology in primary progressive aphasia', *Neurobiology of Aging* **33**:4, 744–52.

Roid, G., Nellis, L. and McLellan, M. 2003. 'Assessment with the Leiter international performance scale-revised and the S-BIT', in R.S. McCallum (ed.), *Handbook of Nonverbal Assessment*, New York: Kluwer Academic/Plenum Publishers, 113–40.

Romero, G., Méndez, I., Tello, A. and Torner, C. 2008. 'Auditory brainstem responses as a clinical evaluation tool in children after perinatal encephalopathy', *International Journal of Pediatric Otorhinolaryngology* **72**:2, 193–201.

Roncero, C. and de Almeida, R.G. 2014. 'The importance of being apt: metaphor comprehension in Alzheimer's disease', *Frontiers in Human Neuroscience* **8**:973.

Rousseaux, M., Vérigneaux, C. and Kozlowski, O. 2010. 'An analysis of communication in conversation after severe traumatic brain injury', *European Journal of Neurology* **17**:7, 922–9.

Roy, N. 2004. 'Functional voice disorders', in R.D. Kent (ed.), *The MIT Encyclopedia of Communication Disorders*, Cambridge, MA: MIT Press, 27–30.

Roy, N., Gray, S.D., Simon, M., Dove, H., Corbin-Lewis, K. and Stemple, J.C. 2001. 'An evaluation of the effects of two treatment approaches for teachers with voice disorders: a prospective randomized clinical trial', *Journal of Speech, Language, and Hearing Research* **44**:2, 286–96.

Royal College of Psychiatrists 2013. *Good Practice Guidelines for the Assessment and Treatment of Adults with Gender Dysphoria*, London: Royal College of Psychiatrists.

Rudolph, J.M. and Wendt, O. 2014. 'The efficacy of the cycles approach: a multiple baseline design', *Journal of Communication Disorders* **47**:1, 1–16.

Rudzinski, L.A., Fletcher, R.M., Dickson, D.W., Crook, R., Hutton, M.L., Adamson, J. and Graff-Radford, N.R. 2008. 'Early onset familial Alzheimer disease with spastic paraparesis, dysarthria, and seizures and N135S mutation in PSEN1', *Alzheimer Disease and Associated Disorders* **22**:3, 299–307.

Rumpf, A.-L., Kamp-Becker, I., Becker, K. and Kauschke, C. 2012. 'Narrative competence and internal state language of children with Asperger syndrome and ADHD', *Research in Developmental Disabilities* **33**:5, 1395–1407.

Rush, P., Blennerhassett, L., Epstein, K. and Alexander, D. 1991. 'WAIS-R verbal and performance profiles of adolescents referred for atypical learning styles', in D.S. Martin (ed.), *Cognition, Education and Deafness*, Washington, DC: Gallaudet University Press, 82–8.

Rustin, L., Botterill, W. and Kelman, E. 1996. *Assessment and Therapy for Young Dysfluent Children*, London: Whurr Publishers.

Saad, A.N., Parina, R.P., Tokin, C., Chang, D.C. and Gosman, A. 2014. 'Incidence of oral clefts among different ethnicities in the state of California', *Annals of Plastic Surgery* **72**:(suppl. 1), S81–S83.

Sabbagh, H.J., Hassan, M.H., Innes, N.P., Elkodary, H.M., Little, J. and Mossey, P.A. 2015. 'Passive smoking in the etiology of non-syndromic orofacial clefts: a systematic review and meta-analysis', *PloS One* **10**:3, e0116963.

Sacks, J.M. and Levy, S. 1959. 'The sentence completion test', in L.E. Abt and L. Bellak (eds.), *Projective Psychology – Clinical Approaches to the Total Personality*, New York: Grove Press, 357–402.

Safaz, I., Alaca, R., Yasar, E., Tok, F. and Yilmaz, B. 2008. 'Medical complications, physical function and communication skills in patients with traumatic brain injury: a single centre 5-year experience', *Brain Injury* **22**:10, 733–9.

Sahlén, B. and Nettelbladt, U. 1993. 'Context and comprehension: a neurolinguistic and interactional approach to the understanding of semantic-pragmatic disorder', *European Journal of Disorders of Communication* **28**:2, 117–40.

St. Louis, K.O. 1996. 'A tabular summary of cluttering subjects in the special edition', *Journal of Fluency Disorders* **21**:(3–4), 337–43.

St. Louis, K.O., Filatova, Y., Coşkun, M., Topbaş, S., Ozdemir, S., Georgieva, D., McCaffrey, E. and George, R.D. 2010. 'Identification of cluttering and stuttering by the public in four countries', *International Journal of Speech-Language Pathology* **12**:6, 508–19.

St. Louis, K.O., Myers, F.M., Bakker, K. and Raphael, L.J. 2007. 'Understanding and treating cluttering', in E.G. Conture and R.F. Curlee (eds.), *Stuttering and Related Disorders of Fluency*, 3rd edn, New York: Thieme, 297–325.

Sainz, M., Skarzynski, H., Allum, J.H.J., Helms, J., Rivas, A., Martin, J., Zarowka, P.G., Phillips, L., Delauney, J., Brockmeyer, S.J., Kompis, M., Korolewa, I., Albegger, K., Zwirner, P., Van de Heyning, P. and D'Haese, P. 2003. 'Assessment of auditory skills in 140 cochlear implant children using the EARS protocol', *ORL: Journal for Oto-Rhino-Laryngology, Head and Neck Surgery* **65**:2, 91–6.

Sakurai, Y., Itoh, K., Sai, K., Lee, S., Abe, S., Terao, Y. and Mannen, T. 2015. 'Impaired laryngeal voice production in a patient with foreign accent syndrome', *Neurocase* **21**:3, 289–98.

Saldert, C., Ferm, U. and Bloch, S. 2014. 'Semantic trouble sources and their repair in conversations affected by Parkinson's disease', *International Journal of Language & Communication Disorders* **49**:6, 710–21.

Saldert, C., Fors, A., Ströberg, S. and Hartelius, L. 2010. 'Comprehension of complex discourse in different stages of Huntington's disease', *International Journal of Language & Communication Disorders* **45**:6, 656–69.

Samamé, C. 2013. 'Social cognition throughout the three phases of bipolar disorder: a state-of-the-art overview', *Psychiatry Research* **210**:3, 1275–86.

Sarant, J., Harris, D., Bennet, L. and Bant, S. 2014. 'Bilateral versus unilateral cochlear implants in children: a study of spoken language outcomes', *Ear and Hearing* **35**:4, 396–409.

Sarant, J., Harris, D. and Bennet, L. 2015. 'Academic outcomes for school-aged children with severe-profound hearing loss and early unilateral and bilateral cochlear implants', *Journal of Speech, Language, and Hearing Research* **58**:3, 1017–32.

Sayal, K., Washbrook, E. and Propper, C. 2015. 'Childhood behavior problems and academic outcomes in adolescence: longitudinal population-based study', *Journal of the American Academy of Child and Adolescent Psychiatry* **54**:5, 360–8.

Schaerlaekens, A., Zink, I. and Van Ommeslaeghe, K. 1993. *Reynell Taalontwikkelingsschalen*, Nijmegen: Berkhout B.V.

Schalén, L. and Andersson, K. 1992. 'Differential diagnosis and treatment of psychogenic voice disorder', *Clinical Otolaryngology & Allied Sciences* **17**:3, 225–30.

Schalén, L., Andersson, K. and Eliasson, I. 1992. 'Diagnosis of psychogenic dysphonia', *Acta Oto-laryngologica* **112**:(suppl. 492), 110–12.

Schenkel, L.S., Chamberlain, T.F. and Towne, T.L. 2014. 'Impaired theory of mind and psychosocial functioning among pediatric patients with Type I versus Type II bipolar disorder', *Psychiatry Research* **215**:3, 740–6.

Schoen, E., Paul, R. and Chawarska, K. 2011. 'Phonology and vocal behavior in toddlers with autism spectrum disorders', *Autism Research* **4**:3, 177–88.

Scholtz, A.W., Fish, J.H., Kammen-Jolly, K., Ichiki, H., Hussl, B., Kreczy, A. and Schrott-Fischer, A. 2001. 'Goldenhar's syndrome: congenital hearing deficit of conductive or sensorineural origin? Temporal bone histopathologic study', *Otology & Neurotology* **22**:4, 501–5.

Schweinfurth, J.M. and Silver, S.M. 2000. 'Patterns of swallowing after supraglottic laryngectomy', *Laryngoscope* **110**:8, 1266–70.

Sciberras, E., Mueller, K.L., Efron, D., Bisset, M., Anderson, V., Schilpzand, E.J., Jongeling, B. and Nicholson, J.M. 2014. 'Language problems in children with ADHD: a community-based study', *Pediatrics* **133**:5, 793–800.

Scott, J.G. 2011. 'Attention/concentration: the distractible patient', in M.R. Schoenberg and J.G. Scott (eds.), *The Little Black Book of Neuropsychology: A Syndrome-Based Approach*, New York: Springer, 149–58.

Sellars, C., Hughes, T. and Langhorne, P. 2005. 'Speech and language therapy for dysarthria due to non-progressive brain damage', *Cochrane Database Systematic Reviews* **3**:CD002088.

Semel, E., Wiig, E.H. and Secord, W.A. 1995. *Clinical Evaluation of Language Fundamentals-3 (CELF-3)*, San Antonio, TX: Psychological Corporation.

  2003. *Clinical Evaluation of Language Fundamentals-4 (CELF-4)*, San Antonio, TX: Psychological Corporation.

Shamay-Tsoory, S.G., Tomer, R. and Aharon-Peretz, J. 2005. 'The neuroanatomical basis of understanding sarcasm and its relationship to social cognition', *Neuropsychology* **19**:3, 288–300.

Sharma, A., Gilley, P.M., Martin, K., Roland, P., Bauer, P. and Dorman, M. 2007. 'Simultaneous versus sequential bilateral implantation in young children: effects on central auditory system development and plasticity', *Audiological Medicine* **5**:4, 218–23.

Sharma, M. and Purdy, S.C. 2007. 'A case study of an 11-year-old with auditory processing disorder', *Australian and New Zealand Journal of Audiology* **29**:1, 40–52.

Sharma, M., Purdy, S.C. and Kelly, A.S. 2009. 'Comorbidity of auditory processing, language, and reading disorders', *Journal of Speech, Language, and Hearing Research* **52**:3, 706–22.

Shaywitz, S.E. and Shaywitz, B.A. 2003. 'Dyslexia (specific reading disability)', *Pediatrics in Review* **24**:5, 147–53.

Shehata, G.A., El Mistikawi, T., Risha, A.S., and Hassan, H.S. 2014. 'The effect of aphasia upon personality traits, depression and anxiety among stroke patients', *Journal of Affective Disorders* **172**, 312–14.

Shekhtman, Y., Kim, I., Riviello Jr, J.J., Milla, S.S. and Weiner, H.L. 2013. 'Focal resection of leptomeningeal angioma in a rare case of Sturge–Weber syndrome without facial nevus', *Pediatric Neurosurgery* **49**:2, 99–104.

Shih, C., Tseng, F.Y., Yeh, T.H., Hsu, C.J. and Chen, Y.S. 2009. 'Ipsilateral and contralateral acoustic brainstem response abnormalities in patients with vestibular schwannoma', *Otolaryngology – Head and Neck Surgery* **141**:6, 695–700.

Shriberg, L.D. 1993. 'Four new speech and prosody-voice measures for genetics research and other studies in developmental phonological disorder', *Journal of Speech and Hearing Research* **36**:1, 105–40.

Shriberg, L.D., Aram, D.M. and Kwiatkowski, J. 1997. 'Developmental apraxia of speech: I. Descriptive and theoretical perspectives', *Journal of Speech, Language, and Hearing Research* **40**:2, 273–85.

Shriberg, L.D., Potter, N.L. and Strand, E.A. 2011. 'Prevalence and phenotype of childhood apraxia of speech in youth with galactosemia', *Journal of Speech, Language, and Hearing Research* **54**:2, 487–519.

Shriberg, L.D., Tomblin, J.B. and McSweeny, J.L. 1999. 'Prevalence of speech delay in 6-year-old children and comorbidity with language impairment', *Journal of Speech, Language, and Hearing Research* **42**:6, 1461–81.

Sices, L., Taylor, H.G., Freebairn, L., Hansen, A. and Lewis, B. 2007. 'Relationship between speech-sound disorders and early literacy skills in preschool-age children: impact of comorbid language impairment', *Journal of Developmental and Behavioral Pediatrics* **28**:6, 438–47.

Siegel, R., Naishadham, D. and Jemal, A. 2013. 'Cancer statistics, 2013', *CA: A Cancer Journal for Clinicians* **63**:1, 11–30.

Sigurdardottir, S. and Vik, T. 2011. 'Speech, expressive language, and verbal cognition of preschool children with cerebral palsy in Iceland', *Developmental Medicine and Child Neurology* **53**:1, 74–80.

Sigurdsson, E., Fombonne, E., Sayal, K. and Checkley, S. 1999. 'Neurodevelopmental antecedents of early-onset bipolar affective disorder', *British Journal of Psychiatry* **174**:2, 121–7.

Simard, E.P., Torre, L.A. and Jemal, A. 2014. 'International trends in head and neck cancer incidence rates: differences by country, sex and anatomic site', *Oral Oncology* **50**:5, 387–403.

Simioni, M., Araujo, T.K., Monlleo, I.L., Maurer-Morelli, C.V. and Gil-da-Silva-Lopes, V.L. 2015. 'Investigation of genetic factors underlying typical orofacial clefts: mutational screening and copy number variation', *Journal of Human Genetics* **60**:1, 17–25.

Sinclair, C.F., Carroll, W.R., Desmond, R.A. and Rosenthal, E.L. 2011. 'Functional and survival outcomes in patients undergoing total glossectomy compared with total laryngoglossectomy', *Otolaryngology – Head and Neck Surgery* **145**:5, 755–8.

Singer, S., Danker, H., Guntinas-Lichius, O., Oeken, J., Pabst, F., Schock, J., Vogel, H.J., Meister, E.F., Wulke, C. and Dietz, A. 2014. 'Quality of life before and after total laryngectomy: results of a multicenter prospective cohort study', *Head & Neck* **36**:3, 359–68.

Singh, T.D., Fugate, J.E., Hocker, S.E. and Rabinstein, A.A. 2015. 'Postencephalitic epilepsy: clinical characteristics and predictors', *Epilepsia* **56**:1, 133–8.

Skahan, S.M., Watson, M. and Lof, G.L. 2007. 'Speech-language pathologists' assessment practices for children with suspected speech sound disorders: results of a national survey', *American Journal of Speech-Language Pathology* **16**:3, 246–59.

Skodda, S., Schlegel, U., Hoffmann, R. and Saft, C. 2014. 'Impaired motor speech performance in Huntington's disease', *Journal of Neural Transmission* **121**:4, 399–407.

Skolarus, L.E., Burke, J.F., Brown, D.L. and Freedman, V.A. 2014. 'Understanding stroke survivorship: expanding the concept of poststroke disability', *Stroke* **45**:1, 224–30.

Skuk, V.G. and Schweinberger, S.R. 2014. 'Influences of fundamental frequency, formant frequencies, aperiodicity, and spectrum level on the perception of voice gender', *Journal of Speech, Language, and Hearing Research* **57**:1, 285–96.

Sluckin, A. 2000. 'Selective mutism', in J. Law, A. Parkinson and R. Tamhne (eds.), *Communication Difficulties in Childhood: A Practical Guide*, Abingdon: Radcliffe Medical Press, 273–80.

Smith Doody, R., Hrachovy, R.A. and Feher, E.P. 1992. 'Recurrent fluent aphasia associated with a seizure focus', *Brain and Language* **42**:4, 419–30.

Smith, A. 1982. *Symbol Digits Modalities Test*, Los Angeles, CA: Western Psychological Services.

Smoski, W.J., Brunt, M.A. and Tannahill, J.C. 1992. 'Listening characteristics of children with central auditory processing disorders', *Language, Speech, and Hearing Services in Schools* **23**:2, 145–52.

Song, A. and Jones, S. 1979. *Wisconsin Behavior Rating Scale*, Central Madison: Central Wisconsin Center for the Developmentally Disabled.

Spantideas, N., Drosou, E., Karatsis, A. and Assimakopoulos, D. 2015. 'Voice disorders in the general Greek population and in patients with laryngopharyngeal reflux. Prevalence and risk factors', *Journal of Voice* **29**:3, 389.e27–389.e32.

Sparreboom, M., Langereis, M.C., Snik, A.F. and Mylanus, E.A. 2015. 'Long-term outcomes on spatial hearing, speech recognition and receptive vocabulary after sequential bilateral cochlear implantation in children', *Research in Developmental Disabilities* **36**, 328–37.

Sparrow, S.S., Balla, D.A. and Cicchetti, D.V. 1984. *Vineland Adaptive Behavior Scales*, Circle Pines, MN: American Guidance Service.

Speleman, K., Kneepkens, K., Vandendriessche, K., Debruyne, F. and Desloovere, C. 2012. 'Prevalence of risk factors for sensorineural hearing loss in NICU newborns', *B-ENT* **8**:1, 1–6.

Staiger, A., Finger-Berg, W., Aichert, I. and Ziegler, W. 2012. 'Error variability in apraxia of speech: a matter of controversy', *Journal of Speech, Language, and Hearing Research* **55**:5, S1544–S1561.

Starosta-Rubinstein, S., Young, A.B., Kluin, K., Hill, G., Aisen, A.M., Gabrielsen, T. and Brewer, G.J. 1987. 'Clinical assessment of 31 patients with Wilson's disease. Correlations with structural changes on magnetic resonance imaging', *Archives of Neurology* **44**:4, 365–70.

Stein, D.J. and Noordzij, J.P. 2013. 'Incidence of chronic laryngitis', *Annals of Otology, Rhinology, and Laryngology* **122**:12, 771–4.

Stemple, J.C., Glaze, L. and Klaben, B.G. 2000. *Clinical Voice Pathology: Theory and Management*, San Diego, CA: Singular.

Stich, H.F., Parida, B.B. and Brunnemann, K.D. 1992. 'Localized formation of micronuclei in the oral mucosa and tobacco-specific nitrosamines in the saliva of "reverse" smokers, Khaini-tobacco chewers and gudakhu users', *International Journal of Cancer* **50**:2, 172–6.

St-Pierre, M.-C., Ska, B. and Béland, R. 2005. 'Lack of coherence in the narrative discourse of patients with dementia of the Alzheimer's type', *Journal of Multilingual Communication Disorders* **3**:3, 211–15.

Strauss, E., Sherman, E.M.S. and Spreen, O. 2006. *A Compendium of Neuropsychological Tests: Administration, Norms, and Commentary*, 3rd edn, New York: Oxford University Press.

Strömland, K., Miller, M., Sjögreen, L., Johansson, M., Joelsson, B.M., Billstedt, E., Gillberg, C., Danielsson, S., Jacobsson, C., Andersson-Norinder, J. and Granström, G. 2007. 'Oculo-auriculo-vertebral spectrum: associated anomalies, functional deficits and possible developmental risk factors', *American Journal of Medical Genetics* **143A**:12, 1317–25.

Stutsman, R. 1948. *Merrill-Palmer Scale of Mental Tests*, New York: Stoelting.

Sudhir, P.M., Chandra, P.S., Shivashankar, N. and Yamini, B.K. 2009. 'Comprehensive management of psychogenic dysphonia: a case illustration', *Journal of Communication Disorders* **42**:5, 305–12.

Sujansky, E. and Conradi, S. 1995. 'Sturge–Weber syndrome: age of onset of seizures and glaucoma and the prognosis for affected children', *Journal of Child Neurology* **10**:1, 49–58.

Suskauer, S.J., Trovato, M.K., Zabel, T.A. and Comi, A.M. 2010. 'Physiatric findings in individuals with Sturge–Weber syndrome', *American Journal of Physical Medicine & Rehabilitation* **89**:4, 323–30.

Swartz, S. and Swartz, L. 1987. 'Talk about talk: metacommentary and context in the analysis of psychotic discourse', *Culture, Medicine and Psychiatry* **11**:4, 395–416.

Tagliaferri, F., Compagnone, C., Korsic, M., Servadei, F. and Kraus, J. 2006. 'A systematic review of brain injury epidemiology in Europe', *Acta Neurochirurgica* **148**:3, 255–68.

Takizawa, C., Thompson, P.L., van Walsem, A., Faure, C. and Maier, W.C. 2015. 'Epidemiological and economic burden of Alzheimer's disease: a systematic literature review of data across Europe and the United States of America', *Journal of Alzheimer's Disease* **43**:4, 1271–84.

Tan, E.E., Hee, K.Y., Yeoh, A., Lim, S.B., Tan, H.K., Yeow, V.K. and Daniel, L.M. 2014. 'Hearing loss in newborns with cleft lip and/or palate', *Annals of the Academy of Medicine, Singapore* **43**:7, 371–7.

Teigland, A. 1996. 'A study of pragmatic skills of clutterers and normal speakers', *Journal of Fluency Disorders* **21**:(3–4), 201–14.

Tellegen, P.J., Laros, J.A. and Petermann, F. 2007. *SON-R 2.5-7 Non-Verbaler Intelligenztest*, Göttingen, Germany: Hogrefe.

Temple, C.M. 1988. 'Developmental dyslexia and dysgraphia persistence in middle age', *Journal of Communication Disorders* **21**:3, 189–207.

Tervo, T., Michelsson, K., Launes, J. and Hokkanen, L. 2016. 'A prospective 30-year follow-up of ADHD associated with perinatal risks', *Journal of Attention Disorders* to appear.

Thacker, R.C. and De Nil, L.F. 1996. 'Neurogenic cluttering', *Journal of Fluency Disorders* **21**:(3–4), 227–38.

Thapar, A., Cooper, M., Jefferies, R. and Stergiakouli, E. 2012. 'What causes attention deficit hyperactivity disorder?', *Archives of Disease in Childhood* **97**:3, 260–5.

Thesing, C.S., Stek, M.L., van Grootheest, D.S., van de Ven, P.M., Beekman, A.T., Kupka, R.W., Comijs, H.C. and Dols, A. 2015. 'Childhood abuse, family history and stressors in older patients with bipolar disorder in relation to age at onset', *Journal of Affective Disorders* **184**, 249–55.

Theunisse, H.J., Mulder, J.J., Pennings, R.J., Kunst, H.P. and Mylanus, E.A. 2014. 'A database system for the registration of complications and failures in cochlear implant surgery applied to over 1000 implantations performed in Nijmegen, the Netherlands', *Journal of Laryngology and Otology* **128**:11, 952–7.

Theys, C., van Wieringen, A., Sunaert, S., Thijs, V. and De Nil, L.F. 2011. 'A one year prospective study of neurogenic stuttering following stroke: incidence and co-occurring disorders', *Journal of Communication Disorders* **44**:6, 678–87.

Thomson, A.M., Taylor, R., Fraser, D. and Whittle, I.R. 1997. 'The utility of the Right Hemisphere Language Battery in patients with brain tumours', *European Journal of Disorders of Communication* **32**:(3 spec. no.), 325–32.

Thurman, D.J. 2015. 'The epidemiology of traumatic brain injury in children and youths: a review of research since 1990', *Journal of Child Neurology* to appear.

Tomasino, B., Marin, D., Maieron, M., Ius, T., Budai, R., Fabbro, F. and Skrap, M. 2013. 'Foreign accent syndrome: a multimodal mapping study', *Cortex* **49**:1, 18–39.

Tomblin, J.B., Records, N.L., Buckwalter, P., Zhang, X., Smith, E. and O'Brien, M. 1997. 'Prevalence of specific language impairment in kindergarten children', *Journal of Speech, Language, and Hearing Research*, **40**:6, 1245–60.

Tompkins, C.A. 2012. 'Rehabilitation for cognitive-communication disorders in right hemisphere brain damage', *Archives of Physical Medicine and Rehabilitation* **93**:(suppl. 1), S61–S69.

Tompkins, C.A., Baumgaertner, A., Lehman, M.T. and Fassbinder, W. 2000. 'Mechanisms of discourse comprehension impairment after right hemisphere brain damage: suppression in lexical ambiguity resolution', *Journal of Speech, Language, and Hearing Research* **43**:1, 62–78.

Tompkins, C.A., Lehman-Blake, M.T., Baumgaertner, A. and Fassbinder, W. 2001. 'Mechanisms of discourse comprehension impairment after right hemisphere brain damage: suppression in inferential ambiguity resolution', *Journal of Speech, Language, and Hearing Research* **44**:2, 400–15.

Tompkins, C.A., Meigh, K., Scott, A.G. and Lederer, L.G. 2009. 'Can high-level inferencing be predicted by Discourse Comprehension Test performance in adults with right hemisphere brain damage?', *Aphasiology* **23**:7, 1016–27.

Tompkins, V. and Farrar, M.J. 2011. 'Mothers' autobiographical memory and book narratives with children with specific language impairment', *Journal of Communication Disorders* **44**:1, 1–22.

Topaloğlu, I., Salturk, Z., Atar, Y., Berkiten, G., Büyükkoc, O. and Çakir, O. 2014. 'Evaluation of voice quality after supraglottic laryngectomy', *Otolaryngology – Head and Neck Surgery* **151**:6, 1003–7.

Topbaş, S. 2006. 'Does the speech of Turkish-speaking phonologically disordered children differ from that of children speaking other languages?', *Clinical Linguistics & Phonetics* **20**:(7–8), 509–22.

Trax, A.X. and Mills, L.D. 2013. 'A case of foreign accent syndrome', *Journal of Emergency Medicine* **45**:1, 26–9.

Trenerry, M.R., Crosson, B., DeBoe, J. and Leber, W.R. 1989. *The Stroop Neuropsychological Screening Test*, Odessa, FL: Psychological Assessment Resources.

Uesugi, H., Shimizu, H., Maehara, T., Arai, N., Kaito, N., Matsuda, H., Nakayama, H. and Onuma, T. 1998. 'Cases of temporal lobe epilepsy following mild encephalitis/meningitis or suspicion of these diseases', *Journal of Epilepsy* **11**:4, 177–81.

Unruh, S.M. and Lowe, P.A. 2007. 'Selective mutism', in C.R. Reynolds and E. Fletcher-Janzen (eds.), *Encyclopedia of Special Education: A Reference for the Education of Children, Adolescents, and Adults with Disabilities and Other Exceptional Individuals*, 3rd edn, Hoboken, NJ: John Wiley & Sons.

Urben, M.L., Jacobson, A.S. and Lazarus, C.L. 2012. 'Comprehensive approach to restoration of function in patients with radiation-induced pharyngoesophageal stenosis: report of 31 patients and proposal of a new classification scheme', *Head & Neck* **34**:9, 1317–28.

Van Borsel, J. and Taillieu, C. 2001. 'Neurogenic stuttering versus developmental stuttering: an observer judgement study', *Journal of Communication Disorders* **34**:5, 385–95.

Van Borsel, J. and Vandermeulen, A. 2008. 'Cluttering in Down syndrome', *Folia Phoniatrica et Logopaedica* **60**:6, 312–17.

Van Borsel, J., Janssens, L. and Santens, P. 2005. 'Foreign accent syndrome: an organic disorder?', *Journal of Communication Disorders* **38**:6, 421–9.

Van der Meulen, B.F. and Smrkovsky, M. 1986. *McCarthy Scales of Children's Abilities*, Lisse: Swets & Zeitlinger B.V.

Van Dongen, H., Van Harskamp, F. and Luteijn, F. 1976. *Token Test*, Nijmegen: Berkhout.

Van Houtte, E., Van Lierde, K., D'haeseleer, E. and Claeys, S. 2010. 'The prevalence of laryngeal pathology in a treatment-seeking population with dysphonia', *Laryngoscope* **120**:2, 306–12.

Van Lierde, K.M., Van Borsel, J. and Van Cauwenberge, P. 2000. 'Speech patterns in Kabuki make-up syndrome: a case report', *Journal of Communication Disorders* **33**:6, 447–62.

Van Lierop, A.C., Basson, O. and Fagan, J.J. 2008. 'Is total glossectomy for advanced carcinoma of the tongue justified?', *South African Journal of Surgery* **46**:1, 22–5.

Van Weissenbruch, R., Kunnen, M., Albers, F.W., Van Cauwenberge, P.B. and Sulter, A.M. 2000. 'Cineradiography of the pharyngoesophageal segment in postlaryngectomy patients', *Annals of Otology, Rhinology, and Laryngology* **109**:3, 311–19.

Vargha-Khadem, F., Carr, L.J., Isaacs, E., Brett, E., Adams, C. and Mishkin, M. 1997. 'Onset of speech after left hemispherectomy in a nine-year-old boy', *Brain* **120**:1, 159–82.

Vega, C., León, X., Cervelli, D., Pons, G., López, S., Fernández, M., Quer, M. and Masià, J. 2011. 'Total or subtotal glossectomy with microsurgical reconstruction: functional and oncological results', *Microsurgery* **31**:7, 517–23.

Velleman, S.L. and Mervis, C.B. 2011. 'Children with 7q11.23 duplication syndrome: speech, language, cognitive, and behavioral characteristics and their implications for intervention', *Perspectives on Language Learning and Education* **18**:3, 108–16.

Venail, F., Vieu, A., Artieres, F., Mondain, M. and Uziel, A. 2010. 'Educational and employment achievements in prelingually deaf children who receive cochlear implants', *Archives of Otolaryngology – Head & Neck Surgery* **136**:4, 366–72.

Verhoeven, J. and Mariën, P. 2010. 'Neurogenic foreign accent syndrome: articulatory setting, segments and prosody in a Dutch speaker', *Journal of Neurolinguistics* **23**:6, 599–614.

Verhoeven, J., Mariën, P., Engelborghs, S., D'Haenen, H. and De Deyn, P. 2005. 'A foreign speech accent in a case of conversion disorder', *Behavioural Neurology* **16**:4, 225–32.

Viana, A.G., Beidel, D.C. and Rabian, B. 2009. 'Selective mutism: a review and integration of the last 15 years', *Clinical Psychology Review* **29**:1, 57–67.

Walder, B., Haller, G., Rebetez, M.M., Delhumeau, C., Bottequin, E., Schoettker, P., Ravussin, P., Brodmann Maeder, M., Stover, J.F., Zürcher, M., Haller, A., Wäckelin, A., Haberthür, C., Fandino, J., Haller, C.S. and Osterwalder, J. 2013. 'Severe traumatic brain injury in a high-income country: an epidemiological study', *Journal of Neurotrauma* **30**:23, 1934–42.

Walz, N.C., Yeates, K.O., Taylor, H.G., Stancin, T. and Wade, S.L. 2012. 'Emerging narrative discourse skills 18 months after traumatic brain injury in early childhood', *Journal of Neuropsychology,* **6**:2, 143–60.

Ward, A., Tardiff, S., Dye, C. and Arrighi, H.M. 2013. 'Rate of conversion from prodromal Alzheimer's disease to Alzheimer's dementia: a systematic review of the literature', *Dementia and Geriatric Cognitive Disorders Extra* **3**:1, 320–32.

Ward, D., Connally, E.L., Pliatsikas, C., Bretherton-Furness, J. and Watkins, K.E. 2015. 'The neurological underpinnings of cluttering: some initial findings', *Journal of Fluency Disorders* **43**, 1–16.

Waring, R. and Knight, R. 2013. 'How should children with speech sound disorders be classified? A review and critical evaluation of current classification systems', *International Journal of Language & Communication Disorders* **48**:1, 25–40.

Watts, C.R., Ronshaugen, R. and Saenz, D. 2015. 'The effect of age and vocal task on cepstral/spectral measures of vocal function in adult males', *Clinical Linguistics & Phonetics* **29**:6, 415–23.

Weatherspoon, D.J., Chattopadhyay, A., Boroumand, S. and Garcia, I. 2015. 'Oral cavity and oropharyngeal cancer incidence trends and disparities in the United States: 2000–2010', *Cancer Epidemiology* **39**:4, 497–504.

Wechsler, D. 1945. 'A standardized memory scale for clinical use', *Journal of Psychology* **19**:1, 87–95.
1976. *Wechsler Intelligence Scale for Children*, rev., Windsor: NFER-Nelson.
1981. *Wechsler Adult Intelligence Scale*, rev., New York: Psychological Corporation.
1992. *Wechsler Intelligence Scale for Children*, 3rd UK edn, London: Psychological Corporation.
2003. *Wechsler Intelligence Scale for Children*, 4th edn, San Antonio, TX: Psychological Corporation.

Weiner, F.F. 1981. 'Systematic sound preference as a characteristic of phonological disability', *Journal of Speech and Hearing Disorders* **46**:3, 281–6.

Weismer, G. 2006. 'Philosophy of research in motor speech disorders', *Clinical Linguistics & Phonetics* **20**:5, 315–49.

Weissman, A.N. and Beck, A.T. 1978. 'Development and validation of the Dysfunctional Attitudes Scale: a preliminary investigation', paper presented at the 62nd Annual Meeting of the American Educational Research Association, Ontario, Canada, March 1978.

Wells, J.E., McGee, M.A., Scott, K.M. and Oakley Browne, M.A. 2010. 'Bipolar disorder with frequent mood episodes in the New Zealand Mental Health Survey', *Journal of Affective Disorders* **126**:(1–2), 65–74.

Wenger, T.L., McDonald-McGinn, D.M. and Zackai, E.H. 2014. 'Genetics of common congenital syndromes of the head and neck', in L.M. Elden and K.B. Zur (eds.), *Congenital Malformations of the Head and Neck*, New York: Springer, 1–22.

Wepman, J.M. 1958. *Auditory Discrimination Test*, Los Angeles: Western Psychological Services.

Wertz, R.T., Collins, M.J., Weiss, D., Kurtze, J.F., Friden, T., Brookshire, R.H., Pierce, J., Holtzapple, P., Hubbard, D.J., Porch, B.E., West, J.A., Davis, L., Matovitch, V., Morley, G.K. and Resurreccion, E. 1981. 'Veterans cooperative study on aphasia: a comparison of individual and group treatment', *Journal of Speech and Hearing Research* **24**:4, 580–94.

West, C., Hesketh, A., Vail, A. and Bowen, A. 2005. 'Interventions for apraxia of speech following stroke', *Cochrane Database of Systematic Reviews* **4**:CD004298.

Weydt, P., Soyal, S.M., Landwehrmeyer, G.B. and Patsch, W. for the European Huntington Disease Network 2014. 'A single nucleotide polymorphism in the coding region of PGC-1a is a male-specific modifier of Huntington disease age-at-onset in a large European cohort', *BMC Neurology* **14**:1.

Whitehouse, A.J.O., Watt, H.J., Line, E.A. and Bishop, D.V.M. 2009a. 'Adult psychosocial outcomes of children with specific language impairment, pragmatic language impairment and autism', *International Journal of Language & Communication Disorders* **44**:4, 511–28.

Whitehouse, A.J.O., Line, E.A., Watt, H.J. and Bishop, D.V.M. 2009b. 'Qualitative aspects of developmental language impairment relate to language and literacy outcome in adulthood', *International Journal of Language & Communication Disorders* **44**:4, 489–510.

Whitworth, A. 1996. *Thematic Roles in Production, TRIP: An Assessment of Word Retrieval at the Sentence Level*, London: Whurr.

Wickremaratchi, M.M., Perera, D., O'Loghlen, C., Sastry, D., Morgan, E., Jones, A., Edwards, P., Robertson, N.P., Butler, C., Morris, H.R. and Ben-Shlomo, Y. 2009. 'Prevalence and age of onset of Parkinson's disease in Cardiff: a community based cross sectional study and meta-analysis', *Journal of Neurology, Neurosurgery & Psychiatry* **80**:7, 805–7.

Wiig, E.H. and Secord, W. 1989. *Test of Language Competence – Expanded Edition*, San Antonio, TX: Psychological Corporation.

  1992. *Test of Word Knowledge*, New York: Psychological Corporation.

Wiig, E.H., Secord, W. and Semel, E. 1992. *Clinical Evaluation of Language Fundamentals – Preschool*, San Antonio, TX: Psychological Corporation.

Williams, A. 2003. *Speech Disorders: Resource Guide for Preschool Children*, Clifton Park, NY: Thomson/Delmar Learning.

Wingate, M.E. 2002. *Foundations of Stuttering*, San Diego, CA: Academic Press.

Winner, E., Brownell, H., Happé, F., Blum, A. and Pincus, D. 1998. 'Distinguishing lies from jokes: theory of mind deficits and discourse interpretation in right hemisphere brain-damaged patients', *Brain and Language* **62**:1, 89–106.

Wit, J., Maassen, B., Gabreëls, F.J.M., Thoonen, G. and de Swart, B. 1994. 'Traumatic versus perinatally acquired dysarthria: assessment by means of speech-like maximum performance tasks', *Developmental Medicine & Child Neurology* **36**:3, 221–9.

World Health Organization 2001. *International Classification of Functioning, Disability and Health*, Geneva: WHO.

Wu, C.M., Lee, L.A., Chao, W.C., Tsou, Y.T. and Chen, Y.A. 2015. 'Paragraph-reading comprehension ability in Mandarin-speaking children with cochlear implants', *Laryngoscope* **125**:6, 1449–55.

Wu, D., Woodson, E.W., Masur, J. and Bent, J. 2015. 'Pediatric cochlear implantation: role of language, income, and ethnicity', *International Journal of Pediatric Otorhinolaryngology* **79**:5, 721–4.

Wulbert, M., Nyman, B.A., Snow, D. and Owen, Y. 1973. 'The efficacy of stimulus fading and contingency management in the treatment of elective mutism: a case study', *Journal of Applied Behavior Analysis* **6**:3, 435–41.

Wyszynski, D.F. and Wu, T. 2002. 'Prenatal and perinatal factors associated with isolated oral clefting', *Cleft Palate-Craniofacial Journal* **39**:3, 370–5.

Xue, S.A., Hao, G.J., Xiu, L. and Moranski, T. 2008. 'Speaking fundamental frequency changes in women over time', *Asia Pacific Journal of Speech, Language, and Hearing* **11**:3, 189–94.

Yairi, E. and Ambrose, N. 2013. 'Epidemiology of stuttering: 21st century advances', *Journal of Fluency Disorders* **38**:2, 66–87.

Yang, Z.H., Zhao, X.Q., Wang, C.X., Chen, H.Y. and Zhang, Y.M. 2008. 'Neuroanatomic correlation of the post-stroke aphasias studied with imaging', *Neurological Research* **30**:4, 356–60.

Yavaş, M. and Hernandorena, C.M. 1991. 'Systematic sound preference in phonological disorders: a case study', *Journal of Communication Disorders* **24**:2, 79–87.

Yuvaraj, R., Murugappan, M., Norlinah, M.I., Sundaraj, K. and Khairiyah, M. 2013. 'Review of emotion recognition in stroke patients', *Dementia and Geriatric Cognitive Disorders* **36**:(3–4), 179–96.

Zanini, S., Bryan, K., De Luca, G. and Bava, A. 2005. 'Italian Right Hemisphere Language Battery: the normative study', *Neurological Sciences* **26**:1, 13–25.

Zarowitz, B.J., O'Shea, T. and Nance, M. 2014. 'Clinical, demographic, and pharmacologic features of nursing home residents with Huntington's disease', *Journal of the American Medical Directors Association* **15**:6, 423–8.

Zhang, D., Zhou, J., Chen, B., Zhou, L. and Tao, L. 2014. 'Gastroesophageal reflux and carcinoma of larynx or pharynx: a meta-analysis', *Acta Oto-Laryngologica* **134**:10, 982–9.

Zheng, Y., Xia, P., Zheng, H.C., Takahashi, H., Masuda, S. and Takano, Y. 2010. 'The screening of viral risk factors in tongue and pharyngolaryngeal squamous carcinoma', *Anticancer Research* **30**:4, 1233–8.

Zimmerman, I.L., Steiner, V.G. and Pond, R.E. 1979. *Preschool Language Scale*, rev. edn, San Antonio, TX: Psychological Corporation.

Index